Marine Polysaccharides
Volume 2

Special Issue Editor
Paola Laurienzo

MDPI • Basel • Beijing • Wuhan • Barcelona • Belgrade

MDPI

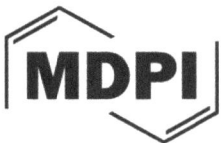

Special Issue Editor
Paola Laurienzo
Institute for Polymers, Composites and Biomaterials, CNR
Italy

Editorial Office
MDPI AG
St. Alban-Anlage 66
Basel, Switzerland

This edition is a reprint of the Special Issue published online in the open access journal *Marine Drugs* (ISSN 1660-3397) from 2010–2017 (available at: http://www.mdpi.com/journal/marinedrugs/special_issues/polysaccharides-2010).

For citation purposes, cite each article independently as indicated on the article page online and as indicated below:

Lastname, F.M.; Lastname, F.M. Article title. *Journal Name* **Year**, *Article number, page range*.

First Edition 2018

Volume 2
ISBN 978-3-03842-899-2 (Pbk)
ISBN 978-3-03842-900-5 (PDF)

Volume 1–3
ISBN 978-3-03842-743-8 (Pbk)
ISBN 978-3-03842-744-5 (PDF)

Table of Contents

About the Special Issue Editor

Paola Laurienzo grew up in Naples, Italy. In 1983, she graduated in Chemistry at "Federico II" University of Naples. This was followed by a Post-doc position at Italian Research National Council. She was appointed as Researcher at the Institute for Polymers, Composites and Biomaterials (IPCB) of CNR in Pozzuoli (Naples, Italy) in 1986. During the first 15 years, her research activity was mainly devoted to polymer and copolymer synthesis with standard and innovative strategies; chemical modification of synthetic polymers; design and chemical–physical characterization of blends; the study of the structure–properties correlations of multiphase polymeric materials. Innovative films for food packaging, new polymers for applications as components in electro-optical devices, and recycling of plastics from waste through reactive blending were developed technologies. Two national patents were obtained in these years. From the year 2000 onwards, her interests have focused on biodegradable polyesters and natural polysaccharides for applications in tissue engineering, drug delivery, and hydrogels for wound healing. Her experience in the synthesis and chemical modification of polymers has now been extended to the realization of novel amphiphilic copolymers for the design of active targeted polymeric micelles for drug delivery, with a focus on cancer therapy.

Preface to "Marine Polysaccharides"

Volume 1: Advancements in the Discovery of Novel Marine Polysaccharides

The field of marine polysaccharides is constantly evolving, due to progress in the discovery and production of new marine polysaccharides. Seaweed remains the most abundant source of polysaccharides, but recent advances in biotechnology have allowed the production of large quantities of polysaccharides from a variety of micro-algae, by controlling growth conditions and tailoring the production of bioactive compounds in a bioreactor. Of particular interest are polysaccharides produced by micro-organisms from extreme marine environments, due to their recognized different biochemistry. Extracellular polysaccharides (EPSs) with unique properties produced by a number of micro-algae are known. The first volume is a collection of papers concerning the identification and characterization of novel marine polysaccharides. It is divided into three chapters; the first two are dedicated to polysaccharides from different marine sources (algae, micro-algae, animals), while the third one gathers information on the isolation, characterization and bioactivity of new EPSs.

Volume 2: Identification of the Methabolic Pathways Involved in the Biological Activity of Marine Polysaccharides

In the second volume, papers reporting on the elucidation of the mechanisms that underlie the biological activity of some marine polysaccharides are collected. The understanding of the underlying mechanisms is an important feature to give a rigorous scientific support to the potential use of many marine polysaccharides as natural drugs in a wide range of therapies. This volume is divided into three chapters, each of them devoted to a specific class of polysaccharides.

Volume 3: Biomedical and Pharmaceutical Applications of Marine Polysaccharides

Recently-developed technology for production of polysaccharides from marine sources makes their potential use as additives in pharmacological formulations, food supplements, and support material for biomedical implants a real possibility. Although development of low-cost and eco-friendly methods remains a challenge, many companies have developed methodologies for extraction and purification of high quantities of polysaccharides from a variety of natural sources, as confirmed by the high number of trademarks that have been registered to date. Moreover, refinements of technological approaches enable further exploitation of available resources. This volume is a collection of papers focusing on the concrete application of polysaccharides in the biomedical field. In the first chapter, review articles illustrating all the potential applications of polysaccharides are presented. The second chapter includes articles on new methodologies for extraction and purification of polysaccharides of different origins, with particular attention on the evaluation of potential toxicity strictly related to the production process. Finally, in the last chapter, papers dealing with specific examples of biomedical applications are reported. The proposals contained within this collection cover a wide range, including food supplements and services in aquaculture, among others.

Paola Laurienzo
Special Issue Editor

marine drugs

MDPI

Article

Molecular Weight-Dependent Immunostimulative Activity of Low Molecular Weight Chitosan via Regulating NF-κB and AP-1 Signaling Pathways in RAW264.7 Macrophages

Bin Zheng [1,2], Zheng-Shun Wen [1,*], Yun-Juan Huang [3], Mei-Sheng Xia [4], Xing-Wei Xiang [2,*] and You-Le Qu [1,*]

1   Zhejiang Provincial Key Engineering Technology Research Center of Marine Biomedical Products, School of Food Science and Pharmaceutics, Zhejiang Ocean University, Zhoushan 316022, China; 6369958@163.com
2   Zhejiang Marine Development Research Institute, Zhoushan 316022, China
3   Zhoushan Hospital (Hospital of Chinese Medicine and Orthopedics), Zhoushan 316000, China; zsdrlz@126.com
4   Ocean College, Zhejiang University, Zhoushan 316021, China; msxia@zju.edu.cn
*   Correspondence: zswenmr@163.com (Z.-S.W.); xxw11086@126.com (X.-W.X.); youle1960@163.com (Y.-L.Q.); Tel./Fax: +86-580-255-4781 (Z.-S.W.)

Academic Editor: Paola Laurienzo
Received: 28 July 2016; Accepted: 13 September 2016; Published: 20 September 2016

Abstract: Chitosan and its derivatives such as low molecular weight chitosans (LMWCs) have been found to possess many important biological properties, such as antioxidant and antitumor effects.   In our previous study, LMWCs were found to elicit a strong immunomodulatory response in macrophages dependent on molecular weight.   Herein we further investigated the molecular weight-dependent immunostimulative activity of LMWCs and elucidated its mechanism of action on RAW264.7 macrophages.   LMWCs (3 kDa and 50 kDa of molecular weight) could significantly enhance the mRNA expression levels of COX-2, IL-10 and MCP-1 in a molecular weight and concentration-dependent manner.   The results suggested that LMWCs elicited a significant immunomodulatory response, which was dependent on the dose and the molecular weight. Regarding the possible molecular mechanism of action, LMWCs promoted the expression of the genes of key molecules in NF-κB and AP-1 pathways, including IKKβ, TRAF6 and JNK1, and induced the phosphorylation of protein IKBα in RAW264.7 macrophage.   Moreover, LMWCs increased nuclear translocation of p65 and activation of activator protein-1 (AP-1, C-Jun and C-Fos) in a molecular weight-dependent manner. Taken together, our findings suggested that LMWCs exert immunostimulative activity via activation of NF-κB and AP-1 pathways in RAW264.7 macrophages in a molecular weight-dependent manner and that 3 kDa LMWC shows great potential as a novel agent for the treatment of immune suppression diseases and in future vaccines.

Keywords: immunostimulative activity; NF-κB/AP-1; molecular weight; low molecular weight chitosans; macrophages

---

1. Introduction

Chitosan is an abundant, natural linear polysaccharide derived from the deacetylation of chitin from crustaceans, insects and fungi. Chitosan is non-toxic ($LD_{50} > 16$ g/kg), and non-immunogenic, biodegradable and can be manufactured reproducibly on the basis of GMP guidelines [1]. Chitosan and its derivatives are widely used as biomedical material with an established safety profile in humans such as an experiment mucosal adjuvant [2–4] and vaccine adjuvant in mice [5]. Recently, chitosan and its derivatives have attracted more and more attention for its commercial applications in the biomedical, food, and chemical industries. The biomedical applications of various forms of chitosan have long been studied. Chitosan derived from chitin is of high molecular weight, has poor solubility and, ultimately, its therapeutic potential. To address these poor physicochemical properties, more active forms, like trimethylated chitosan and low molecular weight chitosans (LMWCs) have been generated. Chitosan and LMWCs interact readily with various cell receptors due to the presence of amine, acetylated amine and hydroxyl groups, and therefore they could trigger a cascade of interconnected reactions in living organisms resulting in anti-diabetic [6], anti-HIV-1 [7], anti-inflammatory [8], anti-oxidant [9], anti-microbial [10], neuroprotective [11] and anti-angiogenic [12] effects. Chitosan and its derivatives have previously been reported to possess immunological enhancement as a novel adjuvant for vaccine. Chitosan has complex and size-dependent effects on innate and adaptive immune responses including mobilization and activation of innate immune cells and production of cytokines and chemokines [13,14]. Suzuki et al. (1986) reported that different molecular weights of chitosan enhanced immune regulation with the increased water-solubility of chitosan in vivo [15].

Chitosan and its derivatives such as low molecular weight chitosans (LMWCs) have been reported to exert many biological activities, such as antioxidant and antitumor effects. Previous studies reported that LMWCs have dual activities, both immunostimulatory activity in non-induced RAW264.7 [16] and anti-inflammatory activity in induced RAW264.7 cells [17]. However, complex and molecular weight-dependent effects of chitosan remain controversial and the mechanisms that mediate these complex effects are still poorly defined. In our previous study, we found that LMWCs (3 kDa and 50 kDa) elicited a immunomodulatory response in macrophages via regulating the secretion and expression of cytokines in macrophage in a molecular weight- and concentration-dependent manner [18]. However, there was no clear information describing the relationship between molecule weight properties and the mechanism of action of LMWCs on RAW264.7 macrophages. Therefore, we hypothesized that LMWCs may have the potential to augment the immunostimulative activity via NF-κB and AP-1 signaling pathways in molecular-weight-dependent manner. Herein, the present study was carried out to investigate the immunostimulative activity and the mechanism of action of LMWCs on RAW264.7 macrophages by determining the effect on the expression of cytokines and activation of NF-κB and AP-1 signaling pathways.

2. Results

2.1. Effects of LMWCs on the mRNA Expression Levels of COX-2, IL-10 and MCP-1 in RAW264.7 Macrophages

Inflammatory factors and their signaling molecules play a prominent role in the maturation and function of macrophages. Herein we evaluated the potential of LMWCs to regulate the expression of these mediators in RAW264.7 cells. As shown in Figure 1A–C, the mRNA expression levels of COX-2, IL-10 and MCP-1 in RAW264.7 cells were analyzed by real-time fluorescent quantitative reverse transcription-polymerase chain reaction (RT-PCR). Following LMWC stimulation, the mRNA expression levels of COX-2 and MCP-1 significantly increased in a molecular weight and concentration-dependent manner and 3 kDa chitosan significantly increased the mRNA expression level of IL-10 comparing with untreated cells ($p < 0.05$), which are consistent with the secretion levels of cytokines in the previous study.

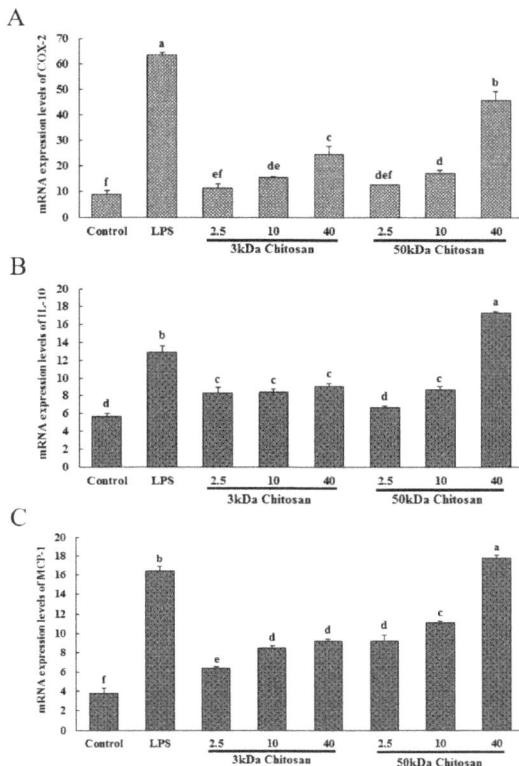

Figure 1. Effect of LMWCs on the mRNA expression levels of COX-2 (**A**), IL-10 (**B**) and MCP-1 (**C**) in RAW264.7 macrophage. Each cell population (1×10^6 cells/mL) was treated with LMWCs (3 kDa and 50 kDa) at the indicated concentrations of 2.5, 10 and 40 μg/mL or LPS (1 μg/mL) for 24 h, respectively. The untreated cells are used as the control. These represent mean values of three independent experiments. Values are presented as means ± SD ($n = 3$, three independent experiments). Bars with different letters (a, b, c, d, e, f) are statistically different ($p < 0.05$).

2.2. Effects of LMWCs on the mRNA Expression Levels of IKKβ in RAW264.7 Macrophages

The effect of LMWCs on the mRNA expression levels of IKKβ in RAW264.7 macrophages was examined by real-time quantitative RT-PCR. As shown in Figure 2, LMWCs (3 kDa, 50 kDa) significantly enhanced the mRNA expression levels of IKKβ of RAW264.7 cells at the dose (40 μg/mL) compared with the control ($p < 0.05$). Meanwhile, we also found that 3 kDa chitosan significantly promoted the mRNA expression levels of IKKβ compared with that at same dose of 50 kDa chitosan, suggesting that LMWCs significantly induced the mRNA expression levels of IKKβ of macrophages in a molecular weight-dependent manner.

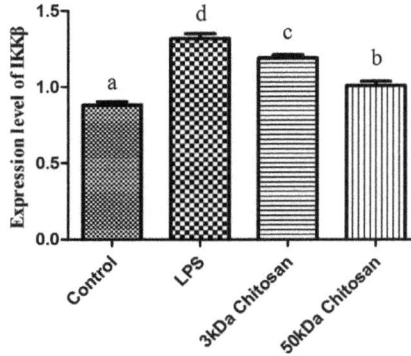

Figure 2. Effects of LMWCs on the mRNA expression levels of IKKβ in RAW264.7 macrophage. Each cell population (4×10^5 cells/mL) was treated with LMWCs (3 kDa and 50 kDa) at the indicated concentrations of 40 μg/mL or LPS (1 μg/mL) for 12 h, respectively. The untreated cells are used as the control. These represent mean values of three independent experiments. Values are presented as means ± SD ($n = 3$). Bars with different letters (a, b, c, d) are statistically different ($p < 0.05$).

2.3. Effect of LMWCs on the mRNA Expression Levels of Key Molecules (TRAF6, JNK1) in RAW264.7 Macrophages

RAW264.7 cells were treated with LMWCs for 12 h, and the mRNA expression levels of key molecules (TRAF6, JNK1) in RAW264.7 macrophages were detected using real-time quantitative RT-PCR. The addition of LMWCs (3 kDa and 50 kDa) resulted in a remarkable increase in expression levels of TRAF6 and JNK1 compared with untreated cells ($p < 0.05$) (Figure 3), but there were no statistically significant differences between 3 kDa and 50 kDa chitosan (Figure 3A,B).

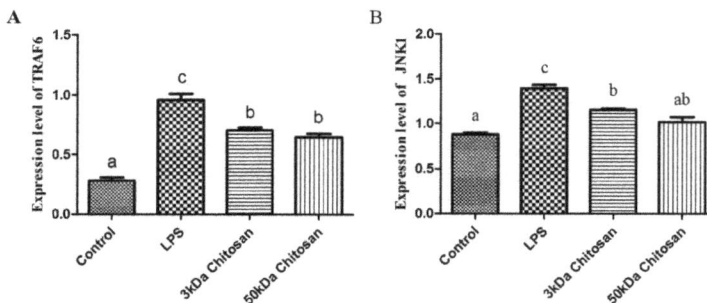

Figure 3. Effects of LMWCs on the mRNA expression levels of key molecules (TRAF6 (**A**), JNK1 (**B**)) from RAW264.7 macrophage. Each cell population (4×10^5 cells/mL) was treated with LMWCs (3 kDa and 50 kDa) at the indicated concentrations of 40 μg/mL or LPS (1 μg/mL) for 12 h, respectively. The untreated cells are used as the control. These represent mean values of three independent experiments. Values are presented as means ± SD ($n = 3$). Bars with different letters (a, b, c) are statistically different ($p < 0.05$).

2.4. Effects of LMWCs on the Phosphorylation of IKBα in the RAW264.7 Cells

As shown in Figure 4, LMWCs affected the phosphorylation of IKBα in the RAW264.7 cells. Compared with the untreated cells, LMWCs significantly increased the phosphorylation of IKBα when RAW264.7 cells were exposed to LMWCs at the indicated concentrations of 40 μg/mL for 12 h (Figure 4A); however, 3 kDa and 50 kDa chitosan did not increase significantly the level of IKBα.

After cells were incubated with the IκB kinase (IKK) inhibitor wedelolactone (20 μmol/L) for 12 h, the results indicated that wedelolactone suppressed the phosphorylation of IKBα compared with untreated cells (Figure 4B), whereas 3 kDa chitosan induced significantly the phosphorylation of IKBα compared with 50 kDa chitosan ($p < 0.05$). Taken together, the results suggested that LMWCs significantly induced the phosphorylation of IKBα from RAW264.7 macrophage cells in a size-dependent manner.

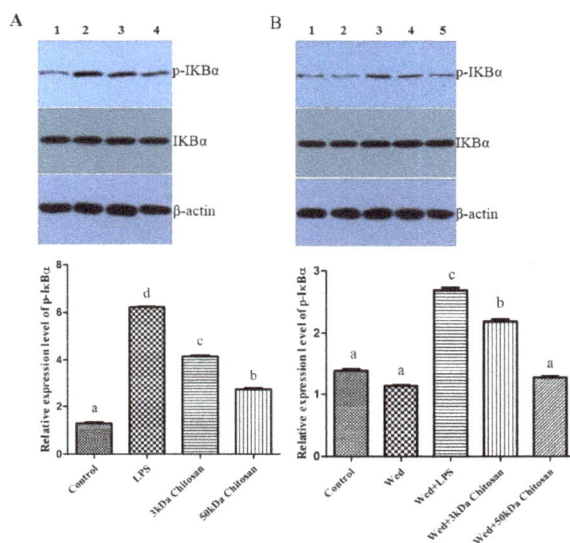

Figure 4. Effect of LMWCs on the phosphorylation of IKBα in RAW264.7 macrophage. (**A**) Each cell population (4×10^5 cells/mL) was treated with LMWCs (3 kDa and 50 kDa) at the indicated concentrations of 40 μg/mL for 12 h, respectively (1: Control; 2: LPS; 3: 3 kDa chitosan; 4: 50 kDa chitosan); (**B**) Each cell population (4×10^5 cells/mL) was treated with LMWCs (3 kDa and 50 kDa) at the indicated concentrations of 40 μg/mL and LPS (1 μg/mL) for 12 h after pre-incubation with 20 μmol/L of wedelolactone (Wed) for 12 h, respectively (1: Control; 2: Wedelolactone (Wed); 3: Wed + LPS; 4: Wed + 3 kDa chitosan; 5: Wed + 50 kDa chitosan). The figures shown are representative of three independent experiments. These represent mean values of three independent experiments. Values are presented as means ± SD ($n = 3$). Bars with different letters (a, b, c, d) are statistically different ($p < 0.05$).

2.5. *Effects of LMWCs on the Protein Expression of p65 in RAW264.7 Macrophages*

In order to examine whether the immunostimulative effects of LMWCs on RAW264.7 macrophages are associated with the translocation of p65 in the nuclear factor kB (NF-κB) pathway, the change in protein levels of NF-κB p65 in the cytoplasm and nucleus were investigated, as seen in Figure 5. As shown in Figure 5, treatment with LMWCs induced significant translocation of nucleic p65 protein and depletion of cytoplasmic p65, which is a subunit of NF-κB ($p < 0.05$). Moreover, the results indicated that treatment with 3 kDa chitosan significantly boosted the levels of nucleic p65 protein compared with 50 kDa chitosan ($p < 0.05$). These results suggested that immunostimulative effects of LMWCs might be associated with the nucleus translocation of p65 in the NF-κB pathway and that LMWCs activate macrophages via NF-κB signaling pathways in a molecular weight-dependent manner.

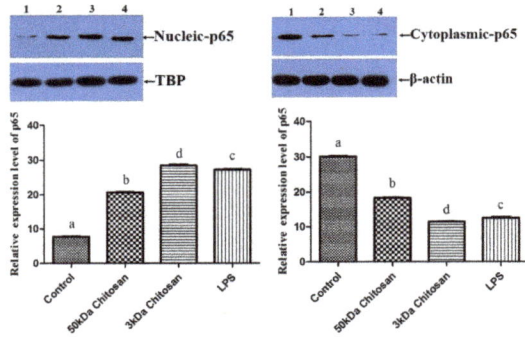

Figure 5. Effect of LMWCs on the nuclear translocation of p65 in the NF-κB pathway in RAW264.7 macrophages. Each cell population (1×10^6 cells/mL) was treated with LMWCs (3 kDa and 50 kDa) at the indicated concentrations of 40 μg/mL for 24 h, respectively (1: Control; 2: 50 kDa chitosan; 3: 3 kDa chitosan; 4: LPS). The figures shown are representative of three independent experiments. These represent mean values of three independent experiments. Values are presented as means ± SD ($n = 3$). Bars with different letters (a, b, c, d) are statistically different ($p < 0.05$).

2.6. Effects of LMWCs on the Expression of AP-1 (C-Jun and C-Fos) in RAW264.7 Macrophages

In order to examine whether immunostimulative effects of LMWCs on RAW264.7 macrophages are associated with the expression of C-Jun and C-Fos proteins in the activator protein-1 (AP-1) pathway, change of protein levels of C-Jun and C-Fos in RAW264.7 macrophages were investigated in Figure 6. As shown in Figure 6, treatment with LMWCs induced significant up-regulation of the expression of C-Jun and C-Fos, which are two subunits of AP-1 ($p < 0.05$). Moreover, the results indicated that treatment with 3 kDa chitosan significantly increased the levels of C-Jun and C-Fos protein compared with 50 kDa chitosan ($p < 0.05$). These results suggested that the immunostimulative effects of 3 kDa chitosan might be associated with the expression activation of C-Jun and C-Fos proteins in RAW264.7 macrophage and LMWCs might activate macrophages via AP-1 signaling pathways in a molecular weight-dependent manner.

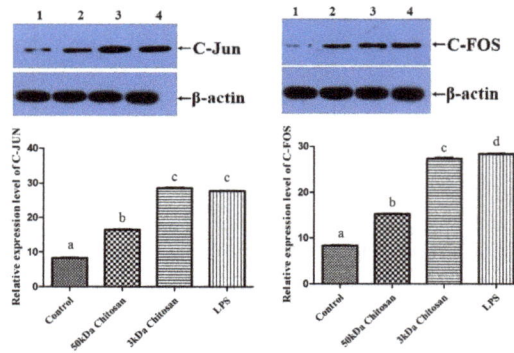

Figure 6. Effect of LMWCs on activator protein-1 (AP-1) in RAW264.7 macrophages. Each cell population (1×10^6 cells/mL) was treated with LMWCs (3 kDa and 50 kDa) at the indicated concentrations of 40 μg/mL for 24 h, respectively (1: Control; 2: 50 kDa chitosan; 3: 3 kDa chitosan; 4: LPS). The figures shown are representative of three independent experiments. These represent mean values of three independent experiments. Values are presented as means ± SD ($n = 3$). Bars with different letters (a, b, c, d) are statistically different ($p < 0.05$).

3. Discussion

Immunomodulatory activities of chitosan and its derivatives have been studied for their potential applications against allergy, infectious diseases or cancer [1,19]. Moreover, previous findings suggested that chitosan and its derivatives induce various inflammatory and pro-inflammatory cytokines upon incubating them with macrophages [20,21]. The immunostimulatory activity of LMWCs in non-induced RAW264.7 vary in a molecular weight-dependent manner because molecular weight might affect their structures and physicochemical properties. Previous studies reported that LMWCs have dual activities, both immunostimulatory activity in non-induced RAW264.7 [16] and anti-inflammatory activity in induced RAW264.7 cells [17]. LMWCs has previously been proved to provoke the immunomodulatory response through up-regulating mRNA expression of pro-inflammatory cytokines and activated RAW264.7 macrophages in a molecular weight-dependent manner [18]. However, its molecular mechanism responsible for regulating immune response is not fully understood. In the present study, the activation effect of LMWCs on the macrophages was investigated and its subsequent intracellular signaling pathways were explored using RAW264.7 macrophages as a cellular model. Our findings have demonstrated that LMWCs elicits an immunostimulative response in RAW264.7 macrophages through the simultaneous activation of the transcription factors NF-κB and AP-1 signaling pathways. Our hypothesized mode of action of LMWCs in this model of RAW264.7 macrophages is presented in Figure 7.

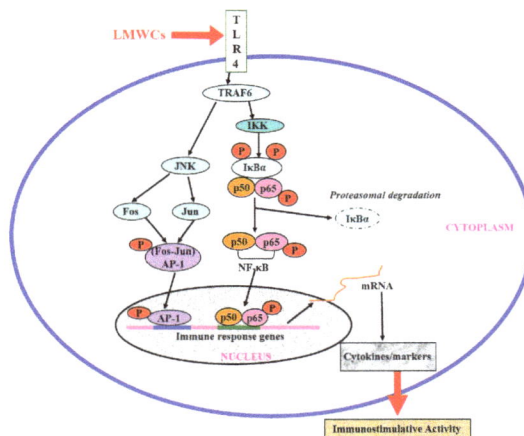

Figure 7. Schematic diagram of the targets of LMWCs.

Macrophages actively participate in immune responses by releasing cytokines such as pro-inflammatory cytokines (TNF-α and IL-1) and inflammatory factors nitric oxide (NO) [22]. In the previous study, we found LMWCs significantly enhanced the pinocytic activity and induce the production of tumor necrosis factor α (TNF-α), interleukin 6 (IL-6), interferon-γ (IFN-γ), NO and inducible nitric oxide synthase (iNOS) in a molecular weight- and concentration-dependent manner [18]. Herein, LMWCs also significantly up-regulated the mRNA expression levels of prostaglandin-endoperoxide synthase 2 (COX-2), IL-10 and monocyte chemotactic protein-1 (MCP-1) in the same manner. The cytokines associated with polarized type I responses of activated M1 phenotypes include TNF-α, moreover, M2 cells typically produce IL-10 [23]. Differential production of chemokines integrates M1 and M2 macrophage in circuits of amplification to attract Th1 and Th2 or T regulatory (Treg) cells for inducing polarized T cell responses [24]. As discussed above, LMWCs significantly promoted the production of TNF-α and IL-10 from RAW264.7 macrophages. Taken together, the results suggested that LMWCs could simultaneously induce Th1- and Th2-type response in a molecular weight-dependent manner.

TNF receptor-associated factor (TRAF) proteins are also key components of activation of the immune system. During activation of macrophages, TRAF molecules autoubiquitinate through the E3 ubiquitin ligase in their RING domain [25]. Ubiquitination of TNF receptor-associated factor 6 (TRAF6) is a key regulatory event and often a target molecule for regulation by inhibitors of NF-κB [26]. TRAF6 may be activated through TLR4, which in turn activates the inhibitor of κB kinase, finally NF-κB will be activated [27]. NF-κB can be stimulated through Toll-like receptors (TLRs) to activate the IKK complex, leading to the translocation of heterodimers of the NF-κB subunits (p65 and p50) to the nucleus [28]. IKKβ is very important molecule for NF-κB activation in response to pro-inflammatory stimuli [29]. Most immune-stimulants activate the function of macrophages through binding specifically with the cell surface receptor proteins. TLR4 is known to be expressed on macrophages and other cells [30,31]. TLR4 signaling pathways may play important roles in immune cell activation. Previous studies reported that TLR4 on the cell membrane might mediate the biological effects of chitosan oligosaccharide on macrophages and the activation of murine spleen CD11c$^+$ dendritic cells [32,33]. Moreover, Muzzarelli RA reported that the structure of chitosan is similar to the saccharide portion of lipid A in LPS, so it can similarly activate macrophages by binding to the surface TLR4 to initiate signal transduction [34]. To further insight into the molecular mechanism on immunomodulatory action of LMWCs, RT-PCR analysis showed that LMWCs directly significantly up-regulated the mRNA expression levels of IKKβ (Figure 2) and TRAF6 (Figure 3). Meanwhile, we also found that 3 kDa chitosan significantly promoted the mRNA expression levels of IKKβ compared with that at the same dose of 50 kDa chitosan, suggesting that LMWCs significantly induced the mRNA expression levels of IKKβ of macrophages dependent on its molecular weight. Our results suggested that the difference in NF-κB activated by LMWCs might be associated with the activation of TRAF6 and IKKβ in a molecular weight-dependent manner.

AP-1 is another important regulatory protein involved in cell growth, differentiation, transformation and apoptosis, moreover may also contribute to inflammatory and immune responses [35,36]. AP-1 is the target of mitogen-activated protein kinase (MAPK) signaling pathways through direct phosphorylation of AP-1 proteins [37,38]. In the immune response, AP-1 can regulate the production of cytokines such as TNF-α, IL-1, and IL-2 [39]. Previous studies suggested that JNK1 regulates the expression of pro-inflammatory cytokines and Nitric Oxide Synthase 2 (NOS2) during LPS and TNF-α activation, is a important molecule in macrophage biology [40,41]. Direct phosphorylation and transcriptional activation of AP-1 components by MAPKs lead to the stimulation of AP-1 activity [42]. Therefore, we further worked to determine whether LMWCs regulate the levels of TRAF6 and JNK1 in the macrophages. RT-PCR analysis showed that LMWCs directly significantly up-regulated the mRNA expression levels of TRAF6 and JNK1 (Figure 3), suggesting that LMWCs significantly induced the mRNA expression levels of TRAF6 of macrophages followed by promoting the expression levels of MAP Kinases JNK1 dependent on its molecule weight. Based on these findings, our results suggested that LMWCs might modulate the transcriptional activities of AP-1 by regulating levels of TRAF6 and JNK1 in macrophages.

Several lines of evidence indicate that LMWC plays an important role in the regulation of inflammatory responses through NF-κB and AP-1 signaling pathway [43–45]. Activation of NF-κB in response to stimuli involves activation of IκBα kinase (IKK), phosphorylation and degradation of IκBα, followed by release of activated NF-κB. The active dimer translocate to the nucleus where it binds to its target DNA sequence and induces the expression of its downstream genes [46,47]. Some of the best characterized substrates of the JNKs are the components of AP-1, a dimeric transcription factor formed by the association of Fos protein (c-Fos, FosB, Fra-1 and Fra-2) with Jun proteins (c-Jun, JunB and JunC). Both the chemical structure and the molecular size of LMWC might affect the NF-κB and AP-1 activation efficacy, followed by the activation of macrophages. Bahar et al. (2012) reported that chitooligosaccharide elicits an acute inflammatory cytokine response in Caco-2 cells through the simultaneous activation of the AP-1 transcription factor pathway [45]. Li et al. (2012) found that all five chitosan oligosaccharides (chitobiose, chitotriose, chitotetraose, chitopentaose, chitohexaose) increased NF-κB-dependent luciferase gene expression and NF-κB downstream genes transcription, and the most significant were chitotetraose and chitohexaose. In addition, they activated the p65 subunit of NF-κB translocating from cytoplasm to nucleus, which suggested that they were the most potent activators of the NF-κB signaling pathway [21,44]. In this regard, this study was carried out to investigate effects of LMWCs on the NF-κB and AP-1 signaling pathways and the expression of its downstream genes. Our data presented here demonstrated that LMWCs (3 kDa and 50 kDa chitosan) were the most potent activators of NF-κB and AP-1 signaling pathway and initiators of their downstream genes transcription. In addition, both of them also activated the p65 subunit of NF-κB p65 and AP-1 translocating from cytoplasm to nucleus in a molecular weight-dependent manner (Figures 5 and 6). Moreover, we assessed whether activation of translocation of the NF-κB p65 subunit is attributed to promoting the phosphorylation of IκBα by LMWCs. The results indicated that LMWCs could increase the phosphorylation of IκBα followed by the activation of degradation of IκBα in the cytoplasm in a molecular weight-dependent manner (Figure 4). Based on these findings, the results suggested that LMWCs activate the p65 subunit of NF-κB p65 translocating from cytoplasm to nucleus by promoting the phosphorylation of IκBα in a molecular weight-dependent manner.

In summary, the results presented in this study suggested that NF-κB and AP-1 signaling pathways were involved in the macrophage activation by two different molecular weights of LMWC. It is assumed that activation of TRAF6, JNK1, IKKβ and IκBα and subsequent activation of transcription factors (NF-κB and AP-1) were the main mechanism involved in the macrophage activation by LMWCs in a molecular weight-dependent manner. Taken together, our findings suggest that molecular weight affects the immuostimulative activity of LMWC via NF-κB and AP-1 pathways and that 3 kDa LMWCs show great potential as a novel agent for the treatment of immune suppression diseases and as an adjuvant in future vaccines.

4. Experimental Section

4.1. Chemicals and Reagents

Dulbecco's modified Eagle's medium (DMEM), penicillin/streptomycin, and the other materials required for culture of cells were purchased from Gibco BRL, Life Technologies (Grand Island, NY, USA). Vitamin C, dimethylsulfox-ide (DMSO), 3-(4,5-dimethylthiazol-2-yl) 2,5-diphenyltetrazolium bromide (MTT), wedelolactone and bovine serum albumin (BSA) were obtained from Sigma (St. Louis, MO, USA). Trizol was from Invitrogen (Carlsbad, CA, USA), revert Aid™ M-MuLV reverse transcriptase was from Fermentas (Amherst, NY, USA), diethylpyrocarbonate (DEPC) and ribonuclease inhibitor were from Biobasic, Canada, oligo (dT)$_{18}$ were from Sangon, China. Power SYBR® Master Mix was from Invitrogen, Carlsbad, CA, USA. Super Signal® West Dura Extended Duration Substrate, NE-PER® Nuclear and cytoplasmic extraction reagents and BCA™ protein assay kit were purchased from Pierce, Rockford, IL, USA. Polyclonal antibodies (Abs) against NF-κB p65 and monoclonal antibody against AP-1 (C-fos and C-jun) and β-actin were from Santa Cruz Biotechnology, Dallas, Texas, USA. Monoclonal antibodies against IκB-α, p-IκB-α and TATA binding protein TBP were from abcam, Cambridge, CB4 0FL, UK. X-ray films were from Kodak, Rochester, NY, USA. All other chemicals were of analytical grade or of the highest grade available commercially.

The low molecular weight chitosans were sterilized by passing it through a 0.22-μm Millipore filter to remove any contaminant and then analyzed for endotoxin level by a gel-clot Limulus amebocyte lysate assay (Zhejiang A and C Biological, Zhejiang, China). The endotoxin level in the stock solution was less than 0.5 EU/mL.

4.2. Cell Culture and Treatment

Mouse macrophages RAW 264.7 cell line was obtained from the Shanghai Institute of Cell Biology (Shanghai, China) and maintained in DMEM, supplemented with heat-inactivated 10% fetal bovine serum, 100 U/mL penicillin, 100 U/mL streptomycin in a humidified atmosphere of 5% CO_2 at 37 °C.

When the cells reached sub-confluence, they were treated for 12 or 24 h with culture medium containing different concentrations of LMWCs, two MW, 3 kDa and 50 kDa (2.5, 10, and 40 µg/mL), and LPS (1 µg/mL) that were tested in the experiments.

4.3. Real-Time Fluorescent Quantitative Reverse Transcription-Polymerase Chain Reaction (RT-PCR) Analysis

After incubation with or without LMWCs, RAW264.7 cells were lysed in 1 mL of Trizol reagent (Invitrogen™, Carlsbad, CA, USA) and the total RNA was isolated according to the manufacture's protocol. The concentration of total RNA was quantified by determining the optical density at 260 nm. The total RNA was used and reverse transcription (RT) was performed using 1st-Strand cDNA Synthesis Kit (Invitrogen™, Carlsbad, CA, USA). Briefly, nuclease-free water was added giving a final volume of 5 µL after mixing 2 µg of RNA with 0.5 µg oligo $(dT)_{18}$ primer in a DEPC-treated tube. This mixture was incubated at 65 °C for 5 min and chilled on ice for 2 min. Then, a solution containing 3 µL of RT buffer Mix, 0.65 µL of RT Enzyme Mix and 1.35 uL Primer Mix, giving a final volume of 10 µL, and the tubes were incubated for 10 min at 30 °C. The tubes then were incubated for 30 min at 42 °C. Finally, the reaction was stopped by heating at 70 °C for 15 min. The samples were stored at −20 °C until further use.

As shown in Table 1, the primers were used to amplify cDNA fragments (144-bp COX2 fragment, 144-bp IL-10 fragment, 101-bp MCP-1 fragment, 73-bp TRAF6 fragment, 109-bp JNK1 fragment, 104-bp IKKβ fragment and 94-bp 18S fragment). Amplification was carried out as previously [18] in total volume of 25 µL containing 1 µL (5 µM) of each target and 18S specific primers, 1 µL of cDNA template, 12.5 µL of Power SYBR® Master Mix (2×) (4 µL of 10× PCR buffer, 4 µL of $MgCl_2$ (25 mM), 4 µL of dNTPs (2.5 mM) and 0.5 µL of Taq DNA polymerase) (Invitrogen, USA), and 10.5 µL of DEPC-treated water was added. Reaction conditions were the standard conditions for the iQTM5 PCR (Bio-Rad, Hercules, CA, USA) (10 s denaturation at 95 °C, 25 s annealing at 63 °C or 64 °C (COX2, IL-10, MCP-1, TRAF6, JNK1, IKKβ, 18S) with 40 PCR cycles. Ct values were obtained automatically using software (Bio-Rad, USA). The comparative Ct method ($2^{-\Delta Ct}$ method) [48] was used to analyze the expression levels of genes, and 18S rRNA was used as the house-keeping gene.

Table 1. Real-Time PCR Primers and Conditions.

Gene	Genbank Accession	Primer Sequence	Product Size (bp)	Annealing (°C)
COX2	NM_011198.3	TCTGGCTTCGGGGAGCACAAC GGTGTTGCACGTAGTCTTCGATCA	144	64
IL-10	NM_010548.2	CAGTCGGCCAGAGCCACAT CTTGGCAACCCAAGTAACCCTT	144	64
MCP-1	NM_011333.3	CTGCATCTGCCCTAAGGTCTTCA AGTGCTTGAGGTGGTTGTGGAA	101	64
TRAF6	D84655.1	GGAGGACAAGGTTGCCGAAAT CCCAAACTTGCCAATCTTCCAA	73	63
JNK1	NM_001310454.1	GCTCTCCAGCACCCATACATCA CCTCTATTGTGTGCTCCCTCTCAT	109	63
IKKβ	AF088910.1	CAGAAGTACACCGTGACCGTTGA CACTGCACAGGCTGCCAGTTA	104	63
18S	NR_003278	CGGACACGGACAGGATTGACA CCAGACAAATCGCTCCACCAACTA	94	64

4.4. Western Blot Analysis

After treated with the various concentrations of LMWCs, RAW264.7 cells were washed three times with cold PBS and lysed with NE-PER™ nuclear and cytoplasmic extraction reagents (Pierce, Rockford, IL, USA). The protein contents were measured with the BCA protein assay kit using bovine serum as a standard. The denatured proteins were separated on 10%–12% sodium dodecyl sulfate polyacrylamide gel electrophoresis (SDS-PAGE), and transferred to PVDF membrane. After blocking the membrane with 5% skim milk in tween-20 containing Tris buffered saline (T-TBS) (20 mM Tris-HCl (pH 7.6), 150 mM NaCl, 0.1% Tween-20) for 1 h at 37 °C, the blots were incubated with mouse monoclonal antibody p-IκBα (1:1000), IκBα (1:2000), TBP (1:800), β-actin (1:1000), C-Fos (1:300) and rabbit polyclonal NF-κB p65 (1:500), C-Jun (1:400) in T-TBS containing 3% skim milk overnight at 4 °C. Subsequently, the membranes were washed with TTBS and incubated with an appropriate secondary antibody (horseradish peroxidase-conjugated goat anti-mouse or anti-rabbit IgG) for 1 h. After washing the membrane with T-TBS five times for 5 min, the signal was visualized with ECL Detection Kit (SuperSignal® West Dura Extended Duration Substrate) and exposed the membranes to X-ray films. The bands were visualized and photographed using JS-680B Gel Documentation and Analysis System. The relative expression levels of the proteins were expressed as 100 (or 10) × the gray value of the target protein band over the gray value of β-actin or TBP in the same sample. Each sample had 3 replicates.

4.5. Statistical Analysis

Data were expressed as mean ± standard deviation (S.D.) and examined for their statistical significance of difference with ANOVA and a Tukey post hoc test by using SPSS 16.0. *p*-values of less than 0.05 were considered statistically significant.

Acknowledgments: This work was supported by grants from National Natural Science Foundation of China (No. 31301982), International Science & Technology Cooperation Program of China (No. 2015DFA30980), Scientific and Technological Project of Zhejiang Ocean University (No. X12M05), Key Scientific and Technological Project of Zhejiang Ocean University (No. X12ZD08) and Zhejiang Provincial Natural Science Foundation of China (No. LQ13C200002).

Author Contributions: The authors contributions were as follows: Bin Zheng: performing of the experiments, data acquisition, analysis and interpretation of data, drafting of manuscript; Zheng-Shun Wen, Xing-Wei Xiang and You-Le Qu: study concept and design, providing guidance on revising the manuscript; Yun-Juan Huang and Mei-Sheng Xia: contribution of reagents/materials/analysis tools.

Conflicts of Interest: The authors declare no conflict of interest.

References

1. Zaharoff, D.A.; Rogers, C.J.; Hance, K.W.; Schlom, J.; Greiner, J.W. Chitosan solution enhances both humoral and cell-mediated immune responses to subcutaneous vaccination. *Vaccine* **2007**, *25*, 2085–2094. [CrossRef] [PubMed]
2. Read, R.C.; Naylor, S.C.; Potter, C.W.; Bond, J.; Jabbal-Gill, I.; Fisher, A.; Illum, L.; Jennings, R. Effective nasal influenza vaccine delivery using chitosan. *Vaccine* **2005**, *23*, 4367–4374. [CrossRef] [PubMed]
3. Mills, K.H.; Cosgrove, C.; McNeela, E.A.; Sexton, A.; Giemza, R.; Jabbal-Gill, I.; Church, A.; Lin, W.; Illum, L.; Podda, A.; et al. Protective levels of diphtheria-neutralizing antibody induced in healthy volunteers by unilateral priming-boosting intranasal immunization associated with restricted ipsilateral mucosal secretory immunoglobulin a. *Infect. Immun.* **2003**, *71*, 726–732. [CrossRef] [PubMed]
4. McNeela, E.A.; Jabbal-Gill, I.; Illum, L.; Pizza, M.; Rappuoli, R.; Podda, A.; Lewis, D.J.; Mills, K.H. Intranasal immunization with genetically detoxified diphtheria toxin induces T cell responses in humans: Enhancement of Th2 responses and toxin-neutralizing antibodies by formulation with chitosan. *Vaccine* **2004**, *22*, 909–914. [CrossRef] [PubMed]
5. Wen, Z.-S.; Xu, Y.-L.; Zou, X.-T.; Xu, Z.-R. Chitosan Nanoparticles Act as an Adjuvant to Promote both Th1 and Th2 Immune Responses Induced by Ovalbumin in Mice. *Mar. Drugs* **2011**, *9*, 1038–1055. [CrossRef] [PubMed]
6. Eun, J.J.; Dal, K.Y.; Shin, H.L.; Hong, K.N.; Jong, G.H.; Prinyawiwatkul, W. Antibacterial activity of chitosans with different degrees of deacetylation and viscosities. *Int. J. Food Sci. Technol.* **2010**, *45*, 676–682.
7. Artan, M.; Karadeniz, F.; Karagozlu, M.Z.; Kim, M.M.; Kim, S.K. Anti-HIV-1 activity of low molecular weight sulfated chitooligosaccharides. *Carbohydr. Res.* **2010**, *345*, 656–662. [CrossRef] [PubMed]

8. Fernandes, J.C.; Spindola, H.; de Sousa, V.; Santos-Silva, A.; Pintado, M.E.; Malcata, F.X.; Carvalho, J.E. Anti-inflammatory activity of chitooligosaccharides in vivo. *Mar. Drugs* **2010**, *8*, 1763–1768. [CrossRef] [PubMed]

9. Ngo, D.N.; Lee, S.H.; Kim, M.; Kim, S.K. Production of chitin-oligosaccharides with different molecular weights and their antioxidant effect in RAW264.7 cells. *J. Funct. Foods* **2009**, *1*, 188–198. [CrossRef]

10. Ju, C.X.; Yue, W.; Yang, Z.H.; Zhang, Q.; Yang, X.; Liu, Z.; Zhang, F. Antidiabetic effect and mechanism of chitooligosaccharides. *Biol. Pharm. Bull.* **2010**, *33*, 1511–1516. [CrossRef] [PubMed]

11. Gong, Y.; Gong, L.; Gu, X.; Ding, F. Chitooligosaccharides promote peripheral nerve regeneration in a rabbit common peronial nerve crush injury model. *Microsurgery* **2009**, *29*, 650–656. [CrossRef] [PubMed]

12. Quan, H.; Zhu, F.; Han, X.; Xu, Z.; Zhao, Y.; Miao, Z. Mechanism of anti-angiogenic activities of chitooligosaccharides may be through inhibiting heparanase activity. *Med. Hypothesis* **2009**, *73*, 205–206. [CrossRef] [PubMed]

13. Lee, C.G.; Da Silva, C.A.; Lee, J.Y.; Hartl, D.; Elias, J.A. Chitin regulation of immune responses: An old molecule with new roles. *Curr. Opin. Immunol.* **2008**, *20*, 684–689. [CrossRef] [PubMed]

14. Li, X.; Min, M.; Du, N.; Gu, Y.; Hode, T.; Naylor, M.; Chen, D.; Nordquist, R.E.; Chen, W.R. Chitin, Chitosan, and Glycated Chitosan Regulate Immune Responses: The Novel Adjuvants for Cancer Vaccine. *Clin. Dev. Immunol.* **2013**, *2013*, 387023. [CrossRef] [PubMed]

15. Suzuki, K.; Mikami, T.; Okawa, Y.; Tokoro, A.; Suzuki, S.; Suzuki, M. Antitumor effect of hexa-*N*-acetylchitohexaose and chitohexaose. *Carbohydr. Res.* **1986**, *151*, 403–408. [CrossRef]

16. Okamoto, Y.; Inoue, A.; Miyatake, K.; Ogihara, K.; Shigemasa, Y.; Minami, S. Effects of chitin/chitosan and their oligomers/monomers on migrations of macrophages. *Macromol. Biosci.* **2003**, *3*, 587–590. [CrossRef]

17. Yang, E.J.; Kim, J.G.; Kim, J.Y.; Kim, S.C.; Lee, N.H.; Hyun, C. Anti-inflammatory effect of chitosan oligosaccharides in RAW264.7 cells. *Cent. Eur. J. Biol.* **2009**, *5*, 95–102.

18. Wu, N.; Wen, Z.; Xiang, X.; Huang, Y.; Gao, Y.; Qu, Y. Immunostimulative activity of low molecular weight chitosans in RAW264.7 macrophages. *Mar. Drugs* **2015**, *13*, 6210–6225. [CrossRef] [PubMed]

19. Chen, Y.L.; Wang, C.Y.; Yang, F.Y.; Wang, B.S.; Chen, J.Y.; Lin, L.T.; Leu, J.D.; Chiu, S.J.; Chen, F.D.; Lee, Y.J.; et al. Synergistic effects of glycated chitosan with high-intensity focused ultrasound on suppression of metastases in a syngeneic breast tumor model. *Cell Death Dis.* **2014**, *5*, e1178. [CrossRef] [PubMed]

20. Da Silva, C.A.; Chalouni, C.; Williams, A.; Hartl, D.; Lee, C.G.; Elias, J.A. Chitin is a size-dependent regulator of macrophage TNF and IL-10 production. *J. Immunol.* **2009**, *182*, 3573–3582. [CrossRef] [PubMed]

21. Bueter, C.L.; Lee, C.K.; Rathinam, V.A.; Healy, G.J.; Taron, C.H.; Specht, C.A.; Levitz, S.M. Chitosan but not chitin activates the inflammasome by a mechanism dependent upon phagocytosis. *J. Biol. Chem.* **2011**, *286*, 35447–35455. [CrossRef] [PubMed]

22. Farias-Eisner, R.; Sherman, M.P.; Aeberhard, E.; Chaudhuri, G. Nitric oxide is an important mediator for tumoricidal activity in vivo. *Proc. Natl. Acad. Sci. USA* **1994**, *91*, 9407–9411. [CrossRef] [PubMed]

23. Rauh, M.J.; Ho, V.; Pereira, C.; Sham, A.; Sly, L.M.; Lam, V.; Huxham, L.; Minchinton, A.I.; Mui, A.; Krystal, G. SHIP represses the generation of alternatively activated macrophages. *Immunity* **2005**, *23*, 361–374. [CrossRef] [PubMed]

24. Mantovani, A.; Sozzani, S.; Locati, M.; Allavena, P.; Sica, A. Macrophage polarization: Tumor-associated macrophages as a paradigm for polarized M2 mononuclear phagocytes. *Trends Immunol.* **2002**, *23*, 549–555. [CrossRef]

25. Bishop, G.A. The multifaceted roles of TRAFs in the regulation of B-cell function. *Nat. Rev. Immunol.* **2004**, *4*, 775–786. [CrossRef] [PubMed]

26. Schneider, M.; Zimmermann, A.G.; Roberts, R.A.; Zhang, L.; Swanson, K.V.; Wen, H.; Davis, B.K.; Allen, I.C.; Holl, E.K.; Ye, Z.; et al. The innate immune sensor NLRC3 attenuates Toll-like receptor signaling via modification of the signaling adaptor TRAF6 and transcription factor NF-κB. *Nat. Immunol.* **2012**, *13*, 823–831. [CrossRef] [PubMed]

27. Yin, Q.; Lin, S.C.; Lamothe, B.; Lu, M.; Lo, Y.C.; Hura, G.; Zheng, L.; Rich, R.L.; Campos, A.D.; Myszka, D.G.; et al. E2 interaction and dimerization in the crystal structure of TRAF6. *Nat. Struct. Mol. Biol.* **2009**, *16*, 658–666. [CrossRef] [PubMed]

28. Hasegawa, M.; Fujimoto, Y.; Lucas, P.C.; Nakano, H.; Fukase, K.; Núñez, G.; Inohara, N. A critical role of RICK/RIP2 polyubiquitination in Nod-induced NF-κB activation. *EMBO J.* **2008**, *27*, 373–383. [CrossRef] [PubMed]

29. Karin, M.; Delhase, M. The IκB kinase (IKK) and NF-κB: Key elements of proinflammatory signaling. *Semin. Immunol.* **2000**, *12*, 85–98. [CrossRef] [PubMed]

30. Beutler, B. Tlr4: Central component of the sole mammalian LPS sensor. *Curr. Opin. Immunol.* **2000**, *12*, 20–26. [CrossRef]

31. Janeway, C.A., Jr.; Medzhitov, R. Innate immune recognition. *Annu. Rev. Immunol.* **2002**, *20*, 197–216. [CrossRef] [PubMed]

32. Zhang, P.; Liu, W.; Peng, Y.; Han, B.; Yang, Y. Toll like receptor 4 (TLR4) mediates the stimulating activities of chitosan oligosaccharide on macrophages. *Int. Immunopharmacol.* **2014**, *23*, 254–261. [CrossRef] [PubMed]

33. Dang, Y.; Li, S.; Wang, W.; Wang, S.; Zou, M.; Guo, Y.; Fan, J.; Du, Y.; Zhang, J. The effects of chitosan oligosaccharide on the activation of murine spleen CD11c+ dendritic cells via Toll-like receptor 4. *Carbohydr. Polym.* **2011**, *83*, 1075–1081. [CrossRef]

34. Muzzarelli, R.A. Human enzymatic activities related to the therapeutic administration of chitin derivatives. *Cell. Mol. Life Sci.* **1997**, *53*, 131–140. [CrossRef] [PubMed]

35. Angel, P.; Karin, M. The role of Jun, Fos and the AP-1 complex in cell-proliferation and transformation. *Biochim. Biophys. Acta* **1991**, *1072*, 129–157. [CrossRef]

36. Shaulian, E.; Karin, M. AP-1 in cell proliferation and survival. *Oncogene* **2001**, *20*, 2390–2400. [CrossRef] [PubMed]

37. Whitmarsh, A.J.; Davis, R.J. Transcription factor AP-1 regulation by mitogen-activated protein kinase signal transduction pathways. *J. Mol. Med.* **1996**, *74*, 589–607. [CrossRef] [PubMed]

38. Pearson, G.; Robinson, F.; Beers Gibson, T.; Xu, B.E.; Karandikar, M.; Berman, K.; Cobb, M.H. Mitogen-activated protein (MAP) kinase pathways: Regulation and physiological functions. *Endocr. Rev.* **2001**, *22*, 153–183. [CrossRef] [PubMed]

39. Giri, R.S.; Thaker, H.M.; Giordano, T.; Williams, J.; Rogers, D.; Sudersanam, V.; Vasu, K.K. Design, synthesis and characterization of novel 2-(2,4-disubstituted-thiazole-5-yl)-3-aryl-3Hquinazoline-4-one derivatives as inhibitors of NF-κB and AP-1 mediated transcription activation and as potential anti-inflammatory agents. *Eur. J. Med. Chem.* **2009**, *44*, 2184–2189. [CrossRef] [PubMed]

40. Sánchez-Tilló, E.; Comalada, M.; Xaus, J.; Farrera, C.; Valledor, A.F.; Caelles, C.; Lloberas, J.; Celada, A. JNK1 Is required for the induction of Mkp1 expression in macrophages during proliferation and lipopolysaccharide-dependent activation. *J. Biol. Chem.* **2007**, *282*, 12566–12573. [CrossRef] [PubMed]

41. Guma, M.; Ronacher, L.M.; Firestein, G.S.; Karin, M.; Corr, M. JNK1 deficiency limits macrophage mediated antigen-induced arthritis. *Arthritis Rheumatol.* **2011**, *63*, 1603–1612. [CrossRef] [PubMed]

42. Wu, H.; Arron, J.R. TRAF6, a molecular bridge spanning adaptive immunity, innate immunity and osteoimmunology. *Bioessays* **2003**, *25*, 1096–1105. [CrossRef] [PubMed]

43. Wu, G.J.; Tsai, G.J. Chitooligosaccharides in Combination with Interferon-γ Increase Nitric Oxide Production via Nuclear Factor-κB Activation in Murine RAW264.7 Macrophages. *Food Chem. Toxicol.* **2007**, *45*, 250–258. [CrossRef] [PubMed]

44. Li, X.; Zhou, C.; Chen, X.; Wang, J.; Tian, J. Effects of Five Chitosan Oligosaccharides on Nuclear Factor-kappa B Signaling Pathway. *J. Wuhan Univ. Technol.—Mater. Sci. Ed.* **2012**, *27*, 276–279. [CrossRef]

45. Bahar, B.; O'Doherty, J.V.; Maher, S.; McMorrow, J.; Sweeney, T. Chitooligosaccharide elicits acute inflammatory cytokine response through AP-1 pathway in human intestinal epithelial-like (Caco-2) cells. *Mol. Immunol.* **2012**, *51*, 283–291. [CrossRef] [PubMed]

46. Moynagh, P.N. The NF-kappaB Pathway. *J. Cell Sci.* **2005**, *118*, 4589–4592. [CrossRef] [PubMed]

47. Hayden, M.S.; Ghosh, S. Shared Principles in NF-κB Signaling. *Cell* **2008**, *132*, 344–362. [CrossRef] [PubMed]

48. Livak, K.J.; Schmittgen, T.D. Analysis of Relative Gene Expression Data Using Real-Time Quantitative PCR and the $2^{-\Delta\Delta Ct}$ Method. *Methods* **2001**, *25*, 402–408. [CrossRef] [PubMed]

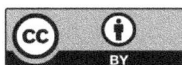

marine drugs

MDPI

Communication

Immunostimulative Activity of Low Molecular Weight Chitosans in RAW264.7 Macrophages

Ning Wu [1], Zheng-Shun Wen [1,*], Xing-Wei Xiang [2], Yan-Na Huang [3], Yang Gao [4] and You-Le Qu [1,*]

[1] Zhejiang Provincial Engineering Technology Research Center of Marine Biomedical Products, Food and Pharmacy College, Zhejiang Ocean University, Zhoushan 316000, China; wun@dxy.cn
[2] Zhejiang Marine Development Research Institute, Zhoushan 316000, China; xxw11086@126.com
[3] College of Animal Science and Technology, Guangxi University, Nanning 530004, China; huangyn@gxu.edu.cn
[4] School of Fishery, Zhejiang Ocean University, Zhoushan, 316000, China; avgy1982@hotmail.com
* Authors to whom correspondence should be addressed; wenzhengshun@zjou.edu.cn (Z.-S.W.); quyoule@zjou.edu.cn (Y.-L.Q.); Tel.: +86-580-2554781(Z.-S.W.); +86-0580-2554536 (Y.-L.Q.); Fax: +86-580-2554781(Z.-S.W.).

Academic Editor: Paola Laurienzo
Received: 2 July 2015; Accepted: 21 September 2015; Published: 30 September 2015

Abstract: Chitosan and its derivatives such as low molecular weight chitosans (LMWCs) have been reported to exert many biological activities, such as antioxidant and antitumor effects. However, complex and molecular weight dependent effects of chitosan remain controversial and the mechanisms that mediate these complex effects are still poorly defined. This study was carried out to investigate the immunostimulative effect of different molecular weight chitosan in RAW264.7 macrophages. Our data suggested that two LMWCs (molecular weight of 3 kDa and 50 kDa) both possessed immunostimulative activity, which was dependent on dose and, at the higher doses, also on the molecular weight. LMWCs could significantly enhance the the pinocytic activity, and induce the production of tumor necrosis factor α (TNF-α), interleukin 6 (IL-6), interferon-γ (IFN-γ), nitric oxide (NO) and inducible nitric oxide synthase (iNOS) in a molecular weight and concentration-dependent manner. LMWCs were further showed to promote the expression of the genes including iNOS, TNF-α. Taken together, our findings suggested that LMWCs elicited significantly immunomodulatory response through up-regulating mRNA expression of proinflammatory cytokines and activated RAW264.7 macrophage in a molecular weight- and concentration-dependent manner.

Keywords: immunostimulative activity; low molecular weight chitosans; cytokines; macrophages

---

1. Introduction

Low immune function of an organism may not only result in the generation and development of a tumor, but may also be one of the most important factors that prevent the tumor patient's recovery. Immunomodulation through natural or synthetic substances may be considered an alternative for the prevention and cure of diseases [1]. Macrophages play a significant role in the host defense mechanism. When activated, they activate phagocytic activity, produce and release reactive oxygen species (ROS) and nitric oxide (NO) in response to stimulation with various agents, and can inhibit the growth of a wide variety of tumor cells and microorganisms [2,3]. Macrophages also secrete cytokines and chemokines, such as tumor necrosis factor (TNF-α), interleukin-1 (IL-1) and interferon-γ (IFN-γ). Moreover, the immunomodulatory activity not only involves effects on cell proliferation and differentiation but also on macrophage activation [4]. Macrophages occupy a unique niche in the immune system, in that they can not only initiate innate immune response, but can also be effector cells that contribute to fight infection and inflammation. Following activation, macrophages can induce expression of accessory and costimulatory molecules that promote sustained stimulatory interactions with T cells and the generation of adaptive immunity. Indeed, the basic mechanisms of the immunostimulatory, anti-tumor, bactericidal and other therapeutic effects of polysaccharides are thought to occur via activation of immune cells resulting in the induction of immune response. Macrophages were thought to be the important target cells of some antitumor and immunomodulatory drug [5].

Polysaccharides obtained from natural sources represent a structurally diverse class of macromolecules, and are known to affect a variety of biological responses, especially the immune response. Chitosan is an abundant, natural linear polysaccharide derived by the deacetylation of chitin from crustaceans, insects and fungi. Chitosan is non-toxic (Lethal Dose $_{50}$ > 16 g/kg), biodegradable, non-immunogenic and can be manufactured reproducibly in accordance with GMP guidelines [6]. Chitosan is a widely used biomaterial with an established safety profile in humans. It is used an experiment mucosal adjuvant [7–9] and vaccine adjuvant in mice [10]. Recently, chitosan has received considerable attention for its commercial applications in the biomedical, food, and chemical industries. The biomedical applications of various forms of chitosan have long been studied. Chitosan derived from chitin is of high molecular weight with poor solubility and, ultimately, unsatisfactory its therapeutic potential. To address these poor physicochemical properties, more active forms, like low molecular weight chitosans (LMWCs) have been generated [11]. In addition, chitosans derivatives seem to activate macrophage secreting cytokines such as interferon-γ (IFN-γ), interleukins [12]. LMWCs, which are more effectively absorbed in the body than high molecular weight chitosan, suitable narrow molecular weight distribution and non-toxicity, could be applied most promisingly to pharmaceutical materials. However, there was no clear information describing the relationship between molecule weight properties and immunostimulative activity of LMWCs. Therefore, we hypothesized that LMWCs may have a potential to augment the immunomodulatory activity in molecular-weight-dependent manner. RAW264.7 cells are commonly accepted as a tool to investigate the molecular mechanisms of macrophages involved in regulating immunity. Herein, we investigated the immunomodulatory activity of LMWCs (3 kDa and 50 kDa) in murine macrophages RAW264.7 cells and to develop a mechanistic understanding on size-dependent effects of chitosan on innate immune responses. The current experiments were designed to investigate the immunomodulatory effects of LMWCs on RAW264.7 macrophages by determining the effect on pinocytic activity, the production of nitric oxide and cytokines and their genes expression.

2. Results

2.1. Effects of LMWCs on the Cell Viability of RAW264.7 Macrophage

LMWCs (3 kDa and 50 kDa) were investigated for their immunostimulative activity in RAW264.7 macrophages. To evaluate possible cytotoxicities of LMWCs on RAW264.7 macrophages, LMWCs at the indicated concentrations of 2.5, 10 and 40 μg/mL were cultured with cells for 24 h, respectively. The results showed that RAW264.7 macrophages viability was not significantly (p > 0.05) influenced by LMWCs at the indicated concentrations of 2.5, 10 and 40 μg/mL (Figure 1). Therefore, LMWCs at the indicated concentrations were selected to conduct assay of immunomodulatory activity.

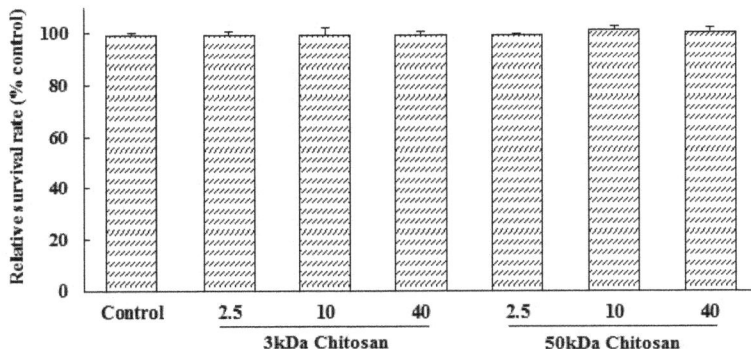

Figure 1. Effects of low molecular weight chitosans (LMWCs) on the cell viability of RAW264.7 macrophage. Each cell population (2×10^4 cells/well) was treated with LMWCs (3 kDa and 50 kDa) at the indicated concentrations of 2.5, 10 and 40 µg/mL for 24 h, respectively. Values are means ± SD ($n =$ 3). Bars with no letters are not statistically different ($p > 0.05$).

2.2. Effects of LMWCs on Pinocytic Activity

The effect of LMWCs on the pinocytic activity of RAW264.7 cells was examined by the uptake of neutral red. As shown in Figure 2, LMWCs (3 kDa and 50 kDa) significantly enhanced the pinocytic activity of RAW264.7 cells in a dose-dependent manner ($p < 0.05$). Meanwhile, we also found that 3 kDa chitosan at doses (10, 40 µg/mL) significantly promoted the pinocytic activity compared with that at same dose of 50 kDa chitosan, suggesting that LMWCs significantly induced the pinocytic activity of macrophages dependent on its size and dose.

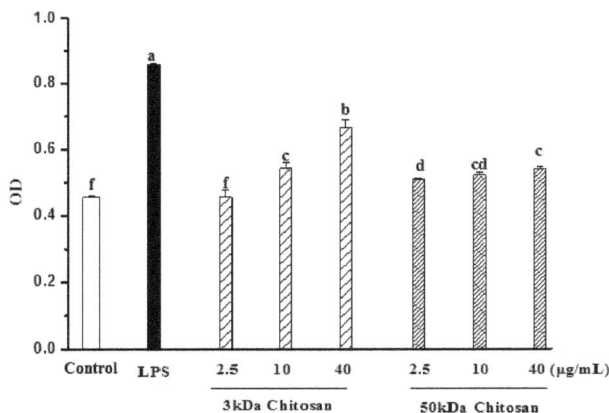

Figure 2. Effects of LMWCs on the pinocytic activity of RAW264.7 macrophage. Each cell population (1×10^4 cells/well) was treated with LMWCs (3 kDa and 50 kDa) at the indicated concentrations of 2.5, 10 and 40 µg/mL for 24 h, respectively. Values are means ± SD ($n = 3$). Bars with different letters (a, b, c, d, e, f) are statistically different ($p < 0.05$).

2.3. Effect of LMWCs on Macrophage Cytokines Production

RAW264.7 cells were treated with LMWCs for 24 h, and the secretion levels of TNF-α, INF-γ and IL-6 in the supernatant were detected using ELISA kits. Untreated RAW264.7 cells secrete a basal level of TNF-α and INF-γ but barely detectable amounts of IL-6 (Figure 3). The addition of LMWCs (3 kDa and 50 kDa) resulted in remarked increase in TNF-α secretion levels in a dose-dependent manner ($p < 0.05$) (Figure 3A). Meanwhile, 3 kDa chitosan also induced remarkably increase in INF-γ and IL-6 ($p < 0.05$) but 50 kDa chitosan did not result in that (Figure 3B,C).

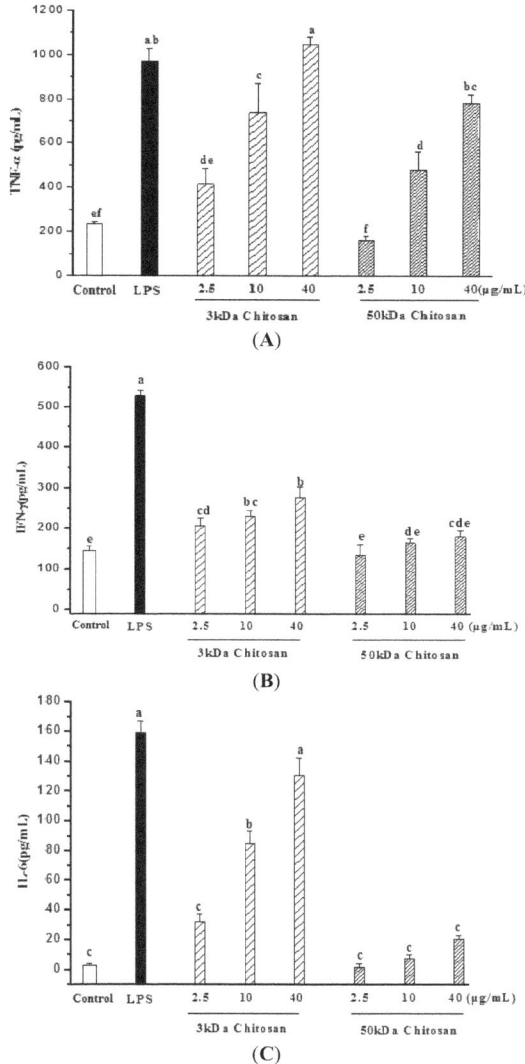

Figure 3. Effects of LMWCs on the production of tumor necrosis factor α (TNF-α) (**A**), interferon-γ (IFN-γ) (**B**) and interleukin 6 (IL-6) (**C**) from RAW264.7 macrophage. Each cell population (1×10^6 cells/mL) was treated with LMWCs (3 kDa and 50 kDa) at the indicated concentrations of 2.5, 10 and 40 μg/mL for 24 h, respectively. Values are means ± SD ($n = 3$). Bars with different letters (a, b, c, d, e, f) are statistically different ($p < 0.05$).

2.4. Effect of LMWCs on Nitric Oxide (NO) Production and Activities of Inducible Nitric Oxide Synthase (iNOS) in RAW264.7 Macrophage

As shown in Figure 4A, a minimum level of NO was released when RAW264.7 cells were exposed to medium alone, whereas Nitric oxide (NO) production increased in a concentration-dependent. The 3 kDa chitosan induced significantly secretion levels of NO compared with 50 kDa chitosan ($p < 0.05$). Taken together, the results suggested that LMWCs significantly induced the production of NO from RAW264.7 macrophage cells in a molecular weight size and concentration-dependent manner.

RAW264.7 cells were treated with LMWCs for 24 h, and the concentration of inducible nitric oxide synthase (iNOS) in the supernatant was detected using ELISA kit (Figure 4B). The addition of LMWCs resulted in remarkable increase of iNOS secretion levels in a concentration-dependent manner ($p < 0.05$).

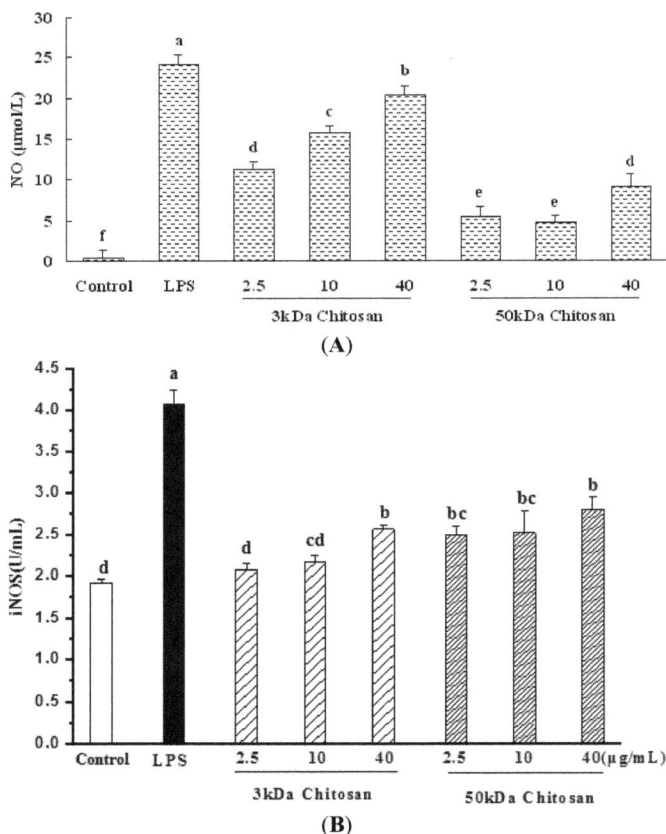

Figure 4. Effect of LMWCs on Nitric oxide (NO) production and activities of inducible nitric oxide synthase (iNOS) in RAW264.7 macrophage. Each cell population (1×10^6 cells/mL) was treated with LMWCs (3 kDa and 50 kDa) at the indicated concentrations of 2.5, 10 and 40 µg/mL for 24 h, respectively. Values are means ± SD ($n = 3$). Bars with different letters (a, b, c, d, e, f) are statistically different ($p < 0.05$).

2.5. Effect of LMWCs on the mRNA Expression Levels of TNF-α and iNOS in RAW264.7 Macrophage

Inflammatory factors and its signaling molecules play the prominent role in the maturation and function of macrophages, the potentials for LMWCs to regulate the expression of these mediators in RAW264.7 cells were investigated. As shown in Figure 5A,B, the mRNA expression levels of TNF-α and iNOS in RAW264.7 cells were evaluated by Q-PCR (Real-time Quantitative PCR Detecting System). Under LMWCs stimulation, the mRNA expression levels of TNF-α and iNOS significantly increased in RAW264.7 cells ($p < 0.05$). Both 3 kDa and 50 kDa chitosan significantly induced the mRNA expression levels of TNF-α and iNOS in a concentration-dependent manner ($p < 0.05$).

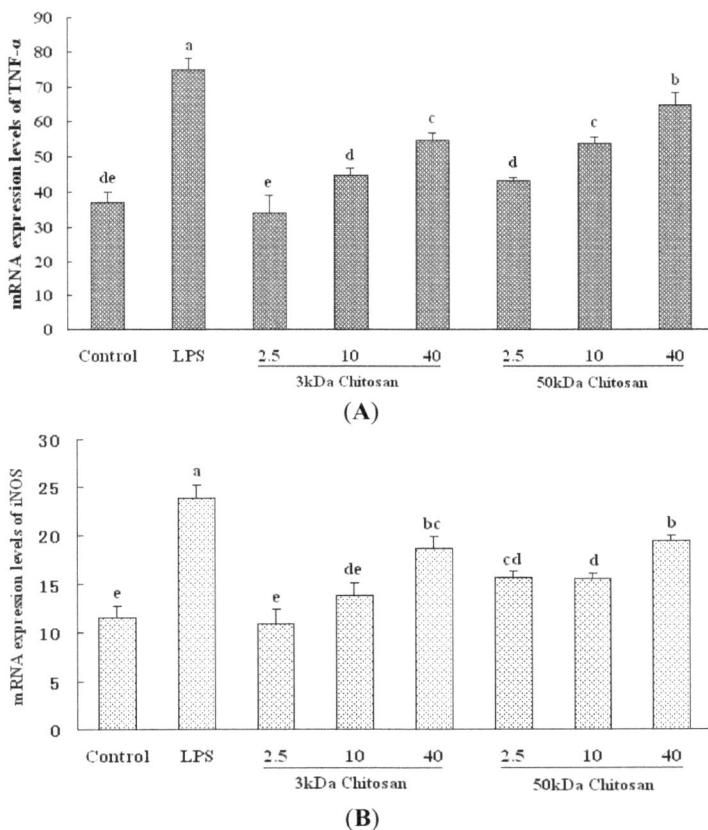

(A)

(B)

Figure 5. Effect of LMWCs on the mRNA expression levels of TNF-α and iNOS in RAW264.7 macrophage. Each cell population (1×10^6 cells/mL) was treated with LMWCs (3 kDa and 50 kDa) at the indicated concentrations of 2.5, 10 and 40 µg/mL for 24 h, respectively. Values are means ± SD ($n = 3$). Bars with different letters (a, b, c, d, e, f) are statistically different ($p < 0.05$).

3. Discussion

Owing to the presence of amine, acetylated amine groups and hydroxyl, chitosan and LMWCs interact readily with various cell receptors that triggers a cascade of interconnected reactions in living organisms resulting in anti-inflammatory [13], anti-diabetic [14], anti-microbial [15], anti-HIV-1 (Human Immunodeficiency Virus) [16], anti-oxidant [17], anti-angiogenic [18] and neuroprotective [19] effects. Chitosan and chitin has previously been reported to possess the immunological enhancement as novel adjuvants for vaccines. Chitin has complex and size-dependent effects on innate and adaptive immune responses, which include the ability to recruit and active innate immune cells and induce cytokine and chemokine production [20,21]. However, relationship between molecule weight properties and immunomodulatory activity, and the exact immune regulatory effects of chitosan remain controversial and the mechanisms that mediate these complex effects are still poorly defined.

One of the most distinguished features of macrophage activation would be an increase in pinocytic activity. Therefore, the effects of LMWCs on the pinocytic activity of RAW264.7 cells were determined using neutral red assay. In the previous studies, given by intravenous administration, significant priming effects of chitosan particles in alveolar macrophages in mice was observed, and the phagocytosable small-sized chitosan activated alveolar macrophage to express cytokines such as tumor necrosis factor-α (TNF-α) [21]. In the present study, the results suggested that LMWCs could significantly prime macrophages for an enhanced pinocytic activity in a concentration- and molecular weight-dependent manner. Our results are in agreement with reports in which phagocytosis could play a role in macrophages polarization since chitosan particles stimulated TGF-β1 and PDGF release from *in vitro* cultured macrophages [22].

Macrophages represent a family of mononuclear leukocytes that are widely distributed throughout the body. As the first defense effector of host body, macrophages can recognize the invading microorganisms and tumor cells, as well as eliminate the invaders. Acticiated Macrophages can produce many kinds of cytokines, such as TNF-α, IL-1β, IL-6, and IL-10, which are involved in the defense functions and inflammation. Macrophages actively participate in immune responses by releasing proinflammatory cytokines (TNF-α, IFN-γ and IL-6) and inflammatory factors such as NO [23]. The different cytokine production is a key feature of acticated and polarized macrophages. The cytokines associated with T helper cell 1 (Th1) immune response include TNF-α and IFN-γ. In contrast, T helper cell 2 (Th2) cytokines include IL-6. Many reports suggest that chitosan can upregulate TNF-α, IL-1β, and NO production in macrophages [24,25]. However, which types of chitosan activate macrophages that lead to different immunological response is not clear. Several factors, such as the administration route, molecular size and particle size, might account for the Th1 *vs.* Th2 response to chitin [26]. In the previous study, water-soluble, low molecular weight chitosan (MW, 21–92 kDa) had specific immunomodulatory effects on Der f-stimulated human MDM (monocyte-derived macrophages) including the shifting of Th2 cytokine polarization, decreasing the production of the inflammatory cytokines IL-6 and TNF-α [27]. In the present study, 3 kDa chitosan significantly promoted the production of TNF-α, IFN-γ and IL-6 from RAW264.7 cells, moreover, 3 kDa chitosan also up-regulated the mRNA expression levels of TNF-α. All these results suggested that 3 kDa chitosan would simultaneously induced Th1- and Th2-type response; however, 50 kDa chitosan promoted the production of TNF-α, which was consistent with a Th1 response elicited when macrophages phagocytose microparticles of chitin [28].

NO is a free radical formed biologically through the oxidation of L-arginine by nitric oxide synthases. Inducible nitric oxide synthase (iNOS) is key enzyme generating nitric oxide (NO) from the amino acid L-arginine in macrophage cells. iNOS-derived NO plays an important role in numerous physiological (e.g., blood pressure regulation, wound repair and host defense mechanisms) and pathophysiological (inflammation, infection, neoplastic diseases, liver cirrhosis, and diabetes) conditions [29]. It is induced in diseases associated with inflammation and oxidative stress [30]. Previously, LMWC (20 kDa chitosan) inhibited NO production in IFN-γ-induced RAW264.7 cells, whereas the chitooligosaccharides (composed of 1–6 sugars) enhanced NO production [31]. Our results are in agreement with reports in what was previously reported in cultured rat peritoneal macrophages where NO was increased by both low (50 kDa) and high molecular weight chitosan stimulation [32,33]. NO generation by iNOS also influences the cytotoxicity of macrophages and tumor-induced immunosuppression. NO production by high molecular weight water-soluble chitosan (WSC, 300 kDa) indicates that it may provide various activities such as anti-microbial, anti-tumoral, and anti-viral activities under specific conditions *in vivo* [34]. In our study, two LMWCs (3 kDa and 50 kDa) significantly promoted the secretion of NO through up-regulating the mRNA expression levels of iNOS in RAW264.7 cells. The results further indicated that LMWCs effectively activated macrophages in a molecule size- and concentration-dependent manner.

Chitosan has three types of reactive functional groups, an amino/acetamido group as well as both primary and secondary hydroxyl groups at the C-2, C-3 and C-6 positions, respectively. The amino contents are the main factors contributing to the differences in their structures and physicochemical properties. Another important characteristic to consider for chitosan is the molecular weight (MW) or chain length [35]. By modulating and improving physicochemical properties, chitosan and its derivatives may provide novel therapeutic applications for the prevention or treatment of chronic diseases [11]. Following activation, macrophages can induce expression of accessory and costimulatory molecules that promote sustained stimulatory interactions with T cells and the generation of adaptive immunity. Indeed, the basic mechanisms of the immunostimulatory, anti-tumor, bactericidal and other therapeutic effects of polysaccharides are thought to occur via activation of immune cells resulting in the induction of immune responses [36]. Macrophages were thought to be the important target cells of some antitumor and immunomodulatory drug [5]. Stimulation of macrophage response is one of the most important mechanisms of all known polysaccharides with immunological competence. Several pathways are usually involved in this process: (1) improving phagocytic activity; (2) increasing NO and reactive oxygen species (ROS) production; and (3) inducing or regulating the secretion of cytokines and chemokines [37]. In the present study, we proved that LMWCs significantly enhanced the abilities of RAW264.7 macrophages to take up neutral red, produce NO, and induce the secretion of cytokines (TNF-α, IFN-γ and IL-6) and regulate their mRNA expression, which indicated that LMWCs could enhance the immune response via macrophages stimulation in a molecular weight- and concentration-dependent manner. Although both the two LMWCs (3 kDa and 50 kDa) are composed of polymerized glucosamine and *N*-acetyl glucosamine, their molecular sizes are greatly different, with the former (3 kDa) being much smaller than the latter (50 kDa). Accordingly, they may have different bioactivities. The molecular size of chitosanous products seems to be crucial for their immune bioactivity, a similarity shared by some polysaccharides from mushrooms and seaweeds [38–40]. Our results showed that the low-MW chitosans (3 kDa) had better immunomodulatory effects than those of higher MW (50 kDa). Zhou *et al.* had reported that λ-carrageenans with MWs of 15 and 9.3 kDa had the best immunomodulatory effects [41]. Lai *et al.* had also reported that low-MW chitosan oligosaccharides had best physiological effects, such as decreasing cholesterol and reinforcing the immune system, which was consistent with our results [42]. LMWCs seem to affect the immune response of macrophages depending upon the molecular weight due to LMWCs with more active amino and hydroxyl groups, but further investigation is necessary to clarify the mechanism of LMWCs.

4. Experimental Section

4.1. Chemicals and Reagents

Dulbecco's modified Eagle's medium (DMEM), penicillin/streptomycin, and the other materials required for culture of cells were purchased from Gibco BRL, Life Technologies (Grand Island, NY, USA). H_2O_2, dimethylsulfoxide (DMSO), 3-(4,5-dimethylthiazol-2-yl)-2,5-diphenyltetrazolium bromide (MTT), lipopolysaccharide (LPS), and bovine serum albumin (BSA) were obtained from Sigma (St. Louis, MO, USA). Trizol was from Invitrogen (Carlsbad, CA, USA), revert Aid™ M-MuLV reverse transcriptase was from Fermentas (Amherst, NY, USA), diethylpyrocarbonate (DEPC) and ribonuclease inhibitor were from BioBasic (Markham, ON, Canada), oligo (dT)$_{18}$ were from Sangon (Shanghai, China). All other chemicals were of analytical grade or of the highest grade available commercially.

The LMWCs were sterilized by passing it through a 0.22-µm Millipore filter (Cat No. SLGP033RB, Billerica, MA, USA) to remove any contaminant and then analyzed for endotoxin level by a gel-clot Limulus amebocyte lysate assay (Zhejiang A and C Biological, Zhejiang, China). The concentration of LMWCs was determined by spectrophotometry with bromocresol green according to Zheng *et al.* [43].

The molecular weights of the chitosan were measured using a gel permeation chromatography system (GPC) (Waters 600E, Waters Co., Milford, MA, USA). The molecular weight range of LMWCs: 46 kDa–54 kDa and 2.4 kDa–3.2 kDa. The endotoxin level in the stock soln. was less than 0.5 EU/mL.

4.2. Cell Culture and Treatment

Mouse macrophages RAW 264.7 cell line was obtained from the Shanghai Institute of Cell Biology (Shanghai, China) and maintained in DMEM, supplemented with heat-inactivated 10% fetal bovine serum, 100 U/mL penicillin, 100 U/mL streptomycin in a humidified atmosphere of 5% CO_2 at 37 °C. When the cells reached sub-confluence, they were treated for 24 h with culture medium containing different concentrations of LMWCs, two MW, 3 kDa and 50 kDa (2.5, 10, and 40 μg/mL), lipopolysaccharide (LPS) (1 μg/mL) that were tested in the experiments.

4.3. Cell Viability Assay of RAW264.7 Macrophages

The effect of LMWCs on the viability of RAW264.7 macrophages was determined by MTT method. RAW264.7 macrophages were seeded at 2×10^4 cells/well in a 96-well plate and incubated at 37 °C in a humidified atmosphere with 5% CO_2. After 24 h, the various concentrations of LMWCs were added into each well and these cells were incubated for 24 h. Each concentration was repeated six wells. The cells were washed with PBS and incubated with MTT (5 mg/mL) in culture medium at 37 °C for another 4 h. After MTT removal, the colored formazan was dissolved in 150 μL of DMSO. The absorption values were measured at 490 nm using a SpectraMax M5 Microplate Reader (Molecular Devices, MDS Analytical Technologies, Sunnyvale, CA, USA). The viability of RAW264.7 macrophages in each well was presented as percentage of control cells.

4.4. Pinocytic Activity Assay

Pinocytic activity assay was measured as previously [20]. Briefly, RAW264.7 cells were seeded at 1×10^4 cells/well in the 96-well plate and incubated at 37 °C in a humidified atmosphere with 5% CO_2. After 24 h, DMEM medium, LPS or the various concentrations of LMWCs were added into each well, and these cells were incubated at 37 °C for 24 h. Each concentration was repeated six wells. Culture media were removed and 100 μL/well of 0.075% neutral red was added, and incubated for 30 min. After washed with PBS for three times, 150 μL of cell lyzing solution were added into each well and cells were put at 37 °C for 1 h. The absorbance was evaluated in a SpectraMax M5 Microplate Reader (Molecular Devices, MDS Analytical Technologies, Sunnyvale, CA, USA) at 570 nm.

4.5. Preparation of Cell Lysates

The cells were seeded at a density of 1×10^6 cells/mL in 6-well plates. When the cells reached sub-confluence, they were treated for 24 h with culture medium containing different concentrations of LMWCs of two MW, 3 kDa and 50 kDa (2.5, 10, and 40 μg/mL), and LPS (1 μg/mL). Upon completion of the incubation studies, the culture supernatant was collected for analysis of NO release and cytokines. The cells were scraped from the plates into ice-cold 1% Triton X-100 lysis buffer and protein concentration was determined by the bicinchoninic acid (BCA) method, using BSA as a reference standard. Aliquots were stored at −80 °C until detection for the activities of iNOS.

4.6. Measurement of Cytokine Levels in RAW264.7 Macrophage Cultures Using an Enzyme Linked Immunosorbent Assay (ELISA)

The RAW264.7 macrophages culture supernatants in each individual treatment were collected to measure pro-inflammatory cytokines TNF-α, IFN-γ and IL-6 levels. The TNF-α, IFN-γ and IL-6 levels were assayed according to the cytokine ELISA protocol from the manufacturer's instructions (Wuhan Boster Biological Engineering Co., Ltd., Wuhan, China).

4.7. Measurement of Nitric Oxide (NO) Release and Intracellular Contents of iNOS

The concentration of nitriles (NO_2^-) and nitrates (NO_3^-), stable end products of nitric oxide (NO), were determined by the reagent kits from the Nanjing Institute of Jiancheng Bioengineering (Nanjing, China). NO production was determined by measuring the optical density at 550 nm and expressed as units per liter. Activity of iNOS in the supernatant was quantified using the iNOS activity assay kit (Nanjing Jiancheng Bioengineering Institute, Nanjing, China) according to the manufacturer's instructions. Values of iNOS level were expressed as activity units per milligram protein.

4.8. Measurement of the mRNA Expression Levels of iNOS and TNF-α by Real-Time PCR

Cells were lysed in 1 mL of Trizol reagent (Invitrogen™, Carlsbad, CA, USA) and the total RNA was isolated according to the manufacture's protocol. The concentration of total RNA was quantified by determining the optical density at 260 nm. The total RNA was used and reverse transcription (RT) was performed using 1st-Strand cDNA Synthesis Kit (Invitrogen, Waltham, MA, USA). Briefly, nuclease-free water was added giving a final volume of 5 μL after mixing 2 μg of RNA with 0.5 μg oligo (dT)$_{18}$ primer in a DEPC-treated tube. This mixture was incubated at 65 °C for 5 min and chilled on ice for 2 min. Then, a solution containing 3 μL of RT buffer Mix, 0.65 μL of RT Enzyme Mix and 1.35 μL Primer Mix, giving a final volume of 10 μL, and the tubes were incubated for 10 min at 30 °C. The tubes then were incubated for 30 min at 42 °C. Finally, the reaction was stopped by heating at 70 °C for 15 min. The samples were stored at −20 °C until further use.

As shown in Table 1, the primers were used to amplify cDNA fragments (141-bp iNOS fragment, 88-bp TNF-α fragment and 94-bp 18S fragment). Amplification was carried out in total volume of 25 μL containing 1 μL (5 μM) of each target and 18S specific primers, 1 μL of cDNA template, 12.5 μL of Power SYBR® Master Mix (2×) (4 μL of 10× PCR buffer, 4 μL of MgCl$_2$ (25 mM), 4 μL of dNTPs (2.5 mM) and 0.5 μL of Taq DNA polymerase) (Invitrogen, Waltham, MA, USA), and 10.5 μL of DEPC-treated water was added. Reaction conditions were the standard conditions for the iQTM5 PCR (Bio-Rad, Hercules, CA, USA) (10 s denaturation at 95 °C, 25 s annealing at 64 °C (TNF-α, iNOS, 18S) with 40 PCR cycles. Ct values were obtained automatically using software (Bio-Rad, Hercules, CA, USA). The comparative Ct method ($2^{-\Delta Ct}$ method) [44] was used to analyze the expression levels of TNF-α.

Table 1. Real-Time Polymerase Chain Reaction (PCR) Primers and Conditions.

Gene	Genbank Accession	Primer Sequence	Product Size (bp)	Annealing (°C)
TNF-α	NM_013693	CGGTGCCTATGTCTCAGCCTCTT GACCGATCACCCCGAAGTTCAGTA	88	64
iNOS	NM_010927.3	TGCCACGGACGAGACGGATA AGGAAGGCAGCGGGCACAT	141	64
18s	NR_003278	CGGACACGGACAGGATTGACA CCAGACAAATCGCTCCACCAACTA	94	64

4.9. Statistical Analysis

Data were expressed as mean ± standard deviation (S.D.) and examined for their statistical significance of difference with ANOVA and a Tukey *post hoc* test by using SPSS 16.0. *p*-Values of less than 0.05 were considered statistically significant.

5. Conclusions

To the best of our knowledge, this is the first report to demonstrate that two important LMWCs (3 kDa and 50 kDa) can induce activation of RAW264.7 macrophages, which may account for their immune-stimulating effects. We observed that two LMWCs significantly enhance the pinocytic activity, and induce the production of tumor necrosis factor α (TNF-α), interleukin 6 (IL-6), interferon-γ (IFN-γ), nitric oxide (NO) and inducible nitric oxide synthase (iNOS) in a concentration-dependent manner. LMWCs were further shown to upregulate the expression of the genes including iNOS and TNF-α. Moreover, 3 kDa chitosan would simultaneously induced Th1- and Th2-type response, and induced stronger immunostimulative activity than that of 50 kDa chitosan. LMWCs seem to affect the balance of the Th1/Th2 immune response of RAW264.7 cells depending upon the molecular weight due to LMWCs with more active amino and hydroxyl groups. In addition, LMWCs, which are more effectively absorbed in the body than that of high molecular weight chitosan, suitable narrow molecular weight distribution and non-toxicity, could be applied most promisingly to pharmaceutical materials. Accordingly, further investigation is necessary to clarify the mechanism of LMWCs as a novel immunomodulator.

Acknowledgments: This work was supported by grant from Zhejiang Provincial Undergraduate Scientific and Technological Innovation Project (2013R411020), Scientific and Technological Project of Zhejiang Ocean University (X12M05), Key Scientific and Technological Project of Zhejiang Ocean University (X12ZD08), Scientific and Technological Project of Department of Education of Zhejiang Province (Y201328199), Zhejiang Provincial Natural Science Foundation of China (No. LQ13C200002), National Natural Science Foundation of China (No. 31301982) and International Science & Technology Cooperation Program of China (2015DFA30980).

Conflicts of Interest: The authors declare that there are no conflicts of interest.

References

1. Guan, D.; Zhang, Z.; Yang, Y.; Xing, G.; Liu, J. Immunomodulatory Activity of Polysaccharide from the Roots of *Actinidia kolomikta* on Macrophages. *Int. J. Biol.* **2011**, *3*. [CrossRef]
2. De Oliveira, C.C.; De Oliveira, S.M.; Godoy, L.M.; Gabardo, J.; Buchi, D.D.F. Canova, Brazilian medical formulation, alters oxidative metabolism of mice macrophages. *J. Infect.* **2006**, *52*, 420–432. [CrossRef] [PubMed]
3. Schepetkin, I.A.; Xie, G.; Kirpotina, L.N.; Klein, R.A.; Jutila, M.A.; Quinn, M.T. Macrophage immunomodulatory activity of polysaccharides isolated from *Opuntia polyacantha*. *Int. Immunopharmacol.* **2008**, *8*, 1455–1466. [CrossRef] [PubMed]
4. Schepetkin, I.A.; Quinn, M.T. Botanical polysaccharides: Macrophage immunomodulation and therapeutic potential. *Int. Immunopharmacol.* **2006**, *6*, 317–333. [CrossRef] [PubMed]
5. Cheng, A.W.; Wan, F.C.; Wang, J.Q.; Jin, Z.Y.; Xu, X.M. Macrophage immunomodulatory activity of polysaccharides isolated from *Glycyrrhiza uralensis* Fish. *Int. Immunopharmacol.* **2008**, *8*, 43–50. [CrossRef] [PubMed]
6. Zaharoff, D.A.; Rogers, C.J.; Hance, K.W.; Schlom, J.; Greiner, J.W. Chitosan solution enhances both humoral and cell-mediated immune responses to subcutaneous vaccination. *Vaccine* **2007**, *25*, 2085–2094. [CrossRef] [PubMed]
7. Read, R.C.; Naylor, S.C.; Potter, C.W.; Bond, J.; Jabbal-Gill, I.; Fisher, A.; Illum, L.; Jennings, R. Effective nasal influenza vaccine delivery using chitosan. *Vaccine* **2005**, *23*, 4367–4374. [CrossRef] [PubMed]
8. Mills, K.H.; Cosgrove, C.; McNeela, E.A.; Sexton, A.; Giemza, R.; Jabbal-Gill, I.; Church, A.; Lin, W.; Illum, L.; Podda, A.; *et al.* Protective levels of diphtheria-neutralizing antibody induced in healthy volunteers by unilateral priming-boosting intranasal immunization associated with restricted ipsilateral mucosal secretory immunoglobulin A. *Infect. Immun.* **2003**, *71*, 726–732. [CrossRef] [PubMed]
9. McNeela, E.A.; Jabbal-Gill, I.; Illum, L.; Pizza, M.; Rappuoli, R.; Podda, A.; Lewis, D.J.; Mills, K.H. Intranasal immunization with genetically detoxified diphtheria toxin induces T cell responses in humans: Enhancement of Th2 responses and toxin-neutralizing antibodies by formulation with chitosan. *Vaccine* **2004**, *22*, 909–914. [CrossRef] [PubMed]
10. Wen, Z.S.; Xu, Y.L.; Zou, X.T.; Xu, Z.R. Chitosan Nanoparticles Act as an Adjuvant to Promote both Th1 and Th2 Immune Responses Induced by Ovalbumin in Mice. *Mar. Drugs* **2011**, *9*, 1038–1055. [CrossRef] [PubMed]
11. Ngo, D.H.; Vo, T.S.; Ngo, D.N.; Kang, K.H.; Je, J.Y.; Pham, H.N.D.; Byun, H.G.; Kim, S.K. Biological effects of chitosan and its derivatives. *Food Hydrocoll.* **2015**, *51*, 200–216. [CrossRef]
12. Park, B.K.; Kim, M.M. Applications of Chitin and Its Derivatives in Biological Medicine. *Int. J. Mol. Sci.* **2010**, *11*, 5152–5164. [CrossRef] [PubMed]

13. Fernandes, J.C.; Spindola, H.; de Sousa, V.; Santos-Silva, A.; Pintado, M.E.; Malcata, F.X.; Carvalho, J.E. Anti-inflammatory activity of chitooligosaccharides *in vivo*. *Mar. Drugs* **2010**, *8*, 1763–1768. [CrossRef] [PubMed]

14. Ju, C.X.; Yue, W.; Yang, Z.H.; Zhang, Q.; Yang, X.; Liu, Z.; Zhang, F. Antidiabetic effect and mechanism of chitooligosaccharides. *Biol. Pharm. Bull.* **2010**, *33*, 1511–1516. [CrossRef] [PubMed]

15. Jung, E.J.; Youn, D.K.; Lee, S.H.; No, H.K.; Ha, J.G.; Prinyawiwatkul, W. Antibacterial activity of chitosans with different degrees of deacetylation and viscosities. *Int. J. Food Sci. Technol.* **2010**, *45*, 676–682. [CrossRef]

16. Artan, M.; Karadeniz, F.; Karagozlu, M.Z.; Kim, M.M.; Kim, S.K. Anti-HIV-1 activity of low molecular weight sulfated chitooligosaccharides. *Carbohydr. Res.* **2010**, *345*, 656–662. [CrossRef] [PubMed]

17. Ngo, D.N.; Lee, S.H.; Kim, M.; Kim, S.K. Production of chitin-oligosaccharides with different molecular weights and their antioxidant effect in RAW264.7 cells. *J. Funct. Foods* **2009**, *1*, 188–198. [CrossRef]

18. Quan, H.; Zhu, F.; Han, X.; Xu, Z.; Zhao, Y.; Miao, Z. Mechanism of anti-angiogenic activities of chitooligosaccharides may be through inhibiting heparanase activity. *Med. Hypotheses* **2009**, *73*, 205–206. [CrossRef] [PubMed]

19. Gong, Y.; Gong, L.; Gu, X.; Ding, F. Chitooligosaccharides promote peripheral nerve regeneration in a rabbit common peroneal nerve crush injury model. *Microsurgery* **2009**, *29*, 650–656. [CrossRef] [PubMed]

20. Lee, C.G.; Da Silva, C.A.; Lee, J.Y.; Hartl, D.; Elias, J.A. Chitin regulation of immune responses: An old molecule with new roles. *Curr. Opin. Immunol.* **2008**, *20*, 684–689. [CrossRef]

21. Li, X.; Min, M.; Du, N.; Gu, Y.; Hode, T.; Naylor, M.; Chen, D.; Nordquist, R.E.; Chen, W.R. Chitin, Chitosan, and Glycated Chitosan Regulate Immune Responses: The Novel Adjuvants for Cancer Vaccine. *Clin. Dev. Immunol.* **2013**, *2013*. [CrossRef] [PubMed]

22. Ueno, H.; Nakamura, F.; Murakami, M.; Okumura, M.; Kadosawa, T.; Fujinag, T. Evaluation effects of chitosan for the extracellular matrix production by fibroblasts and the growth factors production by macrophages. *Biomaterials* **2001**, *22*, 2125–2130. [CrossRef]

23. Sun, H.; Zhang, J.; Chen, F.; Chen, X.; Zhou, Z.; Wang, H. Activation of RAW264.7 macrophages by the polysaccharide from the roots of *Actinidia eriantha* and its molecular mechanisms. *Carbohydr. Polym.* **2015**, *121*, 388–402. [CrossRef] [PubMed]

24. Nishiyama, A.; Tsuji, S.; Yamashita, M.; Henriksen, R.A.; Myrvik, Q.N.; Shibata, Y. Phagocytosis of N-acetyl-D-glucosamine particles, a Th1 adjuvant, by RAW 264.7 cells results in MAPK activation and TNF-α, but not IL-10, production. *Cell. Immunol.* **2006**, *239*, 103–112. [CrossRef] [PubMed]

25. Yu, Z.; Zhao, L.; Ke, H. Potential role of nuclear factor-κB in the induction of nitric oxide and tumor necrosis factor-α by oligochitosan in macrophages. *Int. Immunopharmacol.* **2004**, *4*, 193–200. [CrossRef] [PubMed]

26. Reese, T.A.; Liang, H.R.; Tager, A.M.; Luster, A.D.; van Rooijen, N.; Voehringer, D.; Locksley, R.M. Chitin induces accumulation in tissue of innate immune cells associated with allergy. *Nature* **2007**, *447*, 92–96. [PubMed]

27. Chen, C.L.; Wang, Y.M.; Liu, C.F.; Wang, J.Y. The effect of water-soluble chitosan on macrophage activation and the attenuation of mite allergen-induced airway inflammation. *Biomaterials* **2008**, *29*, 2173–2182. [CrossRef] [PubMed]

28. Shibata, Y.; Metzger, W.J.; Myrvik, Q.N. Chitin particle-induced cell-mediated immunity is inhibited by soluble mannan: Mannose receptor-mediated phagocytosis initiates IL-12 production. *J. Immunol.* **1997**, *159*, 2462–2467. [PubMed]

29. Lechner, M.; Lirk, P.; Rieder, J. Inducible nitric oxide synthase (iNOS) in tumor biology: The two sides of the same coin. *Semin. Cancer Biol.* **2005**, *15*, 277–289. [CrossRef] [PubMed]

30. Sun, J.; Druhan, L.J.; Zweier, J.L. Reactive oxygen and nitrogen species regulate inducible nitric oxide synthase function shifting the balance of nitric oxide and superoxide production. *Arch. Bioch. Biophys.* **2010**, *494*, 130–137. [CrossRef] [PubMed]

31. Wu, G.J.; Tsai, G.J. Chitooligosaccharides in combination with interferon-gamma increase nitric oxide production via nuclear factor-kappaB activation in murine RAW264.7 macrophages. *Food Chem. Toxicol.* **2007**, *45*, 250–258. [CrossRef] [PubMed]

32. Peluso, G.; Petillo, O.; Ranieri, M.; Santin, M.; Ambrosio, L.; Calabro, D.; Avallone, B.; Balsamo, G. Chitosan-mediated stimulation of macrophage function. *Biomaterials* **1994**, *15*, 1215–1220. [CrossRef]

33. Porporatto, C.; Bianco, I.D.; Riera, C.M.; Correa, S.G. Chitosan induces different L-arginine metabolic pathways in resting and inflammatory macrophages. *Biochem. Biophys. Res. Commun.* **2003**, *304*, 266–272. [CrossRef]

34. Jeong, H.J.; Koo, H.N.; Oh, E.Y.; Chae, H.J.; Kim, H.R.; Suh, S.B.; Kim, C.H.; Cho, K.H.; Park, B.R.; Park, S.T.; *et al.* Nitric oxide production by high molecular weight water-soluble chitosan via nuclear factor-κB activation. *Int. J. Immunopharmacol.* **2000**, *22*, 923–933. [CrossRef]

35. Zhang, J.; Xia, W.; Liu, P.; Cheng, Q.; Tahirou, T.; Gu, W.; Li, B. Chitosan modification and pharmaceutical/biomedical applications. *Mar. Drugs* **2010**, *8*, 1962–1987. [PubMed]

36. Beutler, B. Innate immunity: An overview. *Mol. Immunol.* **2004**, *40*, 845–859. [CrossRef] [PubMed]

37. Sun, L.; Wang, L.; Zhou, Y. Immunomodulation and antitumor activities of different-molecular-weight polysaccharides from *Porphyridium cruentum*. *Carbohydr. Polym.* **2012**, *87*, 1206–1210. [CrossRef]

38. Cho, M.; Yang, C.; Kim, S.M.; You, S. Molecular characterization and biological activities of water soluble sulfated polysaccharides from *Enteromorpha prolifera*. *Food Sci. Biotechnol.* **2010**, *19*, 525–533. [CrossRef]

39. Zhang, L.; Li, X.L.; Xu, X.J.; Zeng, F.B. Correlation between antitumor activity, molecular weight, and conformation of lentinan. *Carbohydr. Res.* **2005**, *340*, 1515–1521. [CrossRef] [PubMed]

40. Wu, G.J.; Wu, C.H.; Tsai, G.J. Chitooligosaccharides from the shrimp chitosan hydrolysate induces differentiation of murine RAW264.7 macrophages into dendritic-like cells. *J. Funct. Foods* **2015**, *12*, 70–79. [CrossRef]

41. Zhou, G.F.; Sun, Y.P.; Xin, H.; Zhang, Y.N.; Li, Z.E.; Xu, Z.H. *In vivo* antitumor and immunomodulation activities of different molecular weight λ-carrageenans from *Chondrus ocellatus*. *Pharmacol. Res.* **2004**, *50*, 47–53. [CrossRef] [PubMed]

42. Lai, S.L.; Pan, Z.Y.; Li, X.F. Study on the degradability of chitosan under microwave irradiation. *J. Shanxi Univ. Sci. Technol.* **2005**, *23*, 38–40.

43. Zheng, T.S.; Wang, Y.N.; Zong, A.P. Spectrophotometry of chitosan with Bromocresol Green. *J. China Pharm. Univ.* **2005**, *36*, 543–545.

44. Livak, K.J.; Schmittgen, T.D. Analysis of Relative Gene Expression Data Using Real-Time Quantitative PCR and the $2^{-\Delta Ct}$ Method. *Methods* **2001**, *25*, 402–408. [PubMed]

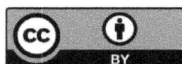

marine drugs

MDPI

Article

Alginate-Derived Oligosaccharide Inhibits Neuroinflammation and Promotes Microglial Phagocytosis of β-Amyloid

Rui Zhou [1], Xu-Yang Shi [2], De-Cheng Bi [1], Wei-Shan Fang [2], Gao-Bin Wei [2] and Xu Xu [1,*]

[1] Shenzhen Key Laboratory of Marine Bioresources and Ecology, Collage of Life Science, Shenzhen University, Shenzhen 518060, China; zhouruiswg@gmail.com (R.Z.); bidecheng@foxmail.com (D.-C.B.)

[2] College of Life Science, Shenzhen Key Laboratory of Microbial Genetic Engineering, Shenzhen University, Shenzhen 518060, China; shixuyang075@gmail.com (X.-Y.S.); fangweishan90@163.com (W.-S.F.); weigaobin@126.com (G.-B.W.)

* Author to whom correspondence should be addressed; xuxu@szu.edu.cn; Tel.: +86-755-26534977; Fax: +86-755-26534274.

Academic Editor: Paola Laurienzo
Received: 17 July 2015; Accepted: 7 September 2015; Published: 16 September 2015

Abstract: Alginate from marine brown algae has been widely applied in biotechnology. In this work, the effects of alginate-derived oligosaccharide (AdO) on lipopolysaccharide (LPS)/β-amyloid (Aβ)-induced neuroinflammation and microglial phagocytosis of Aβ were studied. We found that pretreatment of BV2 microglia with AdO prior to LPS/Aβ stimulation led to a significant inhibition of production of nitric oxide (NO) and prostaglandin E_2 (PGE$_2$), expression of inducible nitric oxide synthase (iNOS) and cyclooxygenase-2 (COX-2) and secretion of proinflammatory cytokines. We further demonstrated that AdO remarkably attenuated the LPS-activated overexpression of toll-like receptor 4 (TLR4) and nuclear factor (NF)-κB in BV2 cells. In addition to the impressive inhibitory effect on neuroinflammation, we also found that AdO promoted the phagocytosis of Aβ through its interaction with TLR4 in microglia. Our results suggested that AdO exerted the inhibitory effect on neuroinflammation and the promotion effect on microglial phagocytosis, indicating its potential as a nutraceutical or therapeutic agent for neurodegenerative diseases, particularly Alzheimer's disease (AD).

Keywords: alginate; β-amyloid; microglia; neuroinflammation; phagocytosis; toll-like receptor 4

1. Introduction

In the last decade, increasing evidence has demonstrated that neuroinflammation is involved in the pathogenesis and progression of various neurodegenerative disorders, including Alzheimer's disease (AD) [1] and Parkinson's disease [2]. The accumulation of β-amyloid (Aβ) and the accompanying neurotoxicity is considered to be one of the most important pathologies of AD [3]. Microglial cells are resident immune cells and act as effectors of various processes in normal and pathological brains. Two of the main functions of microglial cells are mediating neuroinflammation and clearing toxic Aβ aggregates via phagocytosis [4]. Previous reports have proposed that activated microglial cells are induced by pathogen-associated environmental toxins, such as lipopolysaccharide (LPS) or Aβ [5]. LPS/Aβ activates microglial cells via various receptors expressed on the cell surfaces, especially toll-like receptors (TLR) [6]. TLR activation of the microglial cells induce the secretion of a number of inflammatory factors that lead to cytotoxic effects and brain damage, resulting in serious neuroinflammation [7,8]. The TLR4 signaling that triggers the generation of the inflammatory mediators depends on the activation of multiple intracellular signaling pathways, including nuclear factor (NF)-κB and mitogen-activated protein kinases (MAPKs) [6,9]. It has been established that agents that can efficiently attenuate TLR signaling and decrease the inflammatory responses of the activated microglial cells are beneficial in treating AD [10]. In addition, microglia are essentially the macrophages of the brain, and phagocytosis is a key feature of these cells. This function supports brain homoeostasis by clearing neurotoxic substances, including cellular debris and Aβ aggregates. However, it has been found that the clearance of toxic Aβ aggregates by the microglia is impaired in AD [11]. Considering the inflammatory and phagocytotic functions of microglia, one possible therapeutic method for treating AD is to reduce microglia-mediated neuroinflammation and increase microglial clearance of Aβ [12].

Alginate derived from various marine brown algae is an acidic polysaccharide composed of alternating blocks of β-(1-4)-D-mannuronic acid (M) and α-(1-4)-L-guluronic acid (G). Alginate has been widely applied in biotechnology for microencapsulation, drug delivery, and tissue engineering [13,14]. Alginate-derived oligosaccharide (AdO) produced by depolymerizing the polysaccharide using various degradation methods shows a variety of biological activities. Unsaturated AdO depolymerized by enzymatic depolymerization exerts anti-tumor [15], anti-oxidant [16,17], and immunomodulatory effects [18,19], whereas the saturated AdO prepared by acid hydrolysis posses low bioactivities. The anti-inflammatory activities of alginate have been described [20,21]. AdO prepared by oxidative degradation possibly has a carboxyl group at the 1-position of the reducing end, which have been characterized in the previous work (Figure 1) [22]. We have demonstrated that AdO prepared by oxidative degradation suppressed the inflammatory response in LPS-activated marine macrophage RAW 264.7 cells [23], which inspired us to investigate whether AdO could reduce neuroinflammation and subsequently attenuate neuroinflammation-mediated diseases.

In the current study, our aim is to investigate the molecular mechanisms of the inhibitory effect of AdO on LPS/Aβ-stimulated microglial neuroinflammation, and to demonstrate the effect of AdO on the phagocytosis of Aβ by BV2 microglia. Our findings suggested the potential application of AdO as a therapeutic agent for the treatment of AD.

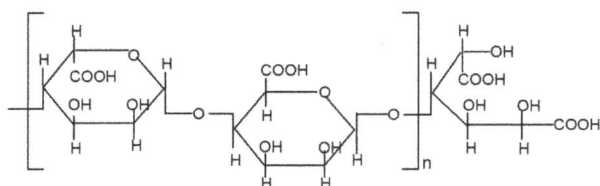

Figure 1. Schematic representation of chemical structures of alginate-derived oligosaccharide (AdO) prepared by oxidative degradation.

2. Results

2.1. AdO Suppresses LPS-Induced Production of Inflammatory Mediators in BV2 Cells

To evaluate the toxicity of AdO to BV2 cells, the cell viability was measured after treatment with AdO. Results showed that AdO with concentrations lower than 500 μg/mL led to little cytotoxic effect in BV2 cells (Figure 2A). Therefore, we investigated the anti-neuroinflammatory effect of 50–500 μg/mL of AdO in LPS-activated BV2 cells in this study. Next, we evaluated the effect of AdO on the production of nitric oxide (NO) and prostaglandin E_2 (PGE$_2$) by LPS-activated BV2 cells. As shown in Figure 2B and C, AdO at various concentrations inhibited the LPS-induced NO and PGE$_2$ levels in BV2 cells in a dose-dependent manner. On the basis that inducible nitric oxide synthase (iNOS) and cyclooxygenase-2 (COX-2) are the key enzymes for production of NO and PGE$_2$, respectively, we performed RT-PCR and Western blot analyses to determine the effects of AdO on the expression of iNOS and COX-2. The results showed that the LPS-induced expression of iNOS and COX-2 was suppressed by AdO treatment at the mRNA level (Figure 2D, E) and at the protein level (Figure 2F,G). These results indicated that AdO reduces NO and PGE_2 production by inhibiting the iNOS and COX-2 expression.

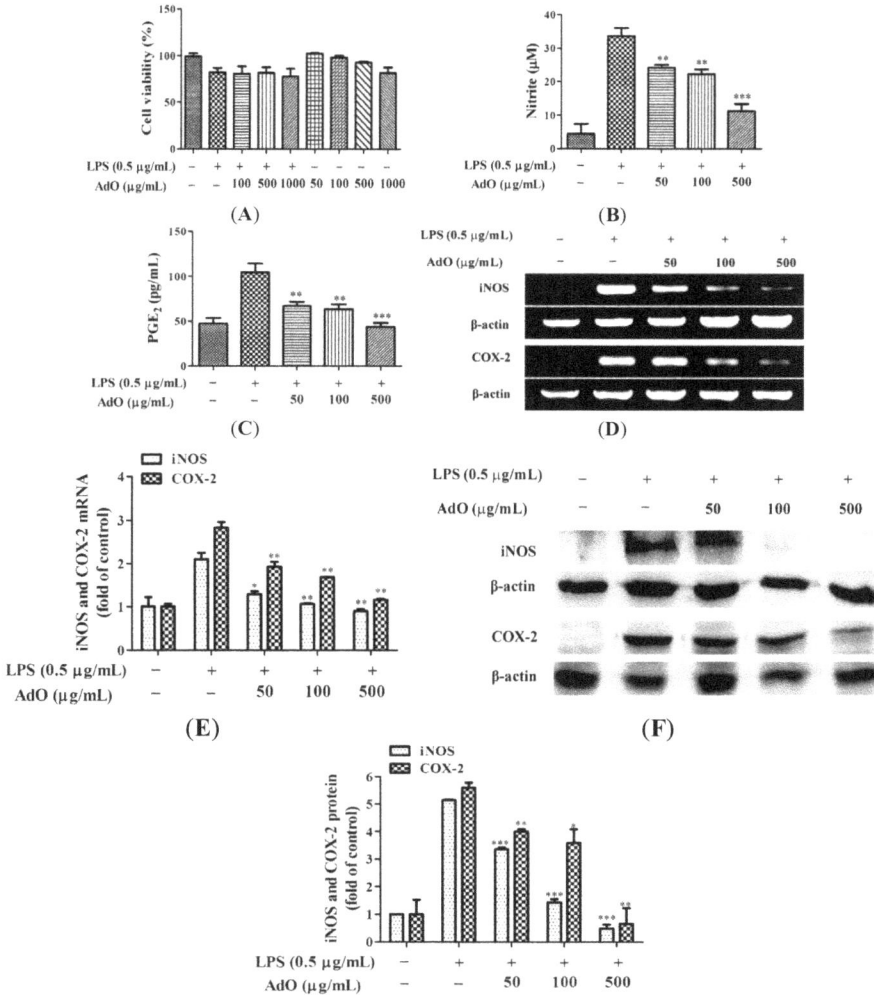

Figure 2. AdO reduced the lipopolysaccharide (LPS)-activated production of nitric oxide (NO) and prostaglandin E_2 (PGE_2) and the expression of inducible nitric oxide synthase (iNOS) and cyclooxygenase-2 (COX-2) in BV2 microglial cells. (**A**) Cell viability was evaluated using the CCK-8 assay for control cells, LPS (0.5 μg/mL) treatment cells, LPS with AdO (100–1000 μg/mL) treatment cells, and AdO (50–1000 μg/mL) treatment cells; (**B**) The nitrite concentration was measured as an indicator of NO production using the Griess reagent; (**C**) PGE_2 production was analyzed using ELISA; (**D**) The expression of the iNOS and COX-2 mRNAs was detected by RT-PCR; (**E**) The relative mRNA levels of iNOS and COX-2 were analyzed with reference to the control group; (**F**) The expression of the iNOS and COX-2 proteins was detected using Western blot analysis; (**G**) The relative levels of the iNOS and COX-2 proteins were analyzed with reference to the control group. The data are presented as the mean ± SD for three independent experiments. * $p < 0.05$, ** $p < 0.01$ and *** $p < 0.001$ indicate significant differences compared with the LPS-treated group.

2.2. AdO Inhibits LPS/Aβ-Activated Secretion of Inflammatory Cytokines in BV2 Cells

As demonstrated in Figure 3, the secretion of tumor necrosis factor-α (TNF-α), interleukin (IL)-1β and IL-6 (Figure 3A) was notably increased with LPS stimulation, but considerably decreased in a dose-dependent manner in the AdO-pretreated cells. Next, we investigated whether AdO could affect the Aβ-activated production of the inflammatory cytokines by the BV2 cells. As expected, the results showed that the AdO treatment remarkably reduced the Aβ-stimulated production of TNF-α, IL-6 and IL-12 (Figure 3B). Interestingly, we demonstrated that Aβ reduced the cell viability to 76.6% ± 3.36%, but pre-treatment with AdO exerted a positive effect on the cell viability (Figure 3C). These results suggest that AdO could effectively suppress the LPS/Aβ-activated inflammatory cytokines secretion by the BV2 cells.

A   B   C

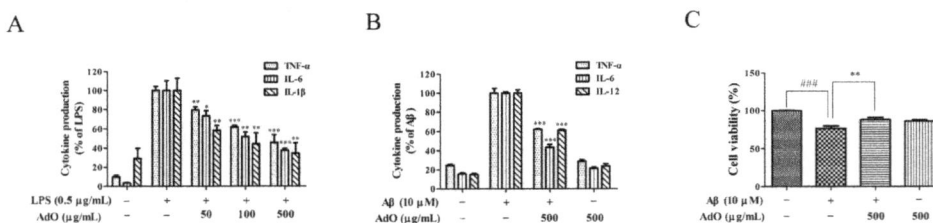

Figure 3. AdO inhibited the LPS/Aβ-activated secretion of proinflammatory cytokines. (**A**) Tumor necrosis factor-α (TNF-α), interleukin (IL)-1β and IL-6 expression in the LPS-activated BV2 cells was measured by ELISA; (**B**) TNF-α, IL-6 and IL-12 production in the Aβ-activated BV2 cells was evaluated by ELISA; (**C**) The cell viability following AdO (500 μg/mL) pretreatment with or without Aβ (10 μM) stimulation was detected by the CCK-8 assay. The data are presented as the mean ± SD for three independent experiments. * $p < 0.05$, ** $p < 0.01$ and *** $p < 0.001$ indicate significant differences compared with the LPS/Aβ-treated group, and ### $p < 0.001$ indicates a significant difference between the control group and the Aβ-treated group.

2.3. AdO Inhibits LPS-Activated Signaling Pathway in BV2 Cells

Next, we evaluated the effect of AdO on the LPS-activated TLR4-NF-κB signaling pathway using immunofluorescence and Western blot analysis. As shown in Figure 4A, TLR4 expression was notably increased by LPS stimulation, and this effect was blocked by the addition of AdO. Similar results were observed in the Western blot analysis (Figure 4B). Figure 4C clearly shows that the translocation of the NF-κB/p65 subunit from the cytoplasm to the cell nucleus was augmented by LPS-stimulation and reduced by AdO treatment. The results of the Western blot analysis agreed well with the immunofluorescence analysis (Figure 4D).

2.4. Effect of AdO on LPS/Aβ-Activated Morphological Changes of the BV2 Cells

Furthermore, it has been demonstrated that anti-inflammatory agents can protect the microglia from LPS or Aβ-activated morphological changes [24,25]. Here, the effect of AdO on the LPS/Aβ-activated cell morphological changes was observed using dark-field microscopy. The enlargement of microglial cell bodies and an amoeboid morphology with retraction of extensions are generally induced by LPS [24]. While these changes were obvious in the LPS-activated BV2 microglia (see white dot arrows in Figure 5A), AdO markedly suppressed those morphological changes (Figure 5A). We analyzed the number of cells with normal (white arrows) or activated (white dot arrows) morphology in ten randomly selected images. The results showed that pretreatment with AdO prevented the LPS-activated morphological changes of the cells in a dose-dependent manner (Figure 5B). In addition, the effect of AdO on the Aβ-activated microglia morphological changes was investigated. As expected, AdO protected the microglia from the Aβ-activated morphological changes (Figure 5C). The analyzed results are shown as histograms (Figure 5D).

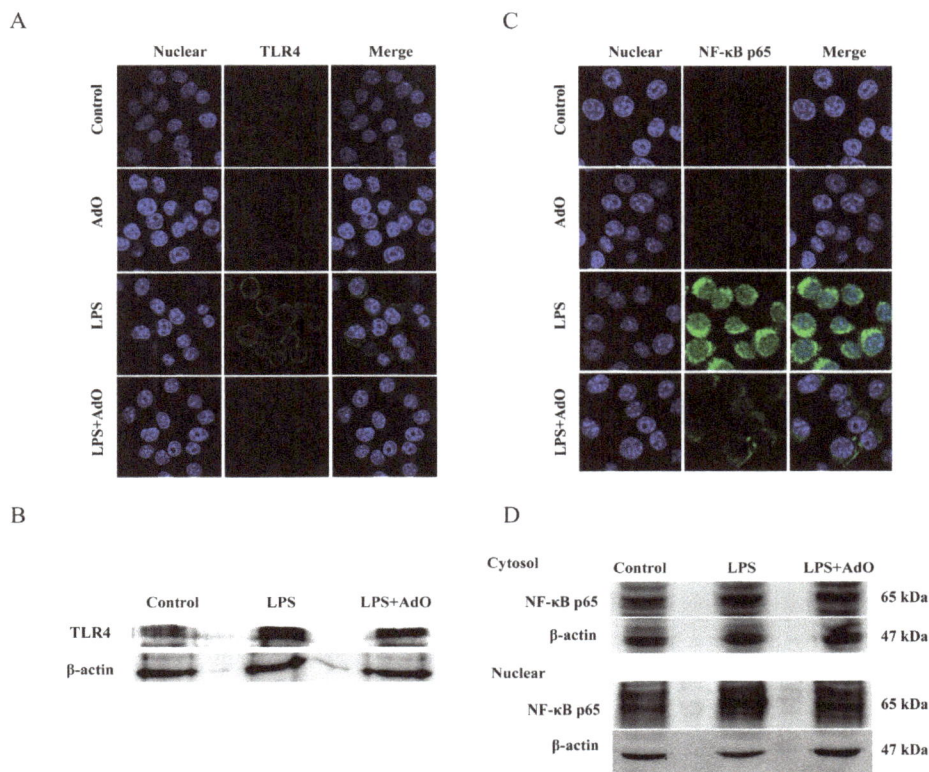

Figure 4. AdO suppressed the LPS-induced toll-like receptor 4 (TLR4) expression and nuclear factor (NF)-κB activation. TLR4 expression was evaluated using immunofluorescence analysis (**A**) and Western blot analysis (**B**); (**C**) NF-κB p65 expression was examined using immunofluorescence analysis; (**D**) The cytoplasm and nuclear proteins were extracted and the NF-κB p65 protein was analyzed by Western blot analysis. The immunofluorescence analysis was carried out by laser scanning confocal microscopy (60×), and the images were processed using ImageJ software. The immunofluorescence analysis and Western blot analysis were performed in three independent experiments.

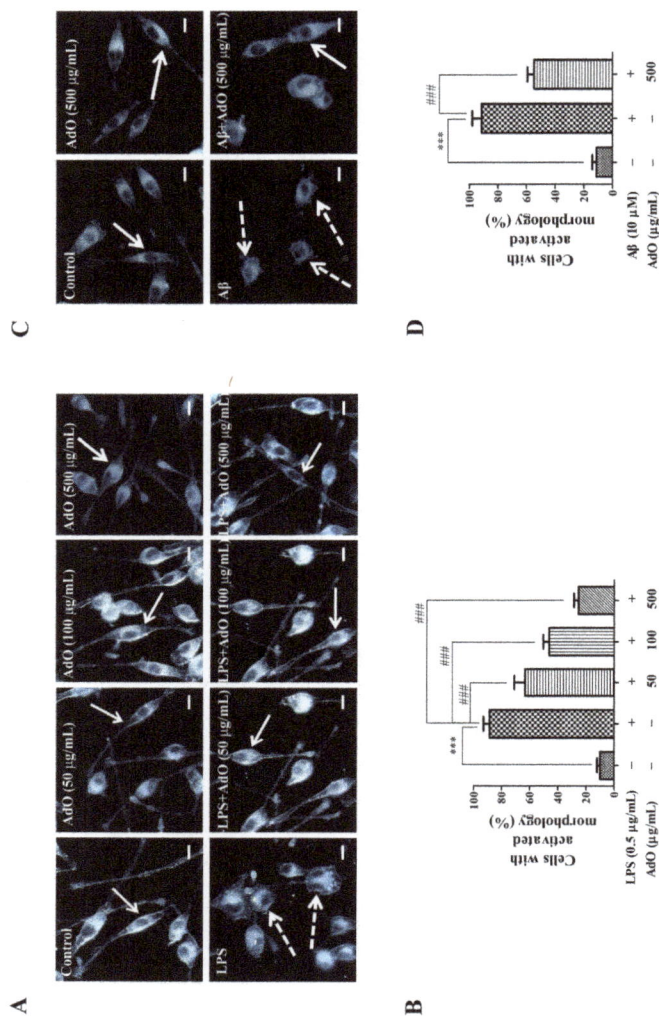

Figure 5. AdO inhibited the morphological changes induced by LPS/β-amyloid (Aβ) in the BV2 cells. (**A**) The cellular morphology of the control group, AdO (50–500 μg/mL)-treated group, LPS (0.5 μg/mL)-treated group and the group treated with AdO prior to LPS are shown in the dark field images; (**B**) The percentage of cells exhibiting the activated morphology was statistically analyzed; (**C**) The cellular morphology of the control group, AdO (500 μg/mL)-treated group, and Aβ (10 μM)-treated group as well as the group treated with AdO prior to Aβ are shown in the dark field images; (**D**) The percentage of cells exhibiting the activated morphology was statistically analyzed. The cellular morphology was observed using dark-field microscopy (40×), and the images were analyzed using ImageJ software (National Institutes of Health, Bethesda, MD, USA). The normal cell morphology is indicated by white arrows, and the activated cell morphology is indicated by white dotted arrows. Scale bar = 20 μm. The images were from three independent experiments. *** $p < 0.001$ indicates significant differences between the control group and the LPS/Aβ-treated group; ### $p < 0.001$ indicates significant differences between the LPS/Aβ-treated group and the group treated with AdO prior to LPS/Aβ.

2.5. AdO Promotes the Phagocytosis of Aβ in BV2 Cells

First, gold nanoparticles (AuNPs) with a 100-nm diameter were used to evaluate the non-specific phagocytic ability of BV2 cells. The BV2 microglia were incubated with AuNPs for the indicated times and observed using dark-field microscopy. The cells with phagocytosed AuNPs are shown in Figure 6A. The intracellular AuNPs were analyzed using ImageJ software. The results showed that BV2 microglia readily accumulated increasing amounts of AuNPs in a time-dependent manner (Figure 6B). Next, the BV2 cells were treated with AdO for 20 h, after which AuNPs were added, and the incubation was continued for an additional 1 h. We found that the BV2 cells treated with AdO accumulated more AuNPs than the untreated cells (Figure 6C). The analyzed results are shown in Figure 6D. AdO treatment increased the phagocytosis of AuNPs in a concentration-dependent manner, suggesting that AdO activated the BV2 microglia and promoted phagocytosis. In addition, the results clearly showed that AdO promoted the uptake of AuNPs in a concentration-dependent manner at the single cell level (Supplementary information Figure S1). These results demonstrated that AdO could promote non-specific phagocytosis in microglia. Next, Hilyte Fluo™ 488-labled β-amyloid (1-42) (FL-Aβ) was used to evaluate the specific phagocytic ability of BV2 cells. We utilized fluorescence analysis to determine the effect of AdO on the microglial phagocytosis of FL-Aβ. As shown in Figure 6E, the control cells engulfed a small amount of FL-Aβ, whereas the AdO-treated cells accumulated a larger amount of FL-Aβ. Compared to the fluorescence (16.6 ± 5.9) of the untreated cells, the AdO treatment of the cells promoted the uptake of FL-Aβ up to two-fold (36.7 ± 8.6) (Figure 6F).

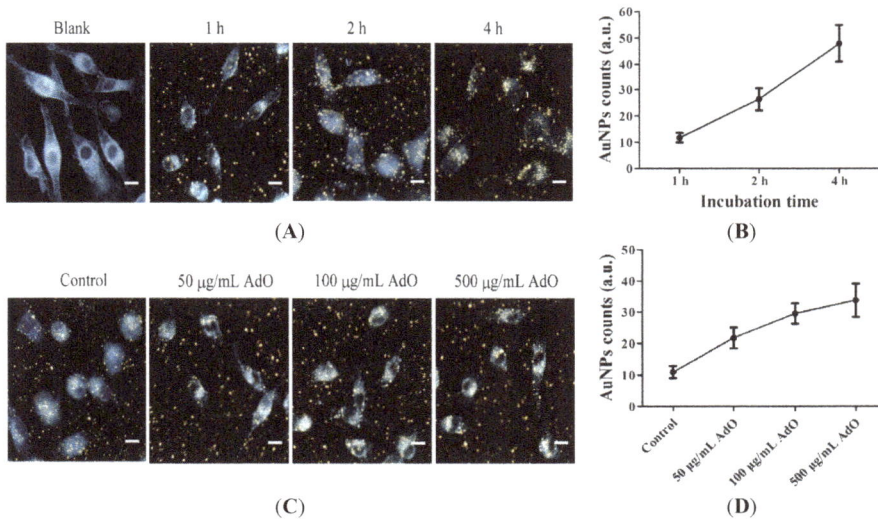

Figure 6. *Cont.*

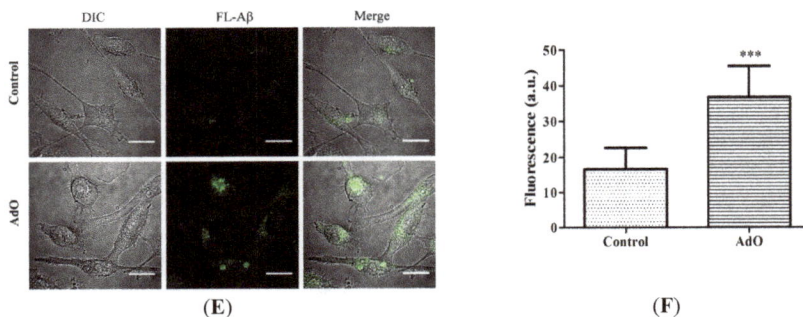

(E)   **(F)**

Figure 6. AdO promoted the phagocytosis of gold nanoparticles (AuNPs) and Hilyte Fluo™ 488-labled β-amyloid (1-42) (FL-Aβ) in the BV2 cells. (**A**) The cells were treated with 1 pM of the AuNPs for indicated incubation times; (**B**) The phagocytosis of the AuNPs by the BV2 cells was evaluated by counting the number of AuNPs in fifty cells using ImageJ software; (**C**) The cells were treated with AdO (50–500 μg/mL) for 20 h and then incubated with 1 pM of the AuNPs for 1 h. (**D**) The average number of phagocytosed AuNPs in fifty cells was analyzed using ImageJ software. The cells with the accumulated AuNPs were examined using dark-field microscopy (40×), scale bar = 20 μm; (**E**) The cells were treated with AdO (50 μg/mL) for 20 h and then incubated with 500 nM FL-Aβ for 4 h. The cells with the accumulated FL-Aβ were examined using laser scanning confocal microscopy (60×), and the morphology of the cells was shown using differential interference contrast (DIC) images, scale bar = 20 μm; (**F**) The average fluorescent intensity of fifty cells was evaluated using ImageJ software. The microscopic images were from three independent experiments. *** $p < 0.001$ indicates significant differences compared with the control group.

2.6. TLR4 Is Involved in the AdO-Promoted Microglial Phagocytosis

TLR4 is the most important receptor for uptake and clearance of Aβ in the BV2 cells [26]. To determine whether TLR4 is involved in the AdO-augmented microglial phagocytosis of Aβ, we used a TLR4 antibody to block TLR4 as mentioned in the previous reports [27,28]. The results indicated that the addition of the anti-TLR4 antibody suppressed the AdO-induced phagocytosis of FL-Aβ (Figure 7A): The incorporation was significantly less than that of the cells treated with AdO alone (Figure 7B). These results indicated that TLR4 is involved in AdO-promoted microglial phagocytosis. In the merged images (Figure 7A), the distribution of FL-Aβ was observed in the cytoplasm and lysosomes, suggesting that the FL-Aβ had already entered the cells. Furthermore, we conducted a flow cytometry assay to verify this involvement. The flow cytometric plots of the phagocytic cell populations are shown in Figure 7C, and the mean fluorescent intensity (MFI) showed a trend that was consistent with the fluorescence microscopic analysis (Figure 7D). Our flow cytometric assay results further confirmed that TLR4 is involved in the AdO-induced promotion of microglial phagocytosis. Finally, because the lysosomes and cytoskeleton participate in the phagocytotic process [29], we evaluated the effect of AdO on the lysosomes and cytoskeleton of the BV2 cells. Unfortunately, these results demonstrated that AdO had little effect on the lysosome production and cytoskeleton formation compared with the untreated cells (Figure S2).

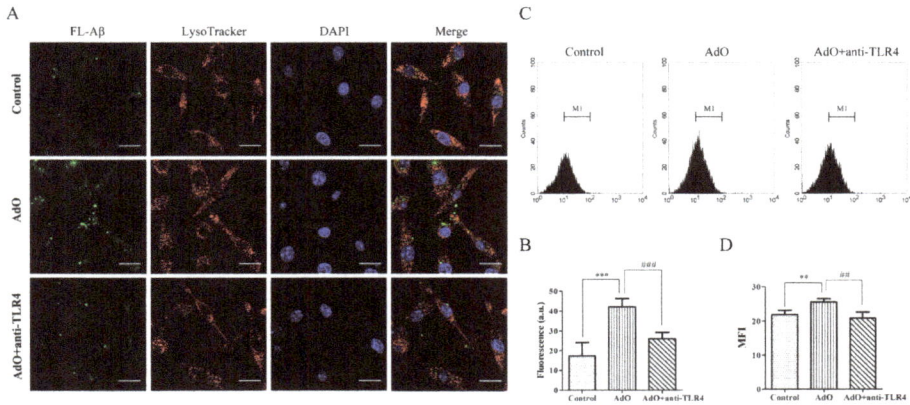

Figure 7. The involvement of TLR4 in the AdO-promoted phagocytosis of Aβ in the BV2 cells. (**A**) The cells were treated with anti-TLR4 (10 μg/mL) for 1 h prior to AdO treatment for 20 h and then incubated with 500 nM FL-Aβ for 4 h. The lysosomes and nuclei of the cells were stained with LysoTracker Red DND-99 and 4′,6-diamidino-2-phenylindole (DAPI), respectively. The cells with the accumulated FL-Aβ were observed using laser scanning confocal microscopy (60×), scale bar = 20 μm; (**B**) The average fluorescence intensity of fifty cells in each group was evaluated using ImageJ software; (**C**) The phagocytosis of FL-Aβ in untreated cells, AdO-treated cells, and anti-TLR4 and AdO-treated cells was analyzed using flow cytometry. The flow cytometric plots show the M1 region of the phagocytic cell populations based on fluorescence intensity; (**D**) The mean fluorescence intensity (MFI) of the cells in the M1 region is shown. The images were from three independent experiments. ** $p < 0.01$ and *** $p < 0.001$ indicate significant differences between the control group and the AdO-treated group, and ## $p < 0.01$ and ### $p < 0.001$ indicate significant differences between the AdO-treated group and the AdO combined with anti-TLR4-treated group.

3. Discussion

Agents that either inhibit the microglia-mediated neuroinflammation or enhance the microglial phagocytosis would be beneficial to AD therapy [5,12,30]. Numerous studies have demonstrated that natural products play important roles in treating or slowing the progression of neurodegenerative disease [30–32]. However, several natural products were found to exert neuroprotection by simultaneously suppressing microglial activation and promoting microglial phagocytosis. Blueberries have been found to significantly attenuate microglial activation and enhance microglial clearance of Aβ [33]. Curcumin exerts excellent neuroprotection through its anti-inflammatory activity and its promotion of phagocytosis [27]. Therefore, it is significant to find more natural products that appropriately inhibit microglial activation and promote the microglial uptake of Aβ. Polysaccharides from natural products exert notable neuroprotective and anti-neuroinflammatory activity [32,34]. Alginate is a natural polysaccharide that is found in various marine brown seaweeds. There have been significant studies in the last few decades that have revealed the bioactivities and broadened the utility of alginate-derived oligosaccharide [13,14]. Previous work has demonstrated that alginate oligosaccharides (1300 Da) prepared by enzymatic depolymerization could easily cross the blood–brain barrier (BBB) [35,36]. We have shown that alginate oligosaccharides prepared by enzymatic and oxidative degradation exhibited similar degree of polymerization (DP) (representative of its molecular mass) using thin-layer chromatography (TLC) analysis in our previous work [18]. The average molecular weight of AdO is about 1500 Da. These findings indicated the accessibility of AdO to the BBB and suggested the potential application of AdO for treating neurodegenerative diseases. In our previous study, we found that AdO could remarkably reduce the production of inflammatory mediators in LPS-activated macrophages [23], which encouraged us to study its anti-neuroinflammatory activity. In the present work, we aimed to evaluate the effects of AdO on the neuroinflammatory responses and microglial phagocytosis of Aβ.

The production of NO and PGE$_2$ and the expression of iNOS and COX-2 are the most important processes involved in LPS-activated neuroinflammation [34]. Here, we found that AdO pretreatment effectively inhibited the LPS-activated production of NO and PGE$_2$ via the suppression of the transcriptional activation of iNOS and COX-2 in BV2 cells (Figure 2). Excessive production of pro-inflammatory cytokines is considered to be an initiator of neuroinflammatory responses, which is a hallmark of neurodegenerative disease [37], and to cause neuronal cytotoxicity and induce nerve cell damage. This study proved that AdO-treatment of BV2 cells remarkably inhibited the LPS-activated production of TNF-α, IL-6 and IL-1β as well as the Aβ-activated production of TNF-α, IL-6 and IL-12 (Figure 3). These results suggest that AdO may be useful in the treatment of neuroinflammation by suppressing microglial activation and attenuating the production of inflammatory mediators.

It has been demonstrated that TLR4-mediated activation of NF-κB signaling pathway plays an important role in the neuroinflammatory responses and various neurodegenerative diseases [9]. The current work showed that pretreatment of BV2 cells with AdO could remarkably suppress the LPS-stimulated TLR4 expression, indicating that the TLR4 signaling pathway was involved in the anti-neuroinflammatory effect of AdO (Figure 4). NF-κB is kept inactive through the binding of IκB proteins in resting microglial cells. Microglial activation with LPS activates NF-κB signaling, leading to IκB phosphorylation and degradation, and the subsequent NF-κB subunit nuclear translocation [38]. Here, we found that the nuclear translocation of the NF-κB p65 subunit was effectively attenuated by AdO treatment (Figure 4). These findings indicate that the inhibitory effects of AdO on TLR4 expression may involve the inactivation of NF-κB signaling in LPS-activated BV2 microglia, subsequently leading to the suppression of inflammatory mediator production. In addition, we found that AdO could protect the microglia from the LPS/Aβ-activated morphological changes (Figure 5). In either case, these results indicated that the neuroprotective effect of AdO is mediated by inactivation the TLR4-NF-κB signaling pathway.

Another key role of microglial cells is their capability to clear toxic Aβ aggregates. Aβ accumulation plays an important role in the progression of AD [3]. Under normal physiological conditions, Aβ aggregates are adequately cleared and degraded by the microglia and macrophages in the brain. Unfortunately, impaired phagocytosis of Aβ by the microglia and macrophages is observed in AD and is considered to be one of the pathological hallmarks of this disease [39]. After demonstrating the excellent inhibitory effect of AdO on microglia-mediated neuroinflammation, we further explored the effect of AdO on the phagocytosis by BV2 cells. Interestingly, we found that AdO treatment promoted the phagocytosis of FL-Aβ (Figure 6). Because TLR4 is directly or indirectly activated to induce the uptake of toxic Aβ aggregates [26,40], we evaluated the involvement of TLR4 in the promotional effect of AdO on the microglial uptake of Aβ. Blocking TLR4 with anti-TLR4 prior to AdO treatment resulted in a decrease in the phagocytosis of Aβ, indicating that AdO promoted phagocytosis through an interaction with TLR4 (Figure 7).

Neuroinflammation and microglial phagocytosis are both important factors to study with respect to the therapeutic intervention for AD [4]. Therefore, the development of natural products that cannot only inhibit the neuroinflammation but that can also enhance the clearance of Aβ is important for the prevention and treatment of AD. It was interesting to find that AdO exhibited remarkably inhibitory effect on neuroinflammation and promoted microglial phagocytosis of Aβ in this study. We demonstrated that AdO inhibited the neuroinflammatory response of LPS-activated BV2 cells, possibly by attenuating TLR4 expression and inactivating the NF-κB signaling pathway. However, the molecular mechanism by which AdO promoted the phagocytosis of Aβ is still uncertain. Our results indicated that the AdO-induced promotion of the uptake of Aβ may directly or indirectly involve TLR4. It has been demonstrated that TLR4 participates in the neuroinflammatory process, suggesting that TLR4 activation aggravates neuroinflammation-mediated diseases [41]. In contrast, studies with mice expressing a mutated form of TLR4 suggested that the activation of microglial TLR4 could reduce Aβ accumulation [42], indicating that TLR4 activation produced the neuroprotective effect. Whether TLR4 activation is neurotoxic or neuroprotective may differ among the various pathological conditions. The present results support the concept that TLR4 activation is tightly controlled to regulate its different roles in neuroinflammation and microglial phagocytosis. Further studies will focus on the molecular mechanisms of the dual effect of AdO on microglial cells in depth and explore the therapeutic potential of AdO in an in vivo model of AD.

4. Materials and Methods

4.1. Materials

Sodium alginate (15-20 cps grade), FITC-phalloidin and 4′,6-diamidino-2-phenylindole (DAPI) were purchased from Sigma-Aldrich (St. Louis, MO, USA). H_2O_2 was supplied by Chengdu Kelong Chemical Co., Ltd. (Chengdu, China). Fetal bovine serum (FBS) was obtained from Biontex (Planegg, Germany). Dulbeco's Modified Eagle's Medium (DMEM) was purchased from Thermo Scientific (Hudson, NH, USA). A CCK-8 kit was supplied from Beyotime Inst Biotech (Jiangsu, China). Aβ oligomers were prepared using amyloid-β 1-42 peptide (ChinaPeptides Co., Ltd., Shanghai, China) as described previously [25]. An ELISA kit for PGE_2 was purchased from Cayman Chemical Co. (Ann Arbor, MI, USA). ELISA kits for tumor necrosis factor (TNF)-α, interleukin (IL)-1β, IL-6 and IL-12 measurement were obtained from Neobioscience Technology Company (Guangdong, China). RNAfast200 Trizol reagent was purchased from Fastagen Biotech (Shanghai, China). The cell lysis buffer was obtained from Biocolors (Shanghai, China). A KeyGEN Nuclear and Cytoplasmic Protein Extraction Kit was purchased from KeyGen Biotech (Nanjing, China). The bicinchoninic acid (BCA) reagent was obtained from Auragene Bioscience Corporation, Inc. (Changsha, China). Antibodies against inducible nitric oxide (iNOS), cyclooxygenase-2 (COX-2) and NF-κB/p65, as well as an Alexa Fluor 488-conjugated secondary anti-mouse antibody, were provided by Cell Signaling Technology (Beverly, MA, USA). Antibody against TLR4 was purchased from Abcam Company (Cambridge, UK). Hilyte Fluo™ 488-labled β-amyloid (1-42) (FL-Aβ) was purchased from AnaSpec, Inc. (San Jose, CA, USA) and LysoTracker Red DND-99 was furnished from Molecular Probes (Invitrogen, MO, USA).

4.2. Preparation of AdO

AdO was prepared from sodium alginate by a reaction with a 5% H_2O_2 solution at 90 °C for 2 h as described in our previous work [23]. The average molecular weight of AdO is about 1500 Da that detected by size exclusion chromatography (SEC) with multi-angle laser light scattering (MALLS).

4.3. Cell Culture

The BV2 microglia were cultured in DMEM supplemented with 10% FBS, 100 U/mL penicillin and 100 μg/mL streptomycin at 37 °C in a humidified incubator with 5% CO_2

4.4. Cytotoxicity Assay

The viability of the BV2 cells treated with AdO was evaluated using the CCK-8 assay. Briefly, the cells were pretreated with AdO (100–1000 μg/mL) for 2 h and then incubated with LPS/Aβ for 24 h or treated with AdO (50–1000 μg/mL) for 24 h. The medium was removed and the cells were incubated with 0.5 mg/mL of the CCK-8 solution. After this incubation, the absorption was measured at 540 nm using a microplate reader (Molecular Devices, LLC, Sunnyvale, CA, USA).

4.5. Measurement of NO and PGE_2

The BV2 microglia were pretreated with AdO (50–500 μg/mL) for 2 h and then stimulated with LPS (0.5 μg/mL) for 24 h. The accumulated nitrite in the culture supernatants was measured using the

Griess reaction method as described in our previous work [23]. PGE_2 production was evaluated using an ELISA kit according to the manufacturer's instructions.

4.6. Reverse Transcription Polymerase Chain Reaction (RT-PCR)

RNA was prepared using RNAfast200 Trizol reagent. Total RNA (1 µg) was used for reverse transcription to produce the cDNAs. The iNOS and COX-2 genes were amplified from the cDNA using PCR. The following PCR primers are used in this work: iNOS: Fwd 5'-CAA CCA GTA TTA TGG CTC CT-3'; Reverse 5'-GTG ACA GCC CGG TCT TTC CA-3'. COX-2: Fwd 5'-CCA CTT CAA GGG AGT CTG GA-3'; Reverse 5'-AGT CAT CTG CTA CGG GAG GA-3'. β-Actin: Fwd 5'-GGA GAA GAT CTG GCA CCA CAC C-3'; Reverse 5'-CCT GCT TGC TGA TCC ACA TCT GCT GG-3'.

4.7. Western Blot Analysis

The BV2 cells were pretreated with AdO for 2 h and then stimulated with LPS (0.5 µg/mL) for 24 h. The cells were lysed in lysis buffer. To determine the effect of AdO on the nuclear translocation of NF-κB p65, the nuclear and cytoplasmic proteins were extracted by a KeyGEN Nuclear and Cytoplasmic Protein Extraction Kit. The protein concentrations were determined using the bicinchoninic acid (BCA) reagent. For Western blot analysis, 50 µg of proteins was separated by 12.5% SDS-PAGE. Then, the proteins were transferred onto a polyvinylidene difluoride (PVDF) membrane (Amersham Pharmacia Biotech, England, UK) and subsequently blocked in 10% skimmed milk in Tris-buffered saline containing 0.1% Tween 20 (TBST). After the membranes were washed adequately, they were incubated with anti-mouse iNOS (1:1000), anti-mouse COX-2 (1:1000), anti-TLR4 (1:1000), or anti-NF-κB/p65 (1:1000) antibodies in 5% skimmed milk in TBST at 4 °C overnight. The membranes were then washed three times with TBST and incubated with a horseradish peroxidase-conjugated secondary antibody at 37 °C for 2 h. All Western blot assays were performed at least three times.

4.8. Measurement of Cytokines

The BV2 microglia were pretreated with AdO (50–500 µg/mL) for 2 h and then treated with LPS (0.5 µg/mL) or Aβ (10 µM) for 24 h. The levels of TNF-α, IL-6, IL-1β and IL-12 were measured using ELISAs according to the manufacturer's protocols.

4.9. Immunofluorescence Analysis

TLR4 expression and nuclear localization of NF-κB/p65 were detected by immunofluorescence analysis. The BV2 cells (4×10^5 cells/well) were cultured on sterile glass coverslips in 6-well culture dishes. After pretreatment with AdO (500 µg/mL) and stimulation with 0.5 µg/mL LPS, the cells were fixed with 4% paraformaldehyde in PBS. Then, the cells were washed with PBS and permeabilized with 0.2% Triton X-100 in PBS. After 60 min of incubation with 1% (w/v) goat serum in PBS, the cells were incubated with anti-TLR4 or anti-NF-κB p65 antibody diluted in PBS (1:200) at 4 °C overnight, washed and then incubated with an Alexa Fluor 488-conjugated secondary anti-mouse antibody for 2 h at 37 °C. The cells were incubated with DAPI (5 µg/mL) for 15 min to reveal the nuclei. The immunofluorescence analysis was carried out by a Fluoview FV1000 laser scanning confocal microscope (Olympus, Tokyo, Japan).

4.10. Cell Morphology

The BV2 cells (4×10^5 cells/well) were seeded onto coverslips placed in 35 mm × 35 mm culture dishes. The cells were pretreated with AdO (50–500 µg/mL) and were stimulated with LPS or Aβ for 24 h. Dark-field microscopy was used to examine the cell morphology of BV2 cells using an Olympus BX51 upright optical microscope (Tokyo, Japan). The morphological changes of the cells were monitored using a 40× objective, and images were captured using a DP70 camera (Olympus,

Tokyo, Japan). Subsequently, the dark field images were analyzed using ImageJ software (National Institutes of Health, Bethesda, USA).

4.11. Phagocytosis Assay

AuNPs were prepared as described in our previous work [43]. Briefly, the cells (4×10^5 cells/well) were treated with AdO (50–500 μg/mL) for 20 h. After three washes, the cells were incubated with a solution of 1 pM AuNPs (100 nm diameter) for the indicated times. The cells were then washed, fixed in 4.0% (w/v) paraformaldehyde and visualized using dark-field microscopy.

In additional studies, the cells (4×10^5 cells/well) were treated with AdO (50 μg/mL) for 20 h and incubated with 500 nM FL-Aβ for 4 h. TLR4 was blocked using anti-TLR4 (10 μg/mL) at 37 °C for 2 h prior to AdO treatment. To reveal the lysosomes and cytoskeleton of the cells, the BV2 cells were fixed and labeled with LysoTracker Red DND-99 (500 nM) and FITC-phalloidin (800 nM) for 1 h. Then, the cells were observed using a Fluoview FV1000 laser scanning confocal microscope (Olympus, Tokyo, Japan). The fluorescence intensity of the cells was analyzed using ImageJ software.

4.12. Flow Cytometric Analysis

The BV2 cells were plated in 24-well culture plates (1×10^5 cells/well). The cells were pretreated with AdO (50 μg/mL) for 20 h and then incubated with FL-Aβ for 4 h. TLR4 was blocked by treating with anti-TLR4 (10 μg/mL) at 37 °C for 2 h prior to the AdO treatment. The flow cytometric measurements were carried out using a fluorescence-activated cell sorting (FACS) system 145 (Becton Deckinson, San Jose, CA, USA). Subsequently, the cells were washed adequately and the fluorescence was compared to untreated controls using a total of 10,000 recorded events for each sample.

4.13. Statistical Analysis

The data for all experiments are presented as the means ± SD. One-way analysis of variance (ANOVA) and Student's t-tests were used to determine any significant differences. *p* values < 0.05 were considered to be significant. Each experiment was repeated at least three times.

5. Conclusions

Alginate is a natural polysaccharide derived from various kinds of marine brown algae. Previous studies demonstrated that AdO exhibits notably diverse pharmacological activities [15,16,18,19]. However, to the best of our knowledge, this is the first work to explore the effect of AdO on microglia-mediated inflammatory responses and microglial phagocytosis of Aβ. The results of this study revealed dual effects of AdO on BV2 microglial cells. First, AdO exerted an inhibitory effect on the LPS/Aβ-activated inflammatory response, and second, AdO promoted the microglial phagocytosis of Aβ. Therefore, the current work proposed that AdO is a potentially therapeutic nutraceutical for treating AD or other neurodegenerative disease.

Acknowledgments: We thank to Jiazuan Ni from Shenzhen University and Zhenqing Zhang from Suzhou University for their kind help. This work was supported by the China Postdoctoral Science Foundation (Grant 2014T70825, Grant 2013M540664), the National Natural Science Foundation of China (Grant 31000770), and the Shenzhen Bureau of Science, Technology and Information (Grant JCYJ20130329111455027 and Grant JCYJ20130408172946974).

Author Contributions: Rui Zhou and Xu Xu conceived and designed the experiments; Rui Zhou, Xu-Yang Shi, De-Cheng Bi, Wei-Shan Fang and Gao-Bin Wei performed the experiments; Rui Zhou, De-Cheng Bi, and Xu Xu analyzed the data; and Rui Zhou and Xu Xu wrote the paper.

Conflicts of Interest: The authors declare no conflicts of interest.

References

1. Maccioni, R.B.; Morales, I.; Guzman-Martinez, L.; Cerda-Troncoso, C.; Farías, G.A. Neuroinflammation in the pathogenesis of Alzheimer's disease. A rational framework for the search of novel therapeutic approaches. *Front. Cell. Neurosci.* **2014**, *8*, 1–9.
2. Tansey, M.G.; Frank-Cannon, T.C.; McCoy, M.K.; Lee, J.K.; Martinez, T.N.; McAlpine, F.E.; Ruhn, K.A.; Tran, T.A. Neuroinflammation in Parkinson's disease: Is there sufficient evidence for mechanism-based interventional therapy? *Front. Biosci.* **2008**, *13*, 709–717. [CrossRef] [PubMed]
3. LaFerla, F.M.; Green, K.N.; Oddo, S. Intracellular amyloid-beta in Alzheimer's disease. *Nat. Rev. Neurosci.* **2007**, *8*, 499–509. [CrossRef] [PubMed]
4. Carret-Rebillat, A.-S.; Pace, C.; Gourmaud, S.; Ravasi, L.; Montagne-Stora, S.; Longueville, S.; Tible, M.; Sudol, E.; Chang, R.C.-C.; Paquet, C.; Mouton-Liger, F.; Hugon, J. Neuroinflammation and Aβ accumulation linked to systemic inflammation are decreased by genetic PKR down-regulation. *Sci. Rep.* **2015**. [CrossRef] [PubMed]
5. Gold, M.; Dolga, A.; Koepke, J.; Mengel, D.; Culmsee, C.; Dodel, R.; Koczulla, A.; Bach, J.-P. α-antitrypsin modulates microglial-mediated neuroinflammation and protects microglial cells from amyloid-β-induced toxicity. *J. Neuroinflammation* **2014**, *11*, 1–15. [CrossRef] [PubMed]
6. Wang, X.X.; Wang, C.M.; Wang, J.M.; Zhao, S.Q.; Zhang, K.; Wang, J.; Zhang, W.; Wu, C.; Yang, J. Pseudoginsenoside-F11 (PF11) exerts anti-neuroinflammatory effects on LPS-activated microglial cells by inhibiting TLR4-mediated TAK1/IKK/NF-κB, MAPKs and Akt signaling pathways. *Neuropharmacology* **2014**, *79*, 642–656. [CrossRef] [PubMed]
7. Gonzalez-Scarano, F.; Baltuch, G. Microglia as mediators of inflammatory and degenerative diseases. *Annu. Rev. Neurosci.* **1999**, *22*, 219–240. [CrossRef] [PubMed]
8. Dheen, S.T.; Kaur, C.; Ling, E.A. Microglial activation and its implications in the brain diseases. *Curr. Med. Chem.* **2007**, *14*, 1189–1197. [CrossRef] [PubMed]
9. Zhao, M.; Zhou, A.; Xu, L.; Zhang, X. The role of TLR4-mediated PTEN/PI3K/AKT/NF-κB signaling pathway in neuroinflammation in hippocampal neurons. *Neurosci.* **2014**, *269*, 93–101. [CrossRef] [PubMed]
10. Moore, A.H.; O'Banion, M.K. Neuroinflammation and anti-inflammatory therapy for Alzheimer's disease. *Adv. Drug. Deliv. Rev.* **2002**, *54*, 1627–1656. [CrossRef]
11. Lucin, K.M.; O'Brien, C.E.; Bieri, G.; Czirr, E.; Mosher, K.I.; Abbey, R.J.; Mastroeni, D.F.; Rogers, J.; Spencer, B.; Masliah, E.; Wyss-Coray, T. Microglial beclin 1 regulates retromer trafficking and phagocytosis and is impaired in Alzheimer's disease. *Neuron* **2013**, *79*, 873–886. [CrossRef] [PubMed]
12. Smith, A.M.; Gibbons, H.M.; Dragunow, M. Valproic acid enhances microglial phagocytosis of amyloid-β1-42. *Neuroscience* **2010**, *169*, 505–515. [CrossRef] [PubMed]
13. Sun, J.C.; Tan, H.P. Alginate-Based Biomaterials for Regenerative Medicine Applications. *Materials.* **2013**, *6*, 1285–1309. [CrossRef]
14. Lee, K.Y.; Mooney, D.J. Alginate: Properties and biomedical applications. *Prog. Polym. Sci.* **2012**, *37*, 106–126. [CrossRef] [PubMed]
15. Iwamoto, Y.; Xu, X.; Tamura, T.; Oda, T.; Muramatsu, T. Enzymatically depolymerized alginate oligomers that cause cytotoxic cytokine production in human mononuclear cells. *Biosci. Biotechnol. Biochem.* **2003**, *67*, 258–263. [CrossRef] [PubMed]
16. Tusi, S.K.; Khalaj, L.; Ashabi, G.; Kiaei, M.; Khodagholi, F. Alginate oligosaccharide protects against endoplasmic reticulum- and mitochondrial-mediated apoptotic cell death and oxidative stress. *Biomaterials* **2011**, *32*, 5438–5458. [CrossRef] [PubMed]
17. Eftekharzadeh, B.; Khodagholi, F.; Abdi, A.; Maghsoudi, N. Alginate protects NT2 neurons against H2O2-induced neurotoxicity. *Carbohydr. Polym.* **2010**, *79*, 1063–1072. [CrossRef]
18. Xu, X.; Wu, X.T.; Wang, Q.Q.; Cai, N.; Zhang, H.; Jiang, Z.; Wan, M.; Oda, T. Immunomodulatory effects of alginate oligosaccharides on murine macrophage RAW264.7 cells and their structure-activity relationships. *J. Agri. Food Chem.* **2014**, *62*, 3168–3176.
19. Xu, X.; Bi, D.-C.; Li, C.; Fang, W.-S.; Zhou, R.; Li, S.-M.; Chi, L.-L.; Wan, M.; Shen, L.-M. Morphological and proteomic analyses reveal that unsaturated guluronate oligosaccharide modulates multiple functional pathways in murine macrophage RAW264.7 cells. *Mar. Drugs* **2015**, *13*, 1798–1818. [CrossRef] [PubMed]

20. Mirshafiey, A.; Khodadadi, A.; Rehm, B.H.; Khorramizadeh, M.R.; Eslami, M.B.; Razavi, A.; Saadat, F. Sodium alginate as a novel therapeutic option in experimental colitis. *Scand. J. Immunol.* **2005**, *61*, 316–321. [CrossRef] [PubMed]

21. Mo, S.-J.; Son, E.-W.; Rhee, D.-K.; Pyo, S. Modulation of tnf-α-induced icam-1 expression, no and h2o2 production by alginate, allicin and ascorbic acid in human endothelial cells. *Arch. Pharm. Res.* **2003**, *26*, 244–251. [CrossRef] [PubMed]

22. Yang, Z.; Li, J.; Guan, H. Preparation and characterization of oligomannuronates from alginate degraded by hydrogen peroxide. *Carbohydr. Polym.* **2004**, *58*, 115–121. [CrossRef]

23. Zhou, R.; Shi, X.Y.; Gao, Y.; Cai, N.; Jiang, Z.D.; Xu, X. Anti-inflammatory activity of guluronate oligosaccharides obtained by oxidative degradation from alginate in lipopolysaccharide-activated murine macrophage RAW 264.7 cells. *J. Agric. Food Chem.* **2015**, *63*, 160–168. [CrossRef] [PubMed]

24. Bi, W.; Zhu, L.H.; Jing, X.N.; Zeng, Z.F.; Liang, Y.R.; Xu, A.D.; Liu, J.; Xiao, S.H.; Yang, L.H.; Shi, Q.Y.; Guo, L.; Tao, E.X. Rifampicin improves neuronal apoptosis in LPS-stimulated co-cultured BV2 cells through inhibition of the TLR-4 pathway. *Mol. Med. Rep.* **2014**, *10*, 1793–1799. [CrossRef] [PubMed]

25. Shukla, S.M.; Sharma, S. Sinomenine inhibits microglial activation by Abeta and confers neuroprotection. *J. Neuroinflammation* **2011**, *8*, 1–11. [CrossRef] [PubMed]

26. Tahara, K.; Kim, H.D.; Jin, J.J.; Maxwell, J.A.; Li, L.; Fukuchi, K. Role of toll-like receptor signalling in Abeta uptake and clearance. *Brain* **2006**, *129*, 3006–3019. [CrossRef] [PubMed]

27. He, G.L.; Liu, Y.; Li, M.; Chen, C.H.; Gao, P.; Yu, Z.P.; Yang, X.S. The amelioration of phagocytic ability in microglial cells by curcumin through the inhibition of EMF-induced pro-inflammatory responses. *J. Neuroinflammation* **2014**, *11*, 169–174. [CrossRef] [PubMed]

28. Iwamoto, M.; Kurachi, M.; Nakashima, T.; Kim, D.; Yamaguchi, K.; Oda, T.; Iwamoto, Y.; Muramatsu, T. Structure-activity relationship of alginate oligosaccharides in the induction of cytokine production from RAW264.7 cells. *FEBS Lett.* **2005**, *579*, 4423–4429. [CrossRef] [PubMed]

29. Underhill, D.M.; Goodridge, H.S. Information processing during phagocytosis. *Nat. Rev. Immunol.* **2012**, *12*, 492–502. [CrossRef] [PubMed]

30. Wu, W.; Wu, Y.; Huang, H.; He, C.; Li, W.; Wang, H.; Chen, H.; Yin, Y. Biochanin A attenuates LPS-induced pro-inflammatory responses and inhibits the activation of the MAPK pathway in BV2 microglial cells. *Int. J. Mol. Med.* **2015**, *35*, 391–398. [PubMed]

31. Essa, M.M.; Vijayan, R.K.; Castellano-Gonzalez, G.; Memon, M.A.; Braidy, N.; Guillemin, G.J. Neuroprotective Effect of Natural Products Against Alzheimer's Disease. *Neurochem. Res.* **2012**, *37*, 1829–1842. [CrossRef] [PubMed]

32. Teng, P.; Li, Y.H.; Cheng, W.J.; Zhou, L.; Shen, Y.; Wang, Y. Neuroprotective effects of Lycium barbarum polysaccharides in lipopolysaccharide-induced BV2 microglial cells. *Mol. Med. Rep.* **2013**, *7*, 1977–1981. [PubMed]

33. Zhu, Y.Y.; Bickford, P.C.; Sanberg, P.; Giunta, B.; Tan, J. Blueberry opposes beta-amyloid peptide-induced microglial activation via inhibition of p44/42 mitogen-activation protein kinase. *Rejuv. Res.* **2008**, *11*, 891–901. [CrossRef] [PubMed]

34. Park, H.Y.; Han, M.H.; Park, C.; Jin, C.-Y.; Kim, G.-Y.; Choi, I.-W.; Kim, N.D.; Nam, T.-J.; Kwon, T.K.; Choi, Y.H. Anti-inflammatory effects of fucoidan through inhibition of NF-κB, MAPK and Akt activation in lipopolysaccharide-induced BV2 microglia cells. *Food Chem. Toxicol.* **2011**, *49*, 1745–1752. [CrossRef] [PubMed]

35. Guo, X.L.; Xin, X.L.; Gan, L.; Nie, Q.; Geng, M.Y. Determination of the accessibility of acidic oligosaccharide sugar chain to blood-brain barrier using surface plasmon resonance. *Biol. Pharm. Bull.* **2006**, *29*, 60–63. [CrossRef] [PubMed]

36. Fan, Y.; Hu, J.F.; Li, J.; Yang, Z.; Xin, X.L.; Wang, J.; Ding, J.; Geng, M.Y. Effect of acidic oligosaccharide sugar chain on scopolamine-induced memory impairment in rats and its related mechanisms. *Neurosci. Lett.* **2005**, *374*, 222–226. [CrossRef] [PubMed]

37. Smith, J.A.; Das, A.; Ray, S.K.; Banik, N.L. Role of pro-inflammatory cytokines released from microglia in neurodegenerative diseases. *Brain. Res. Bull.* **2012**, *87*, 10–20. [CrossRef] [PubMed]

38. Emmanouil, M.; Taoufik, E.; Tseveleki, V.; Vamvakas, S.-S.; Probert, L. A Role for Neuronal NF-κB in Suppressing Neuroinflammation and Promoting Neuroprotection in the CNS. In *Advances in TNF Family Research*; Wallach, D., Kovalenko, A., Feldmann, M., Eds.; Springer: New York, NY, USA, 2011; Volume 691, pp. 575–581.

39. Cherry, J.; Olschowka, J.; O'Banion, M. Neuroinflammation and M2 microglia: The good, the bad, and the inflamed. *J. Neuroinflammation* **2014**, *11*, 1–15. [CrossRef] [PubMed]

40. Michaud, J.P.; Halle, M.; Lampron, A.; Theriault, P.; Prefontaine, P.; Filali, M.; Tribout-Jover, P.; Lanteigne, A.M.; Jodoin, R.; Cluff, C.; *et al.* Toll-like receptor 4 stimulation with the detoxified ligand monophosphoryl lipid A improves Alzheimer's disease-related pathology. *Proc. Natl. Acad. Sci. USA* **2013**, *110*, 1941–1946. [CrossRef] [PubMed]

41. Yao, L.L.; Kan, E.M.; Lu, J.; Hao, A.; Dheen, S.T.; Kaur, C.; Ling, E.-A. Toll-like receptor 4 mediates microglial activation and production of inflammatory mediators in neonatal rat brain following hypoxia: Role of TLR4 in hypoxic microglia. *J. Neuroinflammation* **2013**, *10*, 1–21. [CrossRef] [PubMed]

42. Song, M.; Jin, J.; Lim, J.E.; Kou, J.; Pattanayak, A.; Rehman, J.A.; Kim, H.D.; Tahara, K.; Lalonde, R.; Fukuchi, K. TLR4 mutation reduces microglial activation, increases Abeta deposits and exacerbates cognitive deficits in a mouse model of Alzheimer's disease. *J. Neuroinflammation* **2011**. [CrossRef] [PubMed]

43. Zhou, R.; Zhou, H.Y.; Xiong, B.; He, Y.; Yeung, E.S. Pericellular Matrix Enhances Retention and Cellular Uptake of Nanoparticles. *J. Am. Chem. Soc.* **2012**, *134*, 13404–13409. [CrossRef] [PubMed]

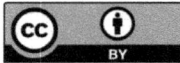

marine drugs

MDPI

Article

λ-Carrageenan Suppresses Tomato Chlorotic Dwarf Viroid (TCDVd) Replication and Symptom Expression in Tomatoes

Jatinder S. Sangha [1], Saveetha Kandasamy [1], Wajahatullah Khan [2], Navratan Singh Bahia [1], Rudra P. Singh [3], Alan T. Critchley [4] and Balakrishnan Prithiviraj [1,*]

[1] Department of Environmental Sciences, Faculty of Agriculture, Dalhousie University, P.O. Box 550, Truro, NS B2N 5E3, Canada; Jatinder.sangha@dal.ca (J.S.S.); skandasamy@dal.ca (S.K.); pulsarsidhu@gmail.com (N.S.B.)

[2] Basic Sciences Department, King Saud Bin Abdul Aziz University for Health Sciences, P.O. Box 22490, Riyadh 11426, Saudi Arabia; Khanmuh@ksau-hs.edu.sa

[3] Agriculture and Agri-Food Canada, 850 Lincoln Rd., Fredericton, NB E3B 4Z7, Canada; singhr@agr.gc.ca

[4] Acadian Seaplants Limited, 30 Brown Avenue, Dartmouth, NS B3B 1X8, Canada; alan.critchley@acadian.ca

* Author to whom correspondence should be addressed; bprithiviraj@dal.ca; Tel.: +1-902-893-6643; Fax: +1-902-895-6734.

Academic Editor: Paola Laurienzo

Received: 27 February 2015; Accepted: 27 April 2015; Published: 8 May 2015

Abstract: The effect of carrageenans on tomato chlorotic dwarf viroid (TCDVd) replication and symptom expression was studied. Three-week-old tomato plants were spray-treated with iota(ι)-, lambda(ι)-, and kappa(κ)-carrageenan at 1 g·L^{-1} and inoculated with TCDVd after 48 h. The λ-carrageenan significantly suppressed viroid symptom expression after eight weeks of inoculation, only 28% plants showed distinctive bunchy-top symptoms as compared to the 82% in the control group. Viroid concentration was reduced in the infected shoot cuttings incubated in λ-carrageenan amended growth medium. Proteome analysis revealed that 16 tomato proteins were differentially expressed in the λ-carrageenan treated plants. Jasmonic acid related genes, allene oxide synthase (AOS) and lipoxygenase (LOX), were up-regulated in λ-carrageenan treatment during viroid infection. Taken together, our results suggest that λ-carrageenan induced tomato defense against TCDVd, which was partly jasmonic acid(JA) dependent, and that it could be explored in plant protection against viroid infection.

Keywords: tomato chlorotic dwarf viroid (TCDVd); carrageenans; induced resistance

---

1. Introduction

Viroids are the smallest (246–400 nucleotides) single-stranded, non-protein-coding circular RNA molecules [1]. Since their initial discovery in 1971 [2,3], almost 30 types of viroids belonging to the Pospiviroidae and Avsunviroidae families have been reported to infect a wide array of plants, and the number may increase with the discovery of additional hosts [4]. The genus *Pospiviroid*, in the family Pospiviroidae, contains about nine viroid species, including tomato chlorotic dwarf viroid (TCDVd) [1], which causes more than 25 diseases in agricultural, horticultural and ornamental plants [5]. Due to their destructive nature, there is growing interest to develop strategies to control viroids. Although considerable advances have been made in the characterization of viroids, mechanisms of viroid pathogenicity and symptom expression [6–9], mechanisms of plant resistance to viroid infection is not understood.

Unlike plant resistance to most other pathogens, natural resistance against viroids is not common [10]. Attempts have been made to protect plant against viroids using different strategies: non-transgenicapproaches such as detection and eradication of viroid-infected plants [11], chemical-induced resistance [12,13], cross protection [14], thermotherapy [15,16], and tissue culture and grafting [15–17] showed variable levels of success in controlling viroid diseases. Crop germplasms have been screened, and resistant clones and cultivars that showed tolerance to viroids have been reported [11,18,19]. Plant breeding techniques offered promising results in some cases such as chrysanthemum stunt viroid (CSVd) resistance in chrysanthemums [20,21], although it may not be possible in other crop species due to lack of resistant germplasms. Recent techniques in molecular biology, such as RNA silencing, showed a reduction in the replication of viroids [17,22], thus suggesting the potential use of this technique in developing viroid resistant varieties through genetic engineering.

Plants deploy a wide range of defense mechanisms against pathogens. These defense mechanisms can be either constitutive or inducible that prevents pathogen ingress [23]. Upon perceiving pathogen attack, usually by the recognition of pathogen-specific elicitors, plants activate defense responses against the pathogen [24]. This may involve a series of molecular events in the pathogen-challenged plants; regulation of the production of plant hormones, secretion of defensive enzymes or accumulation of PR proteins in plant cells [24–26]. Plant defense responses can also be induced by cell wall components of pathogen like chitin, lipo-polysaccharides, bacterial flagellin proteins and other chemicals of natural and synthetic origin like salicylic acid, jasmonic acid, isonicotinic acid and benzothiadiazole [27–29]. Compounds that induce plant defense responses, referred to as elicitors, have been identified in a number of seaweeds. Examples of such compounds include laminarin, fucans, ulvans and carrageenans [28,30,31].

Carrageenans are sulfated polysaccharides that are the major cell wall component of red seaweeds [32]. In some red seaweeds, carrageenans may account for more than 40% by dry weight. Carrageenans are grouped as iota(ι)-, kappa(κ)- and lambda(λ)-carrageenan based on the degree of sulfation, and each one presents its own characteristic bioactivity [31]. An emerging body of literature suggests that carrageenans inhibit binding of viruses like human papillomavirus (HPV) to the animal cells, which is attributed to its structural similarity to heparan sulfate, an HPV cell-attachment factor [33]. Carrageenans have been shown to elicit resistance in plants and animals against pathogens, and this activity depends on the degree of sulfation [28,30,34–36]. In this study, we tested the effect of three types of carrageenans (ι, κ, and λ) on the induction of resistance in tomatoes against TCDVd.

2. Results

2.1. Effect of Carrageenans on TCDVd Infection in Tomatoes

Stunting and bunchy tops are the most characteristic symptoms induced by TCDVd infection in tomatoes. The infected plants showed variable phenotypic symptoms and were positive for TCDVd as confirmed with reverse transcription polymerase chain reaction (RT-PCR). The fruit size was also considerably reduced and roots were thin and fibrous in the infected plants (Figure 1).

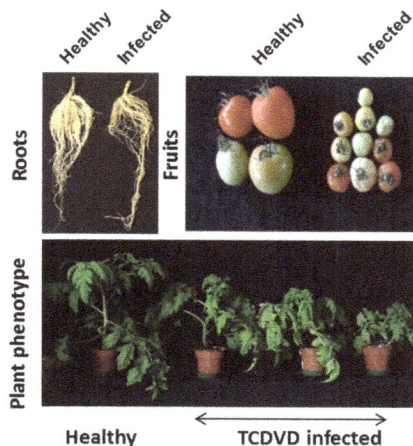

Figure 1. Symptoms of TCDVd infection in tomatoes. Three-week-old tomato plants were inoculated with 10 µL of TCDVd sap and the symptoms were observed at 28 dpi. Infected plants (RT-PCR confirmed) were stunted with bunchy top symptoms, smaller fruits and fewer roots.

To determine if carrageenans reduced TCDVd infection or prevented symptom development in tomatoes, three-week-old tomatoes (cv. Sheyenne) plants were treated with carrageenans (ι, κ, λ) and then inoculated with TCDVd. No difference in viroid replication or symptom development was observed in ι- and κ-carrageenan treated plants. The λ-carrageenan treatment, however, protected the tomatoes from TCDVd infection (Figure 2a) and decreased the replication of TCDVd in the plant tissue as observed with RT-PCR. Based on the phenotype of the plant at 35-days post inoculation (dpi), a higher number (82%) of untreated plants were infected with TCDVd, whereas less than 30% plants that were treated with λ-carrageenan exhibited TCDVd symptoms. Further analysis was performed with RT-PCR using TCDVd specific primers on plants at 0, 14 and 35 dpi. The RT-PCR analysis detected TCDVd transcripts in plants which otherwise appeared normal, particularly at an early stage, *i.e.*, one to two weeks after inoculation. The results indicated that the viroid infection was established in untreated plants by 14 dpi as 46% of plants showed TCDVd transcript at this stage. The number of infected plants in the untreated group increased to 55% at 21 dpi and to 82% at 35 dpi (Figure 2a). In contrast, TCDVd infection was delayed or suppressed in λ-carrageenan treated plants; none of the plants showed TCDVd symptoms at 7 dpi; further, there were no viroid transcripts in the leaves. Fewer plants (12%) developed TCDVd symptoms at 14 dpi and the number of infected plants increased to 20% at 21 dpi, and 28% at 35 dpi. Interestingly, fewer plants were visibly stunted in λ-carrageenan treatment at 35 dpi even though the plants had TCDVd transcripts, suggesting that λ-carrageenan suppressed symptom expression.

To confirm whether the reduction in the severity of symptoms in λ-carrageenan treated plants was associated with the reduction in viroid multiplication, the abundance of TCDVd transcripts was measured using RT-PCR in leaf samples collected at 35 dpi (Figure 2b). The intensity of TCDVd specific bands in the treated plants was quantified using ImageJ software (National Institutes of Health, MD, USA). The result revealed that the average ($n = 10$) band intensity of TCDVd in control plants was higher than in the λ-carrageenan treated plants which conformed with the reduced symptoms in the λ-carrageenan treated plants. These results suggest suppressive effects of λ-carrageenan on TCDVd in-planta.

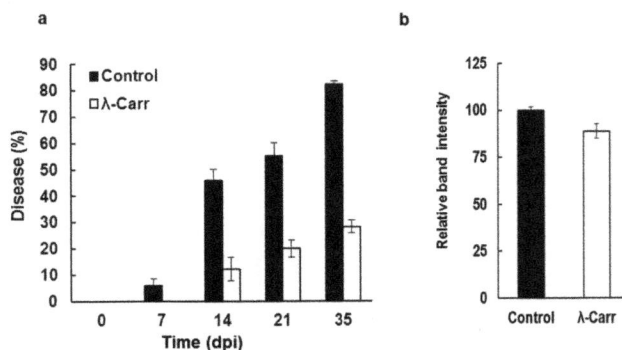

Figure 2. Suppressive effect of λ-carrageenan in tomatoes against TCDVd infection. (a) Percentage of plants showing typical TCDVd symptoms in control and λ-carrageenan (λ-Carr) treated plants. Data represent the mean of percent infected plants from three independent trials (Mean ± SEM, $n = 36$); (b) Relative intensity of TCDVd bands visualized on agarose gel and quantified with ImageJ software in controls and λ-carrageenan (λ-Carr) treated plants at 35 dpi (Mean ± SEM, $n = 10$).

2.2. Effect of Carrageenan Treatments on Plant Height

Viroid infection had a negative effect on the growth and development of plants causing reduced plant height (stunting), short internodes, initiation of new shoots and reduced fruit size. We measured the height of TCDVd-inoculated plants to determine the protective effect of λ-carrageenan against viroid infection. Although the average height of TCDVd infected plants, after one month of infection, was reduced in all treatments compared to non-inoculated plants, the height of λ-carrageenan treated plants was significantly higher ($p < 0.05$) (Figure 3). The average height of TCDVd infected plants treated with λ-carrageenan was ~25 cm compared to ~20 cm in the control. Since viroid infection reduced internode length, we compared the length of the last internode in λ-carrageenan treated and control plants, although the internode length was higher in λ-carrageenan treated plants, the difference was not significant (Figure 3).

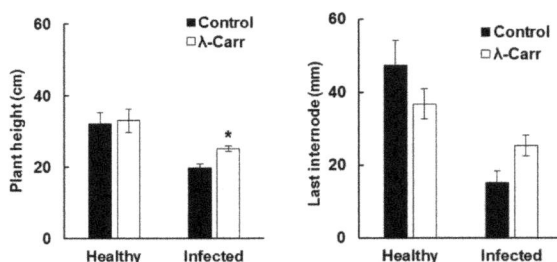

Figure 3. Plant height and last internode length of infected and healthy tomato plants one month after TCDVd inoculation. Bars represent control (black) and λ-carrageenan (λ-Carr, white). Data represent Mean ± SEM ($n = 36$ for healthy plants and $n = 12$ plants for infected plants), student's *t*-test at $p < 0.05$.

2.3. Effect of λ-Carrageenan on TCDVd Replication

To verify if λ-carrageenan had a remedial effect on TCDVd-infected plants that could inhibit the replication of TCDVd, shoot cuttings from TCDVd-infected plants were incubated in the λ-carrageenan amended plant growth medium ($\frac{1}{2}$ strength Murashige & Skoog (MS) medium) for three weeks and the TCDVd concentration in the shoot was determined at weekly intervals by RT-PCR. The viroid concentration in the leaves of the infected shoot gradually reduced in the plant shoot incubated in the λ-carrageenan solution (Figure 4). However, other carageenans, *i.e.*, ι- and κ-carrageenan, did not reduce the concentration of TCDVd concentration in the shoots. Interestingly, ι-carrageenan increased the viroid concentration in the shoot (Figure 4).

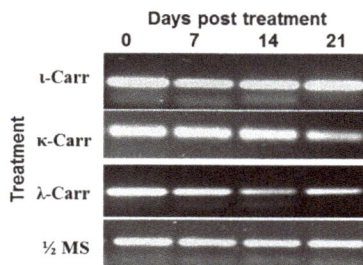

Figure 4. Effect of carrageenans on TCDVd multiplication in tomato determined by RT-PCR. TCDVd concentration in the leaf samples from infected shoots was determined at 0, 7, 14, and 21 days post carrageenan treatment (λ-carrageenan (λ-Carr), ι-carrageenan (ι-Carr), κ-carrageenan (κ-Carr)) with RT-PCR using TCDVd specific primers. The bands were visualized on agarose gel.

2.3.1. λ-Carrageenan Induced Differential Expression of Tomato Proteins

Plant defense response to TCDVd infection was analyzed by a proteomics approach using 2D-gel electrophoresis. The proteome of the leaf tissue of control and λ-carrageenan treated plants inoculated with TCDVd were analyzed. Compared to untreated (control) plants, λ-carrageenan elicited plants showed differential expression of proteins in response to TCDVd infection (Figure 5, Table 1). Seventeen proteins were differentially expressed in control and λ-carrageenan treated tomato plants inoculated with TCDVd. The results showed that 14 proteins increased in abundance in λ-carrageenan treated plant whereas three proteins were reduced. These proteins have different functions, suggesting that TCDVd resistance in tomatoes involved multiple pathways to defend against the infection.

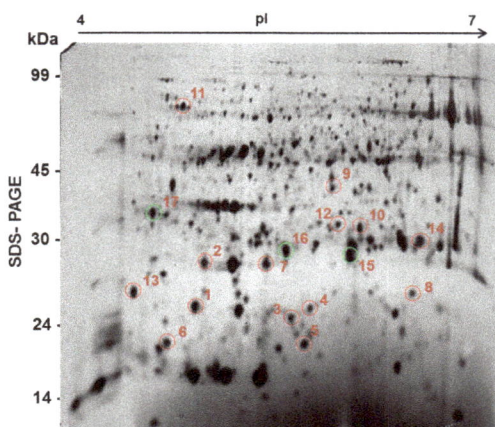

Figure 5. A general proteome map of tomato leaves with TCDVd infection in λ-carrageenan treatment. Proteins were separated first on an IPG strip (pH 4.0–7.0) and then based on molecular weight (kDA) on a 12% SDS-PAGE. Differentially expressed proteins are marked, red circled were increased whereas green circled were decreased.

2.3.2. Effect of λ-Carrageenan on the Expression of Defense Response Genes during Viroid Infection

Plant defense genes are involved in providing protection during challenge by various biotic stresses including pathogens. Some of these genes may be involved in carrageenan-induced defense in tomatoes. We examined the expression of three defense genes (*TomLoxD, TomAOS* and *PR1*) in control and λ-carrageenan-treated tomato plants at different time points after TCDVd inoculation (Figure 6). The results revealed that the λ-carrageenan-elicited defense response against TCDVd is associated with JA-dependent plant defense genes as both *TomAOS* and *TomLoxD* being up-regulated in λ-carrageenan treatment in TCDVd infected plants at 0 and 7 dpi, respectively. In contrast, *PR1* response was not different in λ-carrageenan treated tomato plants as compared to the control group.

Table 1. List of leaf proteins differentially expressed in λ-carrageenan treated tomato with tomato chlorotic dwarf viroid (TCDVd) infection as compared to control plants with TCDVd infection ($p < 0.05$).

Spot ID	Protein Identity	Accession	Molecular Mass (kDa)	Isoelectric Point (pI)	Fold Change	No. of Unique Peptides	Coverage (%)
	Proteins over expressed in λ-carrageenan treated tomato with viroid infection						
1	Cytochrome b6-f complex iron-sulfur subunit	Q69GY7-UCRIA_SOLTU	24.2	4.85	2.39	3	12.6
2	Photo-system II oxygen-evolving complex protein 2	Q7M1Y7-Q7M1Y7_ORYSA	04.0	4.90	2.37	1	35.1
3	Pathogenesis-related protein 10	Q4KYL1_ORYSA	17.5	5.59	2.45	3	6.82
4	17.7 kDa class I small heat-shock protein	A1E463_9ASTR	17.5	5.73	1.92	1	14.3
5	Superoxide dismutase 1	P14830-SODC1_SOLLC	15.2	5.66	2.70	5	23.7
6	17.7 kDa class I heat shock protein	O82011-HSP11_SOLPE	17.7	4.65	2.43	3	18.8
7	Ribulose bisphosphate (RuBP) carboxylase small chain Fragment	A0A3A2_ARTAN	19.7	5.40	2.35	1	4.62
8	Superoxide dismutase	Q6X1D0_SOLLC	27.9	6.45	2.90	4	15.3
9	Cytosolic cysteine synthase	Q9FSZ7_SOLTU	34.2	5.92	1.99	2	7.38
10	Proteasome subunit alpha type	Q93X34_TOBAC	27.1	6.21	2.49	5	18.5
11	Uracil phosphoribosyltransferase	P93394-UPP_TOBAC	24.1	4.73	2.60	3	16.1
12	Cytosolic ascorbate peroxidase 1	B1Q3F7_SOLLC	27.3	6.00	2.85	9	37.6
13	Succinic semialdehyde reductase isoform 2	B1Q3F7_SOLLC	38.2	4.51	1.88	1	2.75
14	Ferredoxin-NADP reductase, leaf-type isozyme, chloroplastic	O04977-FENR1_TOBAC	40.4	6.62	1.73	3	23.8
	Proteins under expressed in λ-carrageenan treated tomato with viroid infection						
15	Carbonic anhydrase	Q5NE20_SOLLC	34.4	6.21	1.79	3	10.6
16	Peptidyl-prolyl *cis-trans* isomerase	A0MTQ0_SOLSG	17.9	5.72	1.97	1	7.02
17	Germin like protein	B9A6I8_TOBAC	21.9	4.68	2.39	1	4.27

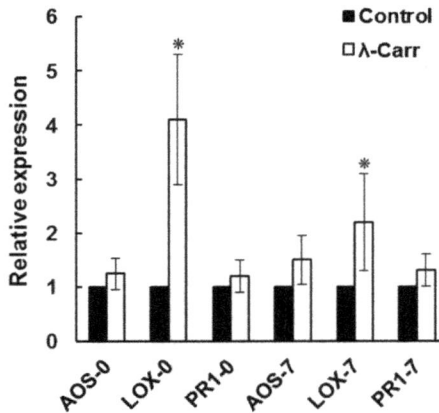

Figure 6. Expression of defense response genes encoding allene oxide synthase (AOS), lipoxygenase (LOX) and pathogenesis related protein 1 (PR1), in tomatoes during TCDVd infection. The expression of genes was analyzed at 0 (AOS-0, LOX-0 and PR1-0) and 7 (AOS-7, LOX-7 and PR1-7) dpi in control and λ-carrageenan (λ-Carr) treated plants. Values with "*" are significantly different ($p < 0.05$). (Mean ± S.E., $n = 3$).

3. Discussion

Viroid RNA has been extensively studied due to their unique structure and infectious nature. However, there are only a few studies on the control of viroid diseases. This study demonstrates the potential use of a sulfated polysaccharide, λ-carrageenan, to induce resistance in tomatoes against TCDVd, a devastating pathogen on a number of plants [37]. The effect of λ-carrageenan appears to be plant-mediated as it did not show a direct effect on viroid RNA *in vitro*; gene expression analysis, and the analysis of the proteomes of the infected plants suggest that λ-carrageenan induced resistance against TCDVd was largely mediated by a jasmonic acid dependent defense pathway.

Use of elicitors to induce plants' resistance against pathogens has been an effective strategy to reduce disease. Elicitors such as INA (2, 6-dichloro-isonicotinic acid), BTH (benzothiadiazole) and BABA (β-aminobutyric acid) induce transcription of specific defense genes [38,39]. Few previous reports suggested the effect of chemicals to protect plants against viroid infection. For example, the use of piperonyl butoxide showed protective effects against potato spindle tuber viroid infection [12]. Antiviral agent ribavirin (300 mg/l), when applied on *Gynura aurantiaca* (Purple Passion) plants infected with citrus exocortis viroid (CEVd), completely suppressed symptoms in newly developed leaves, whereas the application of the same agent three days prior to infection also prevented establishment of infection in the plant [13]. Pretreatment of tomato plants with λ-carrageenan reduced the TCDVd symptom expression, and the progression of the disease was also suppressed. Algal polysaccharides, such as laminarin and carrageenans trigger host defense mechanisms against subsequent pathogenic infections in plants and animals [31,33,36]. The application of κ/β-carrageenan from red marine alga *Tichocarpus crinitus* showed a significant reduction in the number of necrotic lesions on the tobacco leaves inoculated with the mixture of tobacco mosaic virus (TMV) [40]. In the present study, we observed that the highly sulfated λ-carrageenan induced tomato resistance against TCDVd suggesting the role of sulfation in the bioactivity as shown in earlier studies [28,31,41].

TCDVd virulence is dependent on the pathogenicity factors present in the viroid sequence [42]. We also investigated the TCDVd sequence isolated from a number of λ-carrageenan treated plants and did not find any mutational effect that could have caused reduced virulence of the viroid in tomato.

Proteome analysis revealed differential induction of proteins in TCDVd-infected λ-carrageenan treated plants. Several studies have revealed differential responses of plant proteomes in response to disease progression [43]. The proteome changes in plant show that the reduction in infection was primarily mediated by biochemical changes elicited by λ-carrageenan. In a previous study, Itaya *et al.*, [6] showed changes in host gene expression at different stages of the viroid infection and revealed a complex pattern of molecular changes in plant that involve defense responses, metabolic changes in cell wall and proteins and many other miscellaneous functions. Our proteomics results also revealed that tomato proteins involved in various physiological processes were altered indicating a complex nature of viroid-plant interactions. The higher expression of 14 proteins in λ-carrageenan treatment suggests their potential role in tomato defense to TCDVd that should be further investigated.

Results on the expression of lipoxygenase (*LOX*), allene oxide synthase (*AOS*) and pathogenesis-related protein (*PR1*) genes in TCDVd-infected tomatoes suggest a possible role of JA response in plants' resistance against viroid infection. JA response has been important against various biotic stresses in plants. Wang *et al.* [7] investigated the expression of genes in a susceptible and a transgenic (resistant) tomato with potato spindle tuber viroid (PSTVd) infection and revealed several differentially expressed genes in tomatoes and a possible role of jasmonic acid biosynthesis pathway in tomato resistance to viroids. The induction of these two genes (*LOX* and *AOS*) by λ-carrageenan-treated tomatoes support the role of JA dependent signaling pathway in tomato defense against TCDVd. In addition, salicylic acid-inducible *PR1* in control was not different than λ-carrageenan treatment, indicating that jasmonic acid/ethylene is important in viroid-tomato interaction, a finding that needs further understanding.

4. Material and Methods

4.1. Plant and Viroid Culture

Tomato (*Solanum lycopersicum* cv. Sheyenne) seeds and tomato chlorotic dwarf viroid (TCDVd)-infected plants were obtained from the Potato Research Centre, Fredericton, Canada. The viroid culture was maintained on tomatoes (cv. Sheyenne) in a greenhouse at 24 ± 2 °C with a photoperiod of 16 h light and an 8 h dark cycle. For experiments, surface sterilized healthy tomato seeds were planted in 8″ pots containing peat soil (Pro-mix) and maintained in the greenhouse under same conditions as described above.

4.2. Treatments

Three types of carrageenans (iota (ι), kappa (κ) and lambda (λ)) used in this study were provided by Cargill Texturant Solutions (Baupte, France). The carrageenans differed in sulfation, λ-carrageenan (35%) and κ-carrageenan (<30%). Spray solution were prepared by dissolving carrageenans in ultra-pure water (MilliQ) (0.1% w/v) containing 0.02% (v/v) of Tween-20.

4.3. Inoculation of Tomato Plant with TCDVd

Three-week-old tomato plants (8–10 cm tall) with fully expanded third leaves were sprayed with carrageenans until drip using a hand held atomizer. The control plants were treated in a similar manner with water containing Tween-20. Leaves (1 g) from TCDVd infected tomato were ground in 5 mL of 1:10 dilution (w/v) of buffer containing glycine (0.05 M) + dibasic potassium phosphate (0.03 M), pH 9.2 and the resulting sap was used for inoculating plants 48 h after spray treatment. Briefly, 10 µL each of TCDVd sap was rubbed gently over two leaflets of the second leaf for each treatment using a flame sterilized glass rod [37]. Inoculated plants were maintained in the growth chamber at 22 °C, 16 h:8 h for day:night conditions. Data on plant height and internode length were recorded at 21 dpi, whereas the appearance of bunchy top symptoms were observed on plants at 7, 14, 21, and 35 dpi [37].

4.4. Effect of Carrageenans on TCDVd in Infected Shoots

To investigate the effect of carrageenans on viroid multiplication, tomato shoot cuttings (5–6 cm long with 2 internodes) were excised from TCDVd infected plants, washed several times with distilled water and the cut end of the shoot was dipped in a 20 mL glass tube containing half strength Murashige & Skoog (MS) (Sigma, St. Louis, MO, USA) solution and incubated for two days at 24 ± 2 °C with a photoperiod of 16 h light and 8 h dark cycle. The MS medium was removed and replaced with MS solution supplemented with 1 g·L^{-1} carrageenans (ι, κ, λ). TCDVd concentration in the shoots was determined with RT-PCR (as described below) in 20 mm leaf disc excised from upper leaf at 0 (just before treatment), 1, 2, and 3 weeks post-treatment. Each treatment had three replications and the experiment was repeated twice.

4.5. Viroid Nucleic Acid Extraction and RT-PCR

The viroid RNA was extracted from the leaf tissue following published method [37]. Briefly, 100 mg of leaf tissue was homogenized in 500 µL viroid extraction buffer (50 mM NaOH + 2.5 mM EDTA) in a bead beater (Micro Smash MS-100, Tomy Co., Tokyo, Japan), set at 3000 rpm for 2 min. The homogenate was centrifuged 8000× *g* at 4 °C for 20 min and the supernatant (300 µL) was precipitated with 300 µL of isopropanol and 0.1 µL of 3 M sodium acetate (−20 °C overnight). The precipitate was collected by centrifugation (12,000× *g* at 4 °C) for 5 min, washed with 70% ethanol, air-dried, and dissolved in 150 µL of RNAase free water. Two µg RNA was reverse transcribed using High Capacity cDNA Reverse Transcription kit (Applied Biosystems, ON, Canada) with a Pospiviroid reverse primer (5′-AGCTTCAGTTGTTTCCACCGG GT-3′).

Polymerase chain reaction was carried with 2 µL of cDNA using Taq DNA polymerase (Applied Biosystems, Foster City, CA, USA) using the forward primer (5′-ATTAATCCCCGGGGAAACCTGGAG-3′) and reverse primer (5′-AGCTTCAGTTGTTTCCACCGGGT-3′) [44]. PCR was performed with standard conditions, except that 27 cycles were used to avoid saturation of the product. For quantification, ten microliters of amplified product was electrophoresed on 2% agarose gel containing 0.5 µg/mL ethidium bromide and photographed under UV light in a gel documentation system (Quantity One, Gel Doc EQ, Bio-Rad, Hercules, CA, USA). TCDVd band intensities were quantified by ImageJ free software (Version 1.33; http://rsb.info.nih.gov/ij/) and compared relative to the control.

4.6. Carrageenan Induced Defense Gene Expression in Tomatoes

To determine the response of tomato plant to carrageenan treatment following viroid inoculation, the transcript abundance of tomato defense genes *TomLOX* (forward primer, 5′-GGCCACGTTGACCTC CGCAA-3′; reverse primer, 5′-TGCGCTGAAGCCAGCCAGAT-3′, *TomAOS* (forward primer, 5′-ACACGACGCCGTTTTCGAGGTG-3′; reverse primer, 5′-CCGACGAACCGATCGGCGAC-3′ and *PR1* (forward primer, 5′-GACGAGTTGGCGTTGGCCCT-3′; reverse primer, 5′-AGCGGCTAGGTTTTCGCCGT-3′) were analyzed by quantitative real time PCR. Leaf tissues were sampled at 0 and 7 dpi and total RNA was extracted using a plant RNA extraction kit (Qiagen, Mississauga, ON, Canada). The quality and quantity of RNA was assessed with Nanodrop ND-1000 (NanoDrop Technologies Wilmington, DE, USA) and formaldehyde gel electrophoresis. DNAase treated RNA was used to synthesize cDNA using Quantiscript reverse transcriptase kit (Qiagen, Mississauga, ON, Canada) following manufacturer's instructions. Real-time PCR was performed on StepOne™ Real-Time PCR System (Applied Biosystems, Foster City, CA, USA) using SYBR green dye with Rox (Roche Diagnostics, Mississauga, ON, Canada) according to manufacturer instructions. Transcript abundance of each selected gene was normalized to18S ribosomal RNA. Data were analyzed from three independent Real-Time PCR runs.

4.7. Effect of Carrageenan on Tomato Proteomes

Leaf samples from tomato plants spray treated with carrageenans and inoculated with TCDVd as described above were harvested at 3 weeks after viroid inoculation, flash frozen in liquid nitrogen and ground to a fine powder. The total protein was extracted using a solution containing trichloroacetic acid (10%), acetone (89.93%) and dithiothreitol (0.07%). Protein concentration was determined by the Bradford Method [45] and stored in 100 μL aliquots at −80 °C until use.

For protein profiling, 100 μg of total proteins from the control and carrageenan-treated samples were separated with first dimension electrophoresis using 17 cm IPG strips, pH 4–7 at 500 V for 1 h, followed by 1000 V for 1 h and 1750 V for 24 h. The proteins were separated by SDS-PAGE in the second dimension using 12% polyacrylamide gels on a multiphor unit (Amersham Biosciences, Piscataway, NJ, USA). The gels were silver stained following published protocol [46]. The gels were scanned with a GS-700 imaging densitometer (Bio-Rad, Hercules, CA, USA) and analyzed with PD Quest software (Bio-Rad, Hercules, CA, USA).

For protein identification, differentially expressed protein spots were excised from the preparative gels and digested with trypsin using the MassPREP station (Waters, Milford, MA, USA). Protein identification and sequencing were carried out using two-dimensional liquid chromatography ESI MS (Agilent 1100 series 2D nano LC MS). The peptide mass data were subjected to the MASCOT search engine (Agilent, Santa Clara, CA, USA) for analysis. MS/MS spectra were used to search protein identity at NCBI non-redundant protein database using MS/MS Ion Search Engine at http://www.matrixscience.com/search_form_select.html. A single protein, having a higher score than the minimum score for the significance level ($p < 0.05$), was judged as a significant match.

4.8. Statistical Analysis

For data analysis, JMP-IN (Ver. 5) statistical software was used. Data were subjected to analysis of variance (ANOVA) and the means were compared for significance using Tukey's test or student's *t*-test ($p < 0.05$). Each experiment was replicated two to three times in independent trials. Values are represented as mean ± SEM (standard error of the mean).

5. Conclusions

In summary, the results showed that highly sulfated λ-carrageenan suppressed TCDVd in tomatoes by eliciting plant defense responses while less sulfated ι- or κ-carrageenan did not have an effect. The induction of plant resistance with λ-carrageenan could be a novel, cost effective and environmentally friendly approach for the management of this pathogen. Since pospiviroids are replicated in the nucleus by DNA-dependent RNA polymerase II, it remains unclear if λ-carrageenan affected this enzyme *in vivo*, which might have resulted in the reduced viroid concentration in the elicited plants.

Acknowledgments: Balakrishnan Prithiviraj's lab is supported by the grants from Atlantic Canada Opportunities Agency (ACOA), Natural Sciences and Engineering Research Council of Canada (NSERC), Nova Scotia Department of Agriculture and Marketing (NSDAF) and Acadian Seaplants Limited.

Author Contributions: Jatinder S. Sangha (J.S.S.), Balakrishnan Prithiviraj (B.P.), and Rudra P. Singh (R.P.S.) conceived and designed the experiments; J.S.S., Saveetha Kandasamy (S.K.), Wajahat Khan (W.K.), and Navratan S. Bahia (N.S.B.) performed experiments; J.S.S. and B.P. analyzed and interpreted the data; Alan T. Critchley (A.T.C) and R.P.S. contributed reagents and materials; J.S.S. and B.P. wrote the paper.

Conflicts of Interest: The authors declare no conflict of interest.

References

1. Singh, R.P.; Nie, X.; Singh, M. Tomato chlorotic dwarf viroid: An evolutionary link in the origin of pospiviroids. *J. Gen. Virol.* **1999**, *80*, 2823–2828. [PubMed]

2. Diener, T.O. Potato spindle tuber "virus" IV.A replicating, low molecular weight RNA. *Virology* **1971**, *45*, 411–428.

3. Singh, R.P.; Clark, M.C. Infectious low-molecular weight ribonucleic acid from tomato. *Biochem. Biophys. Res. Commun.* **1971**, *44*, 1077–1083. [CrossRef] [PubMed]

4. Tabler, M.; Tsagris, M. Viroids: Petite RNA pathogens with distinguished talents. *Trends Plant Sci.* **2004**, *9*, 339–348. [CrossRef] [PubMed]

5. Singh, R.P.; Teixeria da Silva, J.A. Ornamental plants: Silent carrier of evolving viroids. In *Floriculture, Ornamental and Plant Biotechnology*; Teixeria da Silva, J.A., Ed.; Global Science Books: London, UK, 2006; Volume III, pp. 531–539.

6. Itaya, A.; Matsuda, Y.; Gonzales, R.A.; Nelson, R.S.; Ding, B. Potato spindle tuber viroid strains of different pathogenicity induces and suppresses expression of common and unique genes in infected tomato. *Mol. Plant Microbe Interact.* **2002**, *15*, 990–999. [CrossRef] [PubMed]

7. Wang, Y.; Shibuya, M.; Taneda, A.; Kurauchi, T.; Senda, M.; Owens, R.A.; Sano, T. Accumulation of *Potato spindle tuber viroid*-specific small RNAs is accompanied by specific changes in gene expression in two tomato cultivars. *Virology* **2011**, *413*, 72–83. [CrossRef] [PubMed]

8. Gross, H.J.; Domday, H.; Lossow, C.; Jank, P.; Raba, M.; Alberty, H.; Sänger, H.L. Nucleotide sequence and secondary structure of potato spindle tuber viroid. *Nature* **1978**, *273*, 203–208. [CrossRef] [PubMed]

9. Flores, R.; Serra, P.; Minoia, S.; di Serio, F.; Navarro, B. Viroids: From genotype to phenotype just relying on RNA sequence and structural motifs. *Front. Microbiol.* **2012**, *3*, 1–13. [PubMed]

10. Kovalskaya, N.; Hammond, R.W. Molecular biology of viroid-host interactions and disease control strategies. *Plant Sci.* **2014**, *228*, 48–60. [CrossRef] [PubMed]

11. Singh, R.P.; Crowley, C.F. Evaluation of polyacrylamide gel electrophoresis, bioassay, and dot-blot methods for the survey of potato spindle tuber viroid. *Can. Plant Dis. Surv.* **1985**, *65*, 61–63.

12. Singh, R.P. Piperonyl butoxide as a protectant against Potato spindle tuber viroid infection. *Phytopathology* **1977**, *67*, 933–935. [CrossRef]

13. Bellés, J.M.; Hansen, A.J.; Granell, A.; Conejero, V. Antiviroid effect of ribavirin on citrus exocortis viroid infection in *Gynura aurantiaca* DC. *Physiol. Mol. Plant Pathol.* **1986**, *28*, 61–65. [CrossRef]

14. Niblett, C.L.; Dickson, E.; Fernow, K.H.; Horst, R.K.; Zaitlin, M. Cross protection among four viroids. *Virology* **1978**, *91*, 198–203. [CrossRef] [PubMed]

15. Postman, J.; Hadidi, A. Eliminati on of apple scar skin viroid from pears by *in vitro* thermotherapy and apical meristem culture. *Acta Hortic.* **1995**, *386*, 536–543.

16. Matoušek, J.; Trněná, L.; Svoboda, P.; Oriniaková, P.; Lichtenstein, C.P. The gradual reduction of viroid levels in hop mericlones following heat therapy: A possible role for a nuclease degrading dsRNA. *Biol. Chem. Hoppe Seyler* **1995**, *376*, 715–722. [CrossRef] [PubMed]

17. Kasai, A.; Sano, T.; Harada, T. Scion on a stock producing siRNAs of potato spindle tuber viroid (PSTVd) attenuates accumulation of the viroid. *PLoS ONE* **2013**, *2*, e57736. [CrossRef]

18. Harris, P.S.; Miller-Jones, D.M.; Howell, P.J. Control of potato spindle tuber viroid: The special problems of a disease in plant breeders' material. In *Plant Health: The Scientific Basis for Administrative Control of Plant Parasites*; Ebbels, D.L., King, J.E., Eds.; Blackwell: Oxford, UK, 1979; pp. 232–237.

19. Pfannenstiel, M.A.; Slack, S.A. Response of potato cultivars to infection by potato spindle tuber viroid. *Phytopathology* **1980**, *70*, 922–926. [CrossRef]

20. Matsushita, Y.; Aoki, K.; Sumitomo, K. Selection and inheritance of resistance to *Chrysanthemum stunt* viroid. *Crop Prot.* **2012**, *35*, 1–4. [CrossRef]

21. Omori, H.; Hosokawa, M.; Shiba, H.; Shitsukawa, N.; Murai, K.; Yazawa, S. Screening of chrysanthemum plants with strong resistance to *Chrysanthemum stunt* viroid. *J. Jpn. Soc. Hortic. Sci.* **2009**, *78*, 350–355. [CrossRef]

22. Schwind, N.; Zwiebel, M.; Itaya, A.; Ding, B.; Wang, M.-B.; Krczal, G.; Wassenegger, M. RNAi mediated resistance to *Potato spindle tuber viroid* in transgenic tomato expressing a viroid hairpin RNA construct. *Mol. Plant Pathol.* **2009**, *10*, 459–469. [CrossRef] [PubMed]

23. Pieterse, C.M.J.; Dicke, M. Plant interactions with microbes and insects: From molecular mechanisms to ecology. *Trends Plant Sci.* **2007**, *12*, 564–569. [CrossRef] [PubMed]

24. Jones, J.D.G.; Dangl, J.L. The plant immune system. *Nature* **2006**, *444*, 323–329. [CrossRef] [PubMed]

25. Scheel, D. Resistance response physiology and signal transduction. *Curr. Opin. Plant Biol.* **1998**, *1*, 305–310. [CrossRef] [PubMed]

26. Pieterse, C.M.J.; van Wees, S.C.M.; van Pelt, J.A.; Knoester, M.; Laan, R.; Gerrits, H.; Weisbeek, P.J.; van Loon, L.C. A novel signaling pathway controlling induced systemic resistance in Arabidopsis. *Plant Cell* **1998**, *10*, 1571–1580. [CrossRef] [PubMed]

27. Dixon, R.A.; Harrison, M.J.; Lamb, C.J. Early events in the activation of plant defense responses. *Annu. Rev. Plant Phytopathol.* **1994**, *32*, 479–501. [CrossRef]

28. Mercier, L.; Lafitte, C.; Borderies, G.; Briand, X.; Esquerré-Tugayé, M.T.; Fournier, J. The algal polysaccharide carrageenans can act as an elicitor of plant defence. *New Phytol.* **2001**, *149*, 43–51. [CrossRef]

29. Bektas, Y.; Eulgem, T. Synthetic Plant Defense Elicitors. *Front. Plant Sci.* **2014**, *5*. [CrossRef] [PubMed]

30. Klarzynski, O.; Plesse, B.; Joubert, J.M.; Yvin, J.C.; Kopp, M.; Kloareg, B.; Fritig, B. Linear beta-1, 3 glucans are elicitors of defense responses in tobacco. *Plant Physiol.* **2000**, *124*, 1027–1038. [CrossRef] [PubMed]

31. Sangha, J.S.; Ravichandran, S.; Prithiviraj, K.; Critchley, A.T.; Prithiviraj, B. Sulfated macroalgal polysaccharides λ-carrageenan and ι-carrageenan differentially alter *Arabidopsis thaliana* resistance to *Sclerotinia sclerotiorum*. *Physiol. Mol. Plant Pathol.* **2010**, *75*, 38–45. [CrossRef]

32. Gordon-Mills, E.M.; McCandless, E.L. Carrageenans in the cell walls of *Chondrus crispus* Stack. (Rhodophyceae, Gigartinales). I. Localization with fluorescent antibody. *Phycologia* **1975**, *14*, 275–281.

33. Buck, C.B.; Thompson, C.D.; Roberts, J.N.; Müller, M.; Lowy, D.R.; Schiller, J.T. Carrageenan is a potent inhibitor of papillomavirus infection. *PLoS Pathog.* **2006**, *2*, e69. [CrossRef] [PubMed]

34. Kobayashi, A.; Tai, A.; Kanzaki, H.; Kawazu, K. Elicitor-active oligosaccharides from algal laminaran stimulate the production of antifungal compounds in alfalfa. *Z. Naturforschung* **1993**, *48*, 575–579.

35. Bouarab, K.; Potin, P.; Correa, J.; Kloareg, B. Sulfated oligosaccharides mediate the interaction between a marine red alga and its green algal pathogenic endophyte. *Plant Cell* **1999**, *11*, 1635–1650. [CrossRef] [PubMed]

36. Khan, W.; Rayirath, U.P.; Subramanian, S.; Jithesh, M.N.; Rayorath, P.; Hodges, D.M.; Critchley, A.T.; Craigie, J.S.; Norrie, J.; Prithiviraj, P. Seaweed extracts as biostimulants of plant growth and development. *J. Plant Growth Regul.* **2009**, *28*, 386–399. [CrossRef]

37. Singh, R.P.; Dilworth, A.D.; Singh, M.; Babcock, K.M. An alkaline solution simplifies nucleic acid preparation for RT-PCR and infectivity assays of viroids from crude sap and spotted membrane. *J. Virol. Methods* **2006**, *132*, 204–211. [CrossRef] [PubMed]

38. Bostock, R.M.; Karban, R.; Thaler, J.S.; Weyman, P.D.; Gilchrist, D. Signal interactions in induced resistance to pathogens and insect herbivores. *Eur. J. Plant Pathol.* **2008**, *107*, 103–111. [CrossRef]

39. Zimmerli, L.; Jakab, G.; Métraux, J.P.; Mauch-Mani, B. Potentiation of pathogen-specific defense mechanisms in *Arabidopsis* by beta aminobutyric acid. *Proc. Natl. Acad. Sci. USA* **2000**, *97*, 12920–12925. [CrossRef] [PubMed]

40. Nagorskaia, V.P.; Reunov, A.V.; Lapshina, L.A.; Ermak, I.M.; Barabanova, A.O. Influence of kappa/beta-carrageenan from red alga *Tichocarpus crinitus* on development of local infection induced by tobacco mosaic virus in Xanthi-nc tobacco leaves. *Izv. Akad. Nauk Ser. Biol.* **2007**, *3*, 360–364. [PubMed]

41. Sangha, J.S.; Khan, W.; Ji, X.; Zhang, J.; Mills, A.A.; Critchley, A.T.; Prithiviraj, B. Carrageenans, sulphated polysaccharides of red seaweeds, differentially affect *Arabidopsis thaliana* resistance to *Trichoplusia ni* (Cabbage Looper). *PLoS ONE* **2011**, *6*, e26834. [CrossRef] [PubMed]

42. Singh, R.P.; Dilworth, A.D.; Ao, X.; Singh, M.; Misra, S. Molecular and biological characterization of a severe isolate of Tomato chlorotic dwarf viroid containing a novel terminal right (TR) domain sequence. *Eur. J. Plant Pathol.* **2010**, *127*, 63–72. [CrossRef]

43. Rampitsch, C.; Natalia, V.B. Proteomics and plant disease: Advances in combating a major threat to the global food supply. *Proteomics* **2012**, *12*, 673–690. [CrossRef] [PubMed]

44. Bostan, H.; Nie, X.; Singh, R.P. An RT-PCR primer pair for the detection of *Pospiviroid* and its application in surveying ornamental plants for viroids. *J. Virol. Methods* **2004**, *116*, 189–193. [CrossRef] [PubMed]

45. Bradford, M.M. A rapid and sensitive method for the quantitation of microgram quantities of protein utilizing the principle of protein-dye binding. *Anal. Biochem.* **1976**, *72*, 248–254. [CrossRef] [PubMed]

46. Shevchenko, A.; Wilm, M.; Vorm, O.; Mann, M. Mass spectrometric sequencing of proteins from silver-stained polyacrylamide gels. *Anal. Chem.* **1996**, *68*, 850–858. [CrossRef] [PubMed]

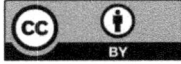

marine drugs

MDPI

Article

Morphological and Proteomic Analyses Reveal that Unsaturated Guluronate Oligosaccharide Modulates Multiple Functional Pathways in Murine Macrophage RAW264.7 Cells

Xu Xu [1], De-Cheng Bi [1,†], Chao Li [1,†], Wei-Shan Fang [1], Rui Zhou [1], Shui-Ming Li [2], Lian-Li Chi [3], Min Wan [4] and Li-Ming Shen [1,*]

[1] College of Life Science, Shenzhen Key Laboratory of Marine Bioresources and Ecology, Shenzhen University, Shenzhen 518060, China; xuxu@szu.edu.cn (X.X.); 215017325@qq.com (D.-C.B.); 611279860@qq.com (C.L.); 1210417703@qq.com (W.-S.F.); zhouruiswg@gmail.com (R.Z.)

[2] College of Life Science, Shenzhen Key Laboratory of Microbial Genetic Engineering, Shenzhen University, Shenzhen 518060, China; msbiotools@gmail.com

[3] National Glycoengineering Research Center, Shandong University, Jinan 250100, China; lianlichi@gmail.com

[4] Division of Physiological Chemistry 2, Department of Medical Biochemistry and Biophysics, Karolinska Institute, Stockholm 17177, Sweden; min.wan@ki.se

* Author to whom correspondence should be addressed; slm@szu.edu.cn; Tel.: +86-755-2601-2653; Fax: +86-755-2653-4237.

† These authors contributed equally to this work.

Academic Editor: Paola Laurienzo

Received: 5 February 2015; Accepted: 20 March 2015; Published: 30 March 2015

Abstract: Alginate is a natural polysaccharide extracted from various species of marine brown algae. Alginate-derived guluronate oligosaccharide (GOS) obtained by enzymatic depolymerization has various pharmacological functions. Previous studies have demonstrated that GOS can trigger the production of inducible nitric oxide synthase (iNOS)/nitric oxide (NO), reactive oxygen species (ROS) and tumor necrosis factor (TNF)-α by macrophages and that it is involved in the nuclear factor (NF)-κB and mitogen-activated protein (MAP) kinase signaling pathways. To expand upon the current knowledge regarding the molecular mechanisms associated with the GOS-induced immune response in macrophages, comparative proteomic analysis was employed together with two-dimensional electrophoresis (2-DE), matrix-assisted laser desorption/ionization time-of-flight mass spectrometry (MALDI-TOF/TOF MS) and Western blot verification. Proteins showing significant differences in expression in GOS-treated cells were categorized into multiple functional pathways, including the NF-κB signaling pathway and pathways involved in inflammation, antioxidant activity, glycolysis, cytoskeletal processes and translational elongation. Moreover, GOS-stimulated changes in the morphologies and actin cytoskeleton organization of RAW264.7 cells were also investigated as possible adaptations to GOS. This study is the first to reveal GOS as a promising agent that can modulate the proper balance between the pro- and anti-inflammatory immune responses, and it provides new insights into pharmaceutical applications of polysaccharides.

Keywords: guluronate oligosaccharide; macrophage activation; nuclear factor-κB; anti-inflammation; antioxidant; cell morphology

1. Introduction

Alginate is currently extracted from marine brown algae and is known to be arranged in homopolymeric α-L-guluronate (G) blocks (polyguluronate, PG), β-D-mannuronate blocks (M)

(polymannuronate, PM) and random heteropolymeric G and M stretches [1]. Alginate is used for biotechnological and medical purposes in a wide range of commercial applications in the pharmaceutical field. Alginate oligosaccharide (AOS), which is obtained by lyase depolymerization of polymer and has a relatively low molecular weight, is regarded as a non-toxic, biocompatible, nonimmunogenic and biodegradable polymer, making it an attractive candidate for biomedical applications [2]. This oligosaccharide has various physiological functions, such as the promotion of bifidobacterial growth [3], the stimulation of endothelial cell growth and migration [4], and human keratinocyte growth [5]. AOS is also involved in the induction of cytokine production in macrophages [6–8], the enhancement of protection against infections by certain pathogens [9], antioxidant [10,11] and neuroprotective activities [12], and the suppression of Th2 development and IgE secretion through the induction of IL-12 secretion [13].

Macrophages play major roles in host defense, immunity and inflammatory responses and help to maintain steady-state tissue homeostasis [14]. The inflammatory response is a self-limiting process and involves the sequential activation of signaling pathways leading to the production of both pro- and anti-inflammatory mediators [15]. Our recent studies have demonstrated that enzymatically depolymerized guluronate oligosaccharide (GOS) from PG could markedly increase phagocytosis of IgG-opsonized *Escherichia coli* and *Staphylococcus aureus* and intracellular bacterial killing by macrophages, resulting in enhancement of the antibacterial activity of macrophages via the activation of several signaling pathways that are related to innate immunity and bacterial clearance in murine acute peritonitis *in vivo* [16]. GOS activates macrophages by binding to Toll-like receptor (TLR) 2/4, causing cytokine production [17]. We have also confirmed that GOS activates the nuclear factor (NF)-κB and mitogen-activated protein (MAP) kinase signaling pathways, elevates inducible nitric oxide synthase (iNOS) expression and, in turn, nitric oxide (NO) production, and induces tumor necrosis factor (TNF)-α secretion and reactive oxygen species (ROS) production [18]. GOS stimulates cellular inflammatory responses and releases factors, which indicates that it could be used in the agriculture, food and drug industries as a potent immunomodulatory agent.

Proteomics is now generally accepted as a useful method due to its high-throughput capability to analyze total protein expression and elucidate cellular processes at the molecular level [19,20]. To gain more information and elucidate specific mechanisms underlying the involvement of GOS involved in phagocytosis and signal transduction pathways, we carried out a proteomic study to identify differentially expressed proteins extracted from control and GOS-treated RAW264.7 cells using two-dimensional electrophoresis (2-DE) and matrix-assisted laser desorption/ionization time-of-flight mass spectrometry (MALDI-TOF/TOF MS). We identified nine proteins with significant changes (fold change $\geq$ 2.0) in expression between the GOS-treated and untreated RAW264.7 cells. These results were confirmed by Western blot, biochemical studies and morphological analyses. Considered together with the findings of our previous studies [16,18], the current results suggest that the functional pathways of activation and negative regulation of the NF-κB signaling pathway, pro- and anti-inflammation, pro- and anti-oxidation, cytoskeletal remodeling and cell proliferation might be involved in GOS-induced macrophage activation and immunomodulation. Notably, the inflammatory response requires the coordinated activation of various signaling pathways that regulate the expression of both pro- and anti-inflammatory mediators [15]. Thus, we provide key insight into the potential mechanisms by which the immune response is modulated by GOS.

2. Results

2.1. Preparation and Structural Analysis of GOS

As shown in Figure 1, IR spectroscopy revealed characteristic peaks at 3457, 2930, 1743, 1621, 1415, 1126, 1103, 1035 and 789 cm^{-1}. The broad absorption band at 3457 cm^{-1} is representative of the stretching frequency of OH groups, and the band at 2930 cm^{-1} is attributable to CH asymmetric stretching. The weak absorption peak at 1743 cm^{-1} indicates the presence of uronic acids, and the absorption peaks at 1621 cm^{-1} and 1415 cm^{-1} are also representative of polysaccharides. The region at 1200–1000 cm^{-1} contained three absorption peaks indicative of a pyranoid saccharide [21]. The very weak absorption peak at 789 cm^{-1} is a unique characteristic of guluronic acid residues.

Furthermore, the molecular weight and degree of polymerization (DP) of GOS, which was enzymatically digested from PG, was determined using ESI-MS. The results indicated (Figure 2) that multiple charged ions, which were associated with different amounts of sodium or potassium adducts, were observed for GOS in the negative mode ESI-MS analysis. The charge states of the ions were deduced based on their isotopic distributions, and their molecular weights were then calculated. The interpretation of the MS peaks (Table 1) revealed that the primary GOS ranged from dimers to octamers (G2–G8).

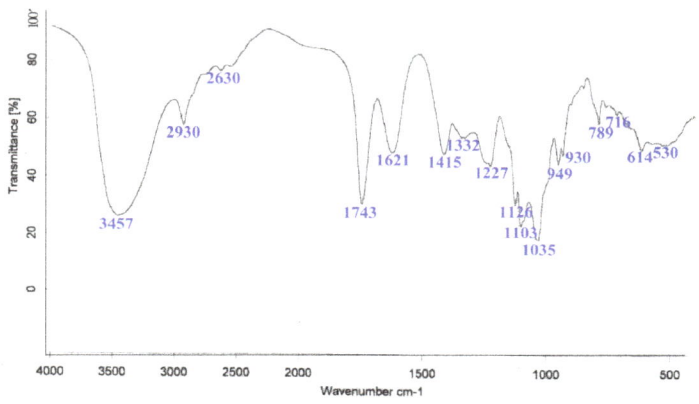

Figure 1. The infrared (IR) spectrum of polyguluronic acid (PG). The spectrum was run in KBr pellets with 1 mg of sample and 200 mg of KBr.

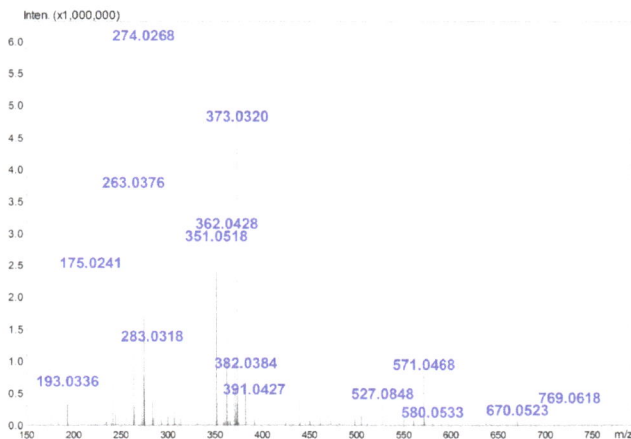

Figure 2. The electrospray ionization mass spectrometry (ESI-MS) of guluronate oligosaccharide (GOS). The spectrum was acquired in the negative ion mode with a high-resolution hybrid time-of-flight mass spectrometer. The ions were present in the form of $[M + xNa(K) - (x + n)H]^{n-}$. The corresponding molecular weights and DP were then calculated using the monoisotopic peaks and charge states of each group of ions.

Table 1. Ions observed in the mass spectrometry (MS) analysis of GOS.

m/z	Charge State	Ion Format	Corresponding DP [a]	MW [b]
351	1	$[M - H]^-$	2	352
263	2	$[M - 2H]^{2-}$	3	528
274	2	$[M + Na - 3H]^{2-}$	3	528
283	2	$[M + K - 3H]^{2-}$	3	528
571	1	$[M + 2Na - 3H]^-$	3	528
362	2	$[M + Na - 3H]^{2-}$	4	704
373	2	$[M + 2Na - 4H]^{2-}$	4	704
382	2	$[M + 2Na - 4H + H_2O]^{2-}$	4	704
439	2	$[M - 2H]^{2-}$	5	880
450	2	$[M + Na - 3H]^{2-}$	5	880
461	2	$[M + 2Na - 4H]^{2-}$	5	880
472	2	$[M + 3Na - 5H]^{2-}$	5	880
481	2	$[M + 3Na-5H + H_2O]^{2-}$	5	880
527	2	$[M - 2H]^{2-}$	6	1056
538	2	$[M + Na - 3H]^{2-}$	6	1056
549	2	$[M + 2Na - 4H]^{2-}$	6	1056
560	2	$[M + 3Na - 5H]^{2-}$	6	1056
571	2	$[M + 4Na - 6H]^{2-}$	6	1056
670	2	$[M + 5Na - 7H]^{2-}$	7	1232
679	2	$[M + 5Na - 7H + H_2O]^{2-}$	7	1232
490	3	$[M + 3Na - 6H]^{3-}$	8	1407
497	3	$[M + 4Na - 7H]^{3-}$	8	1406

[a] DP = degree of polymerization; [b] MW = molecular weight.

2.2. Comparison of Protein Expression Patterns between GOS-Treated and Control Cells

To explore the underlying mechanisms of the effects of GOS on RAW264.7 cells, comparative proteomic analyses were performed. After RAW264.7 cells were incubated with 1 mg/mL GOS in FBS-free culture medium for 24 h, proteins were extracted and separated by 2-DE. Representative silver-stained 2-DE maps are shown in Figure 3. A comparison of these maps with the images revealed that the expression of nine proteins was significantly altered (by ≥2.0-fold), and these proteins were identified by MALDI-TOF/TOF MS analysis, as shown in Table 2. Among them, six proteins were significantly up-regulated, and three were noticeably down-regulated. The up-regulated proteins were identified as 60S acidic ribosomal protein P2 (RPLP2), annexin A5 (ANXA5), cofilin-2 (CFL2), Cu/Zn-superoxide dismutase (SOD1), galectin-1 (LGALS1) and lactoylglutathione lyase (GLO1). The down-regulated proteins were cofilin-1 (CFL1), fructose-bisphosphate aldolase (ALDOART1) and GTP-binding nuclear protein (RAN).

(A)

(B)

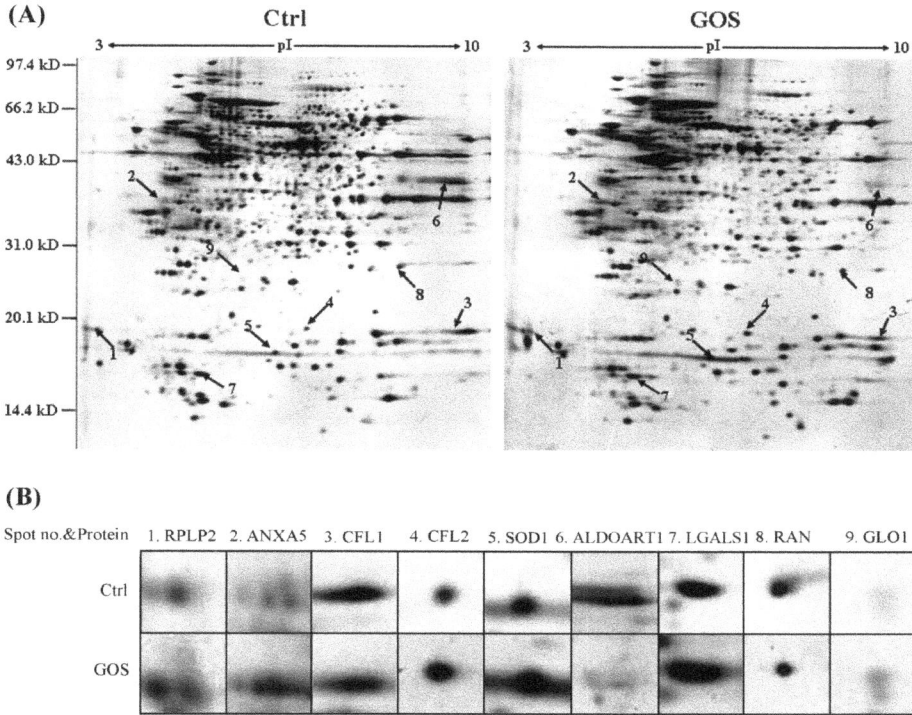

Figure 3. (**A**) A representative two-dimensional electrophoresis (2-DE) gel showing of total proteins from untreated and GOS-treated RAW264.7 cells. Each gel is representative of three independent replicates. Differentially regulated proteins (≥2.0-fold) are indicated by arrows and numbers and are listed in Table 2; (**B**) Magnified image of an identified protein spot.

The proteins could be divided into six functional categories according to the SwissProt database. The first group was related to the NF-κB signaling pathway and included LGALS1 and GLO1. The second group comprising ANXA5 and RAN was related to inflammation. The third group was related to oxidative stress and included SOD1. The fourth group was related to metabolic processes and included ALDOART1. The fifth group, including CFL1 and CFL2, was involved in cytoskeletal processes. The sixth group was related to translational elongation and included RPLP2.

Table 2. Detailed information regarding the differentially expressed proteins detected by MS.

Spot No.	Protein ID	Symbol	Accession Number	MW (kD)/pI	Peptides Matched [a]	Cov (%) [b]	Protein Score	Expr Level [c]	Reported Function
1	60S acidic ribosomal protein P2	RPLP2	P99027	11.65/4.38	3(2)	31	168	+3.3 ± 0.3	Translation
2	Annexin A5	ANXA5	P48036	35.75/4.82	7(6)	30	244	+2.7 ± 0.2	Inflammation
3	Cofilin-1	CFL1	P18760	18.56/8.22	4(3)	26	256	−2.1 ± 0.2	Cell cytoskeleton
4	Cofilin-2	CFL2	P45591	18.71/7.66	1(1)	6	73	+2.4 ± 0.2	Cell cytoskeleton
5	Cu/Zn-superoxide dismutase	SOD1	P08228	15.94/6.02	4(4)	24	315	+2.1 ± 0.2	Antioxidant
6	Fructose-bisphosphate aldolase	ALDOART1	Q9CPQ9	39.35/8.30	5(4)	18	296	−5.9 ± 0.7	Metabolic process
7	Galectin-1	LGALS1	P16045	14.86/5.28	6(6)	43	426	+2.3 ± 0.3	Signal transduction
8	GTP-binding nuclear protein	RAN	P62826	24.42/7.01	6(5)	21	324	−2.2 ± 0.2	Inflammation
9	Lactoylglutathione lyase	GLO1	Q9CPU0	20.81/5.24	2(2)	8	65	+2.4 ± 0.2	Signal transduction

[a] Peptides matched by mass fingerprinting; [b] Protein sequence coverage; [c] Expression level in GOS-treated RAW264.7 cells at 24 h compared with control cells (+, increase; −, decrease).

2.3. Western Blot Analysis for Validation of Differentially Expressed Proteins

Western blot analysis was carried out to confirm the differential expression of ALDOART1, ANXA5, CFL1, CFL2, LGALS1 and SOD1. Figure 4 shows that the expression of ANXA5, CFL2, LGALS1 and SOD1 was significantly up-regulated, whereas the expression of ALDOART1 and CFL1 was clearly down-regulated in GOS-stimulated RAW264.7 cells compared with control cells, which corresponded well with the differences observed in 2-DE analysis.

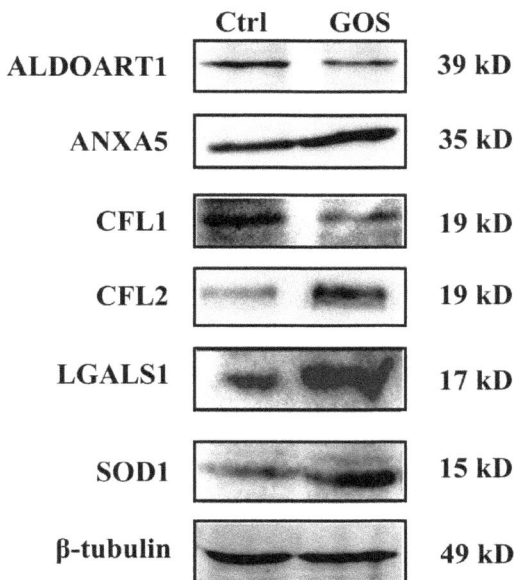

Figure 4. Western blot analysis of altered proteins in GOS-treated RAW264.7 cells. A representative result of three independent experiments is shown. Typical experiment conducted three times with similar results. β-tubulin was used as an internal control.

2.4. Effects of GOS on the Morphology and Actin Cytoskeleton Organization of RAW264.7 Cells

We observed changes in the morphology and actin cytoskeleton organization of GOS-treated RAW264.7 cells compared with control cells under dark-field and confocal microscopy ($\times$40). Figure 5 shows that the GOS treatment induced morphological alterations in the macrophages, including a dramatic increase in cell number, cell size and nucleus size; an increased number of cells with two nuclei; and increased F-actin accumulation compared with untreated cells. As shown in Figure 5A, GOS had an obvious growth-promoting effect on RAW264.7 cells, which was reflected by a marked increase in the total number of cells. Quantitative analysis revealed that GOS treatment caused a 1.25-fold increase in the number of RAW264.7 cells compared with no treatment (Figure 5B). The majority of untreated RAW264.7 cells exhibited a rounded morphology. Treatment with GOS for 24 h stimulated the production of numerous hair-like membrane protrusions or filopodia, which led to an increase in the macrophage cell area, resulting in extended cellular spreading (Figure 5C). The relative cell size and relative nucleus area were measured using ImageJ software. By analyzing the relative cell size distribution of control and GOS-treated RAW264.7 cells, we found that GOS moderately increased the mean cell area to 172.0% $\pm$ 6.6% of the control (100%) (Figure 5D). The GOS-treated RAW264.7 cells also possessed larger nuclei and prominent nucleoli (Figure 5E), and the nuclear areas of the cells treated with GOS were 29.3% $\pm$ 3.5% larger than those of the untreated cells (100%) (Figure 5F). We propose a possible positive correlation between cellular uptake during phagocytosis in macrophages and increases in cell number, cell size and nucleus size in GOS-treated RAW264.7 cells. Furthermore, it is interesting to note that the GOS-treated RAW264.7 cells showed an increase in the number of nuclei (Figure 5G), and quantitative analysis revealed that GOS treatment caused a 2.7-fold increase in the number of cells with dual nuclei compared with the control (no treatment) (Figure 5H). Hence, it appears that GOS facilitates the formation of dual-nuclei cells.

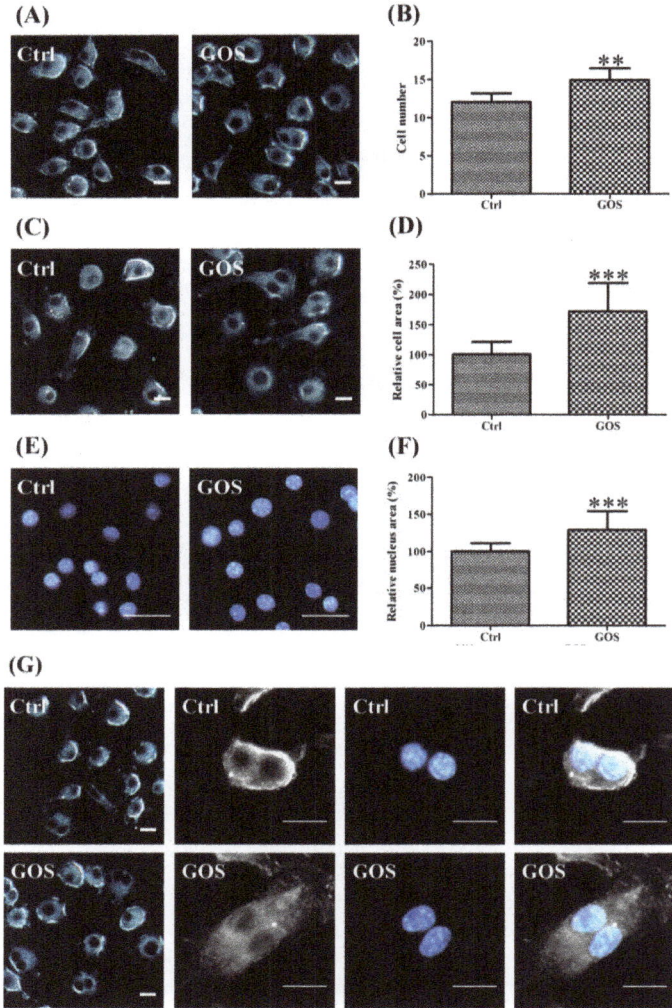

Figure 5. *Cont.*

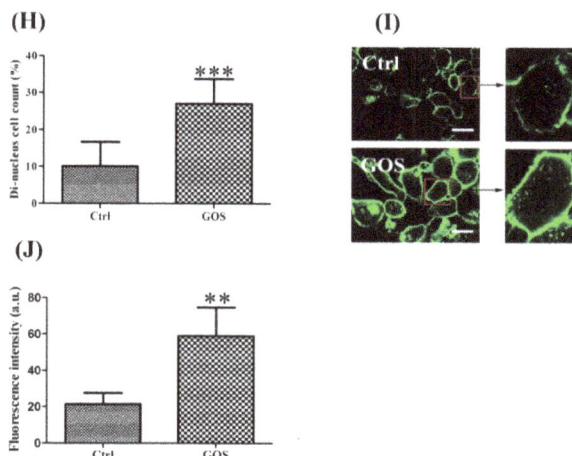

Figure 5. Effects of GOS on the morphology and actin organization of RAW264.7 cells. RAW264.7 cell morphology was observed by dark-field and confocal microscopy (×40). The cells were treated with or without 1 mg/mL GOS for 24 h. Representative dark-field images and analysis results show that GOS induced morphological changes in RAW264.7 cells, including an increase in the cell number (**A,B**), larger cell sizes (**C,D**), extended nucleus areas (**E,F**), and a greater number of dual-nuclei cells (**G,H**), compared with untreated cells (control). F-actin was stained with FITC-phalloidin. GOS-induced F-actin organization was examined using fluorescence images (**I**) and quantitative analysis (**J**). Scale bar, 20 µm. All images were analyzed with ImageJ software. ** $p < 0.01$ and *** $p < 0.001$ indicate significant differences between the control group and the GOS-treated group.

In addition, to determine the cytoskeletal changes in RAW264.7 cells, F-actin was visualized with FITC-phalloidin staining. GOS-treated RAW264.7 cells showed an increase in F-actin expression (Figure 5I). Fluorescence intensity was quantified by ImageJ software. Figure 5J shows that GOS treatment induced a 2.8-fold increase in F-actin fluorescence intensity compared with untreated cells. These results support those of our previous study, showing that cytoskeletal transformation can increase the phagocytosis of bacteria by RAW264.7 cells [16].

2.5. Effects of GOS on Lipopolysaccharide-Activated Morphological Changes in RAW264.7 Cells

Lipopolysaccharide (LPS), a macrophage activator, is known to rapidly activate morphological changes in macrophages. It has been reported that anti-inflammatory agents can generally inhibit the LPS-stimulated cell morphological changes [22,23]. To evaluate the effects of GOS on the morphologies of LPS-stimulated RAW264.7 cells, the cells were monitored under a phase contrast microscope (×40). The normal cells (control) were generally round and smooth with limited cell spreading and finely granulated cytoplasm, whereas the LPS-activated RAW264.7 cells displayed a significantly irregular and rough form with accelerated spreading and the formation of pseudopodia, relatively prominent cytoplasm with increased granularity, and condensed chromatin in the nucleus (Figure 6). Following pretreatment with GOS for 2 h and subsequent stimulation with LPS, the cells became rounded, and the levels of cell spreading and pseudopodia formation were reduced as expected. These results demonstrated that pretreatment with GOS could reduce LPS-stimulated irregular cell morphology, suggesting that GOS might specifically affect macrophage functions.

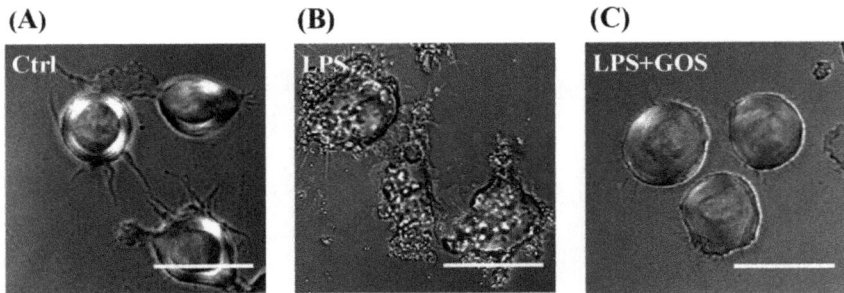

Figure 6. Effects of GOS on the lipopolysaccharide (LPS)-activated morphological changes in RAW264.7 cells. The morphologies of RAW264.7 cells were visualized with a phase contrast microscope ($\times$40). The cells were pretreated with 1 mg/mL GOS for 2 h before incubation with 1 µg/mL LPS for 24 h. (**A**) Control; (**B**) LPS-treated only; and (**C**) LPS-treated with GOS. Scale bar, 20 µm.

3. Discussion

In recent years, many reports have focused on the immunomodulatory effects of AOS [10,18,24]. GOS, which is derived from marine brown seaweed is generally non-toxic and shows a diverse range of beneficial biological activities. Additionally, GOS is regarded as a potential immunotherapeutic agent for the regulation of immune responses in the pharmacological industries [18]. Our previous study indicated that GOS activates the NF-κB signaling pathway, which modulates the expression of various genes involved in immune and inflammatory responses. For example, this pathway stimulates the production of NO, ROS, and TNF-α in macrophages [18]. To further determine the possible underlying biochemical mechanisms associated with GOS-induced immune response in macrophages, we identified differentially expressed proteins using 2-DE. Nine proteins were found to be significantly differentially expressed in GOS-treated cells compared with control cells, and these proteins were considered to be involved in the following processes: signal transduction; inflammatory reactions; antioxidant, metabolic, and cytoskeletal processes; and translational elongation. Further, the results of 2-DE proteomic analysis were validated by Western blot analysis.

The levels of LGALS1 and GLO1, two proteins that participate in signal transduction and are involved in the NF-κB signaling pathway, were increased following GOS treatment. Activation of NF-κB is critical for host defense [25]. However, NF-κB-driven immune responses must not be permanent; they need to be down-regulated and properly terminated [26]. LGALS1, a β-galactoside-binding protein belonging to the galectin family, has been reported to act as an endogenous potent anti-inflammatory factor and form a feedback regulatory loop with NF-κB [27]. NF-κB-activating stimuli increase LGALS1 expression in T cells; however, up-regulation of LGALS1 can inhibit the NF-κB signaling pathway [27–29]. We have reported that GOS activates NF-κB signaling pathway [16,18]. Thus, it could be speculated that GOS promotes NF-κB expression, thereby up-regulating LGALS expression and contributing to the attenuation of NF-κB overactivation. Another protein, GLO1, is involved in regulation of the TNF-induced transcriptional activity of NF-κB. Overexpression of GLO1 contributes to suppress TNF-induced NF-κB-dependent reporter gene expression, whereas a GLO1 specific knockdown significantly increases TNF-induced NF-κB expression [30]. Our results hinted that elevated levels of GLO1 might decrease the transcriptional activities of TNF-induced NF-κB-regulated target genes in GOS-treated RAW264.7 cells. Taken together, the up-regulation of LGALS1 and GLO1 inhibited the overactivation of the NF-κB signaling pathway in GOS-treated cells, which could be considered to be a negative feedback regulatory loop for the maintenance of cell homeostasis. In addition, LGALS1 has been shown to influence Fc gamma receptor (FcγR) expression and FcγR-dependent functions, such as phagocytosis, through active extracellular signal-regulated kinase (ERK)1/2-dependent pathway [31]. Interestingly, our previous reports revealed that GOS treatment enhanced the expression of FcγR II and FcγR III and activated the ERK MAP kinase signaling pathway in macrophages [16,18]. Hence, LGALS1 may play a role in the GOS-induced macrophage phagocytic activity.

ANXA5, a cytosolic Ca^{2+}-binding protein, and RAN, a GTPase-activating protein, play important roles during the immune and inflammatory response [32–34]. ANXA5 decreases the anti-inflammatory cytokines, and ANXA5-knockout animals display increased anti-inflammatory and immunosuppressive potential [34]. RAN appears to be involved in the response to LPS [33], and a high level of RAN overexpression in both macrophages and B cells leads to the down-regulation of LPS signal transduction [35]. In this study, ANXA5 was dramatically up-regulated and RAN was down-regulated in GOS-treated RAW264.7 cells (Figure 4), suggesting that these proteins might contribute to GOS-induced pro-inflammatory effects.

SOD1 is known to be a specific scavenger of the superoxide anion. It is one of the major antioxidant enzymes in mammalian cells and is important for maintaining the balance between $O_2{}^{\cdot-}$ generation and removal [36]. The production of ROS and reactive nitrogen species (RNS) (e.g., H_2O_2, $HO^{\cdot}$, $O_2{}^{\cdot-}$ and NO) by immunocytes is considered to be essential in the destruction of invading pathogens [37]; however, radicals can also cause oxidative stress damage to the host cells. To protect themselves against constant oxidative challenges, cells develop defense mechanisms that ensure a proper balance between pro- and anti-oxidant actions [38]. GOS was able to augment ROS production [18] and up-regulate SOD1 expression in RAW264.7 cells (Figure 4), demonstrating that the activation of SOD1 can protect cells from oxygen radical overaccumulation. Moreover, recent reports have demonstrated that alginate and AOS have potent antioxidant abilities [10,11] and that AOS protects PC12 pheochromocytoma cells against H_2O_2-induced oxidative stress via the activation of antioxidant enzymes, including SOD [12]. Therefore, the increase in SOD1 activity in the GOS-treated cells might also be related to the antioxidant ability of alginate. In addition, the activation of macrophages leads to the secretion of SOD1 via ERK activation, resulting in increased release of TNF-α and the production of ROS, and the overexpression of SOD1 stimulates immune responses, including ROS production and further TNF-α secretion [39].

Oxidative stress, such as that caused by ROS overproduction and the activation of key transcription factors such as NF-κB, can promote aerobic glycolysis and inflammation [40]. It has been reported that glycolysis promotes the proinflammatory activation of macrophages [41], and inflammation can be prevented in mice by blocking the glycolytic metabolic pathway of macrophages [42]. ALDOART1 is a ubiquitous enzyme essential for glycolysis and gluconeogenesis [43]. ALDOART1 was down-regulated in GOS-treated RAW264.7 cells compared with control cells (Figure 4), which may have led to the inhibition of glycolysis and may have impacted cellular metabolism. This result suggests that ALDOART1 may be involved in the negative regulation of GOS-induced pro-inflammatory responses.

Morphological changes constantly occur in macrophages when quiescently surveying environment or after phagocytosis activation. The morphofunctional alterations of cells require active actin cytoskeletal remodeling and metabolic adaptation [14]. In macrophages and dendritic cells, the actin cytoskeleton has been shown to regulate chemotaxis, phagocytosis and antigen presentation [44]. The actin-depolymerizing factor (ADF)/cofilin family of actin binding proteins, which consists of CFL1 (non-muscle cofilin), CFL2 (muscle cofilin) and ADF, are essential regulators of actin filament turnover [45]. CFL1 promotes cytoskeletal dynamics by depolymerizing actin filaments, whereas CFL2 exhibits weaker actin filament depolymerization activity compared to CFL1 and promotes filament assembly [46–48]. Our results showed that GOS induced down-regulation of CFL1 expression and significant up-regulation of CFL2 expression in RAW264.7 cells (Figure 4), implying that GOS elicited synergistic effects on the inhibition of F-actin disassembly and the promotion of actin polymerization. Furthermore, it has been demonstrated that CFL1 is important for cell division, and its inactivation leads to abnormal F-actin accumulation and enhances macrophage phagocytic activity [44]. The depletion of CFL1 results in increases in the cell sizes of different cell types, including macrophages [47], and CFL1-knockdown macrophages contain two or more nuclei [44]. These findings prompted us to investigate the effects of GOS on the morphologies and actin cytoskeleton remodeling of RAW264.7 cells. As expected, after treatment with GOS, the accumulation of F-actin and morphological changes, such as increases in cell size, nucleus area and dual-nuclei cell number, were observed in the RAW264.7 cells. These morphological changes enabled the cells to dynamically adapt to particular stimuli, for example, by enhancing bacterial phagocytosis by GOS-treated RAW264.7 cells, as has been described in our previous report [16]. Moreover, GOS-treated RAW264.7 cells contained more dual-nuclei cells compared with untreated cells, demonstrating that CFL1 does not affect chromosome replication but that it may play an important role in cytokinesis, consistent with a previous report [47].

Furthermore, the total cell number was increased after treatment with GOS, suggesting that it may also promote the proliferation of RAW264.7 cells. Kawada *et al.* have reported that AOS enhances the growth of human endothelial cells and keratinocytes [4,5]. RPLP2 plays an important role in the elongation step of protein synthesis, and enhancement/reduction of RPLP2 expression can affect the rate of protein translation, thereby increasing/decreasing the proliferation rates of cells [49]. Here, we found that GOS stimulated an increase in RPLP2 expression (Figure 4), indicating that it may be responsible for GOS-induced cell proliferation.

It is worth noting that LPS, which is a well-known macrophage activator, is known to inhibit proliferation, induce apoptosis [50], and stimulate macrophage morphological changes [22,23]. LPS-induced apoptosis in macrophages results from two independent mechanisms: first and predominantly, this activity occurs through the autocrine secretion of TNF-α (early apoptotic events), and second, it occurs through the production of NO (late phase of apoptosis) [51]. Although GOS was able to induce TNF-α secretion and NO production [18], apoptotic-like changes were not observed in the GOS-treated macrophages. Furthermore, GOS appeared to protect RAW264.7 cells from cell morphological changes caused by LPS treatment. These findings suggest that different mechanisms or functional pathways might be implicated in the macrophage-activating activities of GOS and LPS. In addition, LPS directed the core metabolism of these cells toward aerobic glycolysis [52], whereas the glycolytic pathway appeared to be down-regulated by GOS in the present study. Furthermore, the changes in cell morphology were different between the LPS- and GOS-treated cells. Therefore, our study indicated that GOS was able to activate macrophages [18], but it could also control the over-inflammatory reaction and cell homeostasis; thus, its function was different from the function of LPS.

4. Materials and Methods

4.1. Materials

Seaweed sodium alginate (20 cps), bacterial lipopolysaccharide (LPS), dithiothreitol (DTT), iodoacetamide (IAA), sodium dodecyl sulfate (SDS) and polyacrylamide were purchased from Sigma-Aldrich (St. Louis, MO, USA). 3-[(3-cholamidopropyl) dimethylammonio]-1-propanesulfonate (CHAPS), Tris base, thiourea and urea were purchased from Amresco (Solon, OH, USA). Immobiline dry strips, immobilized pH gradient (IPG) buffer and IPG cover mineral oil were obtained from GE Healthcare (Fairfield, CT, USA). All reagents for silver-staining were purchased from Guangzhou Chemical Reagent Factory (Guangzhou, China). RPMI 1640 culture medium, fetal bovine serum, penicillin and streptomycin were obtained from Hyclone (Logan, UT, USA).

4.2. Preparation of GOS

PG (DP = 20-24) was prepared from sodium alginate according to Haug *et al.* [53], and its chemical structure was analyzed using a Nicolet 6700 infrared (IR) spectrophotometer (ThermoScientific, Rochester, NY, USA) according to Linker *et al.* [54]. Unsaturated GOS was depolymerized from PG by purified alginate lyase [55]. Before use, GOS was filtered through an endotoxin-removing filter (0.22 μm) (Millipore Co., Billerica, MA, USA).

4.3. Mass Spectrometry Analysis

Electrospray ionization mass spectrometry (ESI-MS) analysis was performed using an ion trap time-of-flight mass spectrometer (Shimadzu, Tokyo, Japan) in the negative mode. GOS was dissolved in 1 mM $NH_3 \cdot H_2O$ in 50% aqueous methanol solution and diluted to a final concentration of 1 mg/mL. The sample was infused into the mass spectrometer using a built-in syringe pump at a flow rate of 10 µL/min. The instrument parameters were set as follows: an interface voltage of −3.0 kV; a nebulizing gas flow rate of 0.5 L/min; a CDL temperature of 200 °C; a heating block temperature of 200 °C; a detector voltage of 1.75 kV; and a scan range of 200–2000.

4.4. Cell Culture

The murine macrophage-like cell line RAW264.7 was obtained from the Shanghai Institute of Biochemistry and Cell Biology (Shanghai, China). RAW264.7 cells were cultured in RPMI 1640 medium plus 10% fetal bovine serum, 100 units/mL penicillin and 100 µg/mL streptomycin. The cells were maintained in a humidified incubator with an atmosphere of 95% air and 5% CO_2 at 37 °C.

4.5. Protein Extraction and 2-DE

RAW264.7 cells were harvested and lysed in lysis buffer (7 M urea, 2 M thiourea, 4% CHAPS, 2% pharmalyte (pH 3–10), 65 mM DTT and 40 mM Tris base), sonicated 10 times each for 5 s each with a 10-s pause between pulses in an ice-water bath and centrifuged at 14,000 rpm for 60 min at 4 °C. The supernatant was used directly for 2-DE analysis. Protein concentrations were determined using the Bradford assay.

Whole cell protein lysates were loaded onto analytical gels (90 µg) and MS-preparative gels (500 µg), and 2-DE was performed as described previously [56]. Briefly, IPG strips were rehydrated for 12 h at 30 V. Isoelectric focusing (IEF) was performed with the following voltage program: 100 V/2 h, 200 V/1 h, 500 V/1 h, linear ramp to 1000 V over 1 h, 8000 V over 3 h, then 8000 V constant for a total focusing time of 50,000 Vh. After IEF, the proteins were reduced and alkylated. The second dimension was carried out using an SE 600 Ruby system (GE Healthcare, Fairfield, CT, USA) by SDS-PAGE with 12.5% polyacrylamide gels. After migration, silver nitrate and Coomassie brilliant blue (CBB) R-250 were used to stain the analytical gels and MS-preparative gels, respectively. For silver staining, the gels were fixed with 40% ethanol and 10% acetic acid overnight, followed by incubated with a buffer solution containing 30% ethanol, 4.1% sodium acetate, 0.2% sodium thiosulfate and 0.125% glutaraldehyde for 30 min. After washing with D. D. H_2O for three times, the gels were stained with 0.1% silver nitrate solution containing 0.02% formaldehyde for 20 min. Then, after washing with D. D. H_2O twice, the gels were developed in 2.5% sodium carbonate containing 0.01% formaldehyde, and the reaction was terminated with 1.5% EDTA (disodium salt) followed by thorough rinsing with water. Subsequently, the gels were imaged using a proXPRESS 2D imaging system (PerkinElmer, Waltham, MA, USA) and analyzed with ImageMaster 2D Platinum software 6.0 (GE Healthcare, Fairfield, CT, USA). Only those spots that changed consistently and significantly (more than 2.0-fold) in three replicates were selected for MS analysis.

4.6. Protein Identification by MS

For protein identification, spots of interest were selected manually, and tryptic in-gel digestion was subsequently performed [56]. MS analysis was achieved with a 5800 MALDI-TOF/TOF mass spectrometer (AB SIEX, Framingham, MA, USA) [57]. Combined MS and MS/MS spectra were searched against the SwissProt database (Release 2013_1) using Mascot (Matrix Science, London, UK). Search parameters were as follows: taxonomy was limited to Mus musculus; trypsin digestion with only one missed cleavage site was accepted; variable modifications allowed for carboxyamidomethylation of cysteine and oxidation of methionine; 100 ppm for precursor ion tolerance and 0.3 Da for fragment ion tolerance.

4.7. Western Blot Analysis

Western blot analysis was carried out using primary antibodies (Abs) against annexin A5 (Boster, Wuhan, China), cofilin-2 (GeneTex, San Antonio, TX, USA), galectin-1, cofilin-1, fructose-bisphosphate aldolase and Cu/Zn-superoxide dismutase (Bioss Biotechnology, Beijing, China), and β-tubulin (Abcam, Cambridge, UK) at optimized dilutions. β-tubulin served as an internal control. Proteins (30 μg/lane) were resolved on 12% SDS-PAGE and transferred onto a PVDF membrane. The blots were incubated overnight at 4 °C with a primary Ab followed by incubation with a horseradish peroxidase (HRP)-conjugated goat anti-rabbit IgG secondary antibody (1:5000, Neobioscience Technology, Shenzhen, China) for 2 h at RT. The blots were then developed using an enhanced chemiluminescence kit (Amersham Pharmacia Biosciences, Buckinghamshire, UK).

4.8. Cell Morphology and Actin Cytoskeleton Organization

RAW264.7 cells (2×10^5) were maintained on sterile glass coverslips (Corning Life Sciences Inc., Tewksbury, MA, USA) in 35×35 mm^2 culture dishes with complete medium. After stimulation with 1 mg/mL GOS for 24 h, stimulation with 1 μg/mL LPS alone for 24 h, or pretreatment with GOS for 2 h followed by stimulation with LPS for 22 h, the cells were washed three times with PBS. Then, they were fixed with 4% paraformaldehyde for 15 min at room temperature (RT) and incubated with DAPI (KeyGEN Biotech, Nanjing, China) for 10 min at RT or with TRITC-labelled phalloidin (1:200) (Sigma-Aldrich, St. Louis, MO, USA) in the dark for 20 min at 4 °C for staining of the F-actin fibers. For examination of cell morphology and the actin cytoskeleton observation, fluorescence and dark-field microscopy were performed using an upright Olympus BX51 optical microscope (Olympus Corporation, Tokyo, Japan), and fluorescence and differential interference contrast microscopy were performed using an Olympus FV1000 confocal scanning laser microscope (Olympus Corporation, Tokyo, Japan).

4.9. Statistical Analysis

All the experiments were repeated at least three times ($n \geq 3$), and all types of samples (treated with GOS and untreated) were prepared in triplicate and run in three different 2-DE gels. The data are expressed as the mean ± standard deviation (SD) and were analyzed using the two-tailed Student's *t*-test to determine any significant differences. *P* values < 0.05 were considered statistically significant.

5. Conclusions

AOS, which play important roles in modulating the immune system, are gaining increasing attention as potential biomaterials. Combining the results from our previous studies [16,18] together with those of the present study, we have broadened the understanding of the mechanism by which GOS maintains a proper balance between the pro- and anti-inflammatory immune responses. Differentially expressed proteins extracted from control and GOS-treated RAW264.7 cells were identified by a proteomic study, which were involved in the functional pathways of activation and negative regulation of the NF-κB signaling pathway, pro- and anti-inflammation, pro- and anti-oxidation, cytoskeletal remodeling and cell proliferation in GOS-induced macrophage activation and immunomodulation. GOS is therefore a promising agent that may be utilized by the pharmacological industries to regulate multiple functional pathways and inflammatory responses.

Acknowledgments: We are grateful to Yong Wang and Qingguo Han from Shenzhen University for their technical assistance, and Jiangxin Wang from Shenzhen University for critical review and helpful suggestions of the manuscript. This work was supported financially by the Project supported by the National Natural Science Foundation of China (Grant No. 31000770), Knowledge Innovation Program in Shenzhen Scientific Research and Development Funding Program (Grant No. JCYJ20130329111455027), and Shenzhen Scientific Research and Development Funding Program (Grant No. JCYJ20130408172946974).

Author Contributions: X.X. and L.-M.S. conceived and designed the experiments; D.-C.B., C.L., W.-S.F., R.Z., S.-M.L., and L.-L.C. performed the experiments; D.-C.B., C.L., X.X. and L.-M.S. analyzed the data; X.X., L.-M.S and M.W. wrote the paper.

Conflicts of Interest: The authors declare no conflict of interest.

References

1. Haug, A. Alginic acid. Isolation and fractionation with potassium chloride and manganous ions. *Methods Carbohydr. Chem.* **1965**, *5*, 69–72.

2. Wan, L.; Heng, P.; Chan, L. Drug encapsulation in alginate microspheres by emulsification. *J. Microencapsul.* **1992**, *9*, 309–316. [CrossRef] [PubMed]

3. Akiyama, H.; Endo, T.; Nakakita, R.; Murata, K.; Yonemoto, Y.; Okayama, K. Effect of depolymerized alginates on the growth of bifidobacteria. *Biosci. Biotechnol. Biochem.* **1992**, *56*, 355. [CrossRef] [PubMed]

4. Kawada, A.; Hiura, N.; Tajima, S.; Takahara, H. Alginate oligosaccharides stimulate VEGF-mediated growth and migration of human endothelial cells. *Arch. Dermatol. Res.* **1999**, *291*, 542–547. [CrossRef] [PubMed]

5. Kawada, A.; Hiura, N.; Shiraiwa, M.; Tajima, S.; Hiruma, M.; Hara, K.; Ishibashi, A.; Takahara, H. Stimulation of human keratinocyte growth by alginate oligosaccharides, a possible co-factor for epidermal growth factor in cell culture. *FEBS Lett.* **1997**, *408*, 43–46. [CrossRef] [PubMed]

6. Iwamoto, Y.; Xu, X.; Tamura, T.; Oda, T.; Muramatsu, T. Enzymatically depolymerized alginate oligomers that cause cytotoxic cytokine production in human mononuclear cells. *Biosci. Biotechnol. Biochem.* **2003**, *67*, 258–263. [CrossRef] [PubMed]

7. Iwamoto, M.; Kurachi, M.; Nakashima, T.; Kim, D.; Yamaguchi, K.; Oda, T.; Iwamoto, Y.; Muramatsu, T. Structure-activity relationship of alginate oligosaccharides in the induction of cytokine production from RAW264.7 cells. *FEBS Lett.* **2005**, *579*, 4423–4429. [CrossRef] [PubMed]

8. Yamamoto, Y.; Kurachi, M.; Yamaguchi, K.; Oda, T. Induction of multiple cytokine secretion from RAW264.7 cells by alginate oligosaccharides. *Biosci. Biotechnol. Biochem.* **2007**, *71*, 238–241. [CrossRef] [PubMed]

9. An, Q.D.; Zhang, G.L.; Wu, H.T.; Zhang, Z.C.; Zheng, G.S.; Luan, L.; Murata, Y.; Li, X. Alginate-deriving oligosaccharide production by alginase from newly isolated Flavobacterium sp. LXA and its potential application in protection against pathogens. *J. Appl. Microbiol.* **2009**, *106*, 161–170. [CrossRef] [PubMed]

10. Ueno, M.; Hiroki, T.; Takeshita, S.; Jiang, Z.; Kim, D.; Yamaguchi, K.; Oda, T. Comparative study on antioxidative and macrophage-stimulating activities of polyguluronic acid (PG) and polymannuronic acid (PM) prepared from alginate. *Carbohydr. Res.* **2012**, *352*, 88–93. [CrossRef] [PubMed]

11. Falkeborg, M.; Cheong, L.Z.; Gianfico, C.; Sztukiel, K.M.; Kristensen, K.; Glasius, M.; Xu, X.; Guo, Z. Alginate oligosaccharides: Enzymatic preparation and antioxidant property evaluation. *Food Chem.* **2014**, *164*, 185–194. [CrossRef] [PubMed]

12. Tusi, S.K.; Khalaj, L.; Ashabi, G.; Kiaei, M.; Khodagholi, F. Alginate oligosaccharide protects against endoplasmic reticulum- and mitochondrial-mediated apoptotic cell death and oxidative stress. *Biomaterials* **2011**, *32*, 5438–5458. [CrossRef] [PubMed]

13. Yoshida, T.; Hirano, A.; Wada, H.; Takahashi, K.; Hattori, M. Alginic acid oligosaccharide suppresses Th2 development and IgE production by inducing IL-12 production. *Int. Arch. Allergy Immunol.* **2004**, *133*, 239–247. [CrossRef] [PubMed]

14. Venter, G.; Oerlemans, F.T.; Wijers, M.; Willemse, M.; Fransen, J.A.; Wieringa, B. Glucose controls morphodynamics of LPS-stimulated macrophages. *PLoS ONE* **2014**, *9*, e96786. [CrossRef] [PubMed]

15. Vallabhapurapu, S.; Karin, M. Regulation and function of NF-κB transcription factors in the immune system. *Annu. Rev. Immunol.* **2009**, *27*, 693–733. [CrossRef] [PubMed]

16. Xu, X.; Bi, D.; Wu, X.; Wang, Q.; Wei, G.; Chi, L.; Jiang, Z.; Oda, T.; Wan, M. Unsaturated guluronate oligosaccharide enhances the antibacterial activities of macrophages. *FASEB J.* **2014**, *28*, 2645–2654. [CrossRef] [PubMed]

17. Kurachi, M.; Nakashima, T.; Miyajima, C.; Iwamoto, Y.; Muramatsu, T.; Yamaguchi, K.; Oda, T. Comparison of the activities of various alginates to induce TNF-α secretion in RAW264.7 cells. *J. Infect. Chemother.* **2005**, *11*, 199–203. [CrossRef] [PubMed]

18. Xu, X.; Wu, X.; Wang, Q.; Cai, N.; Zhang, H.; Jiang, Z.; Wan, M.; Oda, T. Immunomodulatory effects of alginate oligosaccharides on murine macrophage RAW264. 7 cells and their structure-activity relationships. *J. Agric. Food Chem.* **2014**, *62*, 3168–3176. [CrossRef]

19. Van den Bogaerdt, A.J.; El Ghalbzouri, A.; Hensbergen, P.J.; Reijnen, L.; Verkerk, M.; Kroon-Smits, M.; Middelkoop, E.; Ulrich, M.M. Differential expression of CRABP-II in fibroblasts derived from dermis and subcutaneous fat. *Biochem. Biophys. Res. Commun.* **2004**, *315*, 428–433. [CrossRef] [PubMed]

20. Aebersold, R.; Mann, M. Mass spectrometry-based proteomics. *Nature* **2003**, *422*, 198–207. [CrossRef] [PubMed]

21. Jia, W.; Zhang, J.S.; Jiang, Y.; Zheng, Z.Y.; Zhan, X.B.; Lin, C.C. Structure of oligosaccharide F21 derived from exopolysaccharide WL-26 produced by *Sphingomonas* sp. ATCC 31555. *Carbohydr. Polym.* **2012**, *90*, 60–66. [CrossRef] [PubMed]

22. Hong, G.E.; Park, H.S.; Kim, J.-A.; Nagappan, A.; Zhang, J.; Kang, S.; Won, C.; Cho, J.H.; Kim, E.H.; Kim, G.S. Anti-oxidant and anti-inflammatory effects of *Fraxinus rhynchophylla* on lipopolysaccharide (LPS)-induced murine Raw 264.7 cells. *J. Biomed. Res.* **2012**, *13*, 331–338. [CrossRef]

23. Park, E.J.; Kim, S.A.; Choi, Y.M.; Kwon, H.K.; Shim, W.; Lee, G.; Choi, S. Capric acid inhibits NO production and STAT3 activation during LPS-induced osteoclastogenesis. *PLoS ONE* **2011**, *6*, e27739. [CrossRef] [PubMed]

24. Yamamoto, Y.; Kurachi, M.; Yamaguchi, K.; Oda, T. Stimulation of multiple cytokine production in mice by alginate oligosaccharides following intraperitoneal administration. *Carbohydr. Res.* **2007**, *342*, 1133–1137. [CrossRef] [PubMed]

25. Tak, P.P.; Firestein, G.S. NF-κB: A key role in inflammatory diseases. *J. Clin. Investig.* **2001**, *107*, 7–11. [CrossRef] [PubMed]

26. Ruland, J. Return to homeostasis: Downregulation of NF-κB responses. *Nat. Immunol.* **2011**, *12*, 709–714. [CrossRef] [PubMed]

27. Toscano, M.A.; Campagna, L.; Molinero, L.L.; Cerliani, J.P.; Croci, D.O.; Ilarregui, J.M.; Fuertes, M.B.; Nojek, I.M.; Fededa, J.P.; Zwirner, N.W.; *et al.* Nuclear factor (NF)-κB controls expression of the immunoregulatory glycan-binding protein galectin-1. *Mol. Immunol.* **2011**, *48*, 1940–1949. [CrossRef]

28. Rabinovich, G.A.; Toscano, M.A. Turning "sweet" on immunity: galectin-glycan interactions in immune tolerance and inflammation. *Nat. Rev. Immunol.* **2009**, *9*, 338–352. [CrossRef] [PubMed]

29. Koh, H.S.; Lee, C.; Lee, K.S.; Ham, C.S.; Seong, R.H.; Kim, S.S.; Jeon, S.H. CD7 expression and galectin-1-induced apoptosis of immature thymocytes are directly regulated by NF-κB upon T-cell activation. *Biochem. Biophys. Res. Commun.* **2008**, *370*, 149–153. [CrossRef] [PubMed]

30. De Hemptinne, V.; Rondas, D.; Toepoel, M.; Vancompernolle, K. Phosphorylation on Thr-106 and NO-modification of glyoxalase I suppress the TNF-induced transcriptional activity of NF-kappaB. *Mol. Cell. Biochem.* **2009**, *325*, 169–178. [CrossRef]

31. Barrionuevo, P.; Beigier-Bompadre, M.; Ilarregui, J.M.; Toscano, M.A.; Bianco, G.A.; Isturiz, M.A.; Rabinovich, G.A. A novel function for galectin-1 at the crossroad of innate and adaptive immunity: Galectin-1 regulates monocyte/macrophage physiology through a nonapoptotic ERK-dependent pathway. *J. Immunol.* **2007**, *178*, 436–445. [CrossRef] [PubMed]

32. Blackwood, R.A.; Ernst, J.D. Characterization of Ca2(+)-dependent phospholipid binding, vesicle aggregation and membrane fusion by annexins. *Biochem. J.* **1990**, *266*, 195–200. [PubMed]

33. Kang, A.D.; Wong, P.M.; Chen, H.; Castagna, R.; Chung, S.W.; Sultzer, B.M. Restoration of lipopolysaccharide-mediated B-cell response after expression of a cDNA encoding a GTP-binding protein. *Infect. Immun.* **1996**, *64*, 4612–4617. [PubMed]

34. Frey, B.; Munoz, L.E.; Pausch, F.; Sieber, R.; Franz, S.; Brachvogel, B.; Poschl, E.; Schneider, H.; Rodel, F.; Sauer, R.; *et al.* The immune reaction against allogeneic necrotic cells is reduced in Annexin A5 knock out mice whose macrophages display an anti-inflammatory phenotype. *J. Cell. Mol. Med.* **2009**, *13*, 1391–1399. [CrossRef] [PubMed]

35. Zhao, F.; Yuan, Q.; Sultzer, B.M.; Chung, S.W.; Wong, P.M. The involvement of Ran GTPase in lipopolysaccharide endotoxin-induced responses. *J. Endotoxin Res.* **2001**, *7*, 53–56. [CrossRef] [PubMed]

36. Scandalios, J.G. Oxygen Stress and Superoxide Dismutases. *Plant Physiol.* **1993**, *101*, 7–12. [PubMed]

37. Fadeel, B.; Ahlin, A.; Henter, J.I.; Orrenius, S.; Hampton, M.B. Involvement of caspases in neutrophil apoptosis: regulation by reactive oxygen species. *Blood* **1998**, *92*, 4808–4818. [PubMed]

38. Forman, H.J.; Torres, M. Redox signaling in macrophages. *Mol. Aspects Med.* **2001**, *22*, 189–216. [CrossRef] [PubMed]

39. Marikovsky, M.; Ziv, V.; Nevo, N.; Harris-Cerruti, C.; Mahler, O. Cu/Zn superoxide dismutase plays important role in immune response. *J. Immunol.* **2003**, *170*, 2993–3001. [CrossRef] [PubMed]

40. Pavlides, S.; Tsirigos, A.; Vera, I.; Flomenberg, N.; Frank, P.G.; Casimiro, M.C.; Wang, C.; Fortina, P.; Addya, S.; Pestell, R.G.; *et al.* Loss of stromal caveolin-1 leads to oxidative stress, mimics hypoxia and drives inflammation in the tumor microenvironment, conferring the "reverse Warburg effect": A transcriptional informatics analysis with validation. *Cell Cycle* **2010**, *9*, 2201–2219. [CrossRef] [PubMed]

41. Vats, D.; Mukundan, L.; Odegaard, J.I.; Zhang, L.; Smith, K.L.; Morel, C.R.; Wagner, R.A.; Greaves, D.R.; Murray, P.J.; Chawla, A. Oxidative metabolism and PGC-1β attenuate macrophage-mediated inflammation. *Cell Metab.* **2006**, *4*, 13–24. [CrossRef] [PubMed]

42. Cramer, T.; Yamanishi, Y.; Clausen, B.E.; Forster, I.; Pawlinski, R.; Mackman, N.; Haase, V.H.; Jaenisch, R.; Corr, M.; Nizet, V.; *et al.* HIF-1alpha is essential for myeloid cell-mediated inflammation. *Cell* **2003**, *112*, 645–657. [CrossRef] [PubMed]

43. Patron, N.J.; Rogers, M.B.; Keeling, P.J. Gene replacement of fructose-1,6-bisphosphate aldolase supports the hypothesis of a single photosynthetic ancestor of chromalveolates. *Eukaryot. Cell* **2004**, *3*, 1169–1175. [CrossRef] [PubMed]

44. Jonsson, F.; Gurniak, C.B.; Fleischer, B.; Kirfel, G.; Witke, W. Immunological responses and actin dynamics in macrophages are controlled by N-cofilin but are independent from ADF. *PLoS ONE* **2012**, *7*, e36034. [CrossRef] [PubMed]

45. Lappalainen, P.; Drubin, D.G. Cofilin promotes rapid actin filament turnover *in vivo*. *Nature* **1997**, *388*, 78–82. [CrossRef] [PubMed]

46. Bernstein, B.W.; Bamburg, J.R. ADF/cofilin: A functional node in cell biology. *Trends Cell Biol.* **2010**, *20*, 187–195. [CrossRef] [PubMed]

47. Hotulainen, P.; Paunola, E.; Vartiainen, M.K.; Lappalainen, P. Actin-depolymerizing factor and cofilin-1 play overlapping roles in promoting rapid F-actin depolymerization in mammalian nonmuscle cells. *Mol. Biol. Cell* **2005**, *16*, 649–664. [CrossRef]

48. Van Troys, M.; Huyck, L.; Leyman, S.; Dhaese, S.; Vandekerkhove, J.; Ampe, C. Ins and outs of ADF/cofilin activity and regulation. *Eur. J. Cell Biol.* **2008**, *87*, 649–667. [CrossRef] [PubMed]

49. Chen, A.; Kaganovsky, E.; Rahimipour, S.; Ben-Aroya, N.; Okon, E.; Koch, Y. Two forms of gonadotropin-releasing hormone (GnRH) are expressed in human breast tissue and overexpressed in breast cancer: A putative mechanism for the antiproliferative effect of GnRH by down-regulation of acidic ribosomal phosphoproteins P1 and P2. *Cancer Res.* **2002**, *62*, 1036–1044. [PubMed]

50. Vadiveloo, P.K.; Keramidaris, E.; Morrison, W.A.; Stewart, A.G. Lipopolysaccharide-induced cell cycle arrest in macrophages occurs independently of nitric oxide synthase II induction. *Biochim. Biophys. Acta* **2001**, *1539*, 140–146. [CrossRef]

51. Xaus, J.; Comalada, M.; Valledor, A.F.; Lloberas, J.; Lopez-Soriano, F.; Argiles, J.M.; Bogdan, C.; Celada, A. LPS induces apoptosis in macrophages mostly through the autocrine production of TNF-α. *Blood* **2000**, *95*, 3823–3831. [PubMed]

52. Rodriguez-Prados, J.C.; Traves, P.G.; Cuenca, J.; Rico, D.; Aragones, J.; Martin-Sanz, P.; Cascante, M.; Bosca, L. Substrate fate in activated macrophages: A comparison between innate, classic, and alternative activation. *J. Immunol.* **2010**, *185*, 605–614. [CrossRef] [PubMed]

53. Haug, A.; Larsen, B.; Smidsrød, O. A study of the constitution of alginic acid by partial acid hydrolysis. *Acta Chem. Scand.* **1966**, *20*, 183–190. [CrossRef]

54. Linker, A.; Jones, R.S. A new polysaccharide resembling alginic acid isolated from *pseudomonads*. *J. Biol. Chem.* **1966**, *241*, 3845–3851. [PubMed]

55. Xu, X.; Iwamoto, Y.; Kitamura, Y.; Oda, T.; Muramatsu, T. Root growth-promoting activity of unsaturated oligomeric uronates from alginate on carrot and rice plants. *Biosci. Biotechnol. Biochem.* **2003**, *67*, 2022–2025. [CrossRef] [PubMed]

56. Shen, L.; Lan, Z.; Sun, X.; Shi, L.; Liu, Q.; Ni, J. Proteomic analysis of lanthanum citrate-induced apoptosis in human cervical carcinoma SiHa cells. *BioMetals* **2010**, *23*, 1179–1189. [CrossRef] [PubMed]

57. Jamwal, S.; Midha, M.K.; Verma, H.N.; Basu, A.; Rao, K.V.; Manivel, V. Characterizing virulence-specific perturbations in the mitochondrial function of macrophages infected with Mycobacterium tuberculosis. *Sci. Rep.* **2013**, *3*, 1328. [CrossRef] [PubMed]

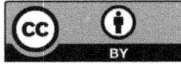

marine drugs

MDPI

Article

Acetylated Chitosan Oligosaccharides Act as Antagonists against Glutamate-Induced PC12 Cell Death via Bcl-2/Bax Signal Pathway

Cui Hao [†], Lixia Gao [†], Yiran Zhang, Wei Wang, Guangli Yu, Huashi Guan, Lijuan Zhang * and Chunxia Li *

Shandong Provincial Key Laboratory of Glycoscience and Glycoengineering, and Key Laboratory of Marine Drugs of Ministry of Education, School of Medicine and Pharmacy, Ocean University of China, Qingdao 266003, China; haocui2010@hotmail.com (C.H.); xialigao1214@163.com (L.G.); zhangyiran_ouc@126.com (Y.Z.); wwwakin@ouc.edu.cn (W.W.); glyu@ouc.edu.cn (G.Y.); hsguan@ouc.edu.cn (H.G.)

* Authors to whom correspondence should be addressed; lijuanzhang@ouc.edu.cn (L.Z.); lchunxia@ouc.edu.cn (C.L.); Tel.: +86-532-8203-2030; Fax: +86-532-8203-3054.

† These authors contributed equally to this work.

Academic Editor: Paola Laurienzo

Received: 1 December 2014; Accepted: 9 February 2015; Published: 12 March 2015

Abstract: Chitosan oligosaccharides (COSs), depolymerized products of chitosan composed of β-$(1{\rightarrow}4)$ D-glucosamine units, have broad range of biological activities such as antitumour, antifungal, and antioxidant activities. In this study, peracetylated chitosan oligosaccharides (PACOs) and N-acetylated chitosan oligosaccharides (NACOs) were prepared from the COSs by chemcal modification. The structures of these monomers were identified using NMR and ESI-MS spectra. Their antagonist effects against glutamate-induced PC12 cell death were investigated. The results showed that pretreatment of PC12 cells with the PACOs markedly inhibited glutamate-induced cell death in a concentration-dependent manner. The PACOs were better glutamate antagonists compared to the COSs and the NACOs, suggesting the peracetylation is essential for the neuroprotective effects of chitosan oligosaccharides. In addition, the PACOs pretreatment significantly reduced lactate dehydrogenase release and reactive oxygen species production. It also attenuated the loss of mitochondrial membrane potential. Further studies indicated that the PACOs inhibited glutamate-induced cell death by preventing apoptosis through depressing the elevation of Bax/Bcl-2 ratio and caspase-3 activation. These results suggest that PACOs might be promising antagonists against glutamate-induced neural cell death.

Keywords: PC12; peracetylated chitosan oligosaccharide; neuroprotective; reactive oxygen species; apoptosis; mitochondrial membrane potential

1. Introduction

Neurodegenerative disease is a general term used to describe a wide range of conditions, such as Alzheimer's disease (AD) and Parkinson's disease, and its occurrence increases with advanced age [1]. A large number of evidence indicates that oxidative stress induced by reactive oxygen species (ROS) plays an important role in neurodegenerative disease. ROS are normal byproducts of aerobic respiration and their level is strictly controlled by various cellular antioxidant compounds and enzymes, while their overproduction leads to cell death [2]. Accordingly, tackling free radicals offers a promising therapeutic target in neurodegenerative disease.

Glutamate is one of the major endogenous excitatory neurotransmitters, which plays an important physiological role in the central nervous system [3]. However, in a variety of pathologic conditions, accumulated high concentrations of glutamate can lead to neuronal injury and cell death through two different mechanisms. One of the mechanisms is that glutamate-induced toxicity is mediated by competitive inhibition of cystine uptake, which leads to oxidative stress [4–6]. Another mechanism is that the excitotoxicity of glutamate is mediated by several types of excitatory amino acid receptors resulting in a massive influx of extracellular Ca^{2+} [7,8]. It is predictable based on both mechanisms that proper antagonists would be able to prevent glutamate-induced neural injury and cell death. It has been reported that high concentration of glutamate induces PC12 cell death [9–12] and different types of classical antidepressants could prevent excitotoxicity of activated glutamate receptors in PC12 cells [13]. Therefore, PC12 cells represent an ideal cell-based system to search for antagonists against glutamate-induced cell death and to study underlying molecular mechanisms.

Chitosan oligosaccharides (COSs) are a degradation product of chitosan, which is derived from deacetylation of chitin, the main component of the exoskeleton of crustaceans. A large number of studies have shown that the COSs have various biological activities, including antioxidant, antimicrobial, and antitumor activities [14]. Recently, it has been reported that the COSs possess good neuroprotective properties such as β-amyloid and acetylcholinesterase inhibitory activities, anti-neuroinflammation, and anti-apoptosis effects [15–18], which suggest the COSs and their derivatives might merit further investigation as novel antagonists against glutamate-induced cell death.

To accomplish this goal, peracetylated chitosan oligosaccharides (PACOs) and N-acetylated chitosan oligosaccharides (NACOs) were prepared and their effects as antagonists against glutamate-induced cell death and underlying molecular mechanisms were investigated in PC12 cells. The results indicated that the PACOs pretreatment markedly inhibited PC12 cell death induced by glutamate exposure in a concentration-dependent manner. Moreover, pretreatment with the PACOs also significantly reduced lactate dehydrogenase (LDH) release and ROS production. It also attenuated the loss of mitochondrial membrane potential (MMP). Further studies indicated that the PACOs inhibited glutamate-induced cell death by preventing apoptosis through depressing the elevation of Bax/Bcl-2 ratio and caspase-3 activation. These results suggest that PACOs might be promising antagonists against glutamate-induced neural cell death.

2. Results and Discussion

2.1. Characterization of Chitosan Oligosaccharides and Its Acetylated Derivatives

Chitosan oligosaccharide COS was prepared by enzymatic hydrolysis of chitosan as described previously [19]. The COSs had the degree of polymerization (DP) of 2, 3, and 4, respectively. They were named COS-2, COS-3 and COS-4 (Figure 1). The acetylated derivatives of COS (N-acetylated chitooligosaccharide (NACO) and peracetylated chitooligosaccharide (PACO)) were prepared using the methods described previously [20]. The structures of Q-2, Q-3, Q-4 (PACOs) and N-2, N-3, and N-4 (NACOs) were also shown in Figure 1. The oligosaccharide structures were confirmed by ^{1}H NMR, ^{13}C NMR, and MS analyses.

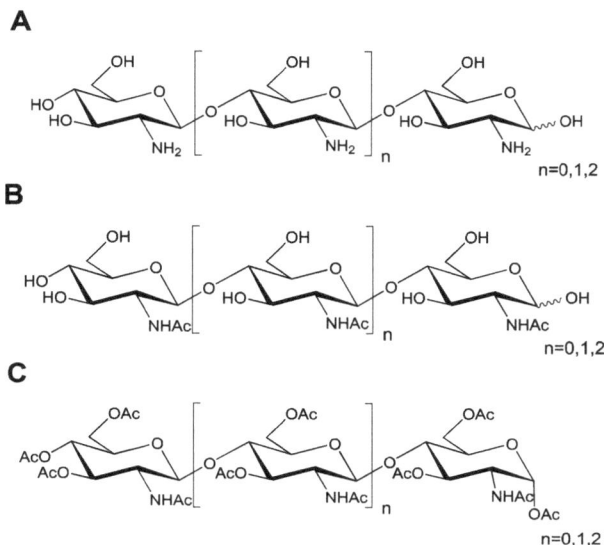

Figure 1. Schematic diagram of the repeating saccharide units in chitosan oligosaccharide and its acetylated derivatives. (A–C) Chemical structure of chitosan oligosaccharides (COS) (**A**), N-acetylated chitosan oligosaccharides (NACO) (**B**), and peracetylated chitosan oligosaccharides (PACO) (**C**). The degree of polymerization (DP) of COS, NACO, and PACO is 2~4.

2.2. Glutamate-Induced PC12 Cell Death

Both undifferentiated and differentiated rat adrenal medullary phenochromocytoma PC12 cells were purchased from the Cell Bank of the Chinese Academy of Sciences (Shanghai, China). Differentiated PC12 cells can form synapses, which are very similar to human neurons. A previously published resazurin assay [21] was used to measure glutamate-induced PC12 cell death. As shown in Figure 2A, glutamate treatment for 24 h could not induce cell death of undifferentiated PC12 cells even when glutamate concentration was as high as 32 mM. However, glutamate induced the death of differentiated PC12 cells in a concentration-dependent manner (Figure 2B), indicating glutamate-induced death was PC12 cell differentiating-dependent.

Glutamate treatment of the differentiated PC12 cells at a concentration of 4 mM led to about 50.0% cell death, thus glutamate at 4 mM was chosen for the subsequent experiments.

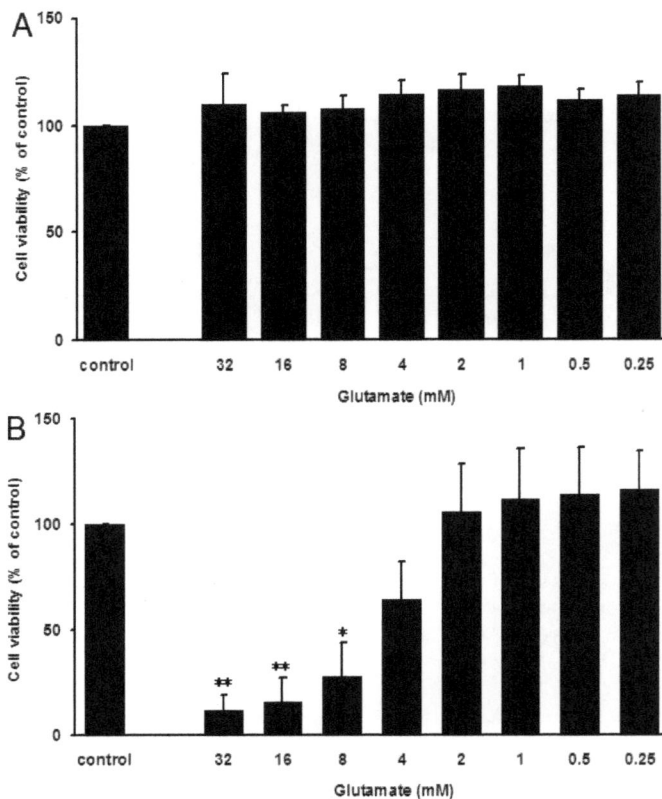

Figure 2. Effect of glutamate on undifferentiated and fully-differentiated PC12 cells. (A–B) The undifferentiated (**A**) and fully-differentiated (**B**) PC12 cells were plated on the cell culture plates at a density of 1×10^5 cells/mL, and then treated with glutamate at different concentrations (0.25, 0.5, 1, 2, 4, 8, 16 and 32 mM) for 24 h. Then the cell viability was evaluated by resazurin assay. The results were presented as a percentage of the normal control group. Values are the mean ± SD ($n = 3$). Significance: * $p < 0.05$, ** $p < 0.01$ *vs.* normal control group without glutamate.

2.3. Oligosaccharides as Antagonists against Glutamate-Induced PC12 Cell Death

Chitosan oligosaccharides and their acetylated derivatives were first tested for their cytotoxicities in fully differentiated PC12 cells by resazurin assay as described previously [21–23], and the results indicated that none of chitosan oligosaccharides and their acetylated derivatives (COSs, PACOs and NACOs) exhibited any significant cytotoxicity even at the concentration of 400 μg/mL (Figure 3). The low cytotoxicity suggested that chitosan oligosaccharides and their acetylated derivatives were ideal compounds to use for screening antagonists against glutamate-induced cell death in PC12 cells.

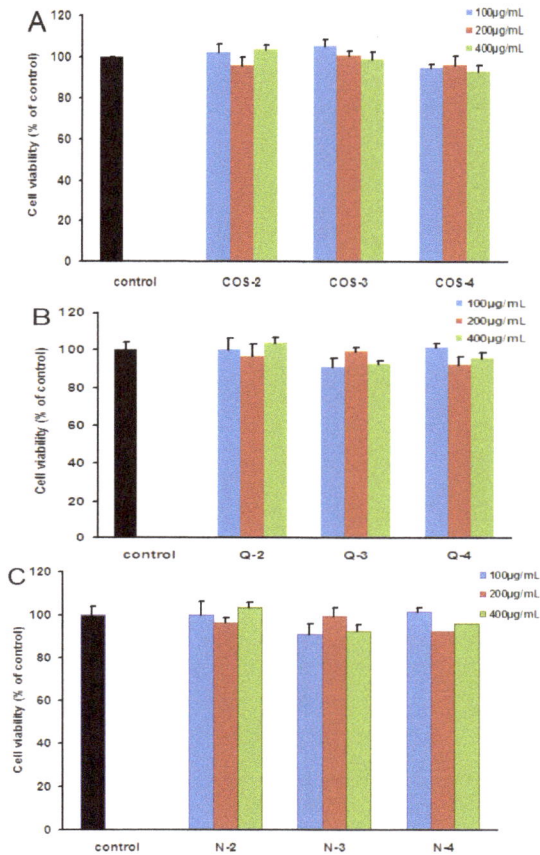

Figure 3. The cytotoxicity of different chitosan oligosaccharides in PC12 cells. PC12 cells were incubated with different chitosan oligosaccharides COS-2~4 (**A**), peracetylated chitosan oligosaccharides Q-2~4 (**B**) and *N*-acetylated chitosan oligosaccharides N-2~4 (**C**) at indicated concentrations (100, 200, 400 µg/mL) for 24 h. Then the cell viability was evaluated by resazurin assay. The results were presented as a percentage of non drug treated normal control group. Values are the mean ± SD (*n* = 3).

These compounds as antagonists against glutamate-induced fully differentiated PC12 cell death were then evaluated by resazurin assay. As shown in Figure 4B, the cells that were exposed to 4 mM L-glutamate showed a significant decrease in cell viability (32% ± 11%, relative to the untreated control group). However, pretreatment with peracetylated chitosan oligosaccharides Q3 or Q4 at 100, 200, and 400 µg/mL for 2 h before L-glutamate exposure significantly restored cell viability, which ranged from about 30% to about 85% as compared to control cells ($p < 0.01$), which was superior to the effect of the positive control drug Huperzine-A (HupA, 100 µM) (about 45%) (Figure 4B). The cell death-preventing effect at 200 µg/mL was greater than the other two concentrations tested (100 and 400 µg/mL) (Figure 4B). In contrast, the non-acetylated chitosan oligosaccharides (COS-2, COS-3, and COS-4) had almost no antagonist effects against glutamate-induced PC12 cell death (Figure 4A). These results indicated that the acetylation modification of chitosan oligosaccharides enhanced their antagonist effects against glutamate-induced PC12 cell death.

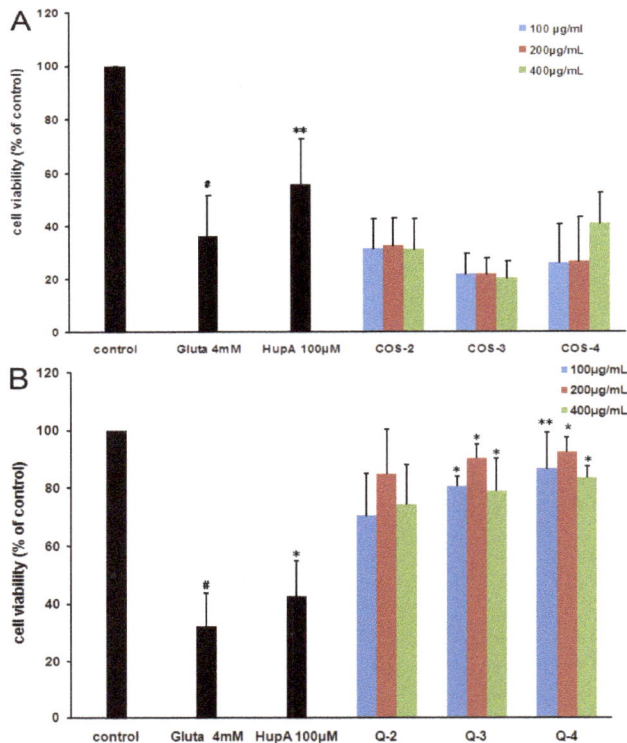

Figure 4. The effect of different chitosan oligosaccharides on glutamate-induced PC12 cell damage. PC12 cells were treated with or without different chitosan oligosaccharides COS-2~4 (**A**) and peracetylated chitosan oligosaccharides Q-2~4 (**B**) at indicated concentrations for 2 h. Then cells were treated with glutamate for another 24 h before performing a resazurin assay. The untreated normal cells (control) were assigned values of 100 and the results presented as mean ± SD (*n* = 4). Significance: # *p* < 0.05 *vs.* normal control group; * *p* < 0.05, ** *p* < 0.01 *vs.* glutamate treated control group.

2.4. The Structure-Activity Relationship of Acetylated Chitosan Oligosaccharides

The influence of molecular weight and the location of the acetylation group on chitosan oligosaccharides were investigated by performing a resazurin assay. As shown in Figure 4B, the peracetylated chitotetraose Q-4 had the best neuroprotective effect among Q-2, Q-3, Q-4, which suggested that the higher molecular weight of peracetylated chitosan oligosaccharides correlated with superior antagonist activity. However, there was no significant difference in the neuroprotective effects of those acetylated chitosan oligosaccharides (*n* = 0, 1, 2) (Figure 4B), which suggested that the degree of polymerization (DP) is not the key factor for their neuroprotective effects. Interestingly, the *N*-acetylated chitosan oligosaccharides with a degree of acetylation of 1.0 had no significant antagonist effect (Figure 5A), which suggested peracetylation was essential for the antagonist effect of chitosan oligosaccharides against glutamate-induced PC12 cell death.

Furthermore, to explore whether the acetyl group was indispensible for the neuroprotective effect of the oligosaccharides, we made another two peracetylated oligosaccharides and evaluated their neuroprotective effects in PC12 cells. As shown in Figure 5B, the acetylated chitobiose Q-2 had the best neuroprotective effect among these acetylated oligosaccharides, and the effect at 200 µg/mL was better than that at other two concentrations tested (100 and 400 µg/mL). Interestingly, the non-acetylated oligosaccharides lactose Lac-2 and cellobiose Cel-2 had no significant antagonist effect against glutamate-induced cell death (Figure 5B) resembling non-acetylated chitosan oligosaccharides. However, after acetylation, the neuroprotective effects of peracetylated lactose Ac-Lac-2 and peracetylated cellobiose Cel-2 were all greater than that of non-acetylated oligosaccharides Lac-2 and Cel-2, and the effect of Ac-Lac-2 at 200 μg/mL was comparable to that of Q-2 (Figure 5B). These results suggested that the acetyl group is indispensible for the neuroprotective effect of the oligosaccharides, and the structure of the sugar backbone might also influence the antagonist effect against glutamate-induced PC12 cell death.

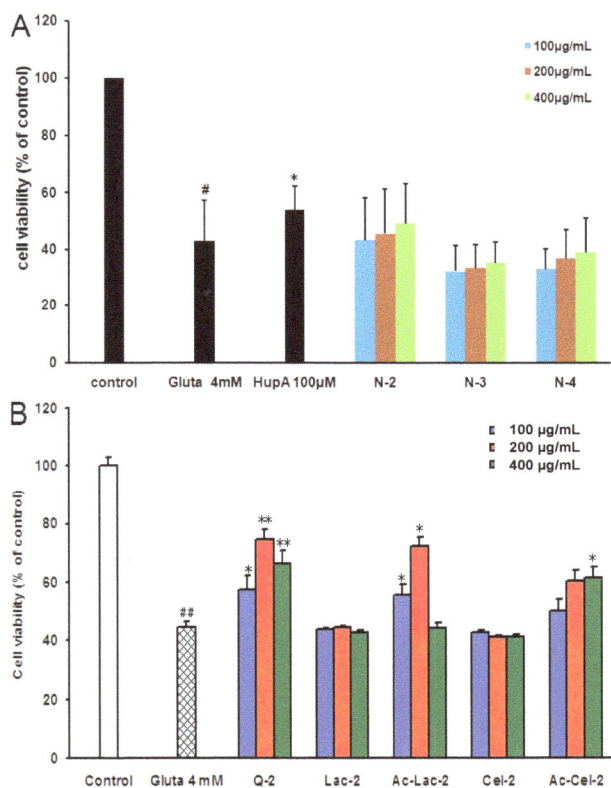

Figure 5. The neuroprotective effects of different acetylated neutral oligosaccharides in PC12 cells. (**A**) PC12 cells were treated with or without different N-acetylated chitosan oligosaccharides N-2~4 at indicated concentrations for 2 h. Then cells were treated with glutamate for another 24 h before performing a resazurin assay. The untreated normal cells (control) were assigned values of 100 and the results presented as mean ± SD ($n = 4$). Significance: # $p < 0.05$ *vs.* normal control group; * $p < 0.05$ *vs.* glutamate treated control group. (**B**) PC12 cells were treated with or without peracetylated chitobiose Q-2, lactose, acetylated lactose, cellobiose, or acetylated cellobiose at indicated concentrations for 2 h. Then cells were treated with glutamate for another 24 h. The untreated normal cells (control) were assigned values of 100 and the results presented as mean ± SD ($n = 3$). Significance: ## $p < 0.01$ *vs.* normal control group; * $p < 0.05$, ** $p < 0.01$ *vs.* glutamate treated control group.

2.5. Effect of Peracetylated Chitosan Oligosaccharides (PACO) on LDH Release and ROS Production

To further investigate the underlying molecular mechanisms of acetylated chitosan oligosaccharides as antagonists against glutamate-induced PC12 cell death, the LDH release assay, another indicator of cell toxicity, was performed. As shown in Figure 6A treatment with glutamate (4 mM) resulted in an increase of LDH release into the medium, which was 161% ± 3% as compared to control cells (Figure 6A). Pre-incubation with peracetylated chitosan oligosaccharides Q3, Q4 at the concentration of 200 μg/mL significantly blocked LDH leakage in the PC12 cell system ($p < 0.01$), which was decreased from 161% to about 105% as compared to control cells (Figure 6A). The inhibition effect of peracetylated chitosan oligosaccharides Q2, Q3, and Q4 on LDH release was greater than that of the positive control drug, huperzine A (HupA, 100 μM) (Figure 6A).

Furthermore, the degree of ROS accumulation after glutamate exposure was also measured to determine the role of ROS in glutamate-induced PC12 cell death. As shown in Figure 6B, treatment with glutamate (4 mM) resulted in an increase of ROS in PC12 cells, which was about 131% ± 5% as compared to control cells. However, pre-treatment with peracetylated chitosan oligosaccharides Q2, Q3, and Q4 at the concentration of 200 μg/mL significantly reduced glutamate induced ROS production from 131% to 103% ($p < 0.01$), which was superior to the effect of positive control drug huperzine A (HupA, 114%) (Figure 6B).

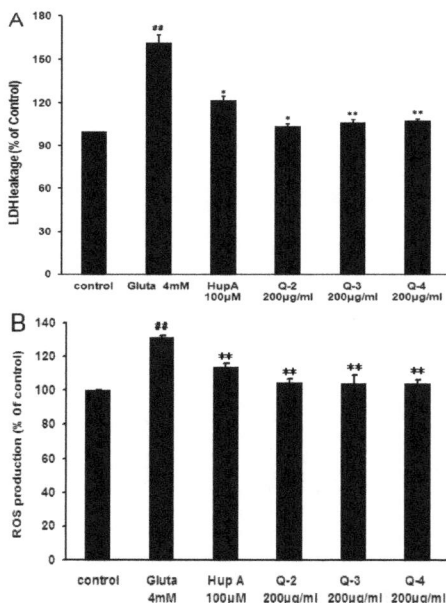

Figure 6. Effect of peracetylated chitosan oligosaccharides on glutamate-induced LDH release and ROS overproduction. (**A**) After the treatment of cells with different PACO monomers Q-2, Q-3 and Q-4 at a concentration of 200 μg/mL for 2 h and 4 mM of glutamate for 24 h, the level of LDH in the culture media was measured using an LDH assay kit. The data were normalized to the activity of LDH released from control cells. Values are the mean ± SD ($n = 4$). Significance: ## $P < 0.01$ *vs.* normal control group; * $P < 0.05$, ** $P < 0.01$ *vs.* glutamate treated control group; (**B**) After the treatment of cells with different PACO monomers Q-2, Q-3 and Q-4 at the concentration of 200 μg/mL for 2 h and 4 mM of glutamate for another 24 h. The fluorescence intensity of DCF was measured in a microplate-reader. Data were expressed as a percentage of non-treated control. Values are the mean ± SD ($n = 4$). Significance: ## $P < 0.01$ *vs.* normal control group; ** $P < 0.01$ *vs.* glutamate treated control group.

2.6. Effects of PACO on Mitochondrial Membrane Potential and the Activation of Caspase-3 and Caspase-9

Since glutamate-induced ROS production was a mitochondria-associated event, the changes in mitochondria induced by glutamate in the presence or absence of the PACOs were then tested. We observed the collapse of mitochondrial membrane potential (MMP) in PC12 cells with the probe JC-1. In brief, after incubation of PC12 cells with glutamate (4 mM) for 24 h, JC-1 uptake was measured by MMP assay kit according to the methods described previously [24]. As shown in Figure 7A, the MMP decreased to 62% ± 2% of control after glutamate treatment. Pretreatment with different PACO monomers (Q-3 and Q-4) at a concentration of 200 µg/mL could significantly protected cells against the glutamate-induced lowering of MMP from 62% to about 90% ($p < 0.05$), which was superior to the effect of the positive control drug, HupA (about 75%) (Figure 7A). The PACO monomer Q-2 could also inhibit the loss of MMP although insignificantly (Figure 7A). These results suggested that the PACOs might protect PC12 cells against glutamate induced apoptosis by attenuating the loss of mitochondrial membrane potential.

Caspases are crucial proteases that drive apoptosis. In our study, caspase-3 was significantly activated in PC12 cells, *i.e.*, 1.3-fold higher than normal control group after treatment with 4 mM of glutamate for 24 h (Figure 7B). However, pretreatment with peracetylated chitosan oligosaccharides (Q-2, Q-3 and Q-4) at the concentration of 200 µg/mL prior to exposure to glutamate could decrease the expression level of caspase 3 proteins from 1.3 to about 0.9, 0.9 and 1.0 fold of normal control group, respectively (Figure 7B,C). Moreover, the activities of caspase-3 and caspase-9 were also evaluated by ELISA assay, and the results indicated that pretreatment with PACOs (Q-2, Q-3 and Q-4) could significantly decrease the activities of both caspase-3 and caspase-9 in PC12 cells ($p < 0.05$), which were superior to the effect of positive control drug HupA (Figure 7D,E). These data suggested that the PACO may inhibit glutamate-induced cell death by down-regulating caspase-3 protein.

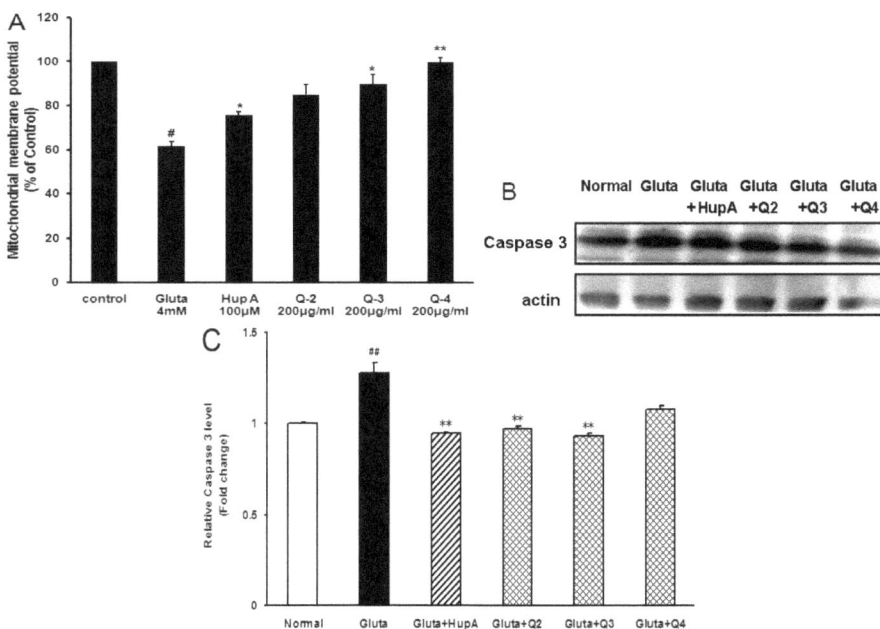

Figure 7. *Cont.*

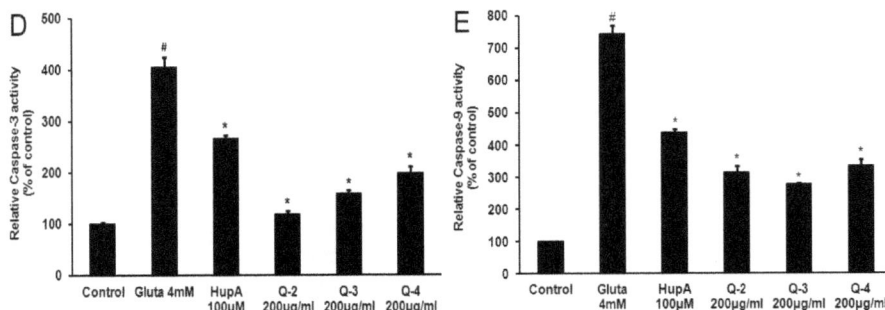

Figure 7. Peracetylated chitosan oligosaccharides protect PC12 cells against glutamate-induced loss of MMP and the activation of Caspase-3 and Caspase-9. (**A**) After being pretreated with 200 µg/mL of different PACO monomers Q-2, Q-3 and Q-4 for 2 h and 4 mM of glutamate for another 24 h, the mitochondrial membrane potential (MMP) in PC12 cells were evaluated with the probe JC-1. Data were expressed as a percentage of non-treated control. Values are the mean ± SD ($n = 3$). Significance: # $p < 0.05$ *vs.* normal control group; * $p < 0.05$, ** $p < 0.01$ *vs.* glutamate treated control group; (**B**) After being pretreated with 200 µg/mL of different PACO monomers Q-2, Q-3 and Q-4 for 2 h and 4 mM of glutamate for another 24 h, the levels of cleaved caspase-3 were measured by western blot. Blots were also probed for β-actin protein as loading controls. The result shown is a representative of three separate experiments with similar results. (**C**) Quantification of immunoblot for the ratio of caspase-3 to β-actin. The ratio for non-treated normal control cells was assigned values of 1.0 and the data presented as mean ± SD ($n = 3$). Significance: ## $p < 0.01$ *vs.* normal control group; ** $p < 0.01$ *vs.* glutamate treated control group. (**D–E**) After treatment, the activities of caspase-3 (**D**) and caspase-9 (**E**) were measured using an ELISA assay kit (Beyotime, China). Data were expressed as a percentage of non-treated control. Values are the mean ± SD ($n = 3$). Significance: # $p < 0.05$ *vs.* normal control group; * $p < 0.05$ *vs.* glutamate treated control group.

2.7. Effects of PACO on the Cytochrome c (Cyto C) Release from Mitochondria

Previous study has shown that cytochrome c (Cyto C) release from mitochondria triggers the apoptotic program [25]. Therefore, we further investigated the possible effect of the PACOs on glutamate-induced cytochrome c release from mitochondria by western blotting assay. As shown in Figure 8A,B, 4 mM glutamate caused significant cytochrome c release, which was 1.7-fold higher than normal control group. However, pretreatment with peracetylated chitosan oligosaccharides (Q-2, Q-3 and Q-4) at a concentration of 200 µg/mL prior to exposure to glutamate could significantly decrease the protein level of Cyto C proteins from 1.7 to about 0.7, 0.6 and 0.8 fold of normal control group, respectively ($p < 0.05$), which was superior to the effect of positive control drug HupA (about 1.4 fold) (Figure 8A,B). These data suggested that the PACO may inhibit cytochrome c release from mitochondria.

To further explore the effects of PACO on Cyto C release from mitochondria, the protein level of cytochrome c in cytoplasm was also measured by immunofluorescence assay. As shown in Figure 8C–H, treatment with glutamate (4 mM) resulted in an increase of cytochrome c in cytoplasm (Figure 8D), while there were nearly no cytochrome c release in normal control cells (Figure 8C). However, pre-treatment with peracetylated chitosan oligosaccharides Q2, Q3, and Q4 at the concentration of 200 µg/mL significantly reduced the protein level of cytochrome c in cytoplasm (Figure 8F–H), which was better than the effect of positive control drug huperzine A (Figure 8E). In summary, PACOs may inhibit glutamate-induced cell death by inhibiting cytochrome c release from mitochondria.

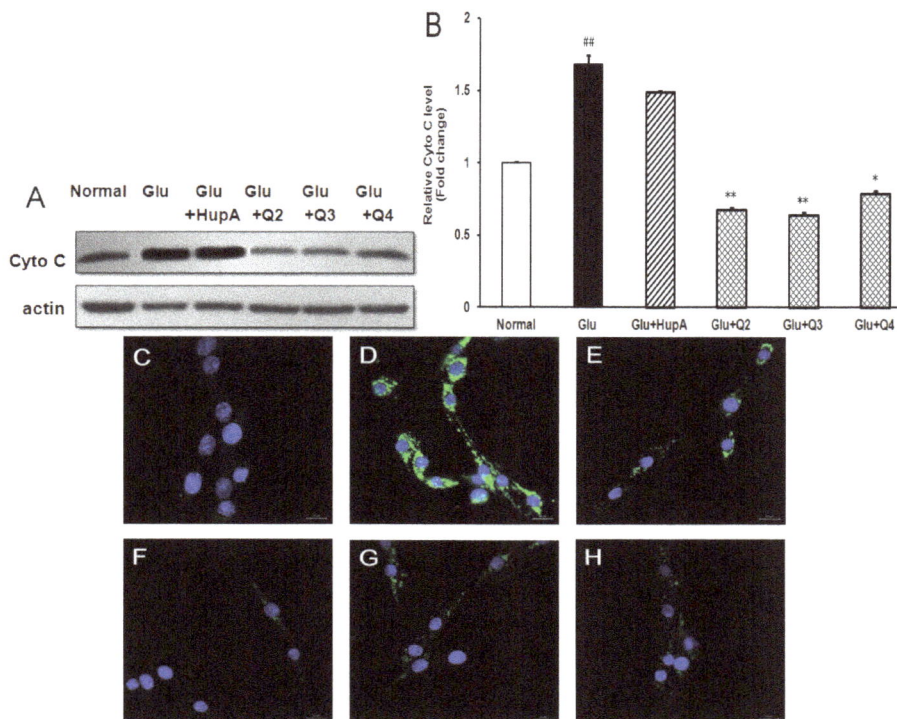

Figure 8. Peracetylated chitosan oligosaccharides protect PC12 cells against glutamate-induced Cyto C release from mitochondria. (**A**) After being pretreated with 200 μg/mL of different PACO monomers Q-2, Q-3 and Q-4 for 2 h and 4 mM of glutamate for another 24 h, the protein levels of Cyto C were evaluated by western blot. Blots were also probed for β-actin as loading controls. The result shown is a representative of three separate experiments with similar results; (**B**) Quantification of immunoblot for the ratio of Cyto C to β-actin. The ratio for non-treated control cells was assigned values of 1.0 and the data presented as mean ± SD (*n* = 3). Significance: ## $p < 0.01$ *vs.* normal control group; * $p < 0.05$, ** $p < 0.01$ *vs.* glutamate treated control group. (**C–H**) After being pretreated with 200 μg/mL of PACO monomers Q-2, Q-3 and Q-4 for 2 h, PC12 cells were exposed to 4 mM glutamate for 24 h. Then the levels of Cyto C in the cytoplasm were detected by immunofluorescence assay using anti-Cyto C antibody. **C**: Normal control, **D**: Glu, **E**: Glu + HupA, **F**: Glu + Q2, **G**: Glu + Q3, **H**: Glu + Q4. Scale bar represents 20 μm.

2.8. Effects of PACO on the Protein Expression of Bcl-2 and Bax

To determine whether Bcl-2 and Bax participated in the process of glutamate-induced PC12 cell death, the cells were treated with or without different drugs and then the expression levels were examined by western blot analysis. As shown in Figure 9A, Bax expression was markedly increased in the glutamate-treated group as compared to normal control group. However, pretreatment with 200 μg/mL of peracetylated chitosan oligosaccharides (Q-2, Q-3 and Q-4) prior to exposure to glutamate significantly decreased the expression level of Bax protein compared to the glutamate-treated control group (Figure 9A). In contrast, the level of Bcl-2 in the glutamate-treated group decreased significantly compared to normal control group (Figure 8B). However, Bcl-2 expression was ameliorated after the PACO treatment in PC12 cells and the effects of Q-2 and Q-3 were better than that of Q-4 and HupA (Figure 9B).

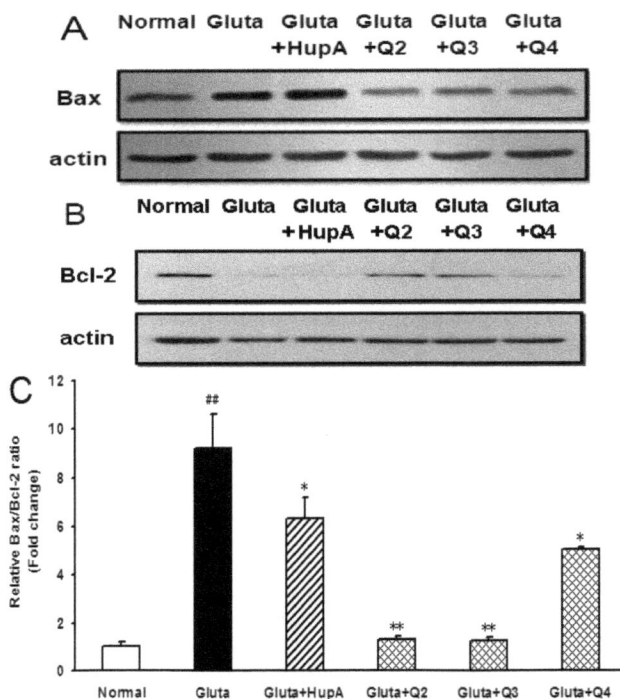

Figure 9. Effect of PACOs on the expression of Bax and Bcl-2 in PC12 cells. (A–B) After being pretreated with 200 µg/mL of different PACO monomers Q-2, Q-3 and Q-4 for 2 h and 4 mM of glutamate for another 24 h, the levels of Bax (**A**) and Bcl-2 (**B**) were measured by western blot. Blots were also probed for β-actin as loading controls. The result shown is a representative of three separate experiments with similar results; (**C**) Quantification of immunoblot for the ratio of Bax and Bcl-2. The ratio for non-treated normal control cells was assigned values of 1.0. Values are the mean ± SD ($n = 3$). Significance: ## $p < 0.01$ *vs.* normal control group; * $p < 0.05$, ** $p < 0.01$ *vs.* glutamate treated control group.

Moreover, the Bax/Bcl-2 ratio after glutamate-treatment increased to levels that were about 9.2-fold higher than normal control group (Figure 9C), suggesting glutamate induced apoptosis of PC 12 cells. Treatment with peracetylated chitosan oligosaccharides (Q-2, Q-3 and Q-4) decreased the Bax/Bcl-2 ratio significantly at a concentration of 200 µg/mL ($p < 0.05$), and they altered the Bax/Bcl-2 ratio from about 9.2 to about 1.3, 1.2 and 5.0, respectively, when compared to that of normal control group (Figure 9C). The inhibition effect of peracetylated chitosan oligosaccharides Q2, Q3, and Q4 on Bax/Bcl-2 ratio was better than that of positive control drug HupA (about 6.0 fold) (Figure 9C). Taken together, these results suggested that the protective effect of the PACO on glutamate-induced apoptosis in PC12 cells might be through Bcl-2/Bax signal pathway.

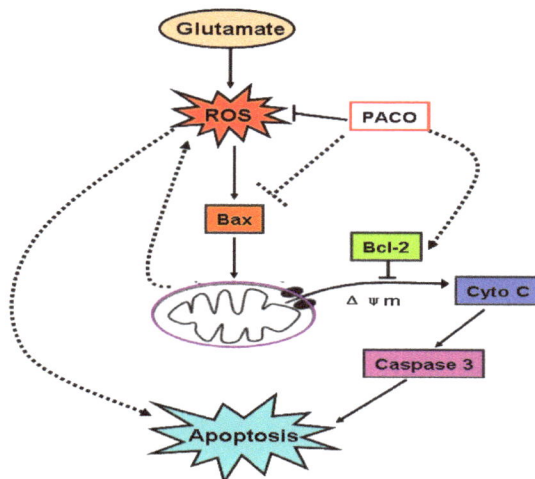

Figure 10. Proposed schemas of the mechanisms by which PACO suppressed glutamate-induced apoptosis in PC12 cells. Glutamate induces intracellular ROS generation in PC12 cells. The resultant oxidative stress triggers the activation of Bax protein, thereby reducing $\Delta\Psi m$, releasing cytochrome c, activating caspase 3, and finally inducing apoptosis. PACO inhibits ROS and suppresses the activity of downstream molecules, such as Bax, Cyto c, and caspase 3, for promoting neuronal survival.

3. Experimental Section

3.1. Reagents

Chitosan with degree of deacetylation of >95% was purchased from Jinhu Crust Product Corp. (Zibo, China). The lactate dehydrogenase (LDH) assay kit, reactive oxygen species (ROS) detection kit, and mitochondrial membrane potential (MMP) detection kit were purchased from the Jiancheng Institute of Biological Engineering (Nanjing, China). Antibodies for detecting Bcl-2, Bax, Cyto C, and cleaved caspase-3 were obtained from Cell Signaling Technology, Inc. (Danvers, MA, USA). FITC labeled secondary antibodies were purchased from Boster (Wuhan, China). All other reagents were from Sigma-Aldrich (St. Louis, MO, USA) unless otherwise stated.

3.2. COSs Production and Purification

The COS mixture was prepared by enzymatic hydrolysis of chitosan according to our previously reported method [19]. In brief, chitosan (50 g) was added to 400 mL distilled water, then 7 mL chitosanase solution (10 U/mL) was added. The mixture was stirred for 24 h in a 50 °C bath, and pH of the reaction mixture was adjusted to 6 by HCl solution (4 mol/L) during the hydrolysis process. The hydrolyzate was adjusted to pH 8~9 with concentrated NaOH and subsequently filtered to remove insoluble parts and the filtrate was concentrated and precipitated by adding four-fold volume of ethanol at 4 °C overnight. The precipitate was collected by centrifugation for 15 min at 8000 rpm then lyophilized to yield powdered products and identified as the COS mixture.

The COS mixture (300 mg) was dissolved in 2 mL of 0.1 M NH_4HCO_3, and then filtered with a microporous membrane (0.45 μm) to obtain a clear solution. The filtrate was loaded on a Bio Gel P6 column (2.6 × 110 cm) that connected to an AKTA UPC100 purification system (Fairfield, GE, USA) equipped with an online refractive index detector. The column was eluted with 0.1 M NH_4HCO_3 solution at a flow rate 0.4 mL/min. Eluents (10 mL/tube) were collected using a fraction collector to afford the pure dimer, trimer and tetramer of COSs. The analysis of each COS was performed by TLC, HPLC, IR, NMR and MS, as reported in previous work [19].

3.3. PACOs and NACOs Preparation and Purification

The acetylation of the COSs mixture to prepare PACOs and NACOs was performed according to the reported methods [20] with some modification.

Dried COSs mixture (5 g) was suspended in acetic anhydride (80 mL) at room temperature with stirring, and 8 mL concentrated H_2SO_4 was added. After stirring for 8 h at 50 °C, a clear dark amber-coloured solution was obtained and TLC (CH_2Cl_2:CH_3OH, 12:1, v/v) indicated the completion of the acetylation. The reaction mixture was added into 100 mL 15% sodium acetate solution at 0 °C and extracted with CH_2Cl_2 (80 mL × 3). The organic layer was then dried over anhydrous sodium sulphate, and concentrated under reduced pressure to give a residue of PACOs mixture. The residue was applied to a silica gel column chromatography (CH_2Cl_2–CH_3OH, 50:1 ~30:1) to give pure dimer, trimer and tetramer of PACOs. The yield of acetylation of COSs mixture was more than 60%.

The pure dimer, trimer or tetramer of PACOs (2 g) was added to methanol (20 mL). Deacetylation was started by adding sodium methoxide until pH 9~10. The resulting reaction mixture was stirred for 20 h at room temperature and monitored by TLC (propanol: water, 2:1, v/v). The reaction was then neutralized by addition of ion-exchange resin (H^+). After filtration, the filtrate was concentrated in vacuum to give pure dimer, trimer or tetramer of NACOs quantitatively.

3.4. MS and NMR Spectroscopy of Isolated PACOs and NACOs

Mass spectra were recorded with Micromass Global Q-TOF Mass Spectrometer (Indian Trail, NC, USA) using the ESI technique to determinate the molecular mass of each oligosaccharide. ^1H and ^{13}C NMR spectra were recorded at 27 °C on a JEOL JNM-ECP 600 MHz and an Agilent 500 MHz DD2 spectrometers with tetramethylsilane (Me$_4$Si) as the internal standard and chemical shifts were recorded as δ values.

Dimer of PACOs (**Q-2**): ^1H-NMR (600 MHz, CDCl$_3$): δ 6.17 (d, 1H, J = 9.2 Hz, N-H'), 6.10 (d, 1H, J = 3.6 Hz, H-1), 5.82 (d, 1H, J = 9.0 Hz, N-H), 5.23 (dd, 1H, J = 11.1, 9.0 Hz, H-3), 5.14 (dd, 1H, J = 9.4, 10.4 Hz, H-3'), 5.07 (t, 1H, J = 9.6 Hz, H-4'), 4.50 (d, 1H, J = 8.4 Hz, H-1'), 4.44 (dd, 1H, J = 12.3, 3.8 Hz, H-6-1), 4.40 (dd, 1H, J = 12.6, 4.1 Hz, H-6-1'), 4.40–4.35 (m, 1H, H-2), 4.21 (dd, 1H, J = 2.1, 12.1Hz, H-6-2), 4.02 (dd, 1H, J = 2.1, 12.4Hz, H-6-2'), 3.97 (app q, 1H, J = 9.2 Hz, H-2'), 3.91 (ddd, 1H, J = 2.2, 3.4, 10.1 Hz, H-5), 3.76 (t, 1H, J = 9.5Hz, H-4), 3.65 (ddd, 1H, J = 2.4, 4.0, 9.9Hz, H-5'), 2.19, 2.15, 2.09, 2.06, 2.01, 2.01,(6s, 18H, 3×-OCOCH$_3$), 1.96, 1.94 (2s, 6H, 2×-NHCOCH$_3$). ^{13}C NMR (150 MHz, CDCl$_3$): δ 171.4, 171.2, 170.7, 170.5 170.4, 170.2, 169.2, 168.9 (8C=O), 101.7 (C-1'), 90.4 (C-1), 75.9 (C-4), 72.5(C-3'), 71.8(C-5'), 70.7 (C-3), 70.6(C-5), 67.8 (C-4'), 61.6 (C-6'), 61.4 (C-6), 54.3 (C-2'), 51.0 (C-2), 23.1, 23.0 (2$\underline{C}$H$_3$CONH), 21.0, 20.9, 20.6, 20.6, 20.5, 20.5 (6$\underline{C}$H$_3$COO). ESI-MS m/z 699.1 [M + Na]$^+$.

Trimer of PACOs (**Q-3**): ^1H-NMR (500 MHz, DMSO-d6): δ 7.97 (d, 1H, J = 9.1 Hz, N-H), 7.91 (d, 1H, J = 9.2 Hz, N-H), 7.91 (d, 1H, J = 9.4 Hz, N-H), 5.81 (d, 1H, J = 3.5 Hz, H-1), 5.12 (t, 1H, J = 9.9 Hz), 5.05–4.97 (m, 2H), 4.81 (t, 1H, J = 9.7 Hz), 4.64 (d, 1H, J = 8.4 Hz, H-1''), 4.55 (d, 1H, J = 8.4 Hz, H-1'), 4.36–4.25 (m, 3H), 4.15–4.10 (m, 1H), 4.05–4.00 (m, 2H, H-2), 3.91–3.77 (m, 4H), 3.72 (t, 1H, J = 9.3 Hz), 3.60–3.48 (m, 3H), 2.15, 2.09, 2.05, 2.00, 1.95, 1.94(2CH$_3$), 1.90 (7s, 24H, 8 × OCOCH$_3$), 1.78, 1.74, 1.73 (3s, 9H, 3 × NHCOCH$_3$); ^{13}C NMR (125 MHz, DMSO-d6): δ 170.1, 170.0, 169.9, 169.8, 169.6, 169.5, 169.4, 169.3, 169.2, 169.1 (11C=O), 100.1, 99.9 (C-1', C-1''), 89.6 (C-1), 75.6, 74.8, 73.3, 72.3, 71.6, 70.4, 70.1(2C), 68.1, 62.6, 61.6, 61.5, 53.8, 53.7, 50.0, 22.6, 22.5, 22.2(3$\underline{C}$H$_3$CONH), 20.8–20.3 (m, 8$\underline{C}$H$_3$COO). ESI-MS m/z 986.2 [M + Na]$^+$.

Tetramer of PACOs (**Q-4**): ^1H-NMR (500 MHz, DMSO-d6): δ 7.96 (d, 1H, J = 9.1 Hz, N-H), 7.92–7.87 (m, 3H, 3NH), 5.81 (d, 1H, J = 3.5 Hz, H-1), 5.12 (t, 1H, J = 9.9 Hz), 5.05–4.94 (m, 3H), 4.81 (t, 1H, J = 9.7 Hz), 4.63 (d, 1H, J = 8.4 Hz, H-1'''), 4.55 (d, 2H, J = 8.4 Hz, H-1'', H-1'), 4.36–4.24 (m, 4H), 4.14–3.99 (m, 4H), 3.90–3.65 (m, 6H), 3.60–3.45 (m, 5H), 2.14, 2.08, 2.07, 2.04, 2.00, 1.95, 1.93(2CH$_3$), 1.89 (8s, 30H, 10 × OCOCH$_3$), 1.78, 1.74, 1.72 (3s, 12H, 4 × NHCOCH$_3$); ^{13}C NMR (125 MHz, DMSO-d6): δ

170.1, 170.1, 170.0, 169.9, 169.8, 169.6, 169.5, 169.4, 169.3, 169.3, 169.2, 169.1 (14C=O), 100.1, 99.9, 99.8 (C-1′, C-1″, C-1‴), 89.6 (C-1), 75.5, 75.2, 74.7, 73.2, 73.1, 72.3, 71.7, 71.5, 70.4, 70.2, 70.1, 68.1, 62.5 (2C), 61.6, 61.5, 53.9, 53.8, 53.7, 50.0, 22.6, 22.6, 22.5, 22.2(4$\underline{C}$H$_3$CONH), 20.8–20.3 (m, 10$\underline{C}$H$_3$COO). ESI-MS *m/z* 1251.6 [M + H]$^+$.

Dimer of NACOs (**N-2**): ^{1}H-NMR (600 MHz, D$_2$O): δ 5.16 (d, 0.6H, *J* = 2.8 Hz, H-1α), 4.66 (d, 0.4H, *J* = 7.9 Hz, H-1β), 4.56 (d, 0.6 H, *J* = 8.5 Hz, H-1′α), 4.55 (d, 0.4 H, *J* = 8.4 Hz, H-1′β), 3.90–3.43 (m, 12H, H-2, H-3, H-4, H-5, H-6-1, H-6-2, H-2′, H-3′, H-4′, H-5′, H-6-1′, H-6-2′), 2.04, 2.00 (2s, 6H, 2 × -NHCOCH$_3$); ^{13}C NMR (150 MHz, D$_2$O): δ 174.9, 174.7 (2C=O), 101.8 (C-1′), 95.1 (C-1β), 90.7 (C-1α), 80.1(C-4α), 79.6 (C-4β), 76.2 (C-5′), 74.8 (C-5β), 73.7 (C-3′), 72.8 (C-3β), 70.2 (C-5α), 70.0 (C-4′), 69.5 (C-3α), 60.8 (C-6′), 60.4 (C-6β), 60.3 (C-6α) 56.3 (C-2β), 55.9 (C-2′), 53.9 (C-2α), 22.4, 22.2 (2CH$_3$). ESI-MS *m/z* 425.2 [M + H]$^+$.

Trimer of NACOs (**N-3**): ^{1}H-NMR (600 MHz, D$_2$O): δ 5.15 (d, 0.65 H, *J* = 2.6 Hz, H-1α), 4.66 (d, 0.36 H, *J* = 7.9 Hz, H-1β), 4.56 (d, 0.65 H, *J* = 8.2 Hz, H-1′), 4.55 (d, 0.65 H, *J* = 8.5 Hz, H-1″), 3.90–3.43 (m, 18H, H-2~H-6, H-2′~H-6′, H-2″~H-6″), 2.03, 2.03 2.01(3s, 9H, 3 × -NHCOCH$_3$). ^{13}C NMR (150 MHz, D$_2$O): δ 174.9, 174.9, 174.7 (3C=O), 101.8(C-1″), 101.6 (C-1′), 95.1 (C-1β), 90.7 (C-1α), 79.9 (C-4α), 79.4 (C-4′, C-4β), 76.2 (C-5″), 74.9 (C-5β), 74.8 (C-5′), 73.7 (C-3″), 72.8 (C-3β), 72.4 (C-3′), 70.3 (C-5α), 70.0 (C-4″), 69.5 (C-3α), 60.8 (C-6″), 60.4 (C-6β), 60.3 (C-6′, C-6α), 56.4 (C-2β), 55.9 (C-2″), 55.3 (C-2′), 53.9 (C-2α), 22.4, 22.4, 22.2 (3CH$_3$). ESI-MS *m/z* 628.1 [M + H]$^+$.

Tetramer of NACOs (**N-4**): ^{1}H-NMR (600 MHz, D$_2$O): δ 5.18 (d, 0.64 H, *J* = 1.7 Hz, H-1α), 4.68 (d, 0.35 H, *J* = 8.1 Hz, H-1β), 4.57 (d, 3 H, *J* = 8.4 Hz, H-1′, H-1″, H-1‴), 3.92–3.44 (m, 24H, H-2~H-6, H-2′~H-6′, H-2″~H-6″, H-2‴~H-6‴), 2.05, 1.05, 2.05, 2.03 (4s, 12H, 4 × -NHCOCH$_3$). ^{13}C NMR (150 MHz, D$_2$O): δ 175.0, 174.9, 174.7 (4C=O), 101.7 (C-1‴), 101.5 (C-1′, C-1″), 95.1 (C-1β), 90.7 (C-1α), 79.9 (C-4α), 79.4 (C-4′, C-4″), 79.2 (C-4β), 76.2 (C-5″), 74.9 (C-5β), 74.8 (C-5′, C-5″), 73.7 (C-3‴), 72.8 (C-3β), 72.4 (C-3′, C-3″), 70.3 (C-5α), 70.0 (C-4‴), 69.5 (C-3α), 60.8 (C-6‴), 60.4 (C-6β), 60.3 (C-6′, C-6″, C-6α), 56.4 (C-2β), 55.9 (C-2‴), 55.3 (C-2′, C-2″), 53.9 (C-2α), 22.5, 22.4, 22.2 (4CH$_3$). ESI-MS *m/z* 831.2 [M + H]$^+$.

3.5. Cell Culture

Both undifferentiated and differentiated rat adrenal medullary phenochromocytoma PC12 cells were purchased from the Cell Bank of the Chinese Academy of Sciences (Shanghai, China). Cells were maintained in Dulbecco's Modified Eagle's medium (DMEM, Gibco, New York, NY, USA) supplemented with 10% FBS (Gibco, New York, NY, USA), 100 U/mL penicillin and 100 µg/mL streptomycin at 37 °C in 5% CO2 atmosphere. Cells were passaged with trypsin every 4 days with the subcultivation ratio of 1:6. All experiments were performed on cells between passages 3–15.

3.6. Determination of Cell Viability

The cell viability of PC12 cells was measured by resazurin assay [21]. In brief, after oligosaccharide treatment for 24 h, 20 µL of resazurin was added to each well at a final concentration of 0.2 mg/mL and incubated for 16 h at 37 °C. Then resazurin fluorescence was measured using a SpectraMax M5 plate reader (Molecular Devices, Sunnyvale, CA, USA) with excitation and emission wavelengths of 544 and 595 nm, respectively. The cell viability was expressed as a percentage of non-treated control.

For the neuroprotective experiments, PC12 cells were seeded into 96-well plates at a density of 5 × 103 cells/well, and cultivated for 24 h. Cells were pretreated with different oligosaccharides at concentrations of 100, 200, 400 µg/mL or 100 µM of Huperzine-A (HupA) for 2 h prior to exposure to 4 mM of glutamate. After 24 h incubation, cell viability was evaluated by resazurin assay.

3.7. LDH Release Assay

The level of lactate dehydrogenase (LDH) released from damaged cells into culture media was measured using an LDH assay kit (Beyotime, Nantong, China) according to the manufacturer's protocol. Briefly, PC12 cells were seeded at a density of 5 × 103 cells/well into 96-well plate. After drug treatment, the cell-free culture supernatants were collected from each well and incubated with the appropriate reagent mixture according to the supplier's instructions at room temperature for 20 min. The absorbance of samples was measured at 440 nm using a micro-plate reader. The data were normalized to the activity of LDH released from control cells. Absorbance of blanks, determined as no-enzyme control, had been subtracted from each value.

3.8. Measurement of Intracellular ROS

Intracellular ROS was monitored using the DCFH-DA fluorescent probe as described previously [26]. In brief, intracellular H_2O_2 or low-molecular-weight peroxides can oxidize DCFH-DA to the highly fluorescent compound dichlorofluorescein (DCF). After drugs treatment, cells were incubated with 10 mM of DCFH-DA at 37 °C for 30 min, and then washed twice with PBS. Finally, the fluorescence intensity of DCF was measured in a micro-plate reader with an excitation wavelength of 485 nm and an emission wavelength of 535 nm. Data were expressed as percentage of non-treated control.

3.9. Measurement of the Mitochondrial Membrane Potential (MMP)

The mitochondrial membrane potential (MMP) of PC12 cells was monitored using the fluorescent, lipophilic and cationic probe, JC-1 (Beyotime, Nantong, China) according to the methods described previously [24]. Briefly, after indicated treatments, cells were cultured in 24-well plates and incubated with JC-1 staining solution (5 μg/mL) for 20 min at 37 °C. Cells were then rinsed twice with JC-1 staining buffer and the fluorescence intensity of both mitochondrial JC-1 monomers (λex 514 nm, λem 529 nm) and aggregates (λex 585 nm, λem 590 nm) were detected using a SpectraMax M5 plate reader (Molecular Devices, USA). The Δψm of PC12 cells in each treatment group was calculated as the fluorescence ratio of red (*i.e.*, aggregates) to green (*i.e.*, monomers).

3.10. Immunofluorescence Assay

The Cyto C release from mitochondria was also evaluated by using indirect immunofluorescence assay. Briefly, after treatment, cells were fixed with 4% Paraformaldehyde for 15 min at room temperature (RT) and further permeabilized by 0.5% Triton X-100 in PBS for 5 min. Then, after being blocked with 2% bovine serum albumin (BSA) in PBS for 1 h at RT, cells were incubated with anti-Cyto C antibody for 1 h. After three washes with PBS, cells were incubated with FITC labeled secondary antibody for 1 h at RT. Then after washing trice, cells were incubated further with DAPI for 10 min. Finally, the fluorescence corresponding to Cyto C and DAPI was observed by using a laser scanning confocal microscopy (Zeiss LSM510, Oberkochen, Germany).

3.11. Western Blot Analysis

Western blot analysis was performed as described previously [27]. Proteins were separated using SDS-PAGE and electrically transferred to a NC membrane (Pall, New York, NY, USA). After that, the membranes were blocked with TBST (50 mM Tris-HCl, pH 7.4, 0.15 M NaCl, 0.1% Tween-20) containing 5% BSA (Sigma, St. Louis, MO, USA) for 2 h. Then the membranes were incubated with primary antibodies against Bax, Bcl-2, or caspase-3 protein diluted at 1:1000 at 4 °C over night. After washing with TBST for three times, the membranes were incubated with goat anti-rabbit IgG labeled with horse radish peroxidase (Santa Cruz, Dallas, TX, USA) diluted at 1:2000 at room temperature for 2 h. Blots were developed using an ECL plus kit (Amersham Bioscience, Aylesbury, UK), exposed to Kodak autoradiographic films and quantified using Image J software.

3.12. Statistical Analysis

All data are represented as the mean ± SD. Comparison between groups was made by one-way analysis of variance (ANOVA) followed by a specific post hoc test to analyze the difference. $p <$

0.05 was considered to indicate statistical significance. The SPSS software package (SPSS program, version 13.0, Chicago, IL, USA) was used for all statistical tests.

4. Conclusions

Chitosan is the universally accepted non-toxic *N*-deacetylated derivative of chitin, one of the most abundant biopolymers on earth. Chitosan oligosaccharides (COSs) have been reported to have a variety of biological activities and widely used in many research fields. The current study demonstrated that the peracetylated chitosan oligosaccharides (PACOs) acted as antagonists against glutamate-induced PC12 cell death in a concentration-dependent manner. PACOs significantly prevented glutamate-induced apoptosis as manifested by depressing the elevation of Bax/Bcl-2 ratio and caspase-3 activation, suggesting its antagonist effect could be partially due to apoptosis regulation. Thus, peracetylated chitosan oligosaccharides might have potential for treating certain neurodegenerative diseases.

The antagonist effects of PACOs were greater than that of non-acetylated COSs and *N*-acetylated oligosaccharides NACOs, suggesting that peracetylation was essential for the neuroprotective effects of chitosan oligosaccharides. In addition, the peracetylated lactose Ac-Lac-2 and peracetylated cellobiose Cel-2 both had greater effects than those of the non-acetylated oligosaccharides Lac-2 and Cel-2, but lesser than those of the acetylated chitosan oligosaccharide Q-2, which suggests that the acetyl groups were indispensible for the neuroprotective effect of neutral oligosaccharides and that the structure of the sugar backbone might also influence the neuroprotective effects observed *in vitro*. It was reported that peracetylation can facilitate passive diffusion of disaccharides across cell membranes, allowing them to enter the Golgi [28]. Thus, the acetylation modification might facilitate the chitosan oligosaccharides to enter the cells to interfere the ROS induced apoptosis in PC12 cells.

Glutamate toxicity is an important mechanism of neuronal death in cerebral ischemia [29,30]. It was reported that glutamate neurotoxicity is considered to have two mechanisms of neuron injury including glutamate receptor-mediated [31] and oxidative stress-mediated [32,33] neurotoxicity. In our study, the PACO treatment potentially reduced LDH release and ROS production, and attenuated the loss of mitochondrial membrane potential (MMP), which suggests that the PACOs displayed their protective effect against glutamate-induced apoptosis in PC12 cells mainly through oxidative stress amelioration [34–36] (Figure 10).

ROS is a well known etiological factor associated with oxidative stress leading to cell death via apoptosis in a variety of cell types [37–40], and such effects can be blocked or delayed by a wide variety of antioxidants [41]. Mitochondria-dependent apoptotic pathways are involved in glutamate-induced cytotoxicity in PC 12 cells [42]. Considering the results indicating that PACOs could reduce ROS production and attenuate the loss of MMP, we suppose that the PACOs may be able to protect PC12 cells against glutamate induced cell apoptosis. As a mitochondrial membrane-associated protein, Bcl-2 exerts its anti-apoptotic effect through inhibition of Bax expression from mitochondria, and inhibition of subsequent activation of the caspase-3 [43]. Moreover, cytochrome c release could be reduced by pretreatment with the PACOs, which suggested the PACOs might influence the Bcl-2/Bax pathway because Bax is believed to be upstream of cytochrome c release in the mitochondria-mediated apoptosis pathway. Taken together, glutamate either significantly up- or down-regulated the expression of Bax, Bcl-2 proteins in PC12 cells. Reversal of these trends by the PACO pretreatment suggests that the anti-apoptosis activity of the PACOs may be mediated through Bcl-2/Bax signal pathway in PC12 cells [15,44,45] (Figure 10).

In conclusion, our study demonstrated that the peracetylated chitosan oligosaccharides PACOs exhibited a protective effect on glutamate-induced PC12 cell death through Bcl-2/Bax signal pathway. Since glutamate-evoked cell injury in neuronal cells is involved in many neuron disorders, it thus raises the possibility of developing PACOs as potential agents for prevention and treatment of neurodegenerative diseases. However, PC12 cells cannot totally represent the characteristics of primary cultured neurons, so further work needs to be done directly on primary neurons *in vitro* and on animal models to test if PACOs are useful in treating glutamate-induced neural injury or death.

Acknowledgments: This study was supported in part by the Program for National Science & Technology Support Program of China (2013BAB01B02), the Natural Science Foundation of China (91129706; 81302811), the NSFC-Shandong Joint Fund (U1406402), the Special Fund for Marine Scientific Research in the Public Interest (201005024), the Shandong Provincial Natural Science Foundation (ZR2011HQ012), and the Innovation Fund Designated for postdoc of Shandong Province (201102030).

Author Contributions: C.X.L., H.S.G. and L.J.Z. conceived and designed the experiments; C.H., L.X.G. and Y.R.Z. performed the experiments; C.H., W.W. and G.L.Y. analyzed the data; W.W., C.X.L. and L.J.Z. wrote the paper.

Conflicts of Interest: The authors declare no conflict of interest.

References

1. Tan, J.W.; Tham, C.L.; Israf, D.A.; Lee, S.H.; Kim, M.K. Neuroprotective effects of biochanin A against glutamate induced cytotoxicity in PC12 cells via apoptosis inhibition. *Neurochem. Res.* **2013**, *38*, 512–518. [CrossRef] [PubMed]
2. Dröge, W. Free radicals in the physiological control of cell function. *Physiol. Rev.* **2002**, *82*, 47–95. [PubMed]
3. Mao, Q.Q.; Zhong, X.M.; Feng, C.R.; Pan, A.J.; Li, Z.Y.; Huang, Z. Protective effects of paeoniflorin against glutamate-induced neurotoxicity in PC12 cells via antioxidant mechanisms and Ca^{2+} antagonism. *Cell Mol. Neurobiol.* **2010**, *30*, 1059–1066. [CrossRef] [PubMed]
4. Choi, D.W. Glutamate neurotoxicity and diseases of the nervous system. *Neuron* **1988**, *1*, 623–634. [CrossRef] [PubMed]
5. Murphy, T.H.; Miyamoto, M.; Sastre, A.; Schnaar, R.L.; Coyle, J.T. Glutamate toxicity in a neuronal cell line involves inhibition of cystine transport leading to oxidative stress. *Neuron* **1989**, *2*, 1547–1558. [CrossRef] [PubMed]
6. Zablocka, A.; Janusz, M. The two faces of reactive oxygen species. *Postep. Hig. Med. Dosw.* **2008**, *62*, 118–124.
7. Monaghan, D.T.; Bridges, R.J.; Cotman, C.W. The excitatory amino acid receptors: Their classes, pharmacology, and distinct properties in the function of the central nervous system. *Annu. Rev. Pharmacol. Toxicol.* **1989**, *29*, 365–402. [CrossRef] [PubMed]
8. Bleich, S.; Romer, K.; Wiltfang, J.; Kornhuber, J. Glutamate and the glutamate receptor system: A target for drug action. *Int. J. Geriatr. Psychiatry* **2003**, *18*, S33–S40. [CrossRef] [PubMed]
9. Penugonda, S.; Mare, S.; Goldstein, G.; Banks, W.A.; Ercal, N. Effects of N-acetylcysteine amide (NACA), a novel thiol antioxidant against glutamate-induced cytotoxicity in neuronal cell line PC12. *Brain Res.* **2005**, *1056*, 132–138. [CrossRef] [PubMed]
10. Penugonda, S.; Mare, S.; Lutz, P.; Banks, W.A.; Ercal, N. Potentiation of lead-induced cell death in PC12 cells by glutamate: Protection by N-acetylcysteine amide (NACA), a novel thiol antioxidant. *Toxicol. Appl. Pharmacol.* **2006**, *216*, 197–205. [CrossRef] [PubMed]
11. Li, N.; Liu, B.; Dluzen, D.E.; Jin, Y. Protective effects of ginsenoside Rg2 against glutamate-induced neurotoxicity in PC12 cells. *J. Ethnopharmacol.* **2007**, *111*, 458–463. [CrossRef] [PubMed]
12. Yan, C.; Wu, L.L.; Pan, Y.; Song, Q.; Ran, C.L.; Liu, S.K. The effect of Jiaweisinisan on cAMP response element binding protein and phosphorylation in PC12 cells injured by Corticosterone and Glutamate. *Chin. Pharmacol. Bull.* **2009**, *25*, 270–274.
13. Li, Y.F.; Zhang, Y.Z.; Liu, Y.Q.; Wang, H.L.; Cao, J.B.; Guan, T.T.; Luo, Z.P. Inhibition of N-methyl-D-aspartate receptor function appears to be one of the common actions for antidepressants. *J. Psychopharmacol.* **2006**, *20*, 629–635. [CrossRef] [PubMed]
14. Zhang, J.; Xia, W.; Liu, P.; Cheng, Q.; Tahi, T.; Gu, W.; Li, B. Chitosan modification and pharmaceutical/biomedical applications. *Mar. Drugs* **2010**, *8*, 1962–1987. [CrossRef] [PubMed]
15. Pangestuti, R.; Kim, S.K. Neuroprotective Properties of Chitosan and Its Derivatives. *Mar. Drugs* **2010**, *8*, 2117–2128. [CrossRef] [PubMed]
16. Lee, S.-H.; Park, J.-S.; Kim, S.-K.; Ahn, C.-B.; Je, J.-Y. Chitooligosaccharides suppress the level of protein expression and acetylcholinesterase activity induced by A[beta]25–35 in PC12 cells. *Bioorganic Med. Chem. Lett.* **2009**, *19*, 860–862. [CrossRef]

17. Yoon, N.Y.; Ngo, D.-N.; Kim, S.-K. Acetylcholinesterase inhibitory activity of novel chitooligosaccharide derivatives. *Carbohydr. Polym.* **2009**, *78*, 869–872. [CrossRef]

18. Zhou, S.; Yang, Y.; Gu, X.; Ding, F. Chitooligosaccharides protect cultured hippocampal neurons against glutamate-induced neurotoxicity. *Neurosci. Lett.* **2008**, *444*, 270–274. [CrossRef] [PubMed]

19. Gao, L.-X.; Li, C.-X.; Wang, S.-X.; Zhao, X.; Guan, H.-S. Preparation and analysis of Chitooligosaccharide isomers with different degree. *Chin. J. Mar. Drugs* **2013**, *32*, 21–27.

20. Wang, J.; Li, Y.-X.; Song, N.; Guan, H.-S. Preparation and Characterization of Chito-oligosaccharide and Peracetylated-chito-oligosaccharides. *Period. Ocean Univers. China* **2005**, *35*, 994–1000.

21. Nociari, M.M.; Shalev, A.; Benias, P.; Russo, C. A novel one-step, highly sensitive fluorometric assay to evaluate cell-mediated cytotoxicity. *J. Immunol. Methods* **1998**, *213*, 157–167. [CrossRef] [PubMed]

22. O'Brien, J.; Wilson, I.; Orton, T.; Pognan, F. Investigation of the Alamar Blue (resazurin) fluorescent dye for the assessment of mammalian cell cytotoxicity. *Eur. J. Biochem.* **2000**, *267*, 5421–5426. [CrossRef] [PubMed]

23. Yin, R.J.; Zhang, M.; Hao, C.; Wang, W.; Qiu, P.J.; Wan, S.B.; Zhang, L.J.; Jiang, T. Different cytotoxicities and cellular localizations of novel quindoline derivatives with or without boronic acid modifications in cancer cells. *Chem. Commun.* **2013**, *49*, 8516–8518. [CrossRef]

24. McElnea, E.M.; Quill, B.; Docherty, N.G.; Irnaten, M.; Siah, W.F.; Clark, A.F.; O'Brien, C.J.; Wallace, D.M. Oxidative stress, mitochondrial dysfunction and calcium overload in human lamina cribrosa cells from glaucoma donors. *Mol. Vis.* **2011**, *17*, 1182–1191. [PubMed]

25. Liu, X.; Kim, C.N.; Yang, J.; Jemmerson, R.; Wang, X. Induction of apoptotic program in cell free extracts: Requirement for dATP and cytochrome c. *Cell* **1996**, *86*, 147–157. [CrossRef] [PubMed]

26. LeBel, C.P.; Ali, S.F.; McKee, M.; Bondy, S.C. Organometal-induced increases in oxygen reactive species: The potential of 2′,7′-dichlorofluorescin diacetate as an index of neurotoxic damage. *Toxicol. Appl. Pharmacol.* **1990**, *104*, 17–24. [CrossRef] [PubMed]

27. Sugawara, T.; Noshita, N.; Lewen, A.; Gashe, Y.; Ferrand-Drake, M.; Fujimura, M.; Morita-Fujimura, Y.; Chan, P.H. Overexpression of copper/zinc superoxide dismutase in transgenic rats protects vulnerable neurons against ischemia damage by blocking the mitochondrial pathway of caspase activation. *J. Neurosci.* **2002**, *22*, 209–217. [PubMed]

28. Brown, J.R.; Fuster, M.M.; Li, R.X.; Varki, N.; Glass, C.A.; Esko, J.D. A Disaccharide-Based Inhibitor of Glycosylation Attenuates MetastaticTumor Cell Dissemination. *Clin. Cancer Res.* **2006**, *12*, 2894–2901. [CrossRef] [PubMed]

29. Kim, J.Y.; Jeong, H.Y.; Lee, H.K.; Kim, S.; Hwang, B.Y.; Bae, K.; Seong, Y.H. Neuroprotection of the leaf and stem of Vitis amurensis and their active compounds against ischemic brain damage in rats and excitotoxicity in cultured neurons. *Phytomedicine* **2011**, *19*, 150–159. [CrossRef] [PubMed]

30. Ma, S.; Liu, H.; Jiao, H.; Wang, L.; Chen, L.; Liang, J.; Zhao, M.; Zhang, X. Neuroprotective effect of ginkgolide K on glutamate-induced cytotoxicity in PC 12 cells via inhibition of ROS generation and Ca^{2+} influx. *NeuroToxicology* **2012**, *33*, 59–69. [CrossRef] [PubMed]

31. Kanki, R.; Nakamizo, T.; Yamashita, H.; Kihara, T.; Sawada, H.; Uemura, K.; Kawamata, J.; Shibasaki, H.; Akaike, A.; Shimohama, S. Effects of mitochondrial dysfunction on glutamate receptor-mediated neurotoxicity in cultured rat spinal motor neurons. *Brain Res.* **2004**, *1015*, 73–81. [CrossRef] [PubMed]

32. Hirata, Y.; Yamamoto, H.; Atta, M.S.; Mahmoud, S.; Oh-Hashi, K.; Kiuchi, K. Chloroquine inhibits glutamate-induced death of a neuronal cell line by reducing reactive oxygen species through sigma-1 receptor. *J. Neurochem.* **2011**, *119*, 839–847. [CrossRef] [PubMed]

33. Chen, J.; Chua, K.W.; Chua, C.C.; Yu, H.; Pei, A.; Chua, B.H.; Hamdy, R.C.; Xu, X.; Liu, C.F. Antioxidant activity of 7,8-dihydroxyflavone provides neuroprotection against glutamate-induced toxicity. *Neurosci. Lett.* **2011**, *499*, 181–185. [CrossRef] [PubMed]

34. Gross, A.; Yin, X.M.; Wang, K.; Wei, M.C.; Jockel, J.; Milliman, C.; Erdjument-Bromage, H.; Tempst, P.; Korsmeyer, S.J. Caspase cleaved BID targets mitochondria and is required for cytochrome c release, while BCL-XL prevents this release but not tumor necrosis factor-R1/Fas death. *J. Biol. Chem.* **1999**, *274*, 1156–1163. [CrossRef] [PubMed]

35. Cory, S.; Adams, J.M. The Bcl2 family: Regulators of the cellular life-or-death switch. *Nat. Rev. Cancer* **2002**, *2*, 647–656. [CrossRef] [PubMed]

36. Liu, X.; Osawa, T. Astaxanthin protects neuronal cells against oxidative damage and is a potent candidate for brain food. *Forum Nutr.* **2009**, *61*, 129–135. [PubMed]

37. Lan, A.P.; Xiao, L.C.; Yang, Z.L.; Yang, C.T.; Wang, X.Y.; Chen, P.X.; Gu, M.F.; Feng, J.Q. Interaction between ROS and p38MAPK contributes to chemical hypoxia-induced injuries in PC12 cells. *Mol. Med. Rep.* **2011**, *5*, 250–255. [PubMed]

38. Tao, L.; Li, X.; Zhang, L.; Tian, J.; Li, X.; Sun, X.; Li, X.; Jiang, L.; Zhang, X.; Chen, J. Protective effect of tetrahydroxystilbene glucoside on 6-OHDA-induced apoptosis in PC12 cells through the ROS-NO pathway. *PLoS One* **2011**, *6*, e26055. [CrossRef] [PubMed]

39. Dong, Y.; Yang, N.; Liu, Y.; Li, Q.; Zuo, P. The neuroprotective effects of phytoestrogen azearalanol on b-amyloid-induced toxicity in differentiated PC-12 cells. *Eur. J. Pharmacol.* **2011**, *670*, 392–398. [CrossRef] [PubMed]

40. Kim, E.K.; Lee, S.J.; Moon, S.H.; Jeon, B.T.; Kim, B.; Park, T.K.; Han, J.S.; Park, P.J. Neuroprotective effects of a novel peptide purified from venison protein. *J. Microbiol. Biotechnol.* **2010**, *20*, 700–707. [CrossRef] [PubMed]

41. Ozkan, O.V.; Yuzbasioglu, M.F.; Ciralik, H.; Kurutas, E.B.; Yonden, Z.; Aydin, M.; Bulbuloglu, E.; Semerci, E.; Goksu, M.; Atli, Y.; *et al.* Resveratrol, a natural antioxidant, attenuates intestinal ischemia/reperfusion injury in rats. *Tohoku J. Exp. Med.* **2009**, *218*, 251–258. [CrossRef] [PubMed]

42. Wang, X.C.; Zhu, G.; Yang, S.; Wang, X.; Cheng, H.; Wang, F.; Li, X.X.; Li, Q.L. Paeonol prevents excitotoxity in rat pheochromocytoma PC12 cells via downregulation of ERK activation and inhibition of apoptosis. *Planta Med.* **2011**, *77*, 1695–1701. [CrossRef] [PubMed]

43. Li, G.; Ma, R.; Huang, C.; Tang, Q.; Fu, Q.; Liu, H.; Hu, B.; Xiang, J. Protective effect of erythropoietin on b-amyloid-induced PC12 cell death through antioxidant mechanisms. *Neurosci. Lett.* **2008**, *442*, 143–147. [CrossRef] [PubMed]

44. Chan, K.C.; Mong, M.C.; Yin, A.C. Antioxidative and anti-inflammatory, neuroprotective effects of astaxanthin and canthaxanthin in nerve growth factor differentiated PC12 cells. *J. Food Sci.* **2009**, *74*, H225–H231. [CrossRef] [PubMed]

45. Wang, C.J.; Hu, C.P.; Xu, K.P.; Yuan, Q.; Li, F.S.; Zou, H.; Tan, G.S.; Li, Y.J. Protective effect of selaginellin on glutamate-induced cytotoxicity and apoptosis in differentiated PC12 cells. *Naunyn Schmiedebergs Arch. Pharmacol.* **2010**, *381*, 73–81. [CrossRef] [PubMed]

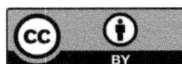

marine drugs

MDPI

Article

Chitosan Nanoparticles Act as an Adjuvant to Promote both Th1 and Th2 Immune Responses Induced by Ovalbumin in Mice

Zheng-Shun Wen, Ying-Lei Xu, Xiao-Ting Zou * and Zi-Rong Xu *

Key Laboratory for Molecular Animal Nutrition of Ministry of Education, Feed Science Institute, College of Animal Science, Zhejiang University (Huajiachi Campus), Qiutao North Road 164, Hangzhou 310029, China; ashun789@yahoo.cn (Z.-S.W.); 106413708@qq.com (Y.-L.X.)

* Authors to whom correspondence should be addressed; xtzou@zju.edu.cn (X.-T.Z.); ashun789@163.com (Z.-R.X.); Tel.: +86-571-86985824; Fax: +86-571-86994963.

Received: 1 May 2011; in revised form: 25 May 2011; Accepted: 7 June 2011; Published: 14 June 2011

Abstract: The study was conducted to investigate the promoted immune response to ovalbumin in mice by chitosan nanoparticles (CNP) and its toxicity. CNP did not cause any mortality or side effects when mice were administered subcutaneously twice with a dose of 1.5 mg at 7-day intervals. Institute of Cancer Research (ICR) mice were immunized subcutaneously with 25 μg ovalbumin (OVA) alone or with 25 μg OVA dissolved in saline containing Quil A (10 μg), chitosan (CS) (50 μg) or CNP (12.5, 50 or 200 μg) on days 1 and 15. Two weeks after the secondary immunization, serum OVA-specific antibody titers, splenocyte proliferation, natural killer (NK) cell activity, and production and mRNA expression of cytokines from splenocytes were measured. The serum OVA-specific IgG, IgG1, IgG2a, and IgG2b antibody titers and Con A-, LPS-, and OVA-induced splenocyte proliferation were significantly enhanced by CNP ($P < 0.05$) as compared with OVA and CS groups. CNP also significantly promoted the production of Th1 (IL-2 and IFN-γ) and Th2 (IL-10) cytokines and up-regulated the mRNA expression of IL-2, IFN-γ and IL-10 cytokines in splenocytes from the immunized mice compared with OVA and CS groups. Besides, CNP remarkably increased the killing activities of NK cells activity ($P < 0.05$). The results suggested that CNP had a strong potential to increase both cellular and humoral immune responses and elicited a balanced Th1/Th2 response, and that CNP may be a safe and efficacious adjuvant candidate suitable for a wide spectrum of prophylactic and therapeutic vaccines.

Keywords: chitosan nanoparticles; adjuvant; immune response; ovalbumin

1. Introduction

Vaccination remains the most effective and cost-efficient means to prevent infectious diseases. The latest trend towards novel and safer vaccines utilizes well-characterized antigens, like purified proteins, peptides, or carbohydrates. These so-called subunit vaccines enable the focusing of the immune response to the desired specificity without the risks associated with vaccines based on whole inactivated or live attenuated pathogens. Unfortunately, such subunit antigens are often poor immunogens when administered alone [1]. Therefore, an adjuvant is required to potentiate the immune response to the coadministered antigen.

However, strong adjuvant activity is often correlated with increased toxicity and adverse effects. The unique capacity of the extract Quil A from the bark of *Quillaja saponaria* and its purified saponin QS-21 to stimulate both the Th1 immune response and the production of cytotoxic T-lymphocyte against exogenous antigens makes them ideal for use in subunit vaccines and vaccines directed against intracellular pathogens as well as for therapeutic cancer vaccines [2,3]. However, in addition to pain on injection, severe local reactions and granulomas, toxicity includes severe haemolysis [4,7] making such adjuvants unsuitable for human uses other than for life threatening diseases, such as HIV infection or cancer [8]. Freund's complete adjuvant (FCA) remains amongst the most potent known adjuvants and a particularly powerful stimulant of both cellular and humoral immunities [9]. Unfortunately, FCA causes severe reactions and is too toxic for human use. Currently, aluminum compounds (Alum) is the only adjuvant in vaccines licensed by the Food and Drug Administration (FDA) for use in humans in the United States [10]. While Alum is safe, it is a relatively weak adjuvant, particularly when used with subunit antigens. Moreover, the Alum is a mild Th2 adjuvant that can effectively enhance IgG1 antibody responses, but it is rarely associated with Th1 type immune responses [11]. Furthermore, Alum is poor at stimulating cell-mediated immune responses, and may actively block activation and differentiation of cytotoxic T-lymphocytes [12]. Hence, there is a major unmet need for a safe and efficacious adjuvant capable of boosting cellular plus humoral immunity [13].

The ability of biodegradable microparticles to promote vaccine-specific immunity has been recognized for more than 80 years [14]. Early studies have demonstrated that the adjuvant potency may be amplified by the formation of nanoparticles with uptake by dendritic cells (DCs) [15,16], and this contributes to their enhancing effects on innate and antigen-specific cellular immunity [17]. Nanoparticles often exhibit significant adjuvant effects in parenteral vaccine delivery since they may be readily taken up by antigent presenting cells. The submicron size of nanoparticles allows them to be taken up by M-cells, in mucosa-associated lymphoid tissue (MALT), *i.e.*, gut-associated, nasal-associated and bronchus-associated lymphoid tissue, initiating sites of vigorous immunological responses [18]. However, the mechanism of action of particulate vaccine adjuvants is not fully understood [19], particularly for polymeric nanoparticles. Possible mechanisms have been suggested: that nanoparticles induce cytokine release by epithelial cells, shift the Th1/Th2 balance, activate macrophages and natural killer cells (NK) and improve the delayed-type hypersensitive reaction, increase cytotoxicity and induce mitosis in cells producing interleukins, breeding factors and interferon, or simply by increased absorption of antigen [20].

Chitosan is a natural nontoxic biopolymer produced by the deacetylation of chitin, a major component of the shells of crustaceans such as crab, shrimp, and crawfish. Recently, chitosan has received considerable attention for its commercial applications in the biomedical, food, and chemical industries [21,23]. The unique character of nanoparticles could make chitosan nanoparticles exhibit more superior activities than chitosan. Chitosan nanoparticles have been synthesized as drug and vaccine delivery carriers as reported in previous studies [24,25]. Due to their bioadhesive, biocompatibility, biodegradability and penetration-enhancement properties, chitosan nanoparticles are most efficiently taken up by phagocytotic cells inducing strong systemic and mucosal immune responses against antigens [20,26,27]. Besides enhancing the immune response by stimulating the uptake by phagocytotic cells, chitosan and its nanoparticles may also stimulate the immune system. Chitosan have been reported to have immune-stimulating activity such as increasing accumulation and activation of macrophage and polymorphonuclear cells, inducing cytokines after intravenous administration [28,33]. Therefore, the use of chitosan nano- and microparticles used as immunological adjuvants to induce both humoral and cell-mediated immunity is promising. However, the evaluation of chitosan nanoparticles as an adjuvant for subcutaneous vaccination has received less attention. Therefore, we hypothesized that chitosan nanoparticles (CNP) may have the adjuvant potential to amplify immune response against vaccination by stimulating the innate immune system. The present study was designed to evaluate the effect of CNP on the immune response induced by a model subunit antigen ovalbumin (OVA) in mice. OVA was used because this protein is considered to be an inert antigen with low capacity to modulate the immune response and is widely used as a model antigen. As a positive control, Quil A is known to be a potent adjuvant for experiment use.

2. Materials and Methods

2.1. Mice

Five-week-old female ICR mice (Grade II) weighing 18–22 g were purchased from Zhejiang Chinese Medical University Animal Research Center (Hangzhou, China) and acclimatized for one week prior to use. Rodent laboratory chow and tap water were provided *ad libitum* and maintained under controlled conditions with a temperature of 24 ± 1 °C, humidity of 50 ± 10%, and a 12/12 h light/dark cycle. All procedures related to the animals and their care conformed to the internationally accepted principles as found in the Guidelines for Keeping Experimental Animals issued by the government of China.

2.2. Chemicals and Cell Line

Chitosan (CS) was obtained from the Chitosan Company of Pan'an, Zhejiang, China (degree of deacetylation, 95%; average molecular weight, 220 kDa). Ovalbumin (OVA), concanavalin A (Con A), 3-(4,5-dimethylthiazol-2-yl)-2,5-diphenyltetrazolium bromide (MTT), lipopolysaccharide (LPS), RPMI-1640 medium, and rabbit anti-mouse IgG peroxidase conjugate were purchased from Sigma Chemical Co., Saint Louis, MO, USA; goat anti-mouse IgG1, IgG2a and IgG2b peroxidase conjugate were from Southern Biotech. Assoc., Birmingham, AL, USA; Quil A was kindly provided by BrenntagNordic A/S, Denmark. Fetal calf serum (FCS) was provided by Hangzhou Sijiqing Corp., Hangzhou, Zhejiang, China. Cytokines (IL-2, IL-10, IFN-γ) detecting ELISA kits were from Rapidbio Lab., West Hills, CA, USA. Trizol was from Invitrogen, China; revert Aid™ M-MuLV reverse transcriptase was from Fermentas, USA; diethylpyrocarbonate (DEPC) and ribonuclease inhibitor were from Biobasic, Canada; oligo (dT)$_{18}$ were from Sangon, China.

Human leukemia K562 cell lines, sensitive to natural killer (NK) cells, were purchased from the Institute of Cell Biology, Chinese Academy Sciences, Shanghai, China. They were maintained in the logarithmic phase of growth in RPMI 1640 medium supplemented with 2 mM L-glutamine (Sigma), 100 IU/mL penicillin, 100 g/mL streptomycin (Sigma), and 10% fetal calf serum at 37 °C under humidified air with 5% CO_2.

2.3. CNP Preparation and Characterization

Chitosan (CS) was obtained from the Chitosan Company of Pan'an (Zhejiang Province, China). The degree of deacetylation was about 95% as determined by elemental analysis, and the average molecular weight of the chitosan was 220 kDa as determined by viscometric methods [34]. Chitosan nanoparticles were prepared and characterized as previously described [35]. Briefly, Chitosan was dissolved at 0.5% (w/v) with 1% (v/v) acetic acid (HOAc) and then raised to pH 4.6–4.8 with 10 N NaOH. CNP were formed by coacervation between positively charged chitosan (0.5%, w/v) and negatively charged sodium tripolyphosphate (0.25%, w/v). Nanoparticles with different mean size were obtained by adjusting the volume ratio of chitosan to tripolyphosphate solution. Nanoparticles were purified by centrifugation at 9000 g for 30 min. Supernatants were discarded and chitosan nanoparticles were extensively rinsed with distilled water to remove any NaOH residues, and freeze dried before further use or analysis. The freeze-dried chitosan nanoparticles were suspended in water for characterization or use for other experiments. Particle size distribution and the zeta potential of chitosan nanoparticles were determined using Zetasizer Nano-ZS90 (Malvern Instruments). The analysis was performed at a scattering angle of 90° at a temperature of 25 °C using samples diluted to different concentration with de-ionized distilled water. Atomic force microscopy (AFM, SPM-9500J3) was used for visualization of the chitosan nanoparticles deposited on silicon substrates operating in the contact mode. AFM imaging was performed using Si_3N_4 probes with a spring constant of 0.06 N/m.

A stock CNP suspension or CS solution with a concentration of 3 mg/mL was prepared. The CNP was sterilized by passing it through a 0.22 μm Millipore filter, CS was autoclaved to remove any contaminant and then analyzed for endotoxin level by a gel-clot *Limulus* amebocyte lysate assay (Zhejiang A and C Biological, Zhejiang, China). The endotoxin level in the stock soln. was less than 0.5 EU/mL.

2.4. Toxicity Assays

Five-week-old female ICR mice were divided into five groups, each consisting of six mice. Animals were injected twice subcutaneously on the back with CNP at a single dose of 0.15, 0.3, 0.75, 1.5 mg in 0.5 mL saline solution at weekly intervals, and monitored daily for 14 days. Saline-treated animals were included as control and the toxicity was assessed by lethality, local swelling and loss of hair at the site of injection.

2.5. Immunization

Five-week-old female ICR mice were divided into six groups, each consisting of six mice. Animals were immunized subcutaneously with OVA (25 µg) alone or with OVA (25 µg) dissolved in saline containing QuilA (10 µg), or CS (50 µg) or CNP (12.5, 50, 200 µg) on day 1. The boosting injection was given 2 weeks later. Saline-treated animals were included as controls. Splenocytes and sera were collected 2 weeks after the secondary immunization for measurement of OVA-specific antibody, natural killer (NK) cell activity and proliferation assay.

2.6. Measurement of OVA-Specific IgG and Subclasses

OVA-specific IgG, IgG1, IgG2a, and IgG2b antibodies in sera were detected by an indirect ELISA. In brief, microtiter plate wells (Nunc) were coated with 100 µL OVA solution (25 µg/mL in 50 mM carbonate–bicarbonate buffer, pH 9.6) for 24 h at 4 °C. The wells were washed three times with PBS containing 0.05% (v/v) Tween 20 (PBS/Tween), and then blocked with 5% FCS/PBS at 37 °C for 2 h. After three washings, 100 µL of a series of diluted sera samples (initial dilution 1:50) or 0.5% FCS/PBS as control were added to triplicate wells. The plates were then incubated for 2 h at 37 °C, and then washed three times. Aliquots of 100 µL of rabbit anti-mouse IgG horseradish peroxidase conjugate diluted 1:10,000, goat anti-mouse IgG1 peroxidase conjugate 1:8000, IgG2a peroxidase conjugate 1:8000, and IgG2b peroxidase conjugate 1:8000 with 0.5% FCS/PBS were added to each plate. The plates were further incubated for 2 h at 37 °C. After washing, the peroxidase activity was assayed as follows: 100 µL of substrate solution (10 mg of O-phenylenediamine and 37.5 µL of 30% H_2O_2 in 25 mL of 0.1 M citrate–phosphate buffer, pH 5.0) was added to each well. The plate was incubated for 10 min at 37 °C, and enzyme reaction was terminated by adding 50 µL/well of 2 N H_2SO_4. The optical density was measured in an ELISA reader at 490 nm, where sets of sera samples have been subjected to within and between group comparisons, ELISA assays were performed on the same day for all of the samples.

2.7. Assay of Natural Killer (NK) Cell Activity

Spleen collected from the OVA-immunized mice under aseptic conditions, in Hank's balanced salt solution (HBSS, Sigma), was minced using a pair of scissors and passed through a fine steel mesh to obtain a homogeneous cell suspension. The erythrocytes were lysed with ammonium chloride (0.8%, w/v). After centrifugation (380× g at 4 °C for 10 min), the pelleted cells were washed three times in PBS, and resuspended in complete medium. Cell numbers were counted with a hemocytometer by trypan blue dye exclusion technique. Cell viability exceeded 95%. The activity of NK cells was measured as previously described [36]. Briefly, K562 cells were used as target cells and seeded in 96-well U-bottom microtiter plate (Costar) at 1×10^5 cells/well in RPMI 1640 complete medium. Splenocytes prepared were used as the effector cells, and were added at 5×10^6 cells/well to give E/T ratio 50:1. The plates were then incubated for 20 h at 37 °C in 5% CO_2 atmosphere. 50 µL of MTT solution (2 mg/mL) was added to each well and the plate was incubated for another 4 h and subjected to MTT assay. Three kinds of control measurements were performed: Target cells control, blank control and effector cells control. NK cell activity was calculated as the following equation: NK activity (%) = (ODT − (ODS − ODE))/ODT × 100, where ODT is the optical density value of target cells control; ODS is the optical density value of test samples; and ODE is the optical density value of effector cells control.

2.8. Splenocyte Proliferation Assay

Spleen collected from the OVA-immunized mice under aseptic conditions, in Hank's balanced salt solution (HBSS, Sigma), was minced using a pair of scissors and passed through a fine steel mesh to obtain a homogeneous cell suspension, and the erythrocytes were lysed with ammonium chloride (0.8%, w/v). After centrifugation (380× g at 4 °C for 10 min), the pelleted cells were washed three times in PBS, and resuspended in complete medium. Cell numbers were counted with a haemocytometer by trypan blue dye exclusion technique. Cell viability exceeded 95%. Splenocyte proliferation was assayed as previously described [37]. Briefly, splenocytes from each mouse were seeded into four wells of a 96-well flat-bottom microtiter plate at 5×10^6 cell/mL in 100 μL of complete medium. Con A (final concentration 5 μg/mL), LPS (final concentration 10 μg/mL), OVA (final concentration 30 μg/mL), or medium were then added, giving a final volume of 200 μL. The plates were incubated at 37 °C in a humid atmosphere with 5% CO_2. After 44 h, 50 μL of MTT solution (2 mg/mL) was added to each well and incubated for further 4 h. The plates were centrifuged (1400× g, 5 min) and the untransformed MTT was removed carefully by pipetting. 150 μL of a DMSO working solution (192 μL DMSO with 8 μL 1 N HCl) was added to each well, and the absorbance was evaluated in an ELISA reader at 570 nm with a 630 nm reference after 15 min. The stimulation index (SI) was calculated based on the following formula: SI = the absorbance value for mitogen-cultures divided by the absorbance value for non-stimulated cultures.

2.9. Cytokine Determination in the Cultured Supernatants of Splenocytes by ELISA

Splenocytes (5×10^5 cells/well) from the immunized mice prepared as described before were incubated with ConA (final concentration 5 μg/mL) in 24-well culture plates at 37 °C in 5% CO_2. After 48 h, the plate was centrifuged at 1400× g for 5 min and culture supernatants were collected for the determination of INF-γ, IL-2, IL-10 levels. The presence of INF-γ, IL-2, IL-10 in the cultured supernatants of splenocytes were determined using the mouse ELISA kits (Rapidbio Lab., West Hills, CA, USA).

2.10. Reversed Transcript-Polymerase Chain Reaction (RT-PCR) for Cytokines Gene Expression

Splenocytes from the immunized mice prepared as described before were seeded into 24-well lat-bottom microtiter plate (Nunc) at 5×10^6 cell/mL in 1 mL complete medium, then ConA (final concentration 5 μg/mL) was added giving a final volume of 2 mL (triplicate wells). The plates were incubated at 37 °C in a humidified atmosphere 5% CO_2. After 12 h treatment, cells were collected by centrifugation (380× g at 4 °C for 10 min), and washed with ice-cold PBS, then subjected to RNA extraction. Cells were lysed in 0.8 mL of Trizol reagent (Invitrogen, China) and the total RNA was isolated according to the manufacture's protocol. The concentration of total RNA was quantified by determining the optical density at 260 nm. The total RNA was used and reverse transcription was performed by mixing 2 μg of RNA with 0.5 μg oligo (dT)$_{18}$ primer in a DEPC-treated tube. Nuclease-free water was added giving a final volume of 12.5 μL. This mixture was incubated at 70 °C for 5 min and chilled on ice for 2 min. Then, a solution containing 4 μL of M-MuLV 5× reaction buffer, 2 μL of 10 mM dNTP, 20 U of ribonuclease inhibitor, and DEPC-treated water was added, giving a final volume of 19 μL, and the tubes were incubated for 5 min at 37 °C. The tubes then received 200 U of M-MuLV reverse transcriptase and were incubated for 60 min at 42 °C. Finally, the reaction was stopped by heating at 70 °C for 10 min. The samples were stored at −20 °C until further use.

As shown in Table 1, the primers were used to amplify cDNA fragments (381-bp IL-2 fragment, 460-bp IFN-γ fragment, 324-bp IL-10 fragment and 564-bp GAPDH fragment). Amplification was carried out in total volume of 50 μL containing 4 μL (10 μM) of each cytokine-specific primers, 5 μL of 10× PCR buffer, 4 μL of MgCl$_2$ (25 mM), 4 μL of dNTPs (2.5 mM), 2 μL of transcribed cDNA, and 0.25 μL of Taq DNA polymerase. PCR was performed for 33 (IL-2), 32 (IFN-γ), 30 (IL-10) or 28 (GAPDH) cycles using a MyCycler (Bio-Rad, Hercules, CA) with the following program of denaturation at 94 °C for 5 min, following by indicated cycles of 94 °C for 30 s, annealing at 58 °C (GAPDH), 60 °C (IL-2), 62 °C (IL-10), 63 °C (IFN-γ) for 30 s, and elongation at 72 °C for 30 s, and a final extension step at 72 °C for 10 min. Semi-quantitative RT-PCR was performed using GAPDH as a house keeping gene to normalize gene expression for the PCR templates. The PCR products were studied on a 1.5% agarose gel and the amplified bands were visualized using Gel DOC2000 (Bio-Rad, USA) after staining with GoldView. The size of the amplification fragments was determined by comparison with a standard DNA marker. The relative level of cytokine expression is calculated for 100 copies of the GAPDH house keeping gene following the formula: $n = 100 \times$ (the intensity of cytokine gene expression band/the intensity of GAPDH band).

Table 1. Sequences of primer used for Reversed Transcript-Polymerase Chain Reaction (RT-PCR). GAPDH, glyceraldehyde-3-phosphate dehydrogenase.

Gene	Primer sequence	Product size (bp)
IL-2	5′-CTCTACAGCGGAAGCACAGC-3′ 5′-CATCTCCTCAGAAAGTCCACCA-3′	381
IFN-γ	5′-TGAACGCTACACACTGCATCTTGG-3′ 5′-CGACTCCTTTTCCGCTTCCTGAG-3′	460
IL-10	5′-CCAGTTTTACCTGGTAGAAGTGATG-3′ 5′-TGTCTAGGTCCTGGAGTCCAGCAGACTCAA-3′	324
GAPDH	5′-CCCACAGTAAATTCAACGGCAC-3′ 5′-CATTGGGGGTTAGGAACACGGA-3′	564

2.11. Statistical Analysis

Data were expressed as mean ± standard deviations (S.D.) and examined for their statistical significance of difference with ANOVA and a Tukey post hoc test by using SPSS 16.0. *P*-values of less than 0.05 were considered statistically significant.

3. Results

3.1. Morphology, Size and Zeta Potential of CNP

As shown in Figure 1, chitosan nanoparticles regularly formed and well distributed in acetic acid (HOAc)/sodium tripolyphosphate solution (pH 5.5) were used in this study. The mean size and size distribution of each batch of nanoparticle suspension was analyzed using the Zetasizer analysis (Figure 1). The size distribution profile represents a typical batch of nanoparticles with a mean diameter of 83.66 nm and a narrow size distribution ranging from 63.16 to 101.70 nm (polydispersity index <1), and shows that the surfaces of chitosan nanoparticles have a positive surface charge of about 35.43 mV. These excellent characteristics are of benefit to the stabilization and penetration capability of CNP, enabling CNP to easily penetrate through capillary and epithelial tissue.

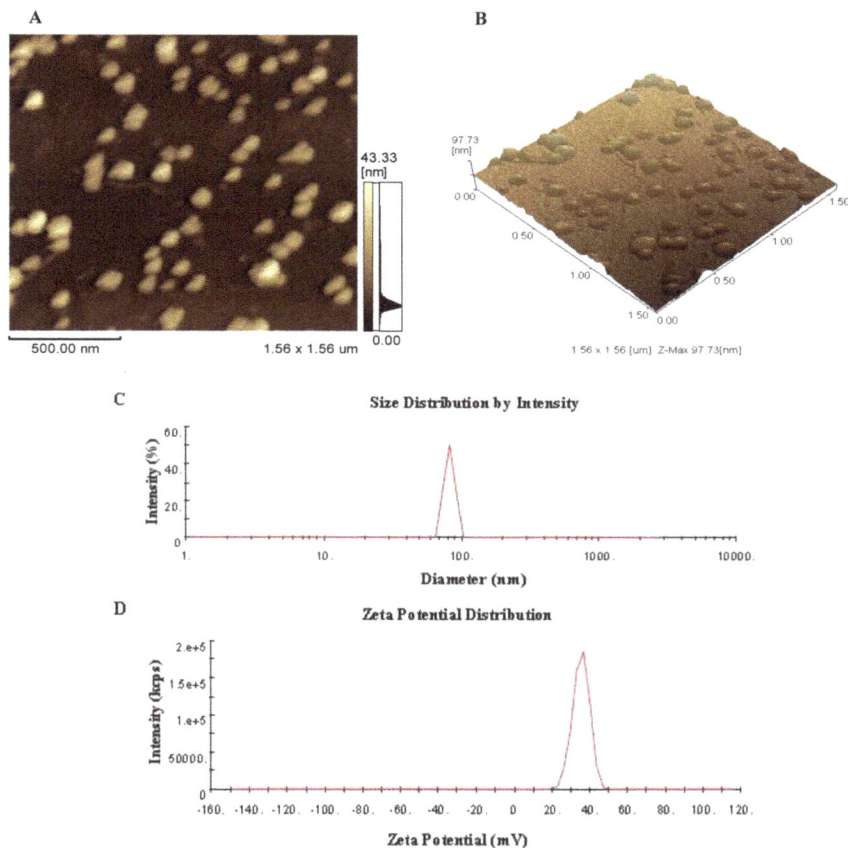

Figure 1. Morphology of chitosan nanoparticles (CNP). (**A**, **B**) atomic force micrographs (AFMs) of CNP; (**C**) the size distribution by intendity of CNP, the size of CNP ranges from 63.16 to 101.70 nm, and the mean of size is about 83.66 nm; (**D**) Zeta potential distribution of CNP, CNP exhibit a zeta potential range from 20.04 to 51.13 mV and have a mean charge with 35.43 mV.

3.2. Toxicity of CNP

The endotoxin level in a stock CNP with a concentration of 3 mg/mL was measured to be less than 0.5 endotoxin units (EU)/mL. Therefore, the CNP samples used in this study were excluded from endotoxin contamination. When the animals were administered subcutaneously twice ranging from 0.15 to 1.5 mg at weekly intervals, no harm was observed. Local swelling or loss of hair was not observed in mice at the test doses. The results suggested that the safety dose of CNP used for animals was at least up to 60 mg/kg.

3.3. Effect of CNP on the OVA-Specific Serum Antibody Response

The OVA-specific IgG, IgG1, IgG2a and IgG2b antibody levels in the serum were measured by the indirect ELISA method two weeks after the last immunization (Figure 2). As a positive control, QuilA elicited the highest IgG and IgG isotypes levels. The serum IgG and IgG1 levels in mice immunized with OVA were significantly enhanced by CNP compared with the control groups (OVA and CS) ($P < 0.05$). Moreover, significant enhancements in OVA-specific IgG2a and IgG2b levels were observed

101

in mice immunized with CNP compared with the OVA and CS control group ($P < 0.05$), and there were significant differences among CNP at all doses and QuilA ($P < 0.05$).

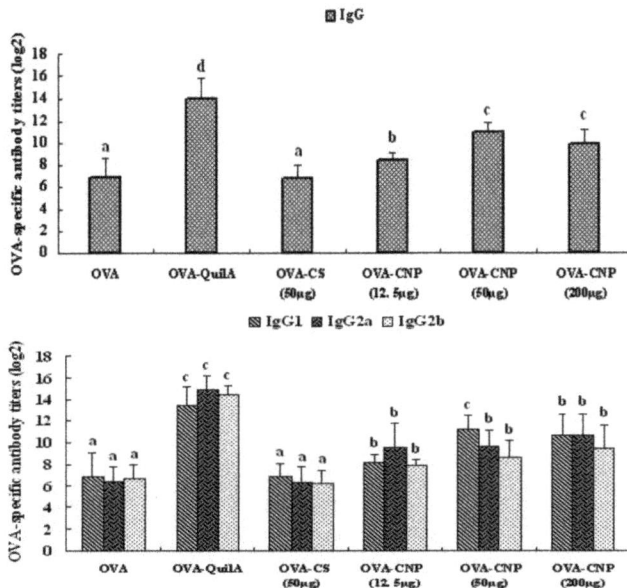

Figure 2. Effect of CNP on OVA-specific IgG, IgG1, IgG2a and IgG2b antibody titers in OVA-immunized mice. Mice ($n = 6$/group) were subcutaneously injected with OVA (25 µg) alone or with OVA 25 (µg) dissolved in saline containing CNP (12.5, 50 or 200 µg), CS (50 µg) or QuilA (10 µg) on days 1 and 15. Sera were collected 2 weeks after the secondary immunizations for analysis these OVA-specific antibodies using indirect ELISA. Bar with different letters are statistically different ($P < 0.05$). Abbreviations: QuilA: mixture of triterpene saponins from the bark of *Quillaja saponaria* Molina.

3.4. Effect of CNP on Natural Killer (NK) Cell Activity in OVA-Immunized Mice

The effects of CNP on natural killer (NK) cell activity in OVA-immunized mice were shown in Figure 3. CNP and Quil A significantly enhanced the killing activity of NK cell in the OVA-immunized mice ($P < 0.05$). The findings indicated that CNP could promote lytic activity of NK cells in mice immunized with OVA.

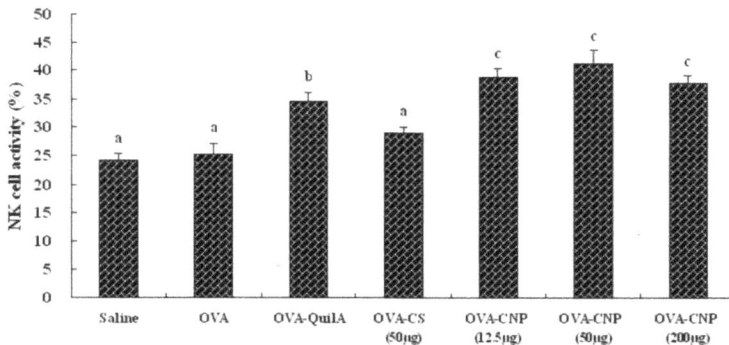

Figure 3. Effect of CNP on NK cell activity in mice immunized with OVA. Mice (*n* = 6/group) were subcutaneously injected with OVA (25 µg) alone or with OVA 25 µg dissolved in saline containing CNP (12.5, 50 or 200 µg), CS (50 µg) or QuilA (10 µg) on days 1 and 15. Bars with different letters are statistically different (*P* < 0.05).

3.5. Effect of CNP on Splenocyte Proliferation in OVA-Immunized Mice

The effects of CNP and QuilA on splenocyte proliferative responses to ConA, LPS and OVA stimulation are shown in Figure 4. Mice immunized with OVA plus CNP or QuilA had higher splenocyte proliferative response to ConA, LPS and OVA than the mice injected with OVA alone (*P* < 0.05). Mice immunized with OVA plus CNP also had higher ConA-, LPS- and OVA-stimulated splenocyte proliferative response than the mice injected with OVA plus CS (*P* < 0.05).

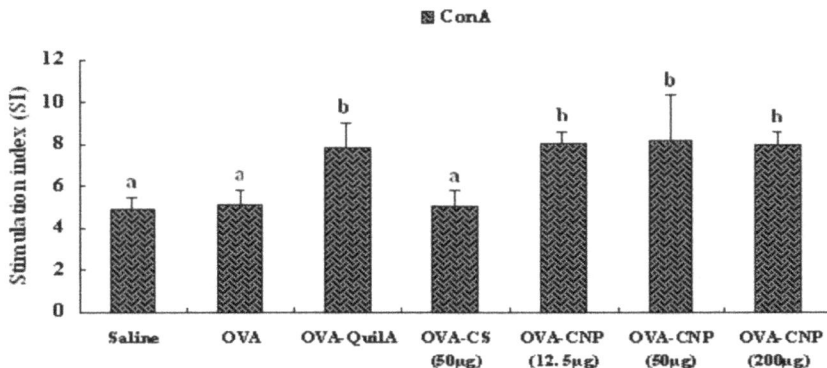

Figure 4. *Cont.*

103

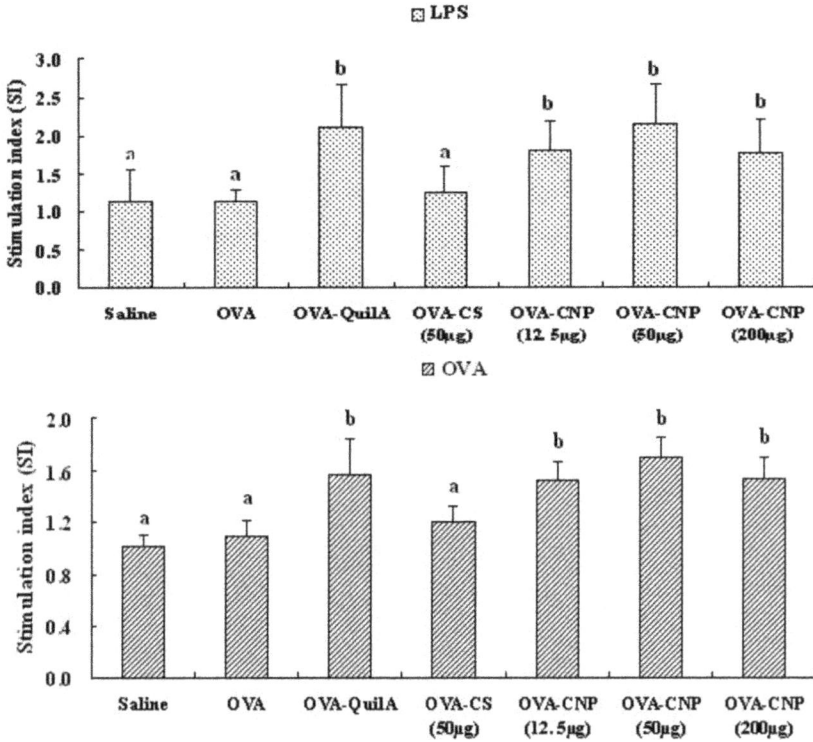

Figure 4. Effect of CNP on mitogen- and OVA-stimulated splenocyte proliferation in the mice immunized with OVA. Bars with different letters are statistically different ($P < 0.05$).

3.6. Effect of CNP on Cytokines Level in Splenocytes from the OVA-Immunized Mice

The contents of cytokines IFN-γ, IL-2 and IL-10 in the supernatants from cultured splenocytes in the mice immunized with OVA-CNP were significantly higher than those in OVA and OVA-CS control mice ($P < 0.05$) (Figure 5). QuilA enhanced significantly the production of cytokine IL-10 (Th 2 type immune response), IFN-γ and IL-2 (Th 1 type immune response) ($P < 0.05$) in the supernatants from cultured splenocytes in the mice immunized with OVA. These results suggested that CNP significantly enhanced the production of the Th1 and Th2 cytokines in OVA-immunized mice, and CNP markedly improved the adjuvant activity of chitosan in the OVA-immunized mice.

☒ IFN-γ ▨ IL-2 ☐ IL-10

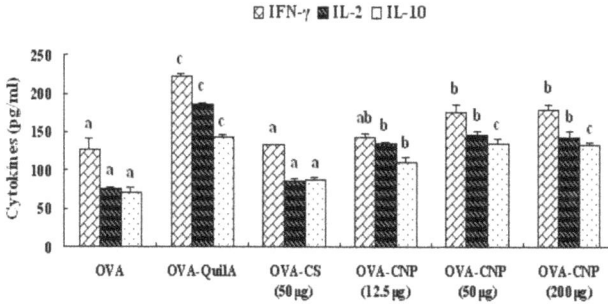

Figure 5. Effects of CNP on cytokine production in splenocytes from the OVA-immunized mice. Splenocytes were prepared and cultured with Con A for 48 h. The levels of IL-2, IFN-γ and IL-10 in the culture supernatants were determined by ELISA as described in the text. Values are expressed as means ± S.D. of six animals. Bars with different letters are statistically different (*P* < 0.05).

3.7. Effect of CNP on mRNA Expression of Cytokines in Splenocytes from the Immunized Mice

As shown in Figure 6 and Table 2, CNP and QuilA not only significantly increased the mRNA expression of Th1 cytokines IL-2 and IFN-γ (*P* < 0.05), but also enhanced that of Th2 cytokines IL-10 in splenocytes from the immunized mice (*P* < 0.05). Therefore, the findings suggested that CNP up-regulated the gene expression of Th1/Th2 cytokines in splenocytes from the immunized mice.

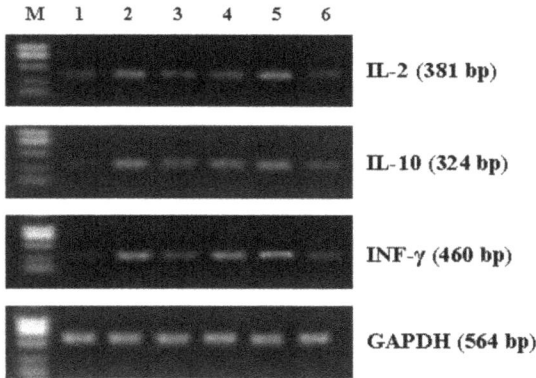

Figure 6. Eeffect of CNP on the mRNA expression of cytokines and GAPDH in splenocytes from the OVA-immunized mice. Lane M, DNA marker; lane 1, OVA; lane 2, QuilA; lane 3, OVA-CNP (12.5 µg); lane 4, OVA-CNP (50 µg); lane 5, OVA-CNP (200 µg); lane 6, OVA-CS (50 µg).

Table 2. The mRNA expression level of cytokines in splenocytes from the OVA-immunized mice.

Gene	OVA	OVA-QuilA	OVA-CNP			OVA-CS
			(12.5 µg)	(50 µg)	(200 µg)	(50 µg)
IL-2	15.0 ± 1.4 [a]	45.6 ± 2.1 [c]	26.6 ± 1.4 [b]	38.8 ± 2.1 [bc]	50.6 ± 2.2 [c]	16.0 ± 1.2 [a]
IFN-γ	15.8 ± 1.6 [a]	40.4 ± 2.3 [c]	29.0 ± 1.4 [b]	38.8 ± 2.3 [bc]	44.0 ± 2.5 [c]	16.0 ± 1.6 [a]
IL-10	15.0 ± 1.4 [a]	45.0 ± 2.7 [c]	22.4 ± 1.8 [ab]	30.4 ± 2.2 [b]	44.8 ± 2.7 [c]	18.2 ± 1.7 [a]

Means within a row with different letters (a, b, c) differ significantly (*P* < 0.05).

4. Discussion

Immunization has been the most effective way to protect individuals and the community against debilitating infectious diseases, thereby preventing the potential economic losses and morbidity associated with such diseases [25]. New generations of vaccines, particularly those based on purified recombinant proteins, synthetic peptides and plasmid DNA, despite their better tolerability, are unfortunately often much less reactogenic and immunogenic. Therefore, there is an urgent need for the development of new and improved vaccine adjuvants [38]. Although a variety of adjuvants have been used in experimental vaccines, most of these materials only elicit an antibody response and/or have undesirable side effects that have limited their potential application in vaccines [39,40].

In the previous studies, chitosan particles could activate components of the nonspecific immune system such as macrophages and NK cells, and could induce nonspecific immunity to bacteria, fungi, and tumors [28,41,42]. In addition, Chitosan particles can also activate dendritic cells (DCs) via the membrane receptors (TLR4 and mannose receptors) [43]. DCs are thought to be the most effective antigen-presenting cells (APCs) in immune response, although macrophages can also function in this role. Activated DCs lead to cytokine production, increase levels of membrane markers, such as major histocompatibility complex class II molecules, and possess the capacity to activate naive T cells. Furthermore, Chitosan micro- and nanoparticles have been reported to have immune-stimulating activity such as increasing accumulation and activation of macrophage and polymorphonuclear cell, promoting resistance to infections by microorganisms, and inducing cytokines [44]. These studies indicated that chitosan particles could stimulate macrophage, DCs, B and T lymphocytes. Therefore, the ability of chitosan nanoparticles used as immunological adjuvants to induce both humoral and cell-mediated immunity seems promising. To further research the safer adjuvant, the present study was undertaken to evaluate the toxicity of CNP and its adjuvant potential on the cellular and humoral immune responses of mice against OVA.

The cellular immune response plays an important role in the host response to intracellular pathogens by limiting replication and accelerating clearance of infected cells as well as in the generation of both humoral and cell-mediated responses to vaccination. Among the T-lymphocytes, helper T cells induce B-lymphocytes to secrete antibodies, and cytotoxic T-lymphocytes help phagocytes to destroy ingested microbes and to kill intracellular microbes. Humoral immunity, however, mediated by antibodies which are produced by B-lymphocytes, functions by neutralizing and eliminating extracellular microbes and microbial toxins. The capacity to elicit an effective T- and B-lymphocyte immunity can be shown by the stimulation of lymphocyte proliferation response. It is generally known that Con A stimulates T cells and LPS stimulates B cell proliferation [45]. We evaluated whether CNP could enhance the cellular immune responses to OVA in mice when given together with OVA. As a positive control, QuilA is known to be a powerful experimental adjuvant, and significantly elicited the mitogen- and OVA-stimulated splenocyte profilerations in OVA-immunized mice [45]. As shown in Figure 4, CNP and QuilA significantly enhanced the mitogen- and OVA-stimulated splenocyte profilerations in OVA-immunized mice as compared with OVA and CS groups, while there was no significant difference between CNP and QuilA. The proliferation assay showed that CNP could significantly promote the Con A-, LPS-, and OVA-stimulated splenocyte proliferation in the immunized mice. The results indicated that CNP could significantly increase the activation potential of T and B cells, and induce the humoral immunity and cell-mediated immune response in the OVA-immunized mice.

Evidence now exists to clearly suggest that Th1 or Th2 responses, generated upon antigenic stimulation, can be modulation *in vivo* depending on the adjuvant used for immunization [46,47]. The different Th1 and Th2 immune response profiles correspond to the activation of two distinct major subsets of T-cells characterized by their pattern of cytokine production [48]. The Th1 immune response is characterized by the production of cytokines IL-2, TNF-β and IFN-γ, and an enhanced production of IgG2a, IgG2b, IgG3 in mice. The Th2 response is characterized by the production of cytokines IL-4, IL-10 and an enhanced production of IgG1 [49]. Immunity to different infectious agents required distinct types of immune responses. The Th1 response, correlated with the induction of cell-mediated immunity [50], is required for protective immunity against intracellular infectious agents, such as certain bacteria, protozoa and presumably against cancer cells [51]. Th2 immunity, which control the humoral immune response through the triggering of B cell proliferation and differentiation [52], is effective for protection against most bacterial as well as certain viral infections [53]. In the present study, the adjuvant activity of CNP on the humoral immune responses to OVA was also evaluated. While OVA alone induced low levels of IgG, IgG1, IgG2a and IgG2b antibodies (Figure 2), the addition of CNP to OVA resulted in dramatic increase in IgG, IgG1, IgG2a and IgG2b antibody titers. Meanwhile, as a positive control group, QuilA could also increase IgG, IgG1, IgG2a and IgG2b antibody titers, resulting in a mixed Th1/Th2 immune response. Thus, in addition to enhancing the magnitude of antibody responses, CNP also modulated the quality of the immune responses, and elicited a balanced Th1/Th2 immune response to OVA in mice as indicated by the significant increases in both IgG1, IgG2a and IgG2b antibody isotypes.

In order to clearly establish that Th cell-derived cytokines were involved in the adjuvant activity of CNP, we analysed the Th1/Th2 cytokines secretion profiles in OVA-immunized mice using ELISA. CNP not only significantly enhanced the production of Th2 cytokine IL-10, but also strongly increased the production of Th1 cytokines IL-2 and IFN-γ from splenocytes in the OVA-immunized mice (Figure 5). To further elucidate the mechanism responsible for the changes in the amounts of Th1/Th2 cytokines, we utilized RT-PCR to analyse the mRNA expression of IL-2 and IFN-γ, the typical Th1 cytokines, and IL-10, the archetypal Th2 cytokine in splenocytes of the immunized mice. CNP not only enhanced the mRNA expression of IL-10, but also increased that of IL-2 and IFN-γ. Cytokines mRNA levels were positively correlated with protein expression of cytokines, *i.e.*, the levels of cytokines. In this study, CNP significantly enhanced the levels of cytokines (IL-2, IFN-γ and IL-10) in OVA-immunized mice. In mice, IL-10 preferentially switch activated B cells to the IgG1 isotype (Th2 type); IFN-γ and IL-2 enhanced IgG2a and IgG2b response (Th1 type) [54]. These results suggested that the effects of CNP on Th1 and Th2 immune response may result, at least in part, from the regulation of mRNA expression of the cytokines.

Natural killer cells (NK cells) are the type of cytotoxic lymphocyte that constitute the major component of the innate immune system. NK cells and CTL play the important role in the defense against tumors and cells infected by viruses [55,57], and moreover, represent two major populations of cytotoxic lymphocytes [58,59]. With spontaneous cell-mediated cytotoxicities, NK cells are also functionally similar to CTLs. NK cells are capable of delivering a response immediately after recognizing specific signals, including stress signals, "danger" signals or signals from molecules of foreign origin [60]. NK cells can react against and destroy a target cell without prior sensitization to it. The target cell could be a cancer cell cultured *in vitro* or from another tissue. NK cell activity assay is a routine method for analysis of a patient's cellular immune response *in vitro*, and can also be used to test the antitumor activities of possible drugs [61]. In this investigation, as shown in Figure 3, CNP significantly enhanced the lytic activity of NK cells in OVA immunized mice, suggesting that CNP could improve cytolytic activities against autologous tumor cells and viruses.

5. Conclusions

Based on the findings presented herein, our data suggested that CNP has immunological adjuvant activity on the specific cellular and humoral immune responses to OVA in mice. Taking account of its natural origin and good biocompatibility, and without lethal toxicity to humans and animals, CNP may be a safe and efficacious adjuvant candidate suitable for a wide spectrum of prophylactic and therapeutic vaccines, for which a balanced and potent stimulation of both the cellular and humoral responses is required. Research on CNP with various types of antigen, including vaccines clinically used in other animal models, verify the adjuvant effect. Moreover, the mechanism of the action of CNP has still not clearly been explained. Therefore, more studies on the mechanism of the adjuvant effect of CNP are needed to elucidate in more detail.

Acknowledgments: We thank Hongxiang Sun for donating the OVA antigen and antibodies for ELISA test, Jun Liu for technical assistance in gene expression, and Mahmoud Azzam for checking language.

References

1. Kammer, AR; Amacker, M; Rasi, S; Westerfeld, N; Gremion, C; Neuhaus, D; Zurbriggen, R. A new and versatile virosomal antigen delivery system to induce cellular and humoral immune responses. *Vaccine* **2007**, *25*, 7065–7074.

2. Kensil, CR; Kammer, R. QS-21: Awater-soluble triterpene glycoside adjuvant. *Expert Opin Investig Drugs* **1998**, *7*, 1475–1482.

3. Skene, CD; Sutton, P. Saponin-adjuvanted particulate vaccines for clinical use. *Methods* **2006**, *40*, 53–59.

4. Gupta, RK; Relyveld, EH; Lindblad, EB; Bizzini, B; Ben-Efraim, S; Gupta, CK. Adjuvants: A balance between toxicity and adjuvanticity. *Vaccine* **1993**, *11*, 293–306.

5. Kensil, CR; Patel, U; Lennick, M; Marciani, D. Separation and characterization of saponins with adjuvant activity from Quillaja saponaria Molina cortex. *J Immunol* **1991**, *146*, 431–437.

6. Kensil, CR; Wu, JY; Soltysik, S. Structural and immunological characterization of the vaccine adjuvant QS-21. *Pharm Biotechnol* **1995**, *6*, 525–541.

7. Waite, DC; Jacobson, EW; Ennis, FA; Edelman, R; White, B; Kammer, R; Anderson, C; Kensil, CR. Three double-blind, randomized trials evaluating the safety and tolerance of different formulations of the saponin adjuvant QS-21. *Vaccine* **2001**, *19*, 3957–3967.

8. Janeway, CA, Jr. The immune system evolved to discriminate infectious nonself from noninfectious self. *Immunol Today* **1992**, *13*, 11–16.

9. Freund, J; Casals, J; Hosmer, E. Sensitization and antibody formation after injection of tubercle bacili and paraffin oil. *Proc Soc Exp Biol Med* **1937**, *37*, 509–513.

10. Pascual, DM; Morales, RD; Gil, ED; Muñoz, LM; López, JE; Casanueva, OLJ. Adjuvants: Present regulatory challenges. *Vaccine* **2006**, *24*, S88–S89.

11. HogenEsch, H. Mechanisms of stimulation of the immune response by aluminum adjuvants. *Vaccine* **2002**, *20*, S34–S39.

12. Schirmbeck, R; Melber, K; Kuhrber, A; Janowicz, ZA; Reimann, J. Immunization with soluble hepatitis B virus surface protein elicits murine H-2 class I-restricted CD8+ cytotoxic T lymphocyte responses *in vivo*. *J Immunol* **1994**, *152*, 1110–1119.

13. Petrovsky, N. Novel human polysaccharide adjuvants with dual Th1 and Th2 potentiating activity. *Vaccine* **2006**, *24*, S26–S29.

14. Glenny, A; Pope, C; Waddington, H; Falacce, U. The antigenic value of toxoid precipitated by potassium alum. *J Pathol Bacteriol* **1926**, *29*, 31–40.

15. Morein, B; Sundquist, B; Hoglund, S; Dalsgaad, K; Osterhaus, A. Iscom, a novel structure for antigenic presentation of membrane proteins from enveloped viruses. *Nature* **1984**, *308*, 457–460.

16. Pearse, MJ; Drane, D. ISCOMATRIX adjuvant for antigen delivery. *Adv Drug Deliv Rev* **2005**, *57*, 465–474.

17. Sharp, FA; Ruane, D; Claass, B; Creagh, E; Harris, J; Malyala, P; Singh, M; O'Hagan, DT; Pétrilli, V; Tschopp, J; et al. Uptake of particulate vaccine adjuvants by dendritic cells activates the NALP3 inflammasome. *Proc Natl Acad Sci USA* **2009**, *106*, 870–875.

18. Sailaja, AK; Amareshwar, P; Chakravarty, P. Chitosan nanoparticles as a drug delivery system. *Res J Pharm Biol Chem Sci* **2010**, *1*, 474–484.

19. Dinarello, CA. Blocking IL-1 in systemic inflammation. *J Exp Med* **2005**, *201*, 1355–1359.

20. van der Lubben, IM; Verhoef, JC; Borchard, G; Junginger, HE. Chitosan and its derivatives in mucosal drug and vaccine delivery. *Eur J Pharm Sci* **2001**, *14*, 201–207.

21. Knorr, D. Use of chitinous polymers in foodda challenge for food research and development. *Food Technol* **1984**, *38*, 85–97.

22. Kurita, K. Chemistry and application of chitin and chitosan. *Polym Degrad Stab* **1998**, *59*, 117–120.

23. Razdan, A; Pettersson, D. Effect of chitin and chitosan on nutrient digestibility and plasma lipid concentrations in broiler chickens. *Br J Nutr* **1994**, *72*, 277–288.

24. van der Lubben, IM; Verhoef, JC; Borchard, G; Junginger, HE. Chitosan microparticles for oral vaccination: Preparation, characterization and preliminary *in vivo* uptake studies in murine Peyer's patches. *Biomaterials* **2001**, *22*, 687–694.

25. De Campos, AM; Sanchez, A; Alonso, MJ. Chitosan nanoparticles: A new vehicle for the improvement of the delivery of drugs to the ocular surface. Application to cyclosporin A. *Int J Pharm* **2001**, *224*, 159–168.

26. Illum, L; Jabbal-Gill, I; Hinchcliffe, M; Fisher, AN; Davis, SS. Chitosan as a novel nasal delivery system for vaccines. *Adv Drug Deliv Rev* **2001**, *51*, 81–96.

27. Zhu, B; Qie, Y; Wang, J; Zhang, Y; Wang, Q; Xu, Y; Wang, H. Chitosan microspheres enhance the immunogenicity of an Ag85B-based fusion protein containing multiple T-cell epitopes of Mycobacterium tuberculosis. *Eur J Pharm Biopharm* **2007**, *66*, 318–326.

28. Nishimura, K; Nishimura, S; Nishi, N; Saiki, I; Tokura, S; Azuma, I. Immunological activity of chitin and its derivatives. *Vaccine* **1984**, *2*, 93–99.

29. Suzuki, K; Mikami, T; Okawa, Y; Tokoro, A; Suzuki, S; Suzuki, M. Antitumor effect of hexa-*N*-acetylchitohexaose and chitohexaose. *Carbohydr Res* **1986**, *151*, 403–408.

30. Tokoro, A; Tatewaki, N; Suzuki, K; Mikami, T; Suzuki, S; Suzuki, M. Growth-inhibitory effect of hexa-*N*-acetylchitohexaose and chitohexaose against meth-A solid tumor. *Chem Pharm Bull* **1988**, *36*, 784–790.

31. Calvo, P; Remunan-Lopez, C; Vila-Jato, JL; Alonso, MJ. Chitosan and chitosan: Ethylene oxide-propylene oxide block copolymer nanoparticles as novel carriers and vaccines. *Pharm Res* **1997**, *14*, 1431–1436.

32. Shimbata, Y; Foster, LA; Metzger, WJ; Myrvik, QN. Alveolar macrophage priming by intravenous administration of chitin particles, polymers of *N*-acetyl-D-glucosamine, in mice. *Infect Immun* **1997**, *65*, 1734–1741.

33. Seferian, PG; Martinez, ML. Immune stimulating activity of two new chitosan containing adjuvant formulations. *Vaccine* **2000**, *19*, 661–668.

34. Qurashi, T; Blair, HS; Alen, SJJ. Studies on modified chitosan membranes. I. Preparation and characterization. *J Appl Polym Sci* **1992**, *46*, 255–261.

35. Qi, L; Xu, Z; Jiang, X; Hu, C; Zou, X. Preparation and antibacterial activity of chitosan nanoparticles. *Carbohydr Res* **2004**, *339*, 2693–2700.

36. Tu, J; Sun, HX; Ye, YP. Immunomodulatory and antitumor activity of triterpenoid fractions from the rhizomes of Astilbe chinensis. *J Ethnopharmacol* **2008**, *119*, 266–271.

37. Sun, HX; Ye, YP; Pan, HJ; Pan, YJ. Adjuvant effect of Panax notoginseng saponins on the immune responses to ovalbumin in mice. *Vaccine* **2004**, *22*, 3882–3889.

38. O'Hagan, DT; MacKichan, ML; Singh, M. Recent developments in adjuvants for vaccines against infectious diseases. *Biomol Eng* **2001**, *18*, 69–85.

39. Aucouturier, J; Dupuis, L; Ganne, V. Adjuvants designed for veterinary and human vaccines. *Vaccine* **2001**, *19*, 2666–2672.

40. Hunter, RL. Overview of vaccine adjuvants: Present and future. *Vaccine* **2002**, *20*(Suppl. 3), S7–S12.

41. Suzuki, K; Okawa, Y; Hashimoto, K; Suzuki, S; Suzuki, M. Protecting effect of chitin and chitosan on experimentally induced murine candidiasis. *Microbiol Immunol* **1984**, *28*, 903–912.

42. Peluso, G; Petillo, O; Ranieri, M; Santin, M; Ambrosio, L; Calabro, D; Avallone, B; Balsamo, G. Chitosan-mediated stimulation of macrophage function. *Biomaterials* **1994**, *15*, 1215–1220.

43. Villiers, C; Chevallet, M; Diemer, H; Couderc, R; Freitas, H; Van Dorsselaer, A; Marche, PN; Rabilloud, T. From secretome analysis to immunology: Chitosan induces major alterations in the activation of dendritic cells via a TLR4-dependent mechanism. *Mol Cell Proteomics* **2009**, *8*, 1252–1264.

44. van der Lubben, IM; Verhoef, JC; Borchard, G; Junginger, HE. Chitosan for mucosal vaccination. *Adv Drug Deliv Rev* **2001**, *52*, 139–144.

45. Sun, HX; Wang, H; Xu, HS; Ni, Y. Novel polysaccharide adjuvant from the roots of Actinidia eriantha with dual Th1 and Th2 potentiating activity. *Vaccine* **2009**, *27*, 3984–3991.

46. Gupta, RK; Siber, GR. Adjuvants for humans vaccines—current status, problems and future prospects. *Vaccine* **1995**, *13*, 1263–1276.

47. Audibert, FM; Lise, LD. Adjuvants: Current status, clinical perspectives and future prospects. *Immunol Today* **1993**, *14*, 281–284.

48. Sedlik, C. Th1 and Th2 subsets of T lymphocytes: Characteristics, physiological role and regulation. *Bull Inst Pasteur* **1996**, *94*, 173–200.

49. Livingston, PO; Adluri, S; Helling, F; Yao, TJ; Kensil, CR; Newman, MJ; Marciani, D. Phase 1 trial of immunological adjuvant QS-21 with a GM2 ganglioside-keyhole limpet haemocyanin conjugate vaccine in patients with malignant melanoma. *Vaccine* **1994**, *12*, 1275–1280.

50. Cher, DJ; Mosmann, TR. Two types of murine helper T-cell clones. II. Delayed-type hypersensitivity is mediated by Th1 clones. *J Immunol* **1987**, *138*, 3688–3694.

51. Mosmann, TR; Sad, S. The expanding universe of T-cells subsets: Th1, Th2 and more. *Immunol Today* **1996**, *17*, 138–146.

52. Coffman, RL; Seymour, BWP; Lebman, DA; Hiraki, DD; Christiansen, JA; Shrader, B; Cherwinski, HM; Savelkoul, HFJ; Finkelman, FD; Bond, MW; *et al.* The role of helper T cell products in mouse B cell differentiation and isotype regulation. *Immunol Rev* **1988**, *102*, 5–28.

53. McKee, AS; Munks, MW; Marrack, P. How do adjuvants work? Important considerations for new generation adjuvants. *Immunity* **2007**, *27*, 687–690.

54. Roitt, I; Brostoff, J; Male, D. *Immunology*; Mosby: London, UK, 2000; pp. 121–135.

55. Boon, T; Cerottini, JC; Van den Eynde, B; van der Bruggen, P; van Pel, A. Tumor antigens recognized by T lymphocytes. *Annu Rev Immunol* **1994**, *12*, 337–365.

56. Moretta, L; Bottino, C; Cantoni, C; Mingari, MC; Moretta, A. Human natural killer cell function and receptors. *Curr Opin Pharmacol* **2001**, *1*, 387–391.

57. Rappuoli, R. Bridging the knowledge gaps in vaccine design. *Nat Biotechnol* **2007**, *25*, 1361–1366.

58. Kos, FJ; Engleman, EG. Immune regulation: A critical link between NK cells and CTLs. *Immunol Today* **1996**, *17*, 174–176.

59. Medzhitov, R; Janeway, CA. Innate immunity: Impact on the adaptive immune response. *Curr Opin Immunol* **1997**, *9*, 4–9.

60. Orange, JS. Formation and function of the lytic NK-cell immunological synapse. *Nat Rev Immunol* **2008**, *8*, 713–725.

61. Zhang, J; Sun, R; Wei, H; Tian, Z. Antitumor effects of recombinant human prolactin in human adenocarcinoma-bearing SCID mice with human NK cell xenograft. *Int Immunopharmacol* **2005**, *5*, 417–425.

Samples Availability: Available from the authors.

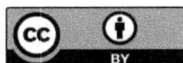

marine drugs

MDPI

Communication

Anti-Inflammatory Activity of Chitooligosaccharides in Vivo

João C. Fernandes [1,*], Humberto Spindola [2], Vanessa de Sousa [2], Alice Santos-Silva [3,4], Manuela E. Pintado [1], Francisco Xavier Malcata [1] and João E. Carvalho [2]

[1] CBQF/Escola Superior de Biotecnologia, Universidade Católica Portuguesa, Rua Dr. António Bernardino de Almeida, P-4200-072 Porto, Portugal; mmpintado@esb.ucp.pt (M.E.P.); fxmalcata@docente.ismai.pt (F.X.M.)

[2] CPQBA/Divisão de Farmacologia e Toxicologia, Universidade Estadual de Campinas, Campinas, São Paulo, Brazil; hmspindola@hotmail.com (H.S.); vanahelena@hotmail.com (V.d.S.); carvalho_je@yahoo.com.br (J.E.C.)

[3] Serviço de Bioquímica, Faculdade de Farmácia da Universidade do Porto, Rua Aníbal Cunha, P-4050-047 Porto, Portugal; assilva@ff.up.pt (A.S.-S.)

[4] Instituto de Biologia Molecular e Celular (IBMC) da Universidade do Porto, Rua do Campo Alegre, P-4169-007 Porto, Portugal

* *Author to whom correspondence should be addressed; jfernandes@email.com; Tel.: +351-96-7892999; Fax: +351-22-5090351.

Received: 15 April 2010; in revised form: 14 May 2010; Accepted: 26 May 2010; Published: 28 May 2010

Abstract: All the reports to date on the anti-inflammatory activity of chitooligosaccharides (COS) are mostly based on *in vitro* methods. In this work, the anti-inflammatory activity of two COS mixtures is characterized *in vivo* (using balb/c mice), following the carrageenan-induced paw edema method. This is a widely accepted animal model of acute inflammation to evaluate the anti-inflammatory effect of drugs. Our data suggest that COS possess anti-inflammatory activity, which is dependent on dose and, at higher doses, also on the molecular weight. A single dose of 500 mg/kg b.w. weight may be suitable to treat acute inflammation cases; however, further studies are needed to ascertain the effect upon longer inflammation periods as well as studies upon the bioavailability of these compounds.

Keywords: chitooligosaccharides; anti-inflammatory; animal model

1. Introduction

Chitooligosaccharides (COS) are partially hydrolyzed products of chitosan, a biopolymer composed of β-(1–4)-linked N-acetyl-D-glucosamine and deacetylated glucosamine units [1]. Several authors have reported the potential of COS as a therapeutic agent against inflammation. These studies were mainly based on *in vitro* tests [2,4]. It has been suggested that this anti-inflammatory action of COS occurs via down-regulation of transcriptional and translational expression levels of TNF-α, IL-6, iNOS and COX-2 [4,6]; furthermore, it depends on the molecular weight of COS [6]. This preliminary study, therefore, intends to investigate the anti-inflammatory activities of COS mixtures with different molecular weights, by studying its effects *in vivo* upon inflammation induced by carrageenan.

2. Results and Discussion

Both COS mixtures administered orally at doses between 50–1,000 mg/kg b.w., didn't generate any significant change in the autonomic or behavioural responses during the observation period. Therefore, the oral LD_{50} value in mice, for both COS, was found to be above 1,000 mg/kg b.w.

Edema induced by phlogistic agents is a widely accepted model for the evaluation of anti-inflammatory effect of drugs [7]. Carrageenan-induced paw edema is a classical model of acute inflammation (used mainly for testing the nonsteroidal anti-inflammatory drugs, as INN) involving various types of chemical mediators of inflammation such as histamine, serotonin, bradykinin and prostaglandins, in which the involvement of the cyclooxygenase products of arachidonic acid metabolism and the production of reactive oxygen species are well established [8]. Development of edema induced by carrageenan is commonly correlated with the early exudative stage of inflammation, one of the important processes of inflammatory pathology [9]. In the beginning of carrageenan injection, there is sudden elevation of paw volume as consequence of histamine liberation from mastocyte cells [10]. After 1 h the inflammation increases gradually and is elevated during the later 3–6 h. This second phase is mediated by prostaglandins, cyclooxygenase products. Continuity between the two phases is provided by kinins [11,12].

To demonstrate the validity of the carrageenan-induced paw edema test, mice were administered INN orally as a positive control at a dosage of 10 mg/kg b.w. 1 h before carrageenan injection. As expected, INN significantly ($p < 0.05$) decreased paw edema at 2, 3 and 6 h after carrageenan injection compared to saline, with inhibition levels of 67.92%, 71.61% and 78.79%, respectively (Figure 1). These results demonstrate that INN, a cyclooxygenase inhibitor, exerts an anti-edematous effect during the second phase of paw edema due to the reduction of prostaglandins, which are second phase inflammatory mediators. Simultaneously, mice were administered various doses of COS3 and COS5 (10–500 mg/kg b.w.) orally 1 h before carrageenan administration. All tested concentrations significantly ($p < 0.05$) decreased the paw volume at 3 and 6 h after carrageenan administration compared to vehicle control (Figure 1). Both COS showed higher action at 500 mg/kg, decreasing the paw volume significantly compared to the other tested concentrations. Also, at this concentration the molecular weight proved to play a major role reducing paw volume, since COS3 showed significant ($p < 0.05$) stronger effect −73.42% and 78.13%, than COS5–63.20% and 71.88% at 3 and 6 h, respectively.

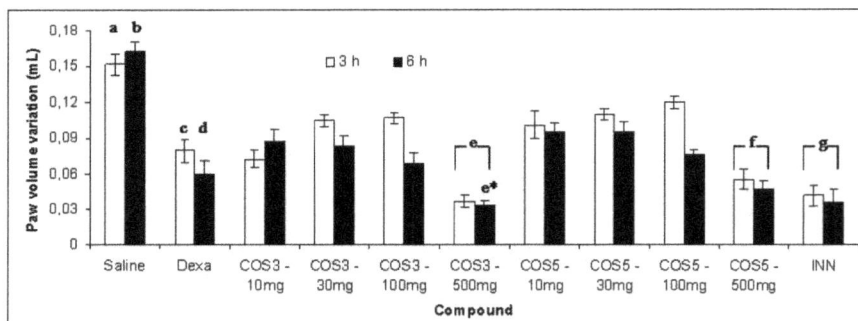

Figure 1. Effect of various doses of both COS, administered orally 60 min prior to injection of carrageenan, on mice paw edema volume (mL), after 3 and 6 h. (Average ± S.E.M.). Legend: (a) statistically different from all other compounds tested ($p < 0.05$), except b; (b) statistically different from all other compounds tested ($p < 0.05$), except a; (c) statistically different ($p < 0.05$) from COS3–500 mg and INN at 3 and 6 h; (d) statistically different from COS3–500 mg and INN at 3 and 6 h; (e) statistically different ($p < 0.05$) from other COS3 concentrations; (e*) statistically different from COS5–500 mg at 6 h ($p < 0.05$); (f) statistically different from other COS5 concentrations; (g) statistically different from COS3 and COS5 concentrations, except 500 mg values ($p < 0.05$).

Overall every dose of COS3 and COS5 tested in this study showed significant reduction of paw edema at 2 h after carrageenan injection, suggesting that COS produces an anti-edematous effect during the second phase, similarly to INN. Therefore, our results suggest that the mechanism of the anti-inflammatory effect of COS may involve the inhibition of the cyclooxygenase pathway; as reported elsewhere [6], COS may exert their anti-inflammatory effect via down-regulation of transcriptional and translational expression levels of COX-2. At this stage, an endpoint was established in order to prevent animals from suffering a severe discomfort resulting from leg ulceration. However, the experiment was extended with the INN group (which showed to be more effective than Dexa as a positive control), and with the most promising COS concentration–500 mg/kg (Figure 2).

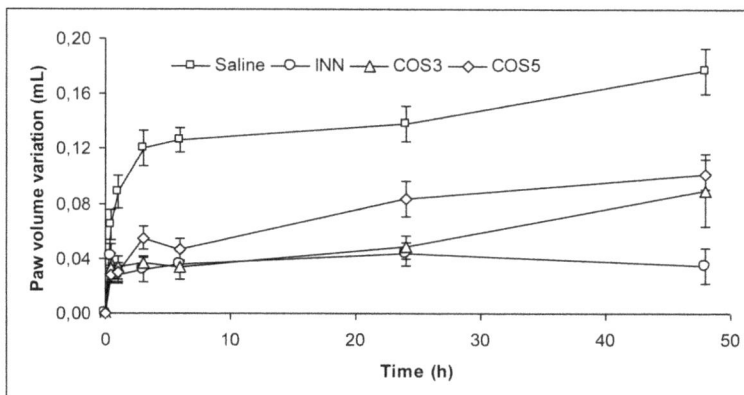

Figure 2. Effect of 500 mg/kg b.w. of both COS, administered orally 60 min prior to injection of carrageenan, on mice paw edema volume (mL), along the time (Average ± S.E.M.).

COS3 continued to exert anti-inflammatory activity, comparable to INN until the 24 h, while COS5 started losing activity around the 15–h which may be related to a lower level of COS5 in the blood circulation, due to its higher MW and concomitant lower absorption rate at intestinal level [1]; by 48 h, both COS mixtures presented a similar effect (between 43–47%), lower than INN (81.81%) but still significantly different from the negative control ($p < 0.05$). After euthanasia, no changes were observed in COS3 and COS5 administered mice. Kidneys, liver, stomach, heart and intestines were analyzed for visible alterations and weighted, presenting no differences compared to control mice; however, the group administered with INN, had considerably inflated and heavier stomachs and intestines–which can be associated to the peptic ulcer inducing effect of INN [13].

3. Experimental Section

3.1. Materials

Chitooligosaccharide mixtures characterized by two distinct average molecular weights 1.2 (COS3)—and 5.3 kDa (COS5)—and possessing a degree of deacetylation in the 80–85% range, were purchased from Nicechem (Shanghai, China). Both compounds were derived from crab shells. All chemicals used in this work were purchased from Sigma-Brazil.

3.2. Animals

Balb/c male mice (6 weeks), weighing between 27 and 32 g, were used in the experiments. The animals were purchased from Centro Multidisciplinar para Investigação Biológica na Área da Ciência em Animais de Laboratório–CEMIB at the University of Campinas (UNICAMP), and were kept in polyethylene boxes (n = 6), in a controlled environment—constant temperature (24 ± 2 °C) with a 12 h light-dark cycle and relative humidity of 40–70%. They were kept without food for 24 h before the experiment and water was *ad libitum*. Groups of six mice were used and the studies were carried out in accordance with current guidelines for the veterinary care of laboratory animals [14], and were performed under the consent and surveillance of Unicamp's Institute of Biology Ethics Committee for Animal Research (1076-1).

3.3. Preliminary screening and acute toxicity assessment

Mice were divided into seven groups, each containing six animals. COS mixtures were administered orally, in varying doses (50, 250 and 1,000 mg/kg b.w.) to these animals, using saline solution as a vehicle. A group of animals treated with the vehicle served as control. They were continuously observed for 4 h to detect changes in their autonomic or behavioural responses viz. alertness, spontaneous activity, irritability, pinna reflex, corneal reflex, urination, salivation and piloerection [15]. Any mortality during this period of experimentation and along the following 14 days was also recorded. Based on the results of this preliminary toxicity test, doses of 10, 30, 100 and 500 mg/kg b.w. were chosen to study the anti-inflammatory activity of COS mixtures.

3.4. Acute inflammation assessment

Anti-inflammatory activity was studied by carrageenan-induced paw edema method [7]. Mice were divided into eleven groups, each containing six animals. COS mixtures were administered orally in different doses (10, 30, 100 and 500 mg/kg b.w.), 60 min prior to carrageenan injection. Two positive control groups [16] were used: one with 10 mg/kg b.w. of indomethacin (INN–a well-known non-steroidal anti-inflammatory drug), and the other with 1 mg/kg b.w. of dexamethasone (Dexa–a potent synthetic member of the glucocorticoid class of steroid hormones). A group of animals treated with the vehicle served as negative control. Edema was induced by injecting 0.02 ml of 2.5% carrageenan in sterile saline into the plantar surface of the right hind paw. The difference of volumes between the basal and sequential measurements in the right hind paw was calculated as the edema formation. The paw volume was measured in an Ugo Basile plethysmometer (Comerio VA, Italy), at 0.5, 1, 2, 3, 4, 6, 8, 24 and 48 h.

3.5. Statistical analysis

The results are expressed as mean $\pm$ SEM ($n = 6$). Statistical significance was determined by analysis of variance and subsequent Duncan's multiple range test ($p < 0.05$). The analysis was performed using Statistical Package for Social Sciences – SPSS statistical software (Chicago, IL, USA).

4. Conclusions

In conclusion, our data suggests that COS are able to induce anti-inflammatory effect mediated by cyclooxygenase inhibition and consequent reduction of prostaglandins. In addition, the efficacy of high-dose COS3 (500 mg/kg b.w.) was comparable to that of indomethacin, but during a shorter period. A single dose of 500 mg/kg b.w. may indeed be suitable to treat acute inflammation cases; however, further studies are needed to ascertain the effect upon longer inflammation periods as well as studies upon the bioavailability of these compounds.

Acknowledgments: Funding for author J.C.F. was via a PhD. fellowship administered by Fundação para a Ciência e a Tecnologia (ref. SFRH/BD/31087/2006). This research was supported by CYTED through project 105PI0274.

References and Notes

1. Fernandes, JC; Eaton, P; Nascimento, H; Belo, L; Rocha, S; Vitorino, R; Amado, F; Gomes, J; Santos-Silva, A; Pintado, ME; Malcata, FX. Effects of chitooligosaccharides on human red blood cell morphology and membrane protein structure. *Biomacromolecules* **2008**, *9*, 3346–3352.
2. Lee, JY; Spicer, AP. Hyaluronan: a multifunctional, megaDalton, stealth molecule. *Curr. Opin. Cell Biol* **2000**, *12*, 581–586.
3. Hwang, SM; Chen, CY; Chen, SS; Chen, JC. Chitinous materials inhibit nitric oxide production by activated RAW 264.7 macrophages. *Biochem. Biophys. Res. Commun* **2000**, *27*, 229–233.
4. Shikhman, AR; Kuhn, K; Alaaeddine, N; Lotz, M. *N*-Acetylglucosamine prevents IL-1ß-mediated activation of human chondrocytes. *J. Immunol* **2001**, *166*, 5155–5160.

5. Lin, CW; Chen, LJ; Lee, PL; Lee, CI; Lin, JC; Chiu, JJ. The inhibition of TNF-α-induced E-selectin expression in endothelial cells via the JNK/NF-kB pathways by highly *N*-acetylated chitooligosaccharides. *Biomaterials* **2007**, *28*, 1355–1366.

6. Lee, SH; Senevirathne, M; Ahn, CB; Kim, SK; Je, JY. Factors affecting anti-inflammatory effect of chitooligosaccharides in lipopolysaccharides-induced RAW264.7 macrophage cells. *Bioorg. Med. Chem. Lett* **2009**, *19*, 6655–6658.

7. Winter, CA; Risley, EA; Nuss, GW. Carregeenan-induced edema in hind paw of the rat as assay for anti-inflammatory drugs. *Proc. Soc. Exp. Biol. Med* **1962**, *11*, 544–547.

8. Lee, KH; Choi, EM. Analgesic and anti-inflammatory effects of *Ligularia fischeri* leaves in experimental animals. *J. Ethnopharmacol* **2008**, *120*, 103–107.

9. Ozaki, Y. Anti-inflammatory effects of *Curcuma xanthorrhiza* Roxb, and its active principle. *Chem. Pharm. Bull* **1990**, *38*, 1045–1048.

10. Geen, KL. Role of endogenous catecholamines in the anti-inflammatory activity of alpha-adrenoceptor blocking agents. *Br. J. Pharmacol* **1964**, *51*, 45–53.

11. Perianayagam, JB; Sharma, SK; Pillai, KK. Anti-inflammatory activity of Trichodesma indicium root extract in experimental animals. *J. Ethnopharmacol* **2006**, *104*, 410–414.

12. Vinegar, R; Scheirber, W; Hugo, R. Biphasic development of carageenin edema in rat. *J. Pharmacol. Exp. Ther* **1969**, *166*, 96–103.

13. Rujjanawate, C; Kanjanapothi, D; Amornlerdpison, D; Pojanagaroon, S. Anti-gastric ulcer effect of *Kaempferia parviflora*. *J. Ethnopharmacol* **2005**, *102*, 120–122.

14. Voipio, HM; Baneux, P; Gomez de Segura, IA; Hau, J; Wolfensohn, S. Joint working group on veterinary care. *Lab. Anim* **2008**, *42*, 1–11.

15. Narayanan, N; Thirugnanasambantham, P; Viswanathan, S; Vijayasekaran, V; Sukumar, E. Antinociceptive, anti-inflammatory and antipyretic effects of ethanol extract of *Clerodendron serratum* roots in experimental animals. *J. Ethnopharmacol* **1999**, *65*, 237–241.

16. Marshall, LA; Chang, JY; Calhoun, W; Yu, J; Carlson, RP. Preliminary studies on phospholipase A$_2$-induced mouse paw edema as a model to evaluate anti-inflammatory agents. *J. Cell. Biochem* **2004**, *40*, 147–155.

Samples Availability: Available from the authors.

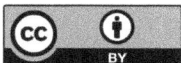

marine drugs

MDPI

Article

Antidiabetic Activity of Differently Regioselective Chitosan Sulfates in Alloxan-Induced Diabetic Rats

Ronge Xing [1,*], Xiaofei He [1,2], Song Liu [1], Huahua Yu [1], Yukun Qin [1], Xiaolin Chen [1], Kecheng Li [1], Rongfeng Li [1] and Pengcheng Li [1,*]

[1] Institute of Oceanology, Chinese Academy of Sciences, Qingdao 266071, China; hexiaofei12@mails.ucas.ac.cn (X.H.); sliu@qdio.ac.cn (S.L.); yuhuahua@qdio.ac.cn (H.Y.); ykqin@qdio.ac.cn (Y.Q.); chenxl@qdio.ac.cn (X.C.); lkc@qdio.ac.cn (K.L.); rongfengli@qdio.ac.cn (R.L.)
[2] College of Earth Science, University of the Chinese Academy of Sciences, Beijing 100049, China
* Authors to whom correspondence should be addressed; xingronge@qdio.ac.cn (R.X.); pcli@qdio.ac.cn (P.L.); Tel.: +86-532-8289-8707; Fax: +86-532-8289-8780.

Academic Editor: Paola Laurienzo
Received: 21 February 2015; Accepted: 4 May 2015; Published: 15 May 2015

Abstract: The present study investigated and compared the hypoglycemic activity of differently regioselective chitosan sulfates in alloxan-induced diabetic rats. Compared with the normal control rats, significantly higher blood glucose levels were observed in the alloxan-induced diabetic rats. The differently regioselective chitosan sulfates exhibited hypoglycemic activities at different doses and intervals, especially 3-*O*-sulfochitosan (3-S). The major results are as follows. First, 3,6-di-*O*-sulfochitosan and 3-*O*-sulfochitosan exhibited more significant hypoglycemic activities than 2-*N*-3, 6-di-*O*-sulfochitosan and 6-*O*-sulfochitosan. Moreover, 3-*S*-treated rats showed a more significant reduction of blood glucose levels than those treated by 3,6-di-*O*-sulfochitosan. These results indicated that $-OSO_3^-$ at the C3-position of chitosan is a key active site. Second, 3-S significantly reduced the blood glucose levels and regulated the glucose tolerance effect in the experimental rats. Third, treatment with 3-S significantly increased the plasma insulin levels in the experimental diabetic rats. A noticeable hypoglycemic activity of 3-S in the alloxan-induced diabetic rats was shown. Clinical trials are required in the future to confirm the utility of 3-S.

Keywords: differently regioselective chitosan sulfates; hypoglycemic activity; glucose tolerance; plasma insulin; alloxan-induced diabetic rats

1. Introduction

Diabetes mellitus (DM) is a common group of metabolic diseases associated with endocrine and metabolic disorders, which are mainly characterized by hyperglycemia, with a genetic predisposition. DM leads to abnormal metabolism of carbohydrates, fats and proteins, sometimes accompanied by the long-term complications of diabetes, including microvascular, macrovascular, and neuropathic disorders [1]. DM affects human eyes, kidneys, hearts, nerves and blood vessels. According to previous reports, diabetes mellitus has become the third most serious threat to human health following malignant tumors and cardiovascular and cerebrovascular disease.

The latest statistical data of the International Diabetes Federation (IDF) showed that at least 382 million people worldwide had diabetes in 2013. Compared with 371 million cases in 2012, the increasing rate reached 8.4 percent, and by 2025, the organization predicts that there will be 592 million cases. Moreover, IDF showed that there are 5.1 million deaths caused by this disease per year, or one death every 6 seconds. The expense for the treatment of diabetes is high: The global diabetes medical costs are $548 billion, accounting for 11% of the global medical expenditure, and this is likely to rise to $627 billion by 2035. It has become a heavy economic burden of the individual, family and society.

In China, 114 million people had diabetes in 2013, which means there is one Chinese patient for every three to four patients with diabetes mellitus in the world, and the amount of patients is expected to increase a few million per year. Therefore, research on the prevention and treatment of diabetes and its complications has become a major public health issue.

Currently available therapies for diabetes include insulin and various oral hypoglycemic agents, such as sulfonylureas, biguanides, metformin, glucosidase inhibitors, troglitazone, *etc.* [2]. In conventional therapy, insulin-dependent diabetes mellitus or type 1 is treated with exogenous insulin while the non-insulin-dependent diabetes mellitus or type 2 is treated with oral hypoglycemic agents [3,4]. However, these drugs have serious side effects. For example, sulfonylureas drugs may cause abnormal liver function and hypoglycemia and are also not recommended for pregnant women because of their teratogenic effects on the fetus. A large dose of biguanide drugs can lead to gastrointestinal reactions, including nausea, vomiting, abdominal pain, diarrhea, and loss of appetite. Patients with lung, liver, and kidney diseases are prone to lactic acidosis after taking biguanide drugs [5–7]. The other classes of antidiabetic drugs, such as insulin sensitizing agents, insulin antagonistic hormone inhibitors, gluconeogenesis inhibitors, insulin like growth factor, ISU (insulin) secretion, and traditional Chinese medicine preparations, including flavonoids, alkaloids and so on, are also not ideal. Therefore, the development of safer, more specific and more effective hypoglycemic agents is important for diabetes treatment.

A previous study found that chitin/chitosan has definite hypoglycemic effects. The presumed mechanism showed that chitosan of a certain molecular weight stimulated the beta-cells proliferation [8], the secretion and release of insulin, and limited the glucagon secretion of islet α cells. Moreover, chitosan was active on the liver: it inhibited hepatic gluconeogenesis and the *in vivo* absorption of sugar; reduced sugar output; enhanced the utilization of sugar by the surrounding tissue, thus reducing the level of blood sugar. Another hypothesis is that chitosan could increase the amounts of insulin and glucose receptors, improve insulin sensitivity, and strengthen the biological activity of the receptor. Subsequently, the intracellular oxidase system was inhibited followed by tissue hypoxia. As a result, glucose metabolism was increased, and the blood sugar decreased.

Some research has shown that differently regioselective sulfate chitosans had varying bioactivities. For example, the anticoagulant activity of 6-*O*-sulfochitosan (6-S) was notably higher than that of 2-*N*-sulfochitosan (2-S) and 3-*O*-sulfochitosan (3-S). However, the selective sulfation at N-2 and/or O-3 had a much higher inhibitory effect on the infection of the AIDS virus *in vitro* than that of the known 6-S [9]. Moreover, many studies showed that diabetes was associated with oxidative stress, which contributed to an increased production of reactive oxygen species (ROS), including superoxide radicals, hydroxyl radicals, lipid peroxidation, and hydrogen peroxide [10,11]. Antioxidants could thus be a potential type of drug for the treatment of diabetes [12]. Non-toxic and natural antioxidants have been shown to prevent oxidative damage in diabetes [13]. Our previous research showed that sulfate chitosans had obvious antioxidant activities [14]. Therefore, the present study investigated the anti-diabetic activity of differently regioselective sulfate chitosans in alloxan-induced diabetic rats. The results showed that 3-S markedly lowered the blood glucose level, improved the glucose tolerance of rats and increased the fasting serum insulin level of alloxan-induced diabetic rats. Based on our study, 3-S could potentially be developed as a new hypoglycemic drug.

2. Results

2.1. Physico-Chemical Parameter of Differently Regioselective Sulfate Chitosans

Table 1 shows the result of differently regioselective sulfate chitosans under the aforementioned reaction conditions. All products have good solubility.

Table 1. Characteristics of differently regioselective chitosan sulfates.

Species	Molecular Weight ($\times 10^4$)	Sulfur Content (%)	Color of Resultant	Solubility
H2,3,6-S	12.4	14.7	Pale yellow	Easily soluble
3,6-S	11.7	12.1	White	Easily soluble
3-S	12.1	5.2	Yellow	Easily soluble
6-S	13.5	7.6	White	Soluble
L2,3,6-S	0.9	14.5	Pale yellow	Easily soluble
CTS	76	0	Pale yellow	Not soluble

2.2. Structural Characterization of All Chitosan Sulfates

In the FTIR (Fourier Transform Infrared) spectrum (as shown in Figure 1), characteristic absorptions at 1222 and 806 cm^{-1}, due to sulfo groups, were assigned to S = O and C–O–S bond stretching, respectively.

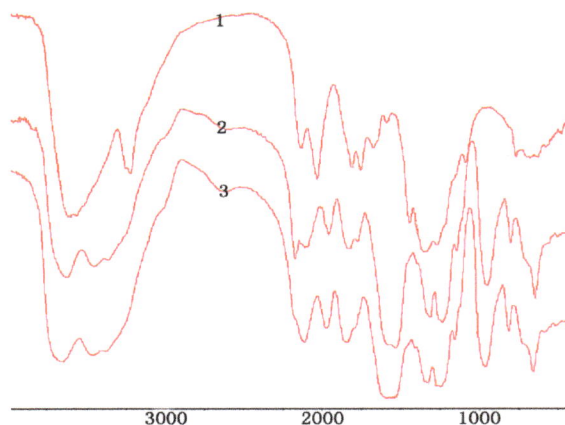

Figure 1. FTIR of H2,3,6-S (1) chitosan; (2) H2,3,6-S under dichloroacetic acid; (3) H2,3,6-S under formic acid.

The structures of 2-phthalimidochitosan, 3,6-S and 3-S were further investigated by means of FTIR spectrum (Figures 2–4). In the FTIR spectrum (as shown in Figure 2), characteristic absorptions at 1712 cm^{-1} and 749 cm^{-1}, due to phthalimido groups, were assigned to C=O and C–H bond stretching, respectively. Figure 3 shows that the phthalimido group was completely eliminated up to 3 h. As shown in Figure 4, the structure of 3-S was exhibited. Characteristic absorptions at 1261 and 805 cm^{-1} were assigned to S=O and C–O–S bond stretching, respectively. In this FTIR spectrum, three characteristic absorptions of the amino group, 1667.46, 1571.16, 1509.30 cm^{-1}, appeared. Moreover, characteristic absorption of CH$_2$ in C6 (2980 cm^{-1}) was determined, which proved the 6-*O*-sulfo group was completely eliminated. Therefore, from the aforementioned result, 3,6-S and 3-S were successfully synthesized.

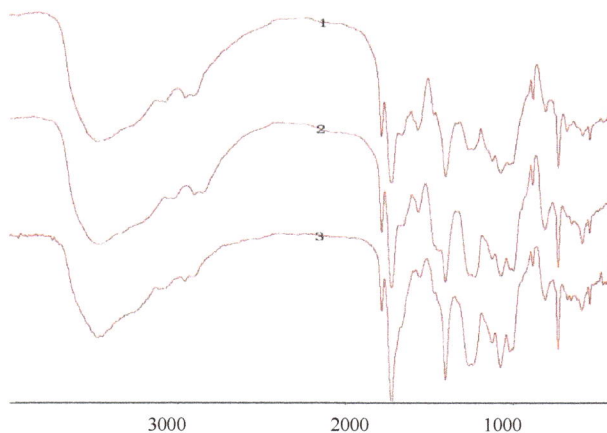

Figure 2. FTIR of 2-phthalimido-chitosan under 90 °C; 1: FTIR of 2-phthalimido-chitosan under 3.5 h; 2: FTIR of 2-phthalimido-chitosan under 3.0 h; 3: FTIR of 2-phthalimido-chitosan under 2.0 h.

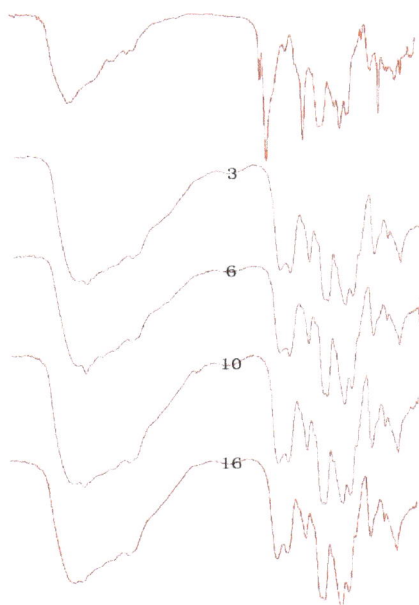

Figure 3. FTIR of 3,6-S; 3: Eliminating the phthalimido group under 3 h; 6: Eliminating the phthalimido group under 6 h; 10: Eliminating the phthalimido group under 10 h; 16: Eliminating the phthalimido group under 16 h.

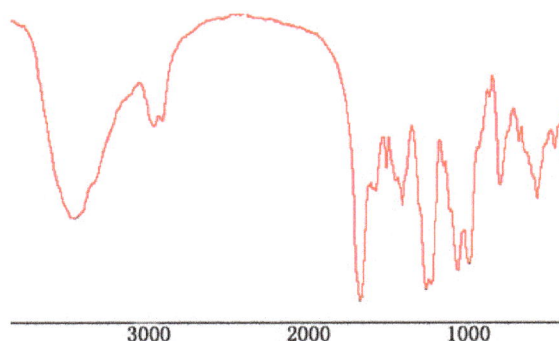

Figure 4. FTIR of 3-S.

The structures of 6-S was investigated by means of FTIR spectrum (Figure 5). In the FTIR spectrum, characteristic absorptions at 1225 cm^{-1} and 805 cm^{-1} were assigned to S=O and C–O–S bond stretching, respectively. Characteristic absorptions of hydroxy group 3440 cm^{-1} did not change in Cu-chitosan chelation and Cu-sulfated chitoan chelation, which proved that the C2-N-group and C3-O-group were completely protected, and a sulfated reaction did not destroy the protection group.

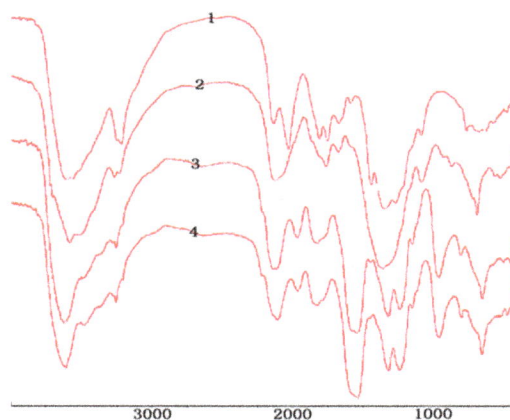

Figure 5. FTIR of 6-S; 1: Chitosan; 2: Cu-chitosan chelation; 3: Cu- sulfated chitoan chelation under formic acid; 4: Cu- sulfated chitoan chelation without formic acid.

In the FTIR spectrum (as shown in Figure 6), characteristic absorptions at 1222 and 806 cm^{-1}, due to sulfo groups, were assigned to S=O and C–O–S bond stretchings, respectively. The peak at 940 cm^{-1}, due to the pyranose units in the polysaccharide, proved that the cyclic pyranosyl rings were not destroyed by microwave radiation.

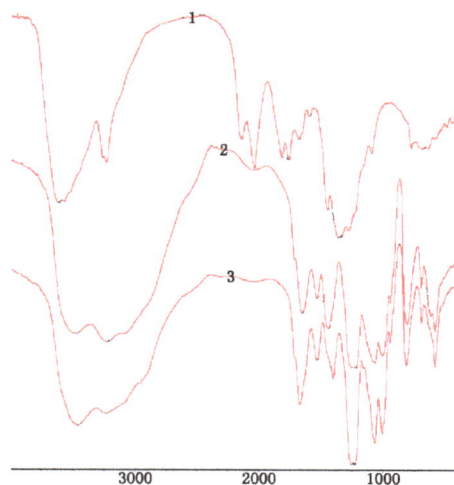

Figure 6. FTIR of L2,3,6-S; 1: Chitosan; 2: L2,3,6-S under traditional heating; 3: L2,3,6-S under microwave radiation (800W).

2.3. The Effects of Differently Regioselective Sulfate Chitosans on Body Weight

As shown in Table 2, compared with the normal control group, the body weight of the diabetic model control group was significantly reduced ($p < 0.05$, $p < 0.01$, $p < 0.01$) on day 12, day 18 and day 30 after alloxan treatment. The body weight of the treatment groups did not significantly change compared to the normal control group. Moreover, the body weight of the 3-S treatment groups almost recovered to the normal level, especially the 150 mg/kg and 50 mg/kg dose groups. These results showed that the differently regioselective sulfate chitosan samples did not affect the rats' body weights and had no negative effect on the rats.

2.4. Determination of Antidiabetic Activity of Differently Regioselective Chitosan Sulfates in Vivo

The effects of the differently regioselective sulfate chitosans on the fasting blood glucose levels of alloxan-induced diabetic rats are shown in Table 3. The administration of a single intraperitoneal injection of 50 mg/kg body weight of alloxan monohydrate induced diabetes in rats after 72 h. The fasting blood glucose levels in alloxan-induced diabetic rats were 21.83–27.01 mmol/L. The fasting blood glucose levels of the diabetic model rats were significantly higher than that of the normal control group. Differently regioselective sulfated chitosans have different hypoglycemic activities. Compared with the diabetic model rats, all doses of H2,3,6-S reduced the blood glucose levels of the rats tested on the 6th, 12th, 18th, 24th and 30th days to different degrees, although the differences were non-significant. Furthermore, we found that the hypoglycemic activity of low molecular weight L2,3,6-S is better than that of high molecular weight H2,3,6-S. A high dose of L2,3,6-S (400 mg/kg) showed a significant reduction ($p < 0.05$, $p < 0.05$) of the blood glucose level of the diabetic rats on the 12th and 18th days post-treatment. Hypoglycemic activities of sulfate chitosans depend on the substitution sites of the sulfate group. First, hypoglycemic activities of the 6-S groups are basically the same as that of the H2,3,6-S groups. Second, hydrazine hydrate could not be treated completely for 3,6-S, treatment with 3,6-S at a dose of 400 mg/kg and 150 mg/kg caused experimental animal mortality. However, treatment with 3,6-S at a low dose of 50 mg/kg in the diabetic rats led to a significant reduction ($p < 0.05$) in the blood glucose level on the 18th day. The results showed that the hypoglycemic activities of sulfate chitosans are enhanced by the introduction of sulfur at site 3. Third, all doses of the 3-S treatment reduced the blood glucose level in the diabetic rats significantly.

121

Treatment with 3-S at a dose of 400 mg/kg caused a significant reduction ($p < 0.05$, $p < 0.05$, $p < 0.05$) in blood glucose levels in the diabetic rats on the 12th, 18th and 24th day post-treatment. Treatment with 3-S at a dose of 50 mg/kg led to a significant reduction ($p < 0.01$, $p < 0.05$) in blood glucose levels on the 12th and 18th day. The highest anti-hyperglycemic activity of 3-S was the 150 mg/kg dose in diabetic rats on the 12th, 18th, 24th and 30th day post-treatment ($p < 0.01$, $p < 0.001$, $p < 0.001$, $p < 0.05$). Therefore, these results indicated that 3-S had the highest hypoglycemic activity, and all of the investigated sulfate chitosans reduced the blood glucose levels in a dose-independent manner.

Table 2. The effects of differently regioselective chitosan sulfates on the body weights of alloxan-induced diabetic rats.

Group	Treatment	0th Day	6th Day	12th Day	18th Day	24th Day	30th Day
1	Normal control	183.9 ± 12.1 (10)	197.1 ± 13.6 (10)	219.0 ± 19.1 (10)	233.3 ± 23.0 (10)	237.9 ± 23.9 (10)	261.3 ± 40.3 (10)
2	Diabetic control (DC)	171.8 ± 25.8 (13)	178.3 ± 34.4 (12)	184.1 ± 39.8 (11) [Δ]	191.4 ± 37.1 (11) [ΔΔ]	203.2 ± 47.9 (10)	201.8 ± 49.4 (10) [ΔΔ]
3	DC + phenformin hydrochloride (100 mg/kg)	175.4 ± 31.4 (12)	181.1 ± 33.2 (10)	189.6 ± 35.0 (9)	199.0 ± 34.5 (9)	199.7 ± 41.8 (9)	208.1 ± 45.2 (8)
4	DC + H2,3,6-S (400 mg/kg)	174.0 ± 14.1 (9)	191.6 ± 11.0 (7)	178.9 ± 22.9 (7)	200.2 ± 21.4 (6)	209.8 ± 22.3 (6)	213.2 ± 20.9 (6)
5	DC + H2,3,6-S (150 mg/kg)	183.3 ± 25.7 (8)	200.4 ± 28.8 (7)	186.1 ± 23.9 (7)	207.4 ± 30.3 (7)	200.5 ± 29.5 (6)	207.7 ± 36.6 (6)
6	DC + H2,3,6-S (50 mg/kg)	185.9 ± 10.5 (8)	201.3 ± 15.1 (7)	198.4 ± 23.4 (7)	218.7 ± 30.6 (7)	224.4 ± 42.9 (7)	223.3 ± 44.5 (7)
7	DC + L2,3,6-S (400 mg/kg)	180.3 ± 14.6 (9)	198.8 ± 8.1 (8)	201.8 ± 11.1 (8)	207.5 ± 31.7 (8)	232.3 ± 27.5 (6)	234.3 ± 41.1 (6)
8	DC + L2,3,6-S (150 mg/kg)	170.8 ± 11.3 (8)	188.9 ± 18.2 (7)	187.9 ± 25.3 (7)	199.0 ± 32.5 (7)	213.1 ± 46.8 (7)	205.9 ± 48.5 (7)
9	DC + L2,3,6-S (50 mg/kg)	178.1 ± 23.7 (9)	200.9 ± 26.0 (7)	204.9 ± 28.3 (7)	217.1 ± 37.4 (7)	228.4 ± 49.1 (7)	228.1 ± 38.8 (7)
10	DC + 6-S (400 mg/kg)	173.4 ± 18.1 (9)	189.5 ± 23.7 (8)	202.4 ± 24.1 (7)	213.0 ± 31.7 (7)	199.0 ± 21.7 (6)	201.6 ± 20.5 (5)
11	DC + 6-S (150 mg/kg)	183.3 ± 13.9 (9)	195.3 ± 18.4 (8)	206.5 ± 23.1 (8)	222.5 ± 36.9 (8)	240.1 ± 43.7 (8)	238.4 ± 41.0 (8)
12	DC + 6-S (50 mg/kg)	179.6 ± 23.1 (8)	189.4 ± 33.9 (8)	196.5 ± 42.4 (8)	201.9 ± 50.1 (8)	222.9 ± 63.6 (8)	223.4 ± 72.9 (8)
13	DC + 3,6-S (400 mg/kg)	170.2 ± 20.1 (9)	‡	‡	‡	‡	‡
14	DC + 3,6-S (150 mg/kg)	168.8 ± 6.11 (9)	‡	‡	‡	‡	‡
15	DC + 3,6-S (50 mg/kg)	167.7 ± 15.2 (7)	175.9 ± 16.3 (7)	188.0 ± 29.4 (7)	193.1 ± 34.8 (7)	196.6 ± 46.9 (7)	211.7 ± 47.3 (6)
16	DC + 3-S (400 mg/kg)	173.8 ± 25.0 (9)	195.9 ± 32.1 (8)	200.5 ± 35.1 (8)	215.5 ± 47.4 (8)	221.0 ± 63.5 (8)	221.9 ± 65.8 (8)
17	DC + 3-S (150 mg/kg)	176.0 ± 28.5 (9)	192.5 ± 41.0 (8)	208.4 ± 38.6 (7)	232.7 ± 42.7 (6)	243.5 ± 48.8 (6)	244.2 ± 59.9 (6)
18	DC + 3-S (50 mg/kg)	189.9 ± 27.1 (8)	207.6 ± 38.3 (7)	221.2 ± 46.4 (6)	230.8 ± 39.2 (6)	245.8 ± 50.8 (6)	247.2 ± 51.9 (6)
19	DC + CTS (400 mg/kg)	183.0 ± 21.2 (9)	200.6 ± 31.7 (7)	207.5 ± 44.6 (6)	214.2 ± 50.4 (5)	221.0 ± 65.9 (5)	236.5 ± 62.7 (4)
20	DC + CTS (150 mg/kg)	174.7 ± 16.4 (9)	188.1 ± 22.2 (8)	201.0 ± 31.5 (7)	215.1 ± 32.5 (7)	224.6 ± 44.7 (7)	219.0 ± 46.9 (7)
21	DC + CTS (50 mg/kg)	184.1 ± 23.6 (9)	197.4 ± 31.1 (7)	194.7 ± 37.6 (7)	198.1 ± 42.9 (7)	203.8 ± 29.7 (5)	212.5 ± 43.2 (4)

Readings are values ± S.E.; (n) = number of animals in each group; $^{\Delta}$ $p < 0.05$, $^{\Delta\Delta}$ $p < 0.01$ vs. normal control.

Table 3. The effects of differently regioselective chitosan sulfates on the fasting blood glucose level of alloxan-induced diabetic rats.

Group	Treatment	0th Day	6th Day	12th Day	18th Day	24th Day	30th Day
1	Normal control	4.94 ± 0.64 (10)	4.96 ± 0.39 (10)	4.97 ± 0.37 (10)	5.84 ± 0.89 (10)	5.74 ± 1.13 (10)	5.70 ± 1.06 (10)
2	Diabetic control (DC)	23.02 ± 6.77 (13) ΔΔΔ	24.22 ± 7.97 (12) ΔΔΔ	26.59 ± 6.77 (11) ΔΔΔ	27.01 ± 7.49 (11) ΔΔΔ	24.06 ± 4.37 (10) ΔΔΔ	21.83 ± 6.66(10) ΔΔΔ
3	DC + phenformin hydrochloride (100 mg/kg)	24.08 ± 5.87 (12)	20.82 ± 7.69 (10)	17.16 ± 7.27 (9) **	14.73 ± 6.23 (9) ***	13.48 ± 4.45 (9) ***	14.84 ± 6.09 (8) *
4	DC + H2,3,6-S (400 mg/kg)	22.60 ± 6.82 (9)	22.84 ± 6.23 (7)	19.74 ± 7.13 (7)	23.88 ± 7.55 (6)	22.12 ± 7.79 (6)	18.12 ± 8.29 (6)
5	DC + H2,3,6-S (150 mg/kg)	23.39 ± 6.96 (8)	24.89 ± 6.11 (7)	23.54 ± 7.03 (7)	27.34 ± 3.79 (7)	21.02 ± 5.22 (6)	22.03 ± 6.78 (6)
6	DC + H2,3,6-S (50 mg/kg)	22.49 ± 6.06 (8)	19.96 ± 7.65 (7)	20.64 ± 8.68 (7)	18.39 ± 10.86 (7)	16.16 ± 10.16 (7)	17.23 ± 9.39 (7)
7	DC + 12,3,6-S (400 mg/kg)	23.23 ± 6.57 (9)	21.41 ± 2.29 (8)	20.28 ± 2.88 (8) *	17.68 ± 6.93 (8) *	15.85 ± 10.59 (6)	15.68 ± 8.39 (6)
8	DC + 12,3,6-S (150 mg/kg)	22.76 ± 6.42 (8)	20.99 ± 7.24 (7)	21.14 ± 6.11 (7)	22.40 ± 6.15 (7)	22.56 ± 5.14 (7)	23.80 ± 6.49 (7)
9	DC + 12,3,6-S (50 mg/kg)	24.11 ± 7.58 (9)	23.76 ± 3.17 (7)	20.56 ± 6.73 (7)	19.50 ± 8.274 (7)	20.26 ± 8.91 (7)	20.73 ± 9.69 (7)
10	DC + 6-S (400 mg/kg)	22.26 ± 5.89 (9)	27.11 ± 7.62 (8)	21.57 ± 8.26 (7)	22.46 ± 10.55 (7)	17.52 ± 9.25 (6)	23.50 ± 10.82 (5)
11	DC + 6-S (150 mg/kg)	22.06 ± 6.88 (9)	20.33 ± 7.93 (8)	20.40 ± 7.06 (8)	18.43 ± 9.35 (8)	20.40 ± 9.53 (8)	16.51 ± 9.60 (8)
12	DC + 6-S (50 mg/kg)	22.98 ± 7.23 (8)	26.98 ± 4.90 (8)	19.99 ± 8.28 (8)	19.53 ± 10.44 (8)	19.64 ± 11.57 (8)	16.58 ± 9.22 (8)
13	DC + 3,6-S (400 mg/kg)	22.59 ± 5.98 (9)	±	±	±	±	±
14	DC + 3,6-S (150 mg/kg)	24.19 ± 7.66 (9)	±	±	±	±	±
15	DC + 3,6-S (50 mg/kg)	26.14 ± 6.50 (7)	22.77 ± 8.32 (7)	20.41 ± 6.25 (7)	19.89 ± 5.27 (7) *	19.73 ± 8.97 (7)	22.08 ± 8.89 (6)
16	DC + 3-S (400 mg/kg)	24.09 ± 7.55 (9)	21.91 ± 9.62 (8)	19.21 ± 7.75 (8) *	20.31 ± 8.96 (8) *	19.50 ± 8.14 (8) *	22.08 ± 8.89 (8)
17	DC + 3-S (150 mg/kg)	23.79 ± 7.77 (9)	22.90 ± 5.10 (8)	18.63 ± 5.22 (7) **	18.22 ± 3.41 (6) **	17.55 ± 3.29 (6) **	16.13 ± 4.36 (6) *
18	DC + 3-S (50 mg/kg)	22.88 ± 7.85 (8)	22.84 ± 6.15 (7)	17.65 ± 4.20 (6) **	18.45 ± 5.14 (6) *	22.43 ± 5.86 (6)	18.70 ± 6.32 (6)
19	DC + CTS (400 mg/kg)	23.94 ± 8.06 (9)	21.37 ± 5.44 (7)	19.75 ± 5.48 (6) *	21.92 ± 7.72 (5)	21.74 ± 9.90 (5)	23.20 ± 8.00 (4)
20	DC + CTS (150 mg/kg)	22.88 ± 7.41 (9)	21.98 ± 7.52 (8)	19.74 ± 6.87 (7)	21.13 ± 9.53 (7)	18.49 ± 8.51 (7)	18.86 ± 9.72 (7)
21	DC + CTS (50 mg/kg)	24.21 ± 8.24 (9)	23.83 ± 7.90 (7)	21.77 ± 7.91 (7)	24.00 ± 8.78 (7)	22.68 ± 9.09 (5)	23.83 ± 4.35 (4)

Readings are values ± S.E.; (n) = number of animals in each group; ΔΔΔ $p < 0.001$ vs. normal control; * $p < 0.05$; ** $p < 0.01$; *** $p < 0.001$ vs. diabetic control.

124

2.5. Effect of 3-S on the Sugar Tolerance of Normal Rats

As described above, 3-S had the highest hypoglycemic activity among all of the selected sulfate chitosans. Therefore, 3-S was further investigated for its activity of increasing the sugar tolerance of the alloxan-induced rats.

Table 4 and Figure 7 showed the fasting blood glucose levels of normal control, and 3-S- and phenformin hydrochloride-treated rats after intraperitoneal administration of glucose (2 g/kg body weight). As shown in Table 4 and Figure 7, in the three groups, the blood glucose concentration peaked 0.5 h after the intraperitoneal administration of glucose. However, compared with the normal control group, the groups treated with 3-S (300 mg/kg) and phenformin hydrochloride (200 mg/kg) exhibited significantly lower blood glucose levels ($p < 0.01$, $p < 0.001$, respectively). After 0.5 h, the blood glucose levels of all of the experimental rats decreased. Moreover, 3-S- and phenformin hydrochloride-treated rats had significantly lower blood glucose concentrations at 1 and 2 h compared to the normal control rats.

Table 4. Glucose tolerance tests in normal and experimental groups.

Group	Dose (mg/kg)	n	Prior to Treatment	After Treatment			
				0 h	0.5 h	1 h	2 h
Normal control		10	4.82 ± 0.50	4.34 ± 1.39	14.95 ± 3.76	9.41 ± 3.63	5.09 ± 1.64
3-S	300	10	4.43 ± 0.44	4.29 ± 0.90	10.94 ± 2.04 **	6.74 ± 0.97 *	4.03 ± 0.70 *
Phenformin hydrochloride	200	10	4.72 ± 1.17	3.19 ± 0.67 *	7.09 ± 2.28 ***	4.84 ± 1.46 **	3.49 ± 0.87 *

* $p < 0.05$; ** $p < 0.01$ *vs.* normal control.

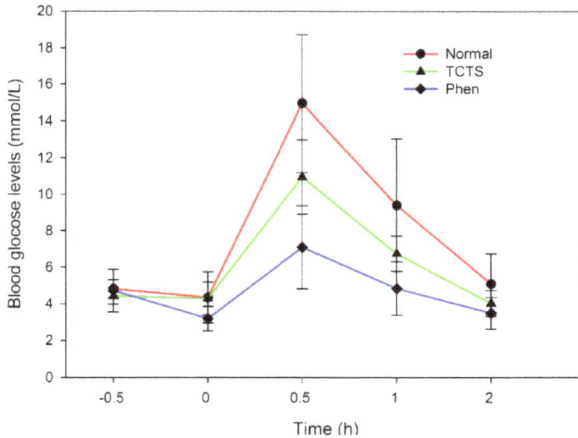

Figure 7. Hypoglycemic effects of 3-S on the fasting blood glucose levels of normal rats during GTT, each value shown in mean ± S.E.; $n = 10$, number of animals in each group.

2.6. The Effect of 3-S on Fasting Blood Glucose and Insulin Levels

Table 5 showed the levels of the fasting blood glucose and plasma insulin in normal control, diabetic control and experimental groups after 14 days of treatment. Compared with the normal control rats, the blood glucose level of the diabetic control rats was significantly increased, whereas the level of plasma insulin was significantly decreased. Treatment with 3-S at doses of 300 and 800 mg/kg caused a significant reduction in blood glucose level and a significant increase in serum insulin level. Moreover, the hypoglycemic activity of 3-S was higher than that of glibenclamide.

Table 5. The effect of 3-S on fasting serum insulin levels of normal and alloxan-induced diabetic rats.

Group	Treatment	n	Blood Glucose Level (mmol/L)		Fasting Serum Insulin Levels µIU/mL
			Before Treatment	After Treatment	
1	Normal control	10	5.17 ± 1.05	5.00 ± 0.81	6.71 ± 1.70
2	Diabetic control (DC)	10	32.10 ± 1.76 ▲▲▲	26.18 ± 5.68 ▲▲▲	3.54 ± 1.93 ▲▲
3	DC + 3-S (800 mg/kg)	10	30.25 ± 5.30	19.76 ± 9.20 *	5.44 ± 1.65 *
4	DC + 3-S (300 mg/kg)	10	29.96 ± 4.94	17.86 ± 7.93 **	5.12 ± 1.50 *
5	DC + 3-S (100 mg/kg)	10	31.78 ± 3.07	20.05 ± 7.28	4.00 ± 1.65
6	DC + Glibenclamide (25 mg/kg)	10	31.92 ± 2.63	26.45 ± 7.00	4.94 ± 1.85

Readings are values $\pm$ S.E.; (*n*) = number of animals in each group; ▲▲ $p < 0.01$; ▲▲▲ $p < 0.001$ *vs.* normal control; * $p < 0.05$; ** $p < 0.01$ *vs.* diabetic control.

3. Discussion

Type I diabetes is an autoimmune disease. Type I diabetics need insulin injections to survive, which sometimes cause a series of complications. The development of safer, more specific and more effective hypoglycemic agents are important. Therefore, this study is the preliminary assessment and comparison of the anti-diabetic activities of differently regioselective chitosan sulfates. The diabetic model was developed by the intraperitoneal injection of alloxan.

Alloxan, a hydrophilic and chemically unstable pyrimidine derivative, is one of the common substances administered to induce diabetes mellitus. Alloxan has a destructive effect on the pancreatic β cells because it can generate a massive amount of oxygen radicals [15,16]. Some studies have shown that free radicals can rapidly accumulate and lead to oxidative stress in diabetic animals, which might impair the function of the liver and kidney, decrease antioxidase activities and increase lipid peroxidation levels [17]. Therefore, the role of oxidative stress/antioxidant balance in diabetes and its complications is an important research topic. Much attention has been focused on the research of antioxidant substances. Based on our previous research, differently regioselective chitosan sulfates have metal chelating and free radical scavenging properties [14]. Therefore, we hypothesized that differently regioselective chitosan sulfates may have hypoglycemic activities.

In the present study, we found that the hypoglycemic activities of regioselective chitosan sulfates are related to the position of their substitute group, though all of the selected sulfated chitosans had hypoglycemic activities. However, substitution degree of sulfate is not a major factor for the effect of hypoglycemic activity *in vivo*. High molecular weight 2-N-3,6-di-O-sulfo chitosan (H2,3,6-S) and 6-O-sulfochitosan (6-S) have equal hypoglycemic activities that were weaker than that of 3,6-si-O-sulfochitosan (3,6-S) and 3-O-sulfochitosan (3-S). Among all of the investigated sulfated chitosans, 3-S has the highest hypoglycemic activity. Treatment with 3-S contributed to a significant reduction of the blood glucose levels in the alloxan-induced diabetic rats. The results indicated that $-OSO_3^-$ at the C3 position is important, as introduction of this substitute group significantly increased the hypoglycemic activity of chitosan. In addition, we found that the hypoglycemic activities of low molecular weight 2-N-3,6-di-O-sulfo chitosan (L2,3,6-S) were obviously higher than that of H2,3,6-S. Therefore, the molecular weight is another important factor influencing hypoglycemic activities of sulfated chitosans. In this study, the hypoglycemic activities of differently regioselective sulfate chitosans are consistent with their antioxidant activity. The ability of 3,6-S and 3-S to scavenge and chelate hydroxyl radicals and their reducing power were stronger than that of H2,3,6-S and 6-S. The antioxidant activity of L2,3,6-S was significantly higher than that of H2,3,6-S. It is noteworthy that the relationship between the dose and the hypoglycemic activities of all of the investigated sulfate chitosans showed a bell-shaped curve. For example, the dose of 3-S (150 mg/kg) exhibited the highest hypoglycemic effect. Its effect was more significant than that of the low (50 mg/kg) or high dose (400 mg/kg) of 3-S. This result suggested that the 150 mg/kg dose may be the effective hypoglycemic dose of 3-S. This result provided a theoretical basis for the pharmacological structure-function relationship among different backbone structures and differently arranged functional groups.

Glucose tolerance is the human tolerance to glucose. Clinical tests usually measure the glucose tolerance of patients suspected of having diabetes. After oral administration of glucose for 2 h, the body reduces the tolerance to glucose if the blood glucose levels range from 7.8 to 11.1 mmol/L. In other words, the sugar uptake and usage of the body are worse than normal. In the present study, 3-S lowered the blood glucose levels and regulated the glucose tolerance effect in experimentally induced rats. 3-S was able to enhance glucose utilization because it significantly decreased the blood glucose level in glucose-loaded rats. This effect may be due to the restoration of a delayed insulin response or the inhibition of the intestinal absorption of glucose. Lazarow *et al.*, [18] and Colca *et al.*, [19] described the mechanism of action of alloxan. According to their studies, alloxan caused a massive reduction in insulin release through the destruction of β cells of the islets of Langerhans.

The pancreas is the primary organ involved in sensing the organism's dietary and energetic states via the glucose concentration in the blood; in response to elevated blood glucose, insulin is secreted [20]. When there are not enough available β cells to supply sufficient insulin to meet the needs of the body, insulin-dependent diabetes occurs [21]. In our study, as shown in Table 5, we observed a significant increase in the plasma insulin level when alloxan diabetic rats were treated with 3-S. At the same time, 3-S, at a dose of 300 mg/kg and 800 mg/kg body weight, was found to have a significant hypoglycemic activity and be more effective than glibenclamide (25 mg/kg). At a dose of 25 mg/kg, glibenclamide did not exhibit any hypoglycemic activity and only slightly increased fasting serum insulin levels. Therefore, the hypoglycemic potential of 3-S may be due to its ability to promote the renewal of β cells in the pancreas, help recover partially destroyed β cells, or stimulate pancreatic insulin secretion. However, the exact mechanism by which 3-S lowered the blood glucose level is not yet clear and needs to be further studied.

4. Materials and Methods

4.1. Materials and Chemicals

Alloxan and the reagents for serum insulin were purchased from Sigma-Aldrich Chemicals Co. (Saint Louis, MS, USA). A glucose analyzer and strips were purchased from Arkray Factory Inc. (Shiga, Japan). Phenformin hydrochloride tablets were purchased from Zhejiang Yatai Pharmaceutical Co. Ltd. (Shaoxing, Zhejiang, China). Glibenclamide tablets were purchased from Tianjin Lisheng Pharmaceutical Co. Ltd. (Tianjin, China). All other chemicals and reagents, unless otherwise specified, were not purified, dried or pretreated.

4.2. Experiment

4.2.1. Preparation of Sulfating Reagent

Five milliliters of HClSO3 were added dropwise and stirred into 30 mL N,N-dimethylformamide (DMF) which was previously cooled at 0–4 °C. The reaction mixture was stirred without cooling until the solution (DMF·SO$_3$) reached room temperature.

4.2.2. The Preparation of Sulfated Chitosan of C2,3,6 Sulfation (H2,3,6-S)

Fifty milliliters of DMF·SO$_3$ was added a 500 mL threenecked bottomed flask containing 50 mL of chitosan solution in a mixture of DMF–DCAA or DMF–formic acid with swirling to get gelatinous chitosan. Then the reaction was run at adequate temperature (40–60 °C) for 1–2.5 h, and 95% of EtOH (300 mL) was added to precipitate the product, giving a white precipitate. The mixture of products was filtered. The precipitate was washed with EtOH, then dissolved in distilled water, and the pH was adjusted to pH 7–8 with 2 M NaOH. The solution was dialyzed against distilled water for 48 h using an 8000 Da MW cut-off dialysis membrane. The product was then concentrated and lyophilized to give chitosan sulfate (2 g chitosan gave 2–3.7 g chitosan sulfates according to different conditions, including time, temperature and acid solvent).

4.2.3. The Preparation of Sulfated Chitosan of C2,3,6 Sulfation (L2,3,6-S)

DMF·SO$_3$ reagent (50 mL) was added to a 300 mL Erlenmeyer flask containing 50 mL of chitosan solution in a mixture of DMF–formic acid with swirling to get gelatinous chitosan. The Erlenmeyer flask containing the mixture of reactant was placed on the center of the turntable of the microwave oven. To control the reaction temperature to ~100 °C, another 50 mL Erlenmeyer flask containing a higher boiling solvent was also placed on the turntable in the microwave oven. Different irradiation powers and radiation times were set. After irradiation ceased, the reaction liquid was immediately poured into 90% EtOH (300 mL), giving a white precipitate. The mixture of products was filtered. The precipitate was washed with EtOH, then dissolved in distilled water, and the pH was adjusted to pH 7–8 with 2 M NaOH. The solution was dialyzed against distilled water for 48 h using a 3600 Da MW cutoff dialysis membrane. The product was then concentrated and lyophilized to give chitosan sulfate (2 g chitosan gave 1.8–3.1 g chitosan sulfated according to different conditions, including radiation power, radiation time, *etc.*).

4.2.4. The Preparation of Sulfated Chitosan of C3,6 Sulfation (3,6-S)

An amount of 4 g of chitosan was suspended in 100 mL dry DMF and stirred, then 5 g phthalic anhydride and 3 mL ethylene glycol was added in this system by stirring. The mixture was stirred for 2 h at 90 °C, and the transparent yellow solution was poured into ice-cold water. The precipitate was filtered off, washed with water, resuspended in EtOH, filtered off again. The product was dried at 60 °C and obtained the 2-phthalimidochitosan. Then 50 mL DMF·SO3 was added dropwise to a 250 mL three-necked bottomed flask containing 2 g 2-phthalimidochitosan and 100 mL DMF. Then the reaction was run at 50 °C for 2 h, and 95% of EtOH (500 mL) was added to precipitate the product, giving a pale yellow precipitate. The mixture of products was filtered and washed with EtOH, then redissolved in distilled water, and the pH was adjusted to 7–8 with 2 M NaOH. The solution was dialyzed against distilled water for 48 h using a 3600 Da MW cut-off dialysis membrane. The product was then concentrated and lyophilized to give pale yellow 3,6-di-*O*-2-*N*-phthalimido-sulfochitosan.

3,6-di-*O*-2-*N*-Phthalimido-sulfochitosan was dissolved in deionized water, and hydrazine hydrate was added. The solution was heated to 70 °C for 3 h. Afterwards, water was added, and the solution evaporated nearly to dryness. This was repeated three to five times to eliminate the remaining hydrazine. Then, the solution was dialyzed against distilled water for 48 h using a 3600 Da MW cut-off dialysis membrane. The product was then concentrated and lyophilized to give pale yellow 3,6-di-*O*-sulfochitosan.

4.2.5. The Preparation of Sulfated Chitosan of C3 Sulfation (3-S)

3,6-di-*O*-Sulfochitosan was dissolved in deionized water, and then the mixture of *N*-methylpyrrolidinone and water was added to the aforementioned solution. The yellow solution was stirred for 3 h at 90 °C. After the reaction, the pH was adjusted to 9.0 by 2 M NaOH. The solution was dialyzed, concentrated and freeze-dried to give yellow 3-*O*-sulfochitosan (TCTS).

4.2.6. The Preparation of Sulfated Chitosan of C6 Sulfation (6-S)

Chitosan was dissolved in 2% formic acid (50 mL), then 1 M CuSO$_4$·5 H$_2$O was added dropwise to the above-mentioned solution at rt. After stirring for 4 h, the PH was adjusted to 6–7 by 2% NH$_3$·H$_2$O, then the reaction was run at rt for 4 h. The resulting precipitate was filtered and washed with water, acetone, and Et$_2$O. This precipitate was dispersed in dry DMF (30 mL) for 16 h, then SO$_3$·DMF was added dropwise to the aforementioned mixture solution, and the reaction was run for 1–3 h at 40–60 °C. After the reaction, the pH was adjusted to 8 by saturated NaHCO$_3$. The solution was dialyzed for 3 days. To eliminate the copper protective group from the complex, the aforementioned solution was passed through an Amberlite IRC 718 column. The eluate was neutralized and then freeze-dried.

4.2.7. Analytical Methods

The degree of deacetylation of chitosan was 87% by potentionmetry and the viscosity average-molecular weight was 7.6×10^5. FTIR spectra was measured by Nicolet Magna-Avatar 360 (American) with KBr disk; Sulfate content % was measured in a SC-132 sulfur meter (LECO), and the average viscometric molecular weight of sulfated chitosan was estimated from the intrinsic viscosity determined in the solvent 0.1 M CH_3COOH/0.2 M NaCl using the Mark-Houwink parameters $\alpha = 0.96$, $K\eta = 1.424$ at 25 °C when the intrinsic viscosity was expressed in $mL \cdot g^{-1}$.

4.3. Animals

Wistar rats, due to their high fecundity, litter size, gentle temperament, strong resistance to infectious diseases, and low incidence of spontaneous tumors, are widely used in various fields of biomedical experimentation. Wistar rats of approximately the same age and a body weight of 180–220 g, half male and half female, were obtained from Tianjin Institute of Pharmaceutical Research and were used after being acclimatized to laboratory conditions for a week. The rats were provided a standard rat pellet diet and water. There were 21 groupsemployed, and each consisted of 5 to 10 animals. The rats were housed in stainless steel cages to provide them with sufficient space and to avoid unnecessary morbidity and mortality. All experimental procedures were performed in strict accordance with the recommendations in the Guide for the Care and Use of Laboratory Animals of the Institutional Animal Ethical Committee, and the protocols were approved by the Committee on the Ethics of Animal Experiments of the Institute of Oceanology, Chinese Academy of Sciences, Shandong, China. All efforts were made to minimize suffering, and the experimental animals were anesthetized using sodium pentobarbital before blood sampling was performed. The animals for the following experiments were pre-fasted overnight, but were allowed free access to water.

4.4. Studies on Alloxan-Induced Diabetic Rats

4.4.1. Induction of Diabetes Mellitus

Diabetes was induced by the intraperitoneal injection of alloxan monohydrate in normal saline to overnight-fasted animals at a dose of 50 mg/kg body weight. After 72 h, the rats were deprived of food for 3 h, and then the blood glucose level was determined. The rats with blood glucose levels above 10 mmol/L were used for the study.

4.4.2. Determination of the Hypoglycemic Effect on Diabetic Rats

Alloxan diabetic rats were divided into 23 groups of 5–10 animals each. Group 1 was the normal group, and Group 2 was the diabetic model control group. The groups were given an equivalent volume of saline (0.5 mL/100 g day body weight) by intragastric administration. For the Group 3 animals, phenformin hydrochloride was applied at a dose of 100 mg/kg body weight/day by intragastric administration. For the Group 4, Group 5 and Group 6 animals, sulfated chitosan of $C_{2,3,6}$ sulfation (H2,3,6-S) was given at a dose of 50, 150 and 400 mg/kg body weight/day by intragastric administration. Group 7, Group 8 and Group 9 animals were treated with low molecular weight sulfated chitosan of $C_{2,3,6}$ sulfation (L2,3,6-S). Group 10, Group 11 and Group 12 were treated with sulfated chitosan of C_6 sulfation (6-S). Group 13, Group 14 and Group 15 were given sulfated chitosan of $C_{3,6}$ sulfation (3,6-S). Group 16, Group 17 and Group 18 were given sulfated chitosan of C_3 sulfation (3-S). Group 19, Group 20 and Group 21 were given chitosan (CTS). The groups were given equivalent doses of H2,3,6-S by intragastric administration, once a day for 30 days. The fasting blood samples (1 mL per rat) were collected on day 6, 12, 18, 24 and 30 to determine the glucose level.

4.4.3. Glucose Tolerance Test

Kunming rats are an outbred rats group. China has the largest production and usage of this rat. After years of breeding, Kunming rats now have a very low rate of spontaneous tumors, strong resistance to disease and resilience, high reproductive rate and survival rate. Therefore, Kunming rats are widely used in various fields of biomedical experiments and account for approximately 70% of the total amount of all the rats. Kunming rats of approximately the same age and with a body weight of 20–30 g, half male and half female, were obtained from the Tianjin Institute of Pharmaceutical Research and were used after being acclimatized to laboratory conditions for a week. They were provided a standard rat pellet diet and water. Three groups were employed, and each consisted of 10 animals. Group 1 was the normal group that received an equivalent volume of saline. For the animals in Group 2, phenformin hydrochloride was administered at a dose of 200 mg/kg body weight/day and in Group 3 animals, 3-S was administered at a dose of 300 mg/kg body weight/day for 14 days. Fifteen days later, after being deprived of food for 15 h, blood was collected from the rat's tail vein for glucose estimation. This value was used as the baseline blood glucose level. Then, Group 2 rats and Group 3 rats were given phenformin hydrochloride and 3-S once by intragastric administration. One hour later, rats of both the control and treated groups were injected intraperitoneally with glucose (2 g/kg body weight). Blood was collected from the rat's tail vein at 30 min intervals up to 2 h [22] for glucose estimation using a glucometer.

4.4.4. Determination of the Plasma Insulin Concentration

Kunming rats were deprived of food and allowed free access to water for 18 h. Then, diabetes was induced by the intraperitoneal injection of alloxan monohydrate at a dose of 50 mg/kg body weight. Seventy-two hours later, the rats were deprived of food for 4 h, and blood was collected from the rat's tail vein for glucose level estimation. The rats with glucose levels above 10 mmol/L were randomly divided into 5 groups. The normal group had 10 normal rats. The normal group and the diabetic model control group were given an equivalent volume of saline by intragastric administration, once a day for 14 days. For the Group 3 animals, phenformin hydrochloride was administered at a dose of 25 mg/kg body weight by intragastric administration, once a day for 14 days. For Group 4, Group 5 and Group 6 animals, 3-S was given at a dose of 100 mg/kg, 300 mg/kg and 800 mg/kg body weight by intragastric administration, once a day for 14 days. On the fourteenth day, after being deprived of food for 12 h, Group 3, Group 4, Group 5 and Group 6 animals were given phenformin hydrochloride and different doses of 3-S by intragastric administration. Two hours later, blood was collected from the rat's eyeballs for glucose level determination. The fasting serum insulin levels were determined using an insulin radioimmunoassay kit [23].

4.5. Statistical Analysis

All of the data were expressed as mean ± standard deviation (SD) of three replicates and were analyzed statistically by one-way analysis of variance using SPSS version 10.0 software. The statistical significance between the means of the experimental and control studies was established by Student's *t*-test. The results were considered to be significant if $p < 0.05$, $p < 0.01$ or $p < 0.001$.

5. Conclusions

The hypoglycemic activity of differently regioselective chitosan sulfates in alloxan-induced diabetic rats was researched in this paper. The conclusions are as follows.

- Differently regioselective chitosan sulfates exhibited hypoglycemic activities.
- Hypoglycemic activity of low molecular weight sulfate chitosan was obviously higher.
- 3-S exhibited significantly hypoglycemic activities in alloxan-induced diabetic rats.
- 3-S could regulate the glucose tolerance effect.
- 3-S could significantly increase the insulin levels in experimentally induced rats.

- $-OSO_3^-$ at the C3-position of chitosan is a key active site.

Acknowledgments: The study was supported by Qingdao science and technology plan (No.14-2-3-47-nsh), the Public Science and Technology Research Funds Projects of Ocean (No. 201305016-2 and No. 201405038-2), the Science and Technology Development Program of Shandong Province (No. 2012GHY11530), and the Action Plan of CAS to Support China's New and Strategic Industries with Science and Technology.

Author Contributions: X.R. and L.P. conceived and designed the experiments; X.R., H.X., L.S. and Y.H. performed the experiments; X.R., Q.Y. and L.K. analyzed the data; C.X. and L.R. contributed reagents/materials/analysis tools; X.R. wrote the paper.

Conflicts of Interest: The authors declare no conflict of interest.

References

1. Triplitt, C.L.; Reasner, C.A.; Isley, W.L. Diabetes Mellitus. In *Pharmacotherapy: A Pathophysiologic Approach*; DiPiro, J.T., Talbert, R.L., Yee, G.C., Matzke, G.R., Wells, B.G., Posey, L.M., Eds.; McGraw-Hill Medical Publishing Division: New York, NY, USA, 2005; p. 1334.
2. Kameswararao, B.; Kesavulu, M.M.; Apparao, C. Evaluation of antidiabetic effect of momordica cymbelaria fruit in alloxan-diabetic rats. *Fitoterapia* **2003**, *74*, 7–13. [CrossRef] [PubMed]
3. Pepato, M.T.; Mori, D.M.; Baviera, A.M.; Harami, J.B.; Vendramini, R.C.; Brunetti, I.L. Fruit of the Jambolan tree and experimental diabetes. *J. Ethnopharmacol.* **2005**, *96*, 43–48. [CrossRef] [PubMed]
4. Rosak, C. The pathophysiologic basis of efficacy and clinical experience with the new oral antidiabetic agents. *J. Diabetes Complicat.* **2002**, *16*, 123–132. [CrossRef] [PubMed]
5. Rahman, Q.; Zaman, K. Medicinal plants with hypoglycaemic activity. *J. Ethnopharmacol.* **1989**, *26*, 1–55. [CrossRef] [PubMed]
6. Shanmugam, K.R.; Mallikarjuna, K.; Nishanth, K.; Kuo, C.H.; Reddy, K.S. Protective effect of dietary ginger on antioxidant enzymes and oxidative damage in experimental diabetic rat tissues. *Food Chem.* **2011**, *124*, 1436–1442. [CrossRef]
7. Suba, V.; Murugesan, T.; Arunachalam, G.; Mardal, S.C.; Sahu, B.P. Anti-diabetic potential of barleria lupilina extract in rats. *Phytomedicine* **2004**, *11*, 202–205. [CrossRef] [PubMed]
8. Bing, L.; Wanshun, L.; Baoqin, H. Antidiabetic effects of Chitooligo-saccharides on pancreatic islet cells and streptozotocin induced diabetic rats. *World J. Gastroenterol.* **2007**, *13*, 725–731. [CrossRef] [PubMed]
9. Nishimura, S.I.; Kai, H.; Shimada, K.; Yoshida, T.; Tokura, S.; Kurita, K. Regioselective syntheses of sulfated polysaccharides: Specific anti-HIV-1 activity of novel chitin sulfates. *Carbohydr. Res.* **1998**, *306*, 427–433. [CrossRef] [PubMed]
10. Rahimi, R.; Nikfar, S.; Larijani, B.; Abdollahi, M. A review on the role of antioxidants in the management of diabetes and its complications. *Biomed. Pharmacother.* **2005**, *59*, 365–373. [CrossRef] [PubMed]
11. Rudge, M.V.C.; Damasceno, D.C.; Volpato, G.T.; Almeida, F.C.G.; Calderon, I.M.P.; Lemonica, I.P. Effect of Ginkgo biloba on the reproductive outcome and oxidative stress biomarkers of streptozotocin-induced diabetic rats. *Braz. J. Med. Biol. Res.* **2007**, *40*, 1095–1099. [CrossRef] [PubMed]
12. Prasad, K. Oxidative stress as a mechanism of diabetes in diabetic BB prone rats: Effect of secoisolariciresinol diglucoside (SDG). *Mol. Cell. Biochem.* **2000**, *209*, 89–96. [CrossRef] [PubMed]
13. Kamalakkannan, N.; Stanely Mainzen Prince, P. Rutin improves the antioxidant status in streptozotocin-induced diabetic rat tissues. *Mol. Cell. Biochem.* **2006**, *293*, 211–219. [CrossRef] [PubMed]
14. Xing, R.E.; Yu, H.H.; Liu, S.; Zhang, W.W.; Zhang, Q.B.; Li, P.C. Antioxidant activity of differently regioselective chitosan sulfates *in vitro*. *Bioorganic Med. Chem.* **2005**, *13*, 1387–1392. [CrossRef]
15. Jelodar, G.; Mohsen, M.; Shahram, S. Effect of walnut leaf, coriander and pomegranate on blood glucose and his topathology of pancreas of alloxan-induced diabetic rats. *Afr. J. Tradit. Complement. Altern. Med.* **2003**, *3*, 299–305.
16. Szkudelski, T. The mechanism of alloxan and streptozotocin action in B cells of the rat pancreas. *Physiol. Res.* **2001**, *50*, 537–546. [PubMed]
17. Hamden, K.; Carreau, S.; Lajmi, S.; Aloulou, D.; Kchaou, D.; Elfeki, A. Protective effect of 17 β-estradiol on hyperglycemia, stress oxidant, liver dysfunction and histological changes induced by alloxan in male rat pancreas and liver. *Steroids* **2008**, *94*, 495–501. [CrossRef]

18. Lazarow, A. Alloxan diabetes and mechanism of β-cell damage by chemical agents. In *Experimental Diabetes*; Lazarow, A., Ed.; Blackwell Scientific Publication: Oxford, UK, 1964; pp. 49–69.

19. Colca, J.R.; Kotagel, N.; Brooks, C.L.; Lacy, P.E.; Landt, M.; Mc Danield, M.L. Alloxan inhibition of a Ca^{2+} and calmodulin-dependent protein kinase in pancreatic islets. *J. Biol. Chem.* **1983**, *25*, 7260–7263.

20. Edem, D.O. Hypoglycemic effects of ethanolic extract of Aligator pear seed (*Persea americana* Mill) in rats. *Eur. J. Sci. Res.* **2009**, *33*, 669–678.

21. Funom, M. Etiology and pathophysiology of diabetes mellitus. Available online: http://ezinearticles.com/?Etiology-and-Pathophysiology-of-Diabetes-Mellitus&id=4353837 (accessed on 24 May 2010).

22. Matteucci, E.; Giampietro, O. Proposal open for discussion: Defining agreed diagnostic procedures in experimental diabetes research. *J. Ethnopharmacol.* **2008**, *115*, 163–172. [CrossRef] [PubMed]

23. Buccolo, G.; David, M. Quantitative determination of serum triglycerides by use of enzyme. *Clin. Chem.* **1973**, *19*, 476–482. [PubMed]

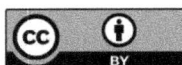

MDPI

Article

Identification of a Pro-Angiogenic Potential and Cellular Uptake Mechanism of a LMW Highly Sulfated Fraction of Fucoidan from *Ascophyllum nodosum*

Nicolas Marinval [1], Pierre Saboural [1], Oualid Haddad [1], Murielle Maire [1], Kevin Bassand [1], Frederic Geinguenaud [2], Nadia Djaker [2], Khadija Ben Akrout [2], Marc Lamy de la Chapelle [2], Romain Robert [1], Olivier Oudar [1], Erwan Guyot [1,3], Christelle Laguillier-Morizot [1,3], Angela Sutton [1,3], Cedric Chauvierre [1], Frederic Chaubet [1], Nathalie Charnaux [1,3] and Hanna Hlawaty [1,*]

[1] Inserm U1148, LVTS, Université Paris 13, Sorbonne Paris Cité, Paris 75018, France; nicolas.marinval@inserm.fr (N.M.); pierre.saboural@univ-paris13.fr (P.S.); haddad.oualid@univ-paris13.fr (O.H.); murielle.maire@univ-paris13.fr (M.M.); bassand.k@gmail.com (K.B.); robert.romain@gmail.com (R.R.); olivier.oudar@univ-paris13.fr (O.O.); erwan.guyot@aphp.fr (E.G.); christelle.laguillier@aphp.fr (C.L.-M.); angela.sutton@aphp.fr (A.S.); cedric.chauvierre@inserm.fr (C.C.); frederic.chaubet@univ-paris13.fr (F.C.); nathalie.charnaux@aphp.fr (N.C.)
[2] Laboratoire CSPBAT, CNRS UMR 7244, UFR SMBH, Université Paris 13, Sorbonne Paris Cité, Bobigny F-93017, France; frederic.geinguenaud@univ-paris13.fr (F.G.); nadia.djaker@univ-paris13.fr (N.D.); khadijabenakrout@hotmail.fr (K.B.A.); marc.lamydelachapelle@univ-paris13.fr (M.L.d.l.C.)
[3] Laboratoire de Biochimie, Hôpital Jean Verdier, Assistance Publique-Hôpitaux de Paris, Bondy 93140, France
* Correspondence: hania.hlawaty@inserm.fr; Tel.: +33-01-48-38-85-14

Academic Editor: Paola Laurienzo
Received: 28 September 2016; Accepted: 10 October 2016; Published: 17 October 2016

Abstract: Herein we investigate the structure/function relationships of fucoidans from *Ascophyllum nodosum* to analyze their pro-angiogenic effect and cellular uptake in native and glycosaminoglycan-free (GAG-free) human endothelial cells (HUVECs). Fucoidans are marine sulfated polysaccharides, which act as glycosaminoglycans mimetics. We hypothesized that the size and sulfation rate of fucoidans influence their ability to induce pro-angiogenic processes independently of GAGs. We collected two fractions of fucoidans, Low and Medium Molecular Weight Fucoidan (LMWF and MMWF, respectively) by size exclusion chromatography and characterized their composition (sulfate, fucose and uronic acid) by colorimetric measurement and Raman and FT-IR spectroscopy. The high affinities of fractionated fucoidans to heparin binding proteins were confirmed by Surface Plasmon Resonance. We evidenced that LMWF has a higher pro-angiogenic (2D-angiogenesis on Matrigel) and pro-migratory (Boyden chamber) potential on HUVECs, compared to MMWF. Interestingly, in a GAG-free HUVECs model, LMWF kept a pro-angiogenic potential. Finally, to evaluate the association of LMWF-induced biological effects and its cellular uptake, we analyzed by confocal microscopy the GAGs involvement in the internalization of a fluorescent LMWF. The fluorescent LMWF was mainly internalized through HUVEC clathrin-dependent endocytosis in which GAGs were partially involved. In conclusion, a better characterization of the relationships between the fucoidan structure and its pro-angiogenic potential in GAG-free endothelial cells was required to identify an adapted fucoidan to enhance vascular repair in ischemia.

Keywords: fucoidan; glycosaminoglycans; glycocalyx; angiogenesis; endocytosis

---

1. Introduction

Glycosaminoglycans (GAGs) are linear and sulfated carbohydrate chains covalently bound to a protein core to form a proteoglycan (PG), including syndecans [1]. The GAGs are shaped of sulfated disaccharide units composed of galactose or glucuronic/iduronic acid and N-acetyl-glucosamine/-galactosamine. As major components of the glycocalyx, GAGs, which cover the luminal outermost endothelial cell layer, are involved in angiogenesis, inflammation, as well as in cell proliferation, adhesion and migration [2,3]. Thus, reorganization of microenvironment, damages and modifications in the endothelial glycocalyx, caused by ischemia are widely studied [4]. Highly sulfated GAGs, such as heparan sulfate, mostly bind the signaling proteins (cytokines, chemokines and growth factors) and allow their retention/release, therefore contributing to glycocalyx and extracellular matrix reorganization [5]. It is known that the interaction of GAGs with signaling proteins involves the negative charges of the sulfates. However, we have previously shown that the relation between GAG expression and their potential in regulation of angiogenesis is difficult to characterize, mainly caused by the heterogeneity of their chain structure, sulfation level and position. Moreover, we also showed that the GAGs expression is subjected to modulation of expression pattern in size and sulfation levels during ischemia, modifying their ability to bind proteins [6].

Fucoidan, a marine sulfated polysaccharide from brown seaweeds that has similar biological activities of heparin, has been shown to promote revascularization in a rat critical hindlimb ischemia [7] and re-endothelialization in rabbit intimal hyperplasia [8]. Its polysaccharidic structure is mainly composed by fucose and uronic acid units, and confers to the fucoidan some properties which are similar in a certain extent to endogenous GAGs. It is noteworthy that this natural GAG mimetic could have comparable affinities for heparin binding proteins, such as chemokines and growth factors [9]. Depending of the type and size of polysaccharide fragments, the fucoidan could have a pro-angiogenic activity by modulating the bioavaibility of angiogenic cytokines in soluble or matrix-associated forms [10,11]. Recently, we demonstrated that the low molecular weight fucoidan (LMWF) modified the heparan sulfate expression pattern in modulating heparanase and syndecans expressions [12]. In addition, we have previously shown that the functionalized fucoidan present in three dimensional porous scaffolds was shown to retain the vascular endothelial growth factor (VEGF) and increased subcutaneous angiogenesis in mouse [13].

Upstream of developing a bio-engineering therapy based on fucoidan to regenerate damaged-vasculature, we propose the structure/function analysis to study its beneficial effect on angiogenesis and the endogenous GAG involvement in this process. Based on recent literature which showed the correlation between low molecular weight sulfated GAG-mimetics and their ability to regenerate damaged tissue [14], we hypothesized that the size and sulfation level of fucoidan could have an influence on cell migration and angiogenesis in glycocalyx-damaged human endothelial cells. We hypothesized that endogenous GAGs expression is altered in cardiovascular diseases and exogenous polysaccharides could modify the GAGs expression that we and others has already shown [12,15].

In our work we analyzed the correlation between the structure of the fucoidans and their functions on in vitro vascular network formation and endothelial cell migration in GAG-free human endothelial cells.

2. Results

2.1. LMWF and MMWF Fractions Collection and Characterization

2.1.1. Fractionation and Composition of ASPHY, MMWF and LMWF

A column of size exclusion chromatography was used to elute the crude fucoidan Ascophyscient (ASPHY, 4100 g/mol) and collect two fractions with different molecular weight (Table 1), a medium molecular weight fucoidan (MMWF, 26,600 g/mol) and a low molecular weight fucoidan (LMWF,

4900 g/mol). Polydispersity analysis showed a very homogeneous population distribution of both polysaccharides LMWF and MMWF, as compared to the heterogeneous crude ASPHY (Table 1 and Figure S1). The composition of the three fucoidans (ASPHY, MMWF and LMWF) was analyzed then to determine sulfate, fucose and uronic acid mass percentage using the colorimetric measurement. The results showed the presence of fucose, sulfate and uronic acid in different percentage rate, 29%, 25%, and 27% for ASPHY, 36%, 29%, and 14% for MMWF and 21%, 23%, and 18% for LMWF, respectively (Table 2). The average density of sulfates for each fucoidan was calculated with a molecular rate of sulfate per fucose unit and showed that all fucoidans displayed a high sulfation rate (>1). The highest sulfation rate was attributed to LMWF (1.55), as compared to MMWF (1.14) and ASPHY (1.22) (Table 2).

Table 1. Molecular weight determination of fractionated fucoidans by HPSEC-MALLS-dRI.

Fucoidans	Mn (g/mol)	M_w (g/mol)	Ip (M_w/Mn)
ASPHY	4100	10800	2.8 ± 0.6
MMWF	26,600	27,400	1.0 ± 1.2
LMWF	4900	5600	1.1 ± 1.2

Table 2. Composition of the fucoidans in fucose, sulfate, uronic acid and expression of the molar ratio sulfate/fucose.

Fucoidans	Fucose	Sulfate	Uronic Acid	Unknown	Ratio Sulfate/Fucose
ASPHY	29%	25%	27%	19%	1.22
MMWF	36%	29%	14%	21%	1.14
LMWF	21%	23%	18%	39%	1.55

2.1.2. Raman and Fourier Transform Infrared Spectroscopy Analysis

Complementary to colorimetric measurement, the spectroscopic analysis of the three polysaccharides (ASPHY, MMWF and LMWF) was performed with Raman and Fourier Transform Infrared (FT-IR) Spectroscopy. The Raman band at 1458 cm^{-1} was assigned to scissoring vibration of CH$_2$ and asymmetric bending vibration of CH$_3$ for absorption at around 1455 cm^{-1}, as suggested previously by Synytsya [16]. The Raman shoulder at 1360 cm^{-1} is originated from symmetric bending vibration of methyl and the FT-IR spectroscopy band at 1389 cm^{-1} could be the corresponding band already described at 1380 cm^{-1} (Figure 1A,B). The main pyranoid ring vibrations (HCC, HCO and COH) were observed in Raman band at 1336 cm^{-1}, while COC stretching of glycosidic bonds and also CC and CO stretching covered the region located at 1200–900 cm^{-1}. In Raman the β-glycosidic linkages between monosaccharide units was described at 890 cm^{-1}. The characteristic band for sulfated polysaccharides attributed to asymmetric O=S=O stretching vibration (with some contribution of carbohydrate vibrations) was founded around 1253 cm^{-1} in FT-IR and 1268 cm^{-1} in Raman, although symmetric O=S=O stretching of sulfate was founded at 1082 cm^{-1} in Raman [17]. The Raman spectra of the three samples of fucoidans showed that LMWF exhibited a strong vibration at 1082 cm^{-1} and 1268 cm^{-1} compared to MMWF. For both LMWF and MMWF spectra, the Raman band at 845 cm^{-1} was attributed to COS bending vibration of sulfate substituents at the axial C2 and the equatorial C4 positions [18], both the 722 cm^{-1} and 820 cm^{-1} bands were attributed to the angular deformations of CH bonds. Otherwise the Raman band at 577 cm^{-1} and 540 cm^{-1} were attributed to the asymmetric and symmetric O=S=O deformation of sulfates [19]. The FT-IR analysis in D$_2$O revealed the intensity of carboxylic groups (COO-) at the band 1609 cm^{-1} for LMWF and MMWF and 1598 cm^{-1} for ASPHY (Figure 1B). The data exhibited stronger intensities in the crude ASPHY and fractionated LMWF, as compared to MMWF.

In the next part of our work, in order to study the structure/function correlation of fucoidans, we analyzed the impact of ASPHY, MMWF and LMWF size and sulfation rate on human endothelial cell viability, angiogenesis and migration.

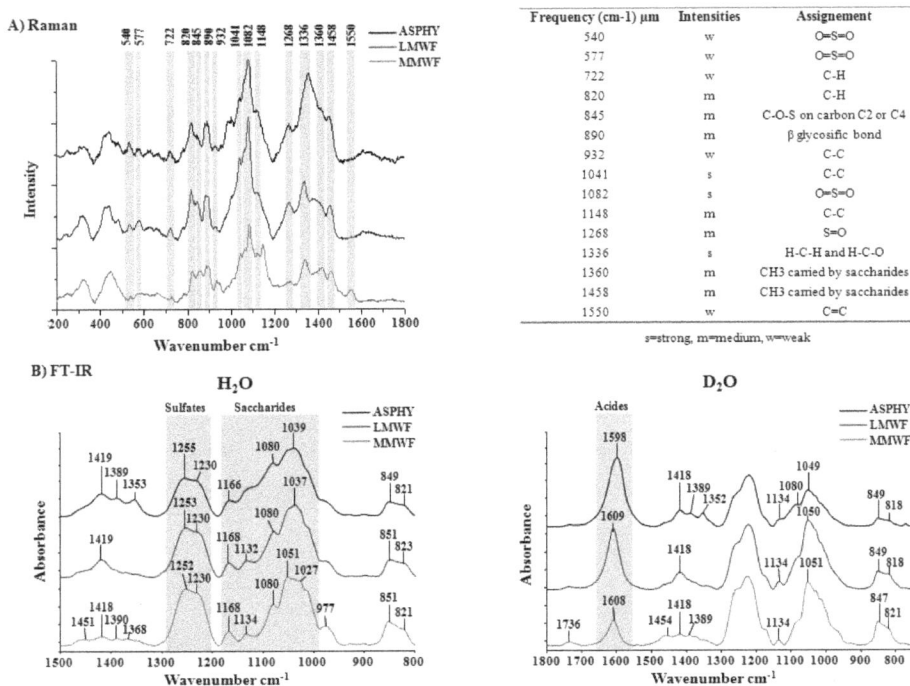

Figure 1. Raman and Fourrier Tansform Infrared (FT-IR) Spectroscopy analysis. Fucoidan spectra are represented in black for crude Ascophyscient (ASPHY), dark grey for the low molecular weight fucoidan (LMWF) and light grey for the medium molecular weight fucoidan (MMWF) for (**A**) Raman and (**B**) FT-IR (in H₂O and in D₂O). The numbers indicates the characteristics bands for polysaccharides.

2.2. Biological Effects of LMWF and MMWF in GAG-Free Endothelial Cells

2.2.1. LMWF and MMWF Affinities towards Heparin-Binding Proteins

We measured and compared the affinity of all the fucoidans towards the heparin-binding proteins (HBP) stromal derived factor-1 (SDF-1/CXCL12), regulated on activation, normal T cell expressed and secreted (RANTES/CCL5) and vascular endothelial growth factor (VEGF) by Surface Plasmon Resonance analysis. We used a low molecular weight heparin (LMWH) and a non-sulfated dextran (Dextran) as positive and negative control, respectively. Our data showed a characteristic model with a rapid association of the polysaccharide to the HBP and a slow dissociation as we have previously described [20] (Figure 2A–C). The results confirmed the direct interaction between fucoidans and HBP, characterized by an affinity KD (Kd/Ka), for SDF-1/CXCL12 (8.2×10^{-11} M for ASPHY, 1.4×10^{-10} M for MMWF and 8.4×10^{-11} M for LMWF) (Figure 2A), for RANTES/CCL5 (5.4×10^{-9} M for ASPHY, 4.7×10^{-9} M for MMWF and 2.1×10^{-9} M for LMWF) (Figure 2B) and for VEGF (8.1×10^{-10} for ASPHY, 2.3×10^{-10} for LMWF and 1.9×10^{-10} for MMWF) (Figure 2C).

There were no significant differences between the affinities of all fucoidans towards SDF-1/CXCL12 and RANTES/CCL5 and the affinities of LMWH (1.0×10^{-10} M, 1.4×10^{-8} M and 5.2×10^{-11} M respectively).

A)

SDF-1/CXCL12	
Name	**KD (M)**
ASPHY	8.2×10^{-11}
LMWF	8.4×10^{-11}
MMWF	1.4×10^{-10}
LMWH	1.0×10^{-10}

B)

RANTES/CCL5	
Name	**KD (M)**
ASPHY	5.4×10^{-9}
LMWF	2.1×10^{-9}
MMWF	4.7×10^{-9}
LMWH	1.4×10^{-8}

C)

VEGF$_{165a}$	
Name	**KD (M)**
ASPHY	8.1×10^{-10}
LMWF	2.3×10^{-10}
MMWF	1.9×10^{-10}
LMWH	5.2×10^{-11}

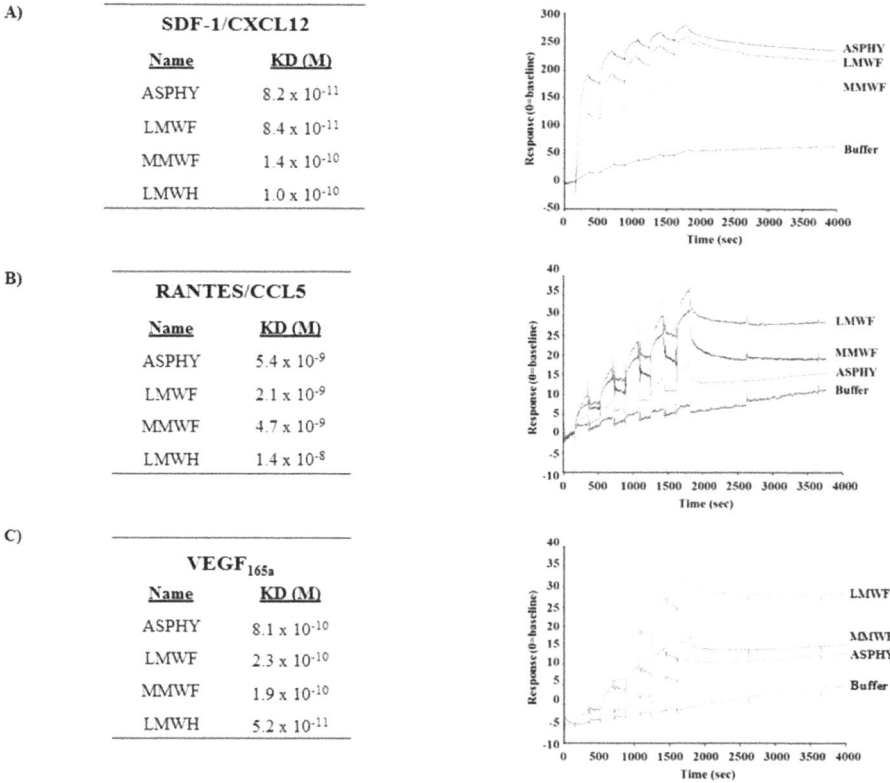

Figure 2. Affinity measurement of fucoidans to SDF-1/CXCL12, RANTES/CCL5 and VEGF. The binding responses of ASPHY, MMWF, LMWF and low molecular weight heparin (LMWH) to SDF-1/CXCL12, RANTES/CCL5 and VEGF were measured by Surface Plasmon Resonance. We immobilized biotinylated SDF-1/CXCL12, RANTES/CCL5 or VEGF on streptavidin chip. Each polysaccharide was injected over flow of a BIAcore sensor chip pre-coated with streptavidin biotinylated SDF-1/CXCL12, RANTES/CCL5 or VEGF. Each set of sensorgrams was obtained by injecting increasing concentration of polysaccharides (1.2, 3.7, 11.1, 33.3, and 100 nM). The response unit (RU) was recorded as a function of time (sec) and the affinities are expressed in molar (M) with the equilibrium dissociation constant KD (Kd/Ka). LMWH was used as a positive control of sulfated polysaccharide whereas non-sulfated dextran was used as a negative control (not shown). Affinity of polysaccharides to (**A**) SDF-1/CXCL12; (**B**) RANTES/CCL5 and (**C**) VEGF, and their corresponding representative sensorgrams.

2.2.2. LMWF and MMWF Effects on Endothelial Cell Viability

We first studied the effects of fucoidans on human umbilical vein endothelial cells (HUVECs) viability using metabolic activity MTT test (Thiazolyl Blue Tetrazolium Bromide) after 24, 48, and 72 h of ASPHY, MMWF and LMWF treatments. Our results demonstrated that all fucoidans showed no toxicity for HUVECs from 1 to 1000 µg/mL, as compared to untreated cells (Figure 3 and data not shown). There was a light increase of cell viability after 24 h of LMWF treatment at 10, 100, and 1000 µg/mL (Figure 3A,C). However, only the highest concentration of MMWF at 1000 µg/mL increased the HUVEC viability (Figure 3B). At 10 µg/mL, LMWF increased the HUVEC viability (Figure 3C), but ASPHY and dextran did not have any effect on HUVEC viability at this concentration

(Figure 2C and data not shown). In addition, there was no increase of HUVEC viability after 48 and 72 h of fucoidan treatment (data not shown). This assay established the viable culture conditions to measure angiogenesis and cell migration assays where we decided to use the fucoidans to analyze its biological activities at 10 µg/mL and up to 24 h of fucoidan treatment.

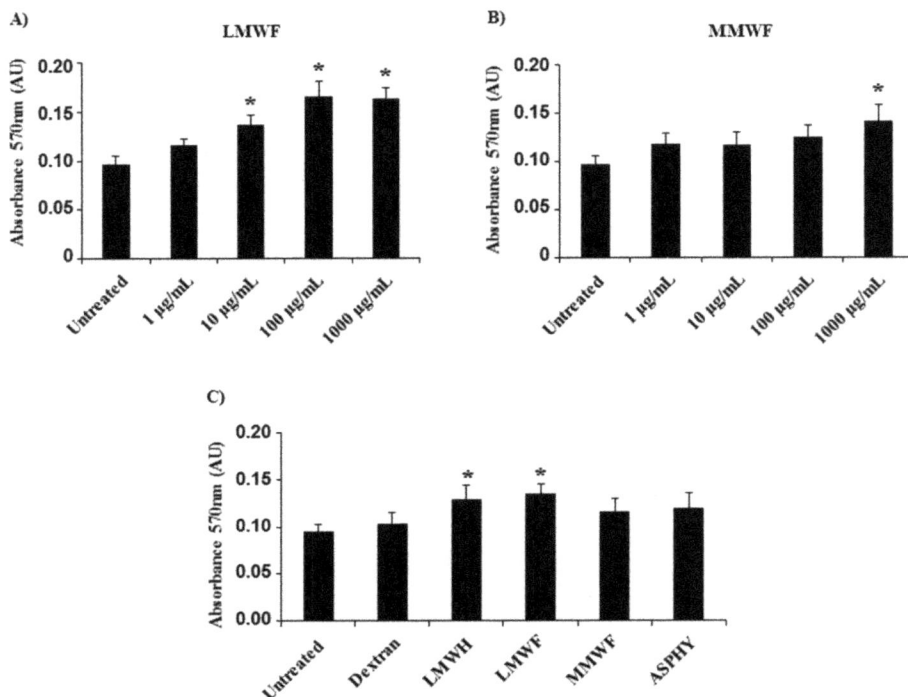

Figure 3. Effect of fucoidans on cell viability. The viability of HUVECs was analyzed by using MTT assay after fucoidan treatment for 24 h. The absorbance was read with a spectrophotometer (at 570 nm). HUVECs were incubated with (**A**) LMWF and (**B**) MMWF at increasing concentration (1, 10, 100, and 1000 µg/mL); (**C**) HUVECs were incubated 24 h with polysaccharides (dextran, LMWH, LMWF, MMWF and ASPHY) at 10 µg/mL. Values are expressed as means $\pm$ SEM ($n \geq 3$). AU-Arbitrary units. * $p < 0.05$ versus Untreated.

2.2.3. LMWF and MMWF Effects on Angiogenesis In Vitro

In order to analyze the fucoidan structure/function relation in the angiogenesis processes, we established a 2-dimensional (2D) vascular network formation assay on Matrigel in vitro. The pro-angiogenic potential of ASPHY, MMWF, and LMWF at 10 µg/mL on HUVECs was analyzed as the percentage of cellular connection resulting in nodes formation per well at 6 h of incubation. Our results showed the significant increase of nodes formation by 56% $\pm$ 16% and by 57% $\pm$ 12%, after LMWF and LMWH treatments, respectively, as compared to control (Figure 4A, black bars). However, dextran, MMWF and ASPHY did not induce any changes in node formation (Figure 4A).

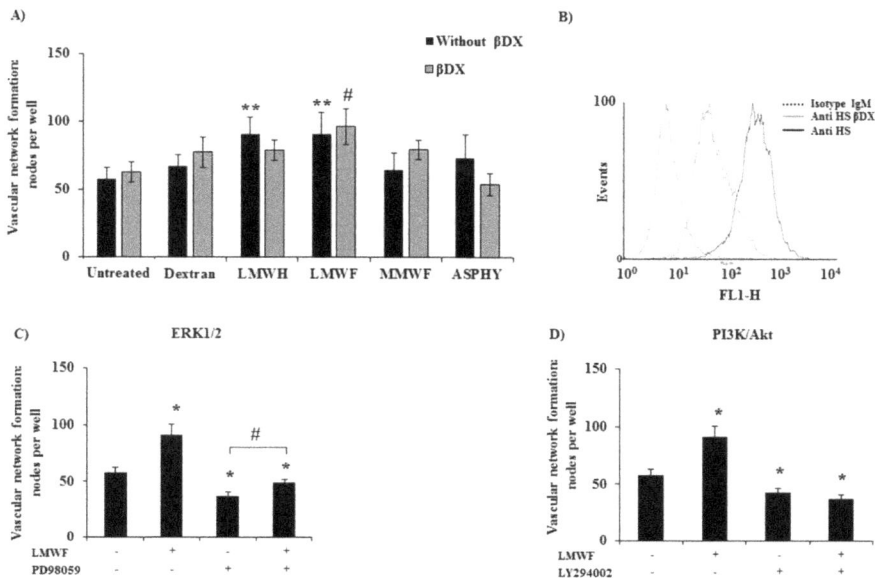

Figure 4. Pro-angiogenic potential of fucoidans on GAG-free HUVECs. (**A**) HUVECs pre-treated or not with βDX (4-Nitrophenyl-β-D-Xylopyranoside) were seeded on Matrigel and incubated with dextran, LMWH, LMWF, MMWF or ASPHY for 6 h. The cells were then stained with Hemalun Mayer's and photographed for analysis. Values are expressed in number of nodes per well. ** $p < 0.01$ LMWF or LMWH versus Untreated (all without βDX). # $p < 0.05$ LMWF versus Untreated (all with βDX); (**B**) Endogenous GAGs expression analyzed by flow cytometry on HUVECs pre-treated or not 48 h with *βDX*; (**C**) PD98059, a pharmacological inhibitor of ERK1/2 and (**D**) LY294002, a pharmacological inhibitor of PI3K/AKT were added in HUVEC culture, then HUVECs were seeded on Matrigel for 6 h and vascular network formation was observed as described before. Values are expressed in nodes per well ($n \geq 3$). * $p < 0.05$ LMWF, PD98059, LY294002, LMWF + PD98059, LY294002 + LMWF versus Untreated; # $p < 0.05$ LMWF + PD98059 versus PD98059.

Recently, Kim et al. [21] reported that fucoidan from *Laminaria japonica* acts synergistically with fibroblast growth factor-2 (FGF-2) in promoting HUVEC angiogenesis by AKT signaling pathways via activation of the p38 and c-Jun N-terminal kinase (JNK) pathways. Based on these results, we performed the Western Blot analysis to verify whether MAPK/Erk1/2 or PI3K/AKT signaling pathways are implied in the pro-angiogenic effect of LMWF. To this aim, we incubated the cells with two pharmacological inhibitors PD98059 (for MAPK/Erk1/2) and LY294002 (for PI3K/AKT) before adding LMWF to cell culture. Our data attested that these two inhibitors significantly reduced the number of LMWF-induced nodes, by 46% ± 4.6% for PD98059 and by 59% ± 5.8% for LY294002, and evidenced the involvement of these signaling pathways in LMWF-induced angiogenesis from *Ascophyllum nodosum* (Figure 4C,D).

We have previously shown that fucoidan treatment can influence the syndecan-1/-4 and the glycosaminoglycan (GAG) expression level in HUVECs [12]. Since GAGs have been demonstrated to play an important role in angiogenesis processes, we studied the endogenous GAGs involvement in LMWF pro-angiogenic response. We established a GAG-free HUVEC model through the 4-nitrophenyl-β-D-Xylopyranoside (βDX) cell treatment for 48 h to inhibit GAG elongation. The efficiency of βDX on endogenous GAG abolition was verified by flow cytometry (Figure 4B). In these conditions, LMWF increased the vascular network formation by 53% ± 13%, whereas ASPHY, MMWF, LMWH and dextran had no effect (Figure 4A, grey bars). These results were similar with those obtained in basic condition with HUVECs expressing GAGs (56% ± 16%), demonstrating that the βDX treatment did not affect LMWF-induced angiogenesis.

These data suggests that endogenous GAGs were not involved in LMWF-induced angiogenesis, highlighting that LMWF had still a pro-angiogenic effect even in GAG-free condition.

2.2.4. LMWF and MMWF Effects on HUVEC Migration In Vitro

To study the LMWF-migratory potential on HUVECs we assessed cell migration in a Boyden chamber. The HUVECs were incubated with ASPHY, MMWF or LMWF in the upper chamber (insert) and allowed to migrate through fibronectin-coated 8 μm-porous membrane to the lower chamber. The results showed a significant increase in HUVEC migration by 35% ± 16% for ASPHY, by 40% ± 11% for LMWF and by 36% ± 7% for LMWH, while MMWF and dextran did not have any effect on HUVEC migration (Figure 5).

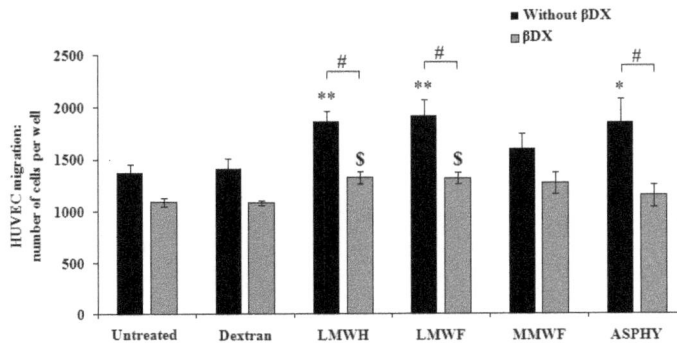

Figure 5. Pro-migratory potential of fucoidans on GAG-free HUVECs. HUVECs were seeded and incubated 24 h in the upper chamber with the polysaccharides dextran, LMWH, LMWF, MMWF or ASPHY at 10 μg/mL. The basal migration was performed in complete medium with 12% FBS. In the aim to remove the GAGs, the cells were pre-treated with βDX for 48 h, then the migration assay was performed with the same treatments as described above. The cells were fixed, stained with Mayer's hemalun solution and counted after migration. Values are expressed as cell number per well. * $p < 0.05$ ASPHY versus Untreated (all without βDX); ** $p < 0.01$ LMWH and LMWF versus Untreated (all without βDX); $ $p < 0.05$ LMWH and LMWF versus Untreated (all with βDX); # $p < 0.05$ LMWH and LMWF and ASPHY (all without βDX) versus LMWH and LMWF and ASPHY (all with βDX).

Then we analyzed the involvement of endogenous GAGs in the pro-migratory effect of fucoidans. HUVECs were treated with βDX for 48 h and seeded in the upper chamber to obtain cell migration in GAG-free conditions. Our result showed that in this GAG-damaged condition, the effects of LMWF and LMWH on cell migration were significantly reduced by 31% ± 4% and 29% ± 4%, respectively. Both, LMWF and LMWH induced the migration in a light manner by 21% ± 5% and 22% ± 5%, respectively (Figure 5), suggesting that GAGs were partially involved in fucoidan-induced endothelial cell mobility.

In summary, LMWF was able to induce endothelial cell migration in Boyden chamber and this activity required the expression of endogenous GAGs to be fully effective.

2.3. Cellular Uptake of LMWF-Alexa in Endothelial Cells

2.3.1. Regulation of LMWF Cell Uptake: Involvement of Endogenous GAGs

Very little is known about fucoidan localization and cellular uptake, which can be involved in HUVEC migration and vascular network formation. The fucoidan's mechanism of action on the cells is still not well understood, however, heparin is known to be accumulated and internalized in endothelial cells by clathrin-mediated endocytosis [22] and it has been shown that the internalization pathway is related to the size of the polysaccharides [23].

A fluorescent LMWF was designed by coupling the LMWF with a red fluorophore Alexa Fluor 555 (LMWF-Alexa). This technique allowed us to analyze the LMWF-Alexa cell uptake at physiological temperature (37 °C) and at low temperature (4 °C) that slow down the cell activity linked to membrane fluidity, dynamics and cell trafficking, thus reducing endocytosis. We measured the LMWF-Alexa accumulation in vesicle-like spots in HUVECs by the quantification of the red fluorescence intensity by confocal microscopy (Figure 6A). These vesicles-like spots reminded membrane movements similar to endocytosis. The control conditions were performed with Dextran-FITC (green fluorescence) and Alexa Fluor 555 (Alexa) alone (red fluorescence). The intracellular fluorescence was detected from 30 min of HUVEC incubation with LMWF-Alexa and reached the maximum of fluorescence intensity at 2 h of incubation at 37 °C. There was a very weak signal of fluorescence intensity detected for Dextran-FITC and Alexa alone at 2 h of incubation at 37 °C (Figure 6A, right panel). In addition, the LMWF-Alexa cell uptake was significantly decreased by 90% ± 2% at 2 h of incubation at low temperature at 4 °C (Figure 6A, left panel). These results evidenced the implication of the molecular chain structure of fucoidan (as compared to non-sulfated-dextran), membrane fluidity and dynamics in HUVEC uptake. The fluorescence intensity did not changed after 2 h of incubation (Figure 6C, black bars and data not shown) showing that the maximum of cell capacity of LMWF-Alexa uptake was reached at 2 h of incubation at 37 °C (Figure 6C, black bars).

We then used the HUVEC GAG-free model and tested the influence of endogenous GAG on LMWF-Alexa cell uptake up to 6 h. We performed an enzymatic degradation of the GAG using the heparinases I, III and chondroitinase ABC mix-solution (H/C) instead of long term culture with βDX treatment which was more appropriate for longer assays (from 6 h up to 24 h). The total endogenous GAG degradation was confirmed by flow cytometry (Figure 6B). Our results showed that the HUVEC pre-treated with H/C solution decreased significantly the fluorescence intensity by 40% ± 10% at 2 h of LMWF-Alexa incubation (Figure 6C, grey bars). Interestingly, H/C treatment (for GAG degradation) slow down the LMWF-Alexa cell uptake and the maximum fluorescence intensity was reached at 6 h of incubation at 37 °C. These results suggested that LMWF-Alexa cell uptake reached the saturable capacity of cells internalization starting from 2 h of incubation and the endogens GAGs are involved but not exclusive to regulate this process. In order to determine the mechanism of LMWF internalization in HUVECs we analyzed the different endocytic pathways.

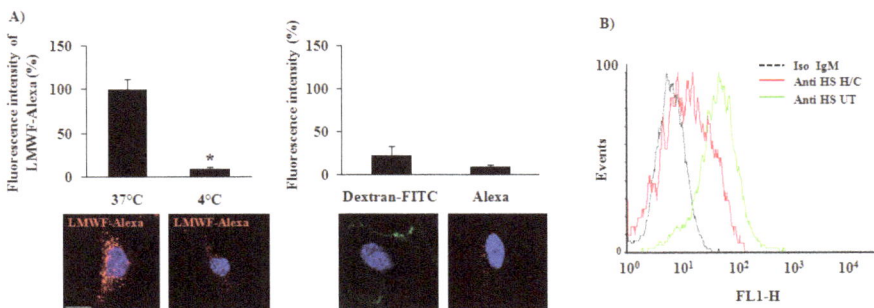

Figure 6. *Cont.*

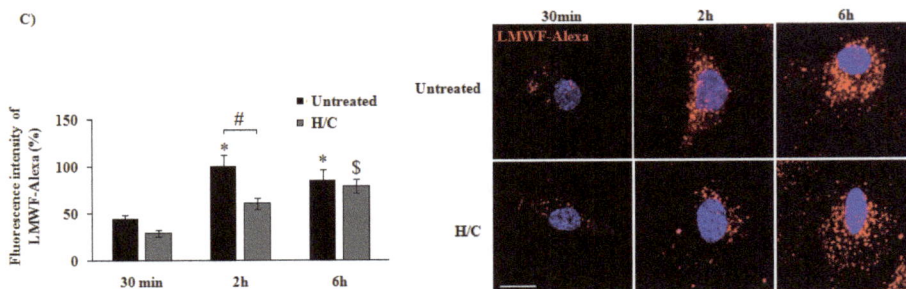

Figure 6. LMWF-Alexa localization in HUVECs by confocal microscopy. LMWF was previously coupled with the fluorophore Alexa Fluor 555. (**A**) LMWF-Alexa was added in HUVEC culture medium at 10 μg/mL during 2 h at 37 °C and 4 °C. Dextran-FITC and Alexa fluor alone (Alexa) were used as negative control. Pictures were taken by confocal microscopy and the intensity of the accumulated fluorescence per cell was quantified by using specific quantification software (DAPI—blue, LMWF-Alexa—red, Dextran-FITC—green, bar = 10 μm). Values are expressed as percentage of the intensity. * $p < 0.01$ 37 °C versus 4 °C; (**B**) Endogenous GAGs expression on HUVECs treated by heparinase I, II, and III and chondroitinase ABC (H/C); (**C**) LMWF-Alexa was incubated with HUVECs (30 min, 2 h, and 6 h) with or without heparinase I, II, and III and chondroitinase ABC (H/C) and the intensity of fluorescence per cell was measured by flow cytometry. Values are expressed as percentage of the intensity normalized on the maximum intensity reached at 2 h. The right panel shows the confocal observation. (DAPI—blue, LMWF-Alexa—red, bar = 10 μm). * $p < 0.05$, 2 h, and 6 h versus 30 min (all Untreated with H/C); \$ $p < 0.05$, 6 h versus 30 min (all treated with H/C); # $p < 0.05$, 2 h of treated with H/C versus 2 h of Untreated.

2.3.2. Mechanism of LMWF Uptake: Implication of Clathrin

In this last part of our work we analyzed the mechanism of LMWF-Alexa endocytosis at 2 h of incubation using two specific markers of the receptor-dependent and receptor-independent endocytic pathways, clathrin and caveolin-1, respectively. We realized a co-localization assay of LMWF-Alexa (red fluorescence) with clathrin or caveolin-1 (green fluorescence) using confocal microscopy. A merge of the green and red fluorescent pictures were performed to see the co-localization of LMWF-Alexa with clathrin or caveolin-1. The fluorescence intensity per cell was quantified and the co-localization level was measured by scoring the proportion of red spots on green spots. The results showed that LMWF-Alexa was co-localized with clathrin at 70% ± 6% (Figure 7A, upper panel, arrows in the merge), but less co-localization was observed with caveolin-1 at 27% ± 7% (Figure 7A, lower panel, merge). This result suggested that LMWF-Alexa was mainly internalized by HUVECs in a clathrin-mediated endocytosis at 2 h of incubation.

To confirm this observation we used specific inhibitors of the major endocytic pathways: (a) the Cytochalasin D (CtyD), inhibitor of F-actin which acts on macropinocytosis/phagocytosis; (b) the dynasore inhibitor of the GTPase activity of dynamin which prevents the clathrin-coated pit formation and (c) the filipin which binds to cholesterol and inhibits the formation of lipid rafts and caveolin-vesicles. Our data demonstrated that at 2 h of incubation, the accumulation of LMWF-Alexa was decreased by 49% ± 6% in presence of dynasore, as compared to control (Figure 7B), however there was no changes of LMWF-Alexa cell uptake after CytD and filipin treatments. The transferrin was used as a positive control of clathrin-mediated endocytosis, and the results showed that the dynasore treatment decreased its cell uptake by 63% ± 4% (Figure S2).

In conclusion, our data evidenced that LMWF was internalized in HUVECs in a clathrin-dependant endocytosis.

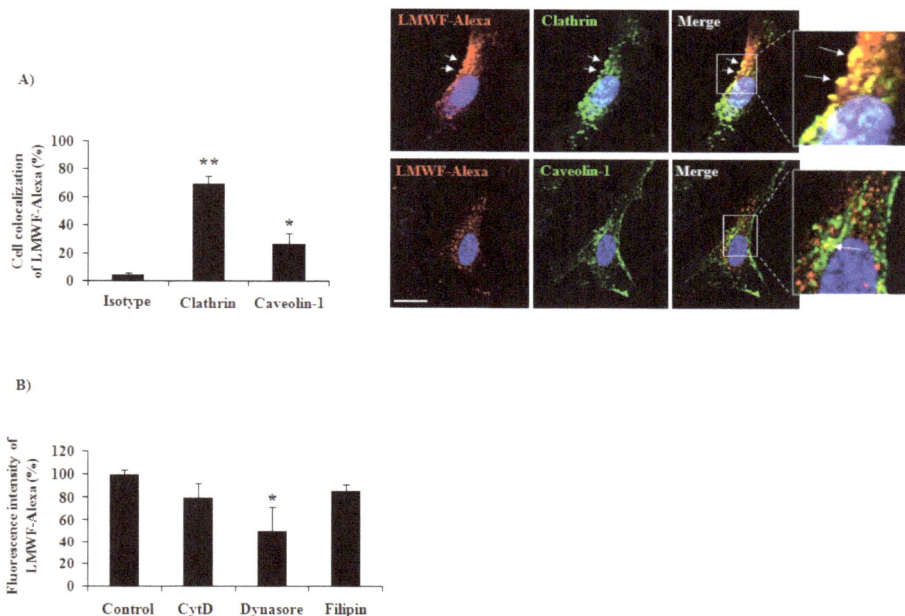

Figure 7. Internalization pathways of LMWF-Alexa in HUVECs analyzed by confocal microscopy. (**A**) HUVECs were incubated 2 h with LMWF-Alexa, fixed, permeabilized and the clathrin or caveolin-1 was revealed by immunofluorescence. A non-specific isotype of immunoglobulin was used as negative control (Isotype). The pictures were taken by confocal microscopy and the staining overlaped in merge (DAPI—blue, LMWF-Alexa—red, Clathrin—green, bar = 10 μm) high view inserts. The intensity of the fluorescence was quantified and the co-localization of markers was measured with the rate red/green represented in the histogram and dot plots. The intensity of fluorescence in HUVECs was quantified using specific software. * $p < 0.05$ Caveolin-1 versus Isotype; ** $p < 0.01$ Clathrin versus Isotype; (**B**) HUVECs were pre-treated or not (control) with specific inhibitors of endocytosis: Cytochalasin D (CytD-inhibits phagocytosis and micropynocytosis), Dynasore (inhibits clathrin mediated endocytosis) and Filipin (inhibits lipid raft formation) before adding LMWF-Alexa in the culture medium for 2 h. The intensity of fluorescence by cells was quantified as described above.* $p < 0.05$ Dynasore versus Control.

3. Discussion

3.1. Structure-Function Correlation

For decades, natural marine sulfated fucanes named fucoidans, demonstrated anti-coagulant [24,25] and anti-thrombotic [9,26] effects comparable to heparin. We have previously shown that the fucoidans have therapeutic potential in cardio-vascular diseases in animal models with an important role in preventing intimal hyperplasia [8,27] and promoting revascularization after ischemia development [7]. We and other studies have shown the therapeutic effects of low molecular weight fucoidans (LMWF) on angiogenesis in vitro and in vivo [10–13,21,28].

Fucoidans are heterogeneous sulfated polysaccharides (size, composition and degree of sulfation), which can be obtained from different brown algaes, such as *Laminaria saccharina*, *L. digitata*, *Fucus evanescens*, *F. serratus*, *F. distichus*, *F. spiralis*, and *Ascophyllum nodosum*. Their structural diversity has been widely analyzed and described, highlighting an average structure based on a linear sulfated poly-fucose backbone with sometimes a few amount of uronic acids and traces of galactose and xylose. Many reports evidenced relationship between the structural features of fucoidans and their most potent biological activity, the widely admitted role of the molecular weight, and the sulfate groups content and distribution closely depending on the starting material and the method of preparation [9,25,29,30]. Thus, to conclude about structure-activity relationships could be tricky when considering different fucoidan fractions from the same origin. This is precisely well illustrated by works about the anti- and pro-angiogenic activity. Pomin et al. evidenced that fucoidans from various origins exhibit an anti-angiogenic activity due to their ability to interfere with Vascular endothelial growth factors (VEGFs) and basic Fibroblast growth factor (FGF-2) [30]. However, Matou et al. showed the pro-angiogenic effect of fucoidans, also extracted from *A. nodosum*, by enhancing the expression of $\alpha6$, $\beta1$ integrin subunits and platelet endothelial cell adhesion molecule 1 (PECAM-1) on the surface of endothelial cells, resulting in an increase of FGF-2-induced angiogenesis [10]. Recently, Nifantiev et al. reviewed numerous studies on the angiogenic activities of fucoidans from different brown algae to highlight structure-activity relationships. They could only conclude that fucoidan fractions from *A. nodosum* with high molecular weight (>30,000 g/mol) exhibited anti-angiogenic activity whereas fucoidan fraction with low molecular weight (<30,000 g/mol) exhibited pro-angiogenic activity [31].

Furthermore, the heterogeneity in structure and composition of fucoidans appeared to correlate with heterogenous activities and the relation between the sulfate content and their anti-coagulant and anti-thrombotic potential was demonstrated by Ustyuzhanina et al. [32]. In this study, a native fucoidan with a degree of sulfation of 1.3 (*Saccharina latissima*) showed stronger activities than higher sulfated fucoidan from the same species, rather than other native fucoidans with a lower sulfation degree of 0.9 or 0.4 (*Fucus vesiculosus* or *Cladosiphon okamuranus*, respectively).

Only few publications presented the fucoidan effects on angiogenesis in endothelial cells or in cancer cells under hypoxic conditions. Chen et al. showed that a low molecular weight fucoidan (LMWF) obtained from *Sargassum hemiphyllum* (M_w = 760 g/mol, 40% sulfate) dose-dependently reduced hypoxia effect on VEGF-induced capillary tube-like structure formation in Human Umbilical Endothelial Cells (HUVEC) in vitro, and did not affect angiogenesis under normoxic condition [33]. In addition, they showed that LMWF treatment inhibited the migration and invasion of hypoxic Human Bladder Cancer Cells (T24). Interestingly, they suggested that under hypoxic conditions, the anti-angiogenic activity of LMWF in bladder cancer may be associated with suppressing Hypoxia-Induced Factor-1 (HIF-1)/VEGF-regulated signaling. Their experiments were performed in presence with both VEGF and fucoidan and it is well established that there are electrostatic interactions between negative charges from fucoidan and positive charges from VEGF, leading to depletion of both molecules that can explain their anti-angiogenic results. Cho et al. investigated the role of a fucoidan obtained from *Fucus vesiculosus* (M_w and composition non mentioned) [34]. They showed the decrease on Hepatocellular Carcinoma Cell (HCC) invasion in normoxic and hypoxic conditions and showed that fucoidan suppressed cells proliferation and invasion in a NDRG-1/CAP43-dependent manner. Teng et al. demonstrated that fucoidan from *Undaria pinnatifida sporophylls* (M_w = 104356 g/mol, 21% sulfate) significantly inhibits cell invasion and lymphatic metastasis in a mouse hepatocarcinoma Hca-F cell line under hypoxic conditions by suppressing HIF-1α/VEGF-C, which attenuates the PI3K/Akt/mTOR signaling pathways [35]. In conclusion, it is very difficult to compare these results with ours, since the experiments of Chen et al., Cho et al. and Teng et al. were performed with the fucoidans prepared from different seaweeds with different molecular weights, compositions and concentrations.

In this study, the characterization using Fourier Transform Infrared (FT-IR) and Raman Spectroscopy indicated that the crude ASPHY and the fractionated low and medium molecular weight fucoidans (LMWF and MMWF, respectively) demonstrated the characteristic bands of the O=S=O stretching vibration of sulfate, as determined through the observation of strong vibrational bands. The observation of the Raman band at 1268 cm^{-1} exhibited variations in intensity between the fucoidans with stronger band for LMWF. The Raman band of both LMWF and MMWF also exhibited vibrations at approximately 845 cm^{-1}, which indicates the presence of sulfate groups at positions 2 and 4, respectively. Bilan et al. [36] obtained similar findings for the fucoidan extracted from *Fucus serratus Linnaeus*.

The FT-IR spectra showed that the intensity of COO- groups is higher in ASPHY and LMWF than in MMWF that can be compared to the amount of uronic acid measured in the fucoidans (27%, 18%, and 14%, respectively).

The spectroscopic data related to sulfate and carboxylic groups of the fucoidans can be correlated to the sulfation rate and uronic acid content obtained with colorimetric measures.

The negative charges carried by these native sulfated polysaccharides allows electrostatic interactions with numerous positively charged proteins, such heparin binding proteins (HBP), shown with stromal derived factor-1 (SDF-1/CXCL12) [37] and growth factors, such as FGF-2 [10,38]. These interactions were thought to induce HUVEC cell migration and lead to new vessels formation in animal models of ischemia [7,13]. In the current paper, we showed that crude (ASHPY) and fractionated fucoidans from *A. nodosum* (MMWF and LMWF) bound to HBP (SDF-1/CXCL12, regulated on activated T cell expressed and secreted RANTES/CCL5 and vascular endothelial growth factor VEGF) with a high affinity. However, our results highlighted a tendency in the affinity between the fractionated fucoidans both highly sulfated (1.55 and 1.14) and two of the HPB SDF-1/CXCL12 and RANTES/CCL5. LMWF presents a higher sulfation rate and relative higher affinity (KD) for both, compared with MMWF, which owns a weaker KD with both. ASPHY and LMWF behave similarly considering the interaction with HBP. This result is in accordance with the hypothesis of the modulation of the affinity by the sulfation rate, however the difference in sulfate degree for LMWF and MMWF was probably not enough significant to distinguish strong variations in the affinity to bind HBP. We hypothesized that the molecular model of interaction of fucoidans with the HBP fixed on the chip was polyvalent and related to the fast association and the slow dissociation phases in accordance with previous study with the GAG-mimetics [20]. The hypothesis was proposed that the amino acids present in the binding site of SDF-1/CXCL12 (BBXB) to heparin can be similar to those which interact with fucoidans. We suggest for the further study the use of adapted sensorgram designed to measure the interaction of fucoidan with the HBP and compete with heparin on the heparin binding-site to validate this model. Structural studies could also evidence that the size of fucoidan is also an important criterion to discriminate its affinity to HBP by using a range of fucoidan owning the same degree of sulfation.

In Boyden chamber migration assay, both LMWF and ASPHY increased the HUVEC migration. The structural analysis of fucoidan could explain the reason why the native fucoidan had a pro-migratory activity similar to LMWF. As shown on the polydispersity measurement, ASPHY contains LMWF populations in majority as its molecular mass was measured at 4100 g/mol. We analyzed distinct effects on HUVEC migration influenced by LMWF and MMWF. These data suggested that the size of LMWF was important, as a high sulfation rate, for the sulfated polysaccharide to have a pro-migratory activity on HUVECs.

The same results were observed in 2 dimensional (2D) vascular network formation on Matrigel with LMWF which shown higher potential to induce nodes formation than MMWF. However the native fucoidan ASPHY did not shown any activity in this assay, demonstrating that the fucoidan activity analyzed in HUVEC migration could act in a different pathway than 2D angiogenesis assay. We also revealed in this study that 2D-angiogenesis induced by LMWF involved PI3K/AKT and the MAPK Erk1/2 pathways, in line with recent study that evidenced the activation of P-38 and JNK pathways [21].

In our studies we evidenced the role of the sulfate groups content and molecular weight of fucoidan fractions on their angiogenic properties, and we proposed some preliminary mechanisms. This is possible because the fractions were obtained from a reliable and reproducible industrial process, that constitued a prerequisite for relevant studies. Anyway these fractions remain complex mixtures of macromolecules and determining a complete structure-activity is a difficult task that we had undertaken.

3.2. Influence of the Endogenous GAGs in Pro-Angiogenic Effect of Fucoidans in GAG-Free HUVEC Migration

Beside, in this study we explored the role of endogenous GAGs fucoidan-induced angiogenesis and HUVEC migration. We hypothesized that in basal condition, fucoidan could act as an intermediate actor between receptors and chemokines by increasing their concentration at the cell surface in co-operation with the endogenous GAGs. This interaction could enhance the formation of co-receptors (proteoglycans) and receptors complexes, their internalization and could lead to an amplification of the cell signal and response. While in absence of GAG expression, fucoidan could substitute the GAG function, prevent glycocalyx degradation and finally restore its function by enhancing the revascularization process. However, other hypothesis assumed that exogenous GAG-mimetics such as fucoidans, as they bind to HBP, could compete with endogenous GAGs for their binding sites leading to the inhibition of HBP activating pathways. Thus, suggesting that the pro-angiogenic activity of LMWF was not linked to its ability to bind HBP but mostly related to intrinsic activity.

We showed that LMWF still has a pro-migratory activity on HUVECs in GAG-free condition but in a lesser extent (40% ± 11% in basal condition versus 21% ± 5% in GAG-free condition). These results were not found for 2D-angiogenesis assay in GAG-free condition, where LMWF still induced nodes formation in the same range than basal condition. Endogenous GAGs shown in this field to be partially required for the fucoidan activity. This suggests that fucoidan could acts independently, depending on the biological effect. Otherwise, it has been proposed that fucoidan acts as a competitor for endogenous GAGs while binding HBP with higher affinity [11]. Considering the high affinity of LMWF to HBP, this model could partially correlate with our results as the tendencies showed that LMWF has stronger effect when the GAGs are expressed.

3.3. Internalization of LMWF

Our results attested that fluorescent LMWF was internalized in 2 h in HUVECs and localized in a perinuclear region. These observations correlated with a previous study focused on the heparin internalization in vascular smooth muscle cells, where the biphasic endocytic pathway of this sulfated polysaccharide was demonstrated [22].

The delay observed in the accumulation of LMWF-Alexa between untreated and Heparinase/Chondroitinase treated HUVECs demonstrated that endogenous GAGs were necessary to internalize the LMWF in 2 h. We evidenced that this internalization was temperature and clathrin-dependent. Proteoglycans are mobilized to induce clathrin-mediated endocytosis, and LMWF, as GAG-mimetic, could also interact with proteoglycan core or HBP at the cell surface and could be internalized and finally induced the biological effects on endothelial cells.

Previous studies have shown the importance of the size of polysaccharide in their cellular fluid internalization pathways with fluorescent low molecular weight dextran (10,000 g/mol) internalized in a clathrin and dynamin mediated micro- and macropinocytosis while medium molecular weight dextran (70,000 g/mol) used the amiloride-sensitive and clathrin-independent macropinocytosis [23]. Lately soluble exogenous GAGs have been demonstrated to improve cellular uptake of coated peptide-DNA complexes and escape from endosomal pathway until final localization in perinuclear region [39]. As suggested by our results, LMWF showed higher pro-angiogenic effect than MMWF. We then chose the LMWF to study its internalization and the potential implication of the GAGs on these mechanisms, which could explain the particular biological effects of LMWF on endothelial cells. Further trafficking studies should be proposed in correlation with cell signaling pathways to determine more accurately the cellular and molecular effects of LMWF on endothelial cells and its role inside the cells (signaling pathways) to induce angiogenesis.

4. Experimental Section

4.1. Reagents

Alexa Fluor Succinimidyl Ester (NHS Ester) was furnished by Molecular Probes (Thermo Fischer Scientific, Waltham, MA, USA). Transferrin-biotin labeled human (Sigma-Aldrich, Saint-Louis, MO, USA) was furnished by Sigma-Aldrich and used as a positive control of clathrin-mediated endocytosis.

4.2. Pharmacological Inhibitors

LY294002 (Sigma-Aldrich), is an inhibitor of the PI3K signaling pathway and was used at 30 µM in cell culture. PD98059 (Sigma-Aldrich) is an inhibitor of the MAPKK MEK1 and MEK2 signaling pathway and was used at 30 µM in cell culture. Cytochalasin D (C8273, Sigma-Aldrich) is an inhibitor of the phagocytosis and micropinocytosis by depolymerizing actin-F and was used at 100 µM in cell culture for 2 h. Filipin (F9765, Sigma-Aldrich) is an inhibitor of the clathrin independent endocytosis which binds to cholesterol and blocking membrane movements. This inhibitor was used at 1 µg/mL in cell culture for 1 h. Dynasore (D7693, Sigma-Aldrich) is an inhibitor of the clathrin mediated endocytosis by bocking the GTPase activity of dynamin and was used at 80 µM in cell culture for 30 min.

4.3. Enzymes and Glycosaminoglycan Substitute

βDX (4-Nitrophenyl β-D-xylopyranoside, Sigma-Aldrich), a substitute of glycosaminoglycans (GAGs) was used as specific inhibitor of the GAG chain elongation. βDX was added at 2 g/mol for 48 h in HUVEC culture to inhibit the endogenous GAGs expression before assays. Heparinase I (5U, 1/100) from *Flavobacterium heparinum* (H2519), Heparinase III (10U, 1/50) from *Flavobacterium heparinum* (H8891), and chondroïtinase ABC (10U, 1/50) from Proteus vulgaris were all obtained from Sigma-Aldrich and used 2 h at 37 °C to depolymerize endogenous GAGs in HUVEC culture before short time assays up to 6 h.

4.4. Antibodies

We used an antibody directed against heparan sulfate chains (Mouse IgM, Clone F58-10E4, AMS Biotechnology, Abingdon, UK) to observe their expression in flow cytometry CLTC is a primary antibody directed against clathrin heavy chain 1 (Mouse IgG1, Everest Biotech, Ramona, CA, USA). CAV-1 is a primary antibody directed against caveolin-1. PA5-17447 was obtained from Pierce (Rabbit IgG, Thermo Scientific, Rockford, IL, USA). The isotype Mouse IgG1 and the isotype Mouse IgM κ was obtained by BD Biosciences (BD Biosciences, Bedford, MA, USA), the isotype Rabbit IgG was produced by R&D (R&D Systems Inc., Minneapolis, MN, USA). The secondary antibodies Goat anti Mouse IgG Alexa fluor 488 was produced by Santa Cruz Biotechnology and Goat anti Rabbit IgG Alexa fluor 488 were produced by Santa Cruz Biotechnology (Santa Cruz Biotechnology, Santa Cruz, CA, USA).

4.5. Polysaccharides

The crude fucoidan (ASPHY) was obtained from the marine alga species *Ascophyllum nodosum* (Algues & Mer, Ascophyscient, batch #ASPHY12399, Ouessant, France). The Ascophyscient fucoidan was previously characterized by our laboratory [40]. A 10,000 g/mol non-sulfated dextran (Dextran T-10, Amersham Pharmacia Biotech, Amersham, UK) and a Dextran-FITC (TdB consultancy, Uppsala, Sweden) were chosen as negative controls. A low molecular weight heparin was used as a positive control (LMWH, M_w = 6300 g/mol, Tinzaparin sodium Innohep, Ballerup, Denmark).

4.6. Fractionation

The crude fucoidan ASPHY was fractionated using size exclusion gel. The column (XK 50/60, GE Life Sciences, Velizy-Villacoublay, France, id: 50 mm, L: 50 cm) was prepared with Bio-Gel P60 (Bio-Rad, Marne-la-Vallée, France). 0.15 M NaCl and 0.02% (w/v) sodium azide were used as carrier after careful filtration through 0.45 µm-filter unit (Millipore, Billerica, MA, USA) at 1.5 mL/min flow rate. 10 mg of Ascophyscient® (30%, w/v) was eluted through the column and 100 mL were collected in several fractions. Then, the fractions were dialyzed five times against water (Spectra/Por, MWCO 1 kDa, Dominique Dutscher, Brumath, France) and freeze-dried. Each fraction was analyzed: fucose, uronic acid and sulfate rate were assessed by colorimetric assay and the molecular weight measured using size-exclusion chromatography with multi-angle laser light scattering-differential refractive index detection (HPSEC/MALLS-DRI) system [40]. We collected and used two fractions from the elution, a low molecular weight fucoidan (LMWF, M_w = 4,900 g/mol) and medium molecular weight fucoidan (MMWF, M_w = 26,600 g/mol).

4.7. Raman Spectroscopy

Raman spectra were recorded with a commercial confocal Raman microspectrometer from 200 to 1800 cm^{-1}. A Horiba Scientific Xplora spectrometer was used at 660 nm excitation wavelength with 3 cm^{-1} spectral resolution. The Raman measurements were carried out in backscattering configuration through a 10× objective (NA = 0.25). The incident laser power was measured at the sample position and set at 20 mW. Raman spectra were acquired during 60 s acquisition time and baseline corrected using Labspec software (HJY, Kyoto, Japan).

4.8. Fourier Transform Infrared Spectroscopy

Fourier Transform Infrared Spectroscopy (FT-IR) spectra of the samples diluted either in D_2O (>99.8% purity, Euriso-Top, CEA, Saclay, France) or in H_2O solution were recorded on a Tensor 27 spectrophotometer (Bruker, Karlsruhe, Germany). Solutions were deposited between two ZnSe windows at a concentration of 333 µg/µL. Experiments were performed by drying the samples and dissolving them in solution at pH ~7. Twenty scans were accumulated (spectral region 4000–400 cm^{-1}, resolution 1 cm^{-1}). Data treatment was performed using the opus software and consisted of multiple point base line correction.

4.9. Surface Plasmon Resonance

Affinity of fucoidans for SDF-1/CXCL12, RANTES/CCL5 or VEGF$_{165}$ was assessed with a BIAcore X100 (GE Healthcare, Freïburg, Germany). Biotinylated-SDF-1/CXCL12, -RANTES/CCL5 or VEGF$_{165}$ was coupled to the surface of a SA sensor chip (carboxymethylated dextran with immobilized streptavidin for capture of biotinylated ligand). Biotinylated-SDF-1 (20 µL of 5 µg/mL in HEPES buffer saline-50 mM HEPES, pH 7.4, 150 mM NaCl, 3 mM EDTA, and 0.05% surfactant P-20) was then injected, at 5 µL/min flow rate, of the streptavidin-coated sensor chip to a resonance unit (RU) value of 110 for SDF1/CXCL12 and 235 for RANTES/CCL5. VEGF$_{165}$ was immobilized on a CM5 sensorchip with the BIAcore amine kit at 1913 RU. Non coupled surfaces were used as controls, 1 M NaCl was used to regenerate the sensor surface. Samples were diluted in running buffer (50 mM HEPES pH 7.4, 150 mM NaCl, 3 mM EDTA, and 0.05% P-20). We selected with the BIAcore control software: temperature (25 °C), flow rate (30 µL/min), contact time (180 s), and sample volume (GE Healthcare) in single cycle method. Samples were injected consecutively at 1.2, 3.7, 11.1, 33.3, and 100 nM. The affinities of fucoidan for SDF-1/CXCL12, RANTES/CCL5 or VEGF$_{165}$ were determined using a 1:1 Langmuir model by analysis the kinetic of the association and dissociation with the BIAcore evaluation software.

4.10. Endothelial Cell Culture

Human umbilical vascular endothelial cells (HUVECs, CRL-1730, ATCC, LGC Molsheim, France) were cultured in endothelial cell basal medium 2 (ECBM2, PromoCell, Heidelberg, Germany) supplemented with 12% fetal bovine serum, EGF (epidermal growth factor, 5.0 ng/mL), hydrocortisone (0.2 µg/mL), VEGF (vascular endothelial growth factor, 0.5 ng/mL), bFGF (basic fibroblast growth factor, 10 ng/mL), R3 IGF-1 (insulin like growth factor, 20 ng/mL), ascorbic acid (1 µg/mL) and antibiotics (penicillin-streptomycin, 1%, Invitrogen, Cergy, France) at 37 °C in 5% CO_2. HUVECs were cultured at 60%–90% of confluence. The media were changed twice a week. The presence of growth factors such as VEGF, EGF, bFGF and IGF-1 in the culture medium of HUVECs, mimics the angiogenic conditions of in vitro cultures. We removed the heparin from the supplemented kit when the fucoidan treatment was performed, since heparin as a sulfated polysaccharide, could be considered as a competitor of fucoidan because of its structural and functional homologies.

4.11. Flow Cytometry

The level of heparan sulfate on HUVEC cell surface was quantified by fluorescence-activated cell sorting (FACS). Cells were pre-incubated for 1 h at 4 °C with anti-heparan sulfate antibody (10 μg/mL, Clone 10E4) or with isotypes (IgM). After washing, cells were labeled for 30 min at 4 °C with streptavidin-Alexa Fluor 488 complex (1/200, Molecular Probes, Invitrogen). Cells were fixed in 1% paraformaldehyde and analyzed with a FACScan (Becton Dickinson, Le Pont de-Claix, France).

4.12. Cell Viability Assay

The viability of HUVECs was demonstrated using MTT (3-[4.5-Dimethylthiazol-2-yl]-2.5-diphenyltetrazolium bromide) assay (Thiazolyl Blue Tetrazolium Bromide, Sigma-Aldrich). 5000 cells/well were incubated in a 96-wells plate for 24, 48, and 72 h with or without polysaccharides (LMWF, MMWF and ASPHY) at increasing concentration (1 μg/mL, 10 μg/mL, 100 μg/mL and 1000 μg/mL). LMWH and dextran were used as a control at 10 μg/mL. MTT solution at 1 mg/mL was added to the medium for 2 h and coloration was revealed in DMSO. The metabolic activity was correlated by the absorbance read at 570 nm with a photometer (Bio-rad$^©$ Microplate reader, Model 680).

4.13. Cell Migration Assay

HUVEC migration was performed with Bio-coat cell migration chambers (Becton Dickinson, Franklin Lakes, NJ, USA) as described [26]. Briefly, inserts were coated with fibronectin (100 μg/mL, BD Biosciences). The polysaccharides (LMWF, MMWF, ASPHY, Dextran or LMWH) were added directly in the upper chamber at 10 μg/mL with 40×104 cell/wells in 500 μL of complete medium for 24 h. The lower chamber was filled with 500 μL of complet medium. The cytokines naturally contained in the complet medium were considered as basal inducer of chemotaxis migration. To test the role of endogenous GAGs, the cells were pre-incubated 48 h with βDX, and kept in inhibition condition for the experiment. Twenty-four hours later, medium and cells in the upper chamber were gently removed. Migrated cells in the lower chamber were fixed with methanol and stained with Mayer's hemalun solution (Carl Roth GmbH + Co. KG, Karlsruhe, Germany). The cells were counted manually by two different observers who performed the blind data acquisition. HUVECs were photographed with phase contrast microscopy (Nikon$^©$ Coolpix 8400, Nikon Corporation, Tokyo, Japan) at objective ×4 and quantified by using the Image J software (Rasband, W.S., ImageJ, U.S. National Institutes of Health, Bethesda, MD, USA).

4.14. 2D Vascular Network Formation Assay

The 2 dimensional (2D)-vascular network formation assay was performed with HUVECs cultured on Matrigel-coated (Corning, Bedford, MA, USA) 16-wells Labtek or 96 wells microplate. 1×10^4 cells/well and incubated for 6 h at 37 °C in complete culture medium with or without 10 μg/mL of polysaccharides (LMWF, MMWF, ASPHY, Dextran or LMWH). The microvascular network was photographed using a phase contrast microscopy coupled camera (Nikon$^©$ Coolpix 8400). The pictures were analyzed with 5 parameters: the total length network, the number of nodes (cell interactions), the number, the perimeter and the area of the generated meshes. The measures were estimated for each experimental condition using Image J analysis system. All measures showed same tendencies and we chose to exhibit the number of nodes that demonstrated higher differences between the treatments.

4.15. Labeling of the LMWF with a Fluorophore

LMWF was first aminated on the terminal aldehyde group of fucose chain by a reductive amination [41]. In this study, 50 mg of LMWF were solved in 0.54 mL solution of diaminopropan 1.5 M in glacial acetic acid and heated for 3 h at 90 °C, then a reduction was performed by adding

0.15 mL of dimethylboran 3 M in the solution and heated 3 h at 90 °C. Samples were dialyzed (cut-off 1000 Da) and freeze-dried. LMWF was then coupled with a red fluorophore (Alexa Fluor® 555 NHS Ester, Thermo Fisher scientific, Waltham, MA, USA). 1 mg of Alexa-Fluor 555 NHS was dissolved in 100 µL of dimethyl sulfoxide (DMSO, VWR BDH Prolabo, Fontenay-sous-Bois, France), beside, 10 mg of Aminated-LMWF was dissolved in 1 mL of carbonate buffer 0.1 M at pH 8.3 and 50 µL of the solution carrying the label was added to the solution stirred in darkness for 1 h at room temperature. The labeled compound was precipitated in ethanol to remove the free labels and eluted two times in column PD-10 (GE Healthcare Life Sciences).

4.16. Kinetic of the Cellular Localization of LMWF

Fluorescents LMWF-Alexa or Dextran-FITC (negative control) were added in HUVECs culture medium at 10 µg/mL in kinetic (30 min, 2 h and, 6 h) at 37 °C and 4 °C. The heparinases and chondroitinase were added to HUVECs culture. Cells were then fixed in paraformaldehyde 4%, stained with Dapi and observed under confocal microscopy (Leica SP8 tandem, Wetzlar, Germany) An average of 30 cells per condition was photographed in stack in the Z axe and the intensity of the accumulated fluorescence per cell was quantified by using specific quantification software (Imaris, Bitplane, Belfast, UK). The intensity gain was normalized on the auto fluorescence of the cells.

4.17. Co-Localization Assay of LMWF with Clathrin and Caveolin-1

HUVECs were incubated in presence of the fluorescent LMWF-Alexa for 2 h in the same conditions as described above, then fixed and permeabilized with saponine 0.1% (Fluka, Sigma-Aldrich). Cells were stained with Dapi and antibodies directed against light chain of clathrin (CLTC), caveolin-1 (CAV-1) or isotypes (Mouse IgG1; Rabbit IgG), then revealed by secondary antibodies (Goat anti mouse Alexa Fluor 488 and Goat anti goat Alexa Fluor 488) coupled with fluorophore. The colocalization assay was performed by using the specific quantification software Imaris.

4.18. Statistical Analysis

For the determination of statistical significance, an ANOVA test was performed with the Statview software (StatView 4.5 Abacus Concepts, Berkeley, USA). A p value of <0.05 was used as the criterion of statistical significance.

5. Conclusions

In summary, we showed in this study that from the heterogeneous crude fucoidan ASPHY collected from *A. nodosum*, we could distinguish two different fucoidans, LMWF and MMWF in their composition and through their pro-angiogenic effects. LMWF showed a higher activity to induce vascular network formation and endothelial cell migration than MMWF and ASPHY. These variations observed in their biological activities are mostly related to the size of the polysaccharide rather than their sulfation rate which were not enough different to distinguish significant variations in the affinity to chemokines SDF-1/CXCL12 and RANTES/CCL5. In addition, we demonstrated that the ability of LMWF to increase the vascular network formation at 6 h was regulated by Erk1/2 and PI3K/AKT cell signaling pathways. Localization study of LMWF-Alexa showed that the endothelial cells responded to fluorescent fucoidan presence by its uptake in a clathrin-mediated endocytosis and reached the maximum of cell capacity in 2 h with its accumulation in a perinuclear region.

Interestingly, we highlighted that the endogenous GAGs which were expressed at the surface of HUVECs, were partially involved in the pro-angiogenic activity of LMWF in vascular network formation and endothelial cell migration. LMWF activities were stronger when the endogenous GAGs were expressed, however in their absence LMWF has still an effect and showed that it could act as a substitute to induce angiogenesis and endothelial cell migration. The internalization of LMWF-Alexa was not inhibited but slowed down in GAG-free HUVECs. This work opens the way to use the most pro-angiogenic fucoidan as therapeutic GAGs substitute after glycocalyx injuries.

Supplementary Materials: The following are available online at www.mdpi.com/1660-3397/14/10/185/s1, Figure S1: Polydispersity analysis, Figure S2: Transferrin endocytosis.

Acknowledgments: This work was supported by the Direction de la Recherche et des Enseignements Doctoraux (Ministère de l'Enseignement Supérieur et de la Recherche), the University Paris 13 and Inserm. N.M. was supported by a fellowship from the Ministère de l'Enseignement Supérieur et de la Recherche. We would like to particularly thank Samira Benadda from Inserm U1149 for her technical assistance with confocal microscopy.

Author Contributions: N.M., H.H. and N.C. conceived and designed the experiments; N.M., P.S., O.H., M.M., K.B., K.B.A., F.G. and R.R. performed the experiments; N.M., H.H., N.C., O.H., F.G., N.D. and M.L.C. analyzed the data; A.S., E.G., O.O., C.L.M., F.C. and C.C. contributed reagents/materials/analysis tools; N.M., H.H. and N.C. wrote the paper.

Conflicts of Interest: The authors declare no conflict of interest.

References

1. Tkachenko, E.; Rhodes, J.M.; Simons, M. Syndecans: New kids on the signaling block. *Circ. Res.* **2005**, *96*, 488–500. [CrossRef] [PubMed]
2. Sutton, A.; Friand, V.; Papy-Garcia, D.; Dagouassat, M.; Martin, L.; Vassy, R.; Haddad, O.; Sainte-Catherine, O.; Kraemer, M.; Saffar, L.; et al. Glycosaminoglycans and their synthetic mimetics inhibit RANTES-induced migration and invasion of human hepatoma cells. *Mol. Cancer Ther.* **2007**, *6*, 2948–2958. [CrossRef] [PubMed]
3. Koo, A.; Dewey, C.F.; Garcia-Cardena, G. Hemodynamic Shear Stress Characteristic of Atherosclerosis-Resistant Regions Promotes Glycocalyx Formation in Cultured Endothelial Cells. *AJP Cell Physiol.* **2012**, *304*, C137–C146. [CrossRef] [PubMed]
4. Chappell, D.; Dörfler, N.; Jacob, M.; Rehm, M.; Welsch, U.; Conzen, P.; Becker, B.F. Glycocalyx protection reduces leukocyte adhesion after ischemia/reperfusion. *Shock* **2010**, *34*, 133–139. [CrossRef] [PubMed]
5. Peysselon, F.; Ricard-Blum, S. Heparin-protein interactions: From affinity and kinetics to biological roles. Application to an interaction network regulating angiogenesis. *Matrix Biol.* **2014**, *35*, 73–81. [CrossRef] [PubMed]
6. Chevalier, F.; Arnaud, D.; Henault, E.; Guillevic, O.; Siñeriz, F.; Ponsen, A.C.; Papy-Garcia, D.; Barritault, D.; Letourneur, D.; Uzan, G.; et al. A fine structural modification of glycosaminoglycans is correlated with the progression of muscle regeneration after ischaemia: Towards a matrix-based therapy? *Eur. Cells Mater.* **2015**, *30*, 51–68.
7. Luyt, C.; Ho-tin-noe, B.; Colliec-jouault, S.E.A.M.; Jacob, M.; Osborne-pellegrin, M.; Guezennec, J.; Louedec, L.; Herv, E.; Letourneur, D.; Michel, J. Low-Molecular-Weight Fucoidan Promotes Therapeutic Revascularization in a Rat Model of Critical Hindlimb Ischemia. *J. Pharmacol. Exp. Ther.* **2003**, *305*, 24–30. [CrossRef] [PubMed]
8. Deux, J.F.; Meddahi-Pellé, A.; le Blanche, A.F.; Feldman, L.J.; Colliec-Jouault, S.; Brée, F.; Boudghène, F.; Michel, J.B.; Letourneur, D. Low molecular weight fucoidan prevents neointimal hyperplasia in rabbit iliac artery in-stent restenosis model. *Arterioscler. Thromb. Vasc. Biol.* **2002**, *22*, 1604–1609. [CrossRef] [PubMed]
9. Berteau, O.; Mulloy, B. Sulfated fucans, fresh perspectives: Structures, functions, and biological properties of sulfated fucans and an overview of enzymes active toward this class of polysaccharide. *Glycobiology* **2003**, *13*, 29–40. [CrossRef] [PubMed]
10. Matou, S.; Helley, D.; Chabut, D.; Bros, A.; Fischer, A. Effect of fucoidan on fibroblast growth factor-2-induced angiogenesis in vitro. *Thromb. Res.* **2002**, *106*, 213–221. [CrossRef]
11. Boisson-Vidal, C.; Zemani, F.; Calliguiri, G.; Galy-Fauroux, I.; Colliec-Jouault, S.; Helley, D.; Fischer, A.-M.; Caligiuri, G.; Galy-Fauroux, I.; Colliec-Jouault, S.; et al. Neoangiogenesis induced by progenitor endothelial cells: Effect of fucoidan from marine algae. *Cardiovasc. Hematol. Agents Med. Chem.* **2007**, *5*, 67–77. [CrossRef] [PubMed]
12. Haddad, O.; Guyot, E.; Marinval, N.; Chevalier, F.; Maillard, L.; Gadi, L.; Laguillier-Morizot, C.; Oudar, O.; Sutton, A.; Charnaux, N.; et al. Heparanase and Syndecan-4 Are Involved in Low Molecular Weight Fucoidan-Induced Angiogenesis. *Mar. Drugs* **2015**, *13*, 6588–6608. [CrossRef] [PubMed]
13. Purnama, A.; Aid-launais, R.; Haddad, O.; Maire, M.; Letourneur, D.; le Visage, C. Fucoidan in a 3D scaffold interacts with vascular endothelial growth factor and promotes neovascularization in mice. *Drug Deliv. Transl. Res.* **2013**, *2*, 187–197. [CrossRef] [PubMed]

14. Ikeda, Y.; Charef, S.; Ouidja, M.O.; Barbier-Chassefière, V.; Sineriz, F.; Duchesnay, A.; Narasimprakash, H.; Martelly, I.; Kern, P.; Barritault, D.; et al. Synthesis and biological activities of a library of glycosaminoglycans mimetic oligosaccharides. *Biomaterials* **2011**, *32*, 769–776. [CrossRef] [PubMed]

15. Barbosa, I.; Morin, C.; Garcia, S.; Duchesnay, A.; Oudghir, M.; Jenniskens, G.; Miao, H.; Guimond, S.; Carpentier, G.; Cebrian, J.; et al. A synthetic glycosaminoglycan mimetic (RGTA) modifies natural glycosaminoglycan species during myogenesis. *J. Cell Sci.* **2005**, *118*, 253–264. [CrossRef] [PubMed]

16. Synytsya, A.; Choi, D.J.; Pohl, R.; Na, Y.S.; Capek, P.; Lattová, E.; Taubner, T.; Choi, J.W.; Lee, C.W.; Park, J.K.; et al. Structural Features and Anti-coagulant Activity of the Sulphated Polysaccharide SPS-CF from a Green Alga Capsosiphon fulvescens. *Mar. Biotechnol.* **2015**, *17*, 718–735. [CrossRef] [PubMed]

17. Pereira, L.; Amado, A.M.; Critchley, A.T.; van de Velde, F.; Ribeiro-Claro, P.J.A. Identification of selected seaweed polysaccharides (phycocolloids) by vibrational spectroscopy (FTIR-ATR and FT-Raman). *Food Hydrocoll.* **2009**, *23*, 1903–1909. [CrossRef]

18. Qiu, X.; Amarasekara, A.; Doctor, V. Effect of oversulfation on the chemicaland biological properties of fucoidan. *Carbohydr. Polym.* **2006**, *63*, 224–228. [CrossRef]

19. Sekkal, M.; Legrand, P. A spectroscopic investigation of the carrageenans and agar in the 1500–100 cm^{-1} spectral range. *Spectrochim. Acta* **1993**, *49*, 209–221. [CrossRef]

20. Friand, V.; Haddad, O.; Papy-Garcia, D.; Hlawaty, H.; Vassy, R.; Hamma-Kourbali, Y.; Perret, G.-Y.; Courty, J.; Baleux, F.; Oudar, O.; et al. Glycosaminoglycan mimetics inhibit SDF-1/CXCL12-mediated migration and invasion of human hepatoma cells. *Glycobiology* **2009**, *19*, 1511–1524. [CrossRef] [PubMed]

21. Kim, B.S.; Park, J.Y.; Kang, H.J.; Kim, H.J.; Lee, J. Fucoidan/FGF-2 induces angiogenesis through JNK- and p38-mediated activation of AKT/MMP-2 signalling. *Biochem. Biophys. Res. Commun.* **2014**, *450*, 1333–1338. [CrossRef] [PubMed]

22. Castellot, J.J.; Wong, K.; Herman, B.; Hoover, R.L.; Albertini, D.F.; Wright, T.C.; Caleb, B.L.; Karnovsky, M.J. Binding and internalization of heparin by vascular smooth muscle cells. *J. Cell. Physiol.* **1985**, *124*, 13–20. [CrossRef] [PubMed]

23. Li, L.; Wan, T.; Wan, M.; Liu, B.; Cheng, R.; Zhang, R. The effect of the size of fluorescent dextran on its endocytic pathway. *Cell Biol. Int.* **2015**, *39*, 531–539. [CrossRef] [PubMed]

24. Mauray, S.; de Raucourt, E.; Chaubet, F.; Maïga-Revel, O.; Sternberg, C.; Fischer, A.M. Comparative anticoagulant activity and influence on thrombin generation of dextran derivatives and of a fucoidan fraction. *J. Biomater. Sci. Polym.* **1998**, *9*, 373–387. [CrossRef]

25. Cumashi, A.; Ushakova, N.; Preobrazhenskaya, M.; D'Incecco, A.; Piccoli, A.; Totani, L.; Tinari, N.; Morozevich, G.E.; Berman, A.E.; Bilan, M.I.; et al. A comparative study of the anti-inflammatory, anticoagulant, antiangiogenic, and antiadhesive activities of nine different fucoidans from brown seaweeds. *Glycobiology* **2007**, *17*, 541–552. [CrossRef] [PubMed]

26. Thorlacius, H.; Vollmar, B.; Seyfert, U.T.; Vestweber, D.; Menger, M.D. The polysaccharide fucoidan inhibits microvascular thrombus formation independently from P- and L-selectin function in vivo. *Eur. J. Clin. Investig.* **2000**, *30*, 804–810. [CrossRef]

27. Hlawaty, H.; Suffee, N.; Sutton, A.; Oudar, O.; Haddad, O.; Ollivier, V.; Laguillier-morizot, C.; Gattegno, L.; Letourneur, D.; Charnaux, N. Low molecular weight fucoidan prevents intimal hyperplasia in rat injured thoracic aorta through the modulation of matrix metalloproteinase-2 expression. *Biochem. Pharmacol.* **2011**, *81*, 233–243. [CrossRef] [PubMed]

28. Lake, A.C.; Vassy, R.; di Benedetto, M.; Lavigne, D.; le Visage, C.; Perret, G.Y.; Letourneur, D. Low molecular weight fucoidan increases VEGF165-induced endothelial cell migration by enhancing VEGF165 binding to VEGFR-2 and NRP1. *J. Biol. Chem.* **2006**, *281*, 37844–37852. [CrossRef] [PubMed]

29. Patankars, M.S.; Oehningerq, S.; Barnett, T.; Williams, R.L.; Clark, G.F. A Revised Structure for Fucoidan May Explain Some of Its Biological Activities. *J. Biol. Chem.* **1993**, 21770–21776.

30. Pomin, V.H. Fucanomics and galactanomics: Current status in drug discovery, mechanisms of action and role of the well-defined structures. *Biochim. Biophys. Acta* **2012**, *1820*, 1971–1979. [CrossRef] [PubMed]

31. Ustyuzhanina, N.E.; Bilan, M.I.; Ushakova, N.A.; Usov, A.I.; Kiselevskiy, M.V.; Nifantiev, N.E. Fucoidans: pro- or antiangiogenic agents? *Glycobiology* **2014**, *24*, 1265–1274. [CrossRef] [PubMed]

32. Ustyuzhanina, N.E.; Ushakova, N.A.; Zyuzina, K.A.; Bilan, M.I.; Elizarova, A.L.; Somonova, O.V.; Madzhuga, A.V.; Krylov, V.B.; Preobrazhenskaya, M.E.; Usov, A.I.; et al. Influence of fucoidans on hemostatic system. *Mar. Drugs* **2013**, *11*, 2444–2458. [CrossRef] [PubMed]

33. Chen, M.C.; Hsu, W.L.; Hwang, P.A.; Chou, T.C. Low Molecular Weight Fucoidan Inhibits Tumor Angiogenesis through Downregulation of HIF-1/VEGF Signaling under Hypoxia. *Mar. Drugs* **2015**, *13*, 4436–4451. [CrossRef] [PubMed]

34. Cho, Y.; Cho, E.J.; Lee, J.H.; Yu, S.J.; Kim, Y.J.; Kim, C.Y.; Yoon, J.H. Fucoidan-induced ID-1 suppression inhibits the in vitro and in vivo invasion of hepatocellular carcinoma cells. *Biomed. Pharmacother.* **2016**, *83*, 607–616. [CrossRef] [PubMed]

35. Teng, H.; Yang, Y.; Wei, H.; Liu, Z.; Liu, Z.; Ma, Y.; Gao, Z.; Hou, L.; Zou, X. Fucoidan Suppresses Hypoxia-Induced Lymphangiogenesis and Lymphatic Metastasis in Mouse Hepatocarcinoma. *Mar. Drugs* **2015**, *13*, 3514–3530. [CrossRef] [PubMed]

36. Bilan, M.I.; Grachev, A.A.; Ustuzhanina, N.E.; Shashkov, A.S.; Nifantiev, N.E.; Usov, A.I. Structure of a fucoidan from the brown seaweed *Fucus evanescens* C.Ag. *Carbohydr. Res.* **2002**, *337*, 719–730. [CrossRef]

37. Fermas, S.; Gonnet, F.; Sutton, A.; Charnaux, N.; Mulloy, B.; Du, Y.; Baleux, F.; Daniel, R. Sulfated oligosaccharides (heparin and fucoidan) binding and dimerization of stromal cell-derived factor-1 (SDF-1/CXCL 12) are coupled as evidenced by affinity CE-MS analysis. *Glycobiology* **2008**, *18*, 1054–1064. [CrossRef] [PubMed]

38. Nakamura, S.; Nambu, M.; Ishizuka, T.; Hattori, H.; Kanatani, Y.; Takase, B.; Kishimoto, S.; Amano, Y.; Aoki, H.; Kiyosawa, T.; et al. Effect of controlled release of fibroblast growth factor-2 from chitosan/fucoidan micro complex-hydrogel on in vitro and in vivo vascularization. *J. Biomed. Mater. Res. A* **2008**, *85*, 619–627. [CrossRef] [PubMed]

39. Naik, R.J.; Sharma, R.; Nisakar, D.; Purohit, G.; Ganguli, M. Exogenous chondroitin sulfate glycosaminoglycan associate with arginine-rich peptide-DNA complexes to alter their intracellular processing and gene delivery efficiency. *Biochim. Biophys. Acta Biomembr.* **2015**, *1848*, 1053–1064. [CrossRef] [PubMed]

40. Saboural, P.; Chaubet, F.; Rouzet, F.; Al-Shoukr, F.; Azzouna, R.B.; Bouchemal, N.; Picton, L.; Louedec, L.; Maire, M.; Rolland, L.; et al. Purification of a Low Molecular Weight Fucoidan for SPECT Molecular Imaging of Myocardial Infarction. *Mar. Drugs* **2014**, *12*, 4851–4867. [CrossRef] [PubMed]

41. Bachelet, L.; Bertholon, I.; Lavigne, D.; Vassy, R.; Jandrot-Perrus, M.; Chaubet, F.; Letourneur, D. Affinity of low molecular weight fucoidan for P-selectin triggers its binding to activated human platelets. *Biochim. Biophys. Acta Gen. Subj.* **2009**, *1790*, 141–146. [CrossRef] [PubMed]

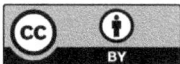

marine drugs

MDPI

Article

Anticancer Effect of Fucoidan on DU-145 Prostate Cancer Cells through Inhibition of PI3K/Akt and MAPK Pathway Expression

Gang-Sik Choo, Hae-Nim Lee, Seong-Ah Shin, Hyeong-Jin Kim and Ji-Youn Jung *

Department of Companion and Laboratory Animal Science, Kongju National University, Yesan 340-702, Korea; chu_0602@naver.com (G.-S.C.); lhn2726@naver.com(H.-N.L.); shinsaya@naver.com(S.-A.S.); tigershout@kongju.ac.kr(H.-J.K.)
* Correspondence: wangza@kongju.ac.kr; Tel.: +82-41-330-1526; Fax: +82-421-330-1529

Academic Editor: Paola Laurienzo
Received: 20 May 2016; Accepted: 29 June 2016; Published: 7 July 2016

Abstract: In this study, we showed that PI3K/Akt signaling mediates fucoidan's anticancer effects on prostate cancer cells, including suppression of proliferation. Fucoidan significantly decreased viability of DU-145 cancer cells in a concentration-dependent manner as shown by MTT [3-(4,5-dimethylthiazol-2-yl)-2,5-diphenyltetrazolium bromide] assay. The drug also significantly increased chromatin condensation, which indicates apoptosis, in a concentration-dependent manner as shown by DAPI (4′,6-diamidino-2-phenylindole) staining. Fucoidan increased expression of Bax, cleaved poly-ADP ribose polymerase and cleaved caspase-9, and decreased of the Bcl-2, p-Akt, p-PI3K, p-P38, and p-ERK in a concentration-dependent manner. In vivo, fucoidan (at 5 and 10 mg/kg) significantly decreased tumor volume, and increased apoptosis as assessed by the TUNEL (terminal deoxynucleotidyl transferase dUTP nick end labeling) assay, confirming the tumor inhibitory effect. The drug also increased expression of p-Akt and p-ERK as shown by immunohistochemistry staining. Therefore, fucoidan may be a promising cancer preventive medicine due to its growth inhibitory effects and induction of apoptosis in human prostate cancer cells.

Keywords: apoptosis; fucoidan; human prostate cancer; phosphoinositide 3-kinase; Akt; mitogen-activated protein kinases

1. Introduction

Cancer is a life-threatening disease that occurs worldwide; in particular, prostate cancer is the most common cancer affecting men in America and is the second leading cause of cancer-related death [1]. Its incidence and mortality in Korea has also increased because of westernized eating habits and an aging population [2,3]. Prostate cancer is initially androgen-dependent and is limited to local or regional stages for which androgen-ablative therapy is applied to suppress the cancer, but in most cases it progresses to androgen-independent disease [4,5]. Complementary and alternative medicine is used to treat prostate cancer by exploiting various nutritional products, in addition to drugs and dietary supplements [6]. Fucoidan is extremely sticky and it has a high molecular weight. Also, it is a sulfated polysaccharide found in the cell wall matrix of brown seaweeds, such as *Undaria pinnatifida, Laminaria angustata, Fucus vesiculosus,* and *Fucus evanescens* [7]. Fucoidan is water-soluble polysaccharides having sulfuric acid groups and consist of D-galactose, D-mannose, D-xylose, D-fucose, and sulfate being structurally divided into galacto fucan sulfate. Fucoidan was reported to induce cell death through apoptosis in colon, breast, and liver cancer cells and also inhibits cancer cell growth by blocking cell cycle progression [8–12]. Furthermore, fucoidan's anti-inflammatory [13], antiviral [14] and anticoagulant [15] effects have received much attention.

More recent studies indicate that chemotherapies based on naturally available marine seaweeds suppress the pathways of mitogen-activated protein kinases (MAPK) and phosphoinositide 3-kinase/protein kinase B (PI3K/Akt) [16,17]. According to the previous study, fucoidan induced apoptosis by the inactivation of p38 MAPK and PI3K/Akt in the PC-3 human prostate cancer cells [18].

MAPK signaling is divided into three subtypes, ERK (extracellular signal-regulated protein kinase), P38 MAPK, and JNK/SAPK (c-Jun *N*-terminal kinase/stress-activated protein kinase), and is known to play a key role in modulating bioactivities such as intracellular responses [19]. ERK, which comprises two isoenzymes, $p44^{ERK1}$ and $p42^{ERK2}$, was the first MAPK to be discovered; when ERKs receive the signal from Ras present in the plasma membrane, they are translocated from the cytoplasm to the nucleus and activate c-Fos and c-Jun and induce the activation of cyclin D1, involved in the cell cycle. Such ERKs are known to be significantly involved in the regulation of various cellular responses, including cell division, proliferation, differentiation, and survival [20].

Akt, also called protein kinase B, is a serine/threonine kinase that was first discovered as a viral oncogene (v-Akt) and exists as three types—Akt1 (PKBα), Akt2 (PKBβ), and Akt3 (PKBγ)—that plays a key role in cell growth and survival [21]. Akt is activated by phosphoinositide 3-kinase (PI3K) and is involved in many processes of intracellular signal transduction such as cell proliferation, differentiation, and angiopoiesis through phosphorylation and activation in the cell membrane [22]. A high level of Akt activation has been found in many cancer cells, including breast and prostate cancer cells, and mutations in Akt or alterations in the activating mechanism of PI3K drive cancer cell growth and resistance to apoptosis, thus acting as a key factor that initiates cancer [23]. Experiments both in vitro and in vivo have validated that the suppression of Akt signaling inhibits proliferation of cancer cells and induces apoptosis; therefore, blocking the Akt signaling pathway can serve to inhibit the abnormal proliferation and growth of tumor cells [24].

In this study, in vitro experiments were performed using androgen-independent DU-145 human prostate carcinoma cells to verify whether fucoidan is effective in inducing apoptosis and has an effect on MAPK and PI3K/Akt signaling. In addition, in vivo experiments to establish the apoptotic effect of fucoidan in prostate cancer has not been reported yet, so we performed in vivo experiment to determine whether fucoidan suppresses tumor growth.

2. Results and Discussion

2.1. Effect of Fucoidan on the Viability of DU-145 Cancer Cells

In this study, the survival rate of cancer cells was measured by the MTT [3-(4,5-dimethylthiazol-2-yl)-2,5-diphenyltetrazolium bromide] assay to explore the effect of fucoidan against DU-145 prostate cancer cells lines. When DU-145 cells were treated with 0, 250, 500, 750, or 1000 μg/mL fucoidan for 24 h, the survival rates of the DU-145 cells were 75.1%, 62.2%, 47.7%, and 39.1%, respectively, all significantly reduced compared with the control group (Figure 1). Boo et al. [18] also reported similar result that after treatment of focoidan, the cell viability of PC-3 prostate cancer cells were significantly reduced in dose dependent manner. Yamasaki et al. [11] reported that the survival rate of MCF-7 breast cancer cells was 25.0% following 1000 μg/mL fucoidan treatment for 24 h, while Yang et al. [12] found a similar effect, with 24 h fucoidan treatment decreasing survival of SMMC-7721 liver cancer cells in a concentration-dependent manner to 40.0% at 500 μg/mL fucoidan. The present results are in agreement with these, though inhibition of survival was slightly less at the same concentrations of fucoidan. Thus, fucoidan suppresses the proliferation of DU-145 prostate cancer cells in a concentration-dependent manner.

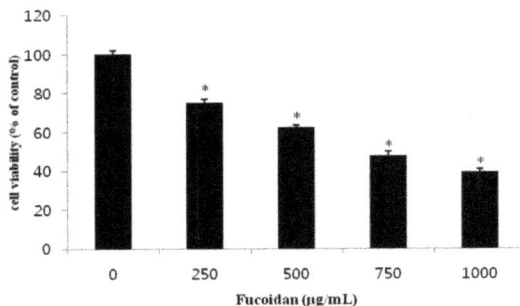

Figure 1. Effect of fucoidan on the cell viability of DU-145 cells. DU-145 cells (2×10^4 cells/mL) were treated with 0, 250, 500, 750, 1000 μg/mL fucoidan in RPMI-1640 medium containing 5% FBS for 24 h. The growth inhibition was measured by the MTT assay. Data are mean standard deviation (SD) for three samples. The significance was determined by Student's *t*-test ($* p < 0.05$ compared with untreated control).

2.2. The Morphological Changes of DU-145 Cancer Cells by the Fucoidan

To investigate whether fucoidan's suppression of DU-145 cells proliferation is attributable to apoptosis, DU-145 prostate cancer cells were treated with 500 or 1000 μg/mL fucoidan, and then chromosomal condensation was observed by DAPI (4′,6-diamidino-2-phenylindole) staining and fluorescence microscopy (Figure 2A). Increased apoptosis elicited by the cells was observed in the fucoidan-treated group, and, consistent with the MTT assay, DAPI staining showed a reduction in the number of cancer cells in the fucoidan-treated group compared with the control group. Furthermore, fucoidan increased cytoplasmic shrinkage and apoptotic body formation compared with the control group by $7.0 \pm 1.5\%$, $22.4 \pm 1.2\%$, and $36.0 \pm 1.3\%$ at 0, 500, and 1000 μg/mL fucoidan, respectively (Figure 2B). These rates were calculated by evaluating of 100 cells by fluorescence microscopy at a magnification of ×200 after selecting five regions randomly. According to the study by Park et al. [23], apoptosis was observed after AGS gastric cancer cells were treated with 100 μg/mL fucoidan; a higher concentration of fucoidan yielded a greater apoptosis effect. These results suggest that DU-145 prostate cancer cells were killed by fucoidan by induction of apoptosis.

2.3. Effect of Fucoidan on the Apoptosis-Related Proteins of DU-145 Cancer Cells

The Bcl-2 family, which comprises proteins that change mitochondrial membrane permeability, plays a key role in regulating apoptosis [24]. Among the Bcl-2 family proteins, Bcl-2 hinders apoptosis, whereas Bax promotes it [25]. When these two signals are out of balance, Bax releases cytochrome c by changing the electric potential of the mitochondrial membrane, which, in turn, triggers the formation of the apoptosome complex including cytochrome c/Apaf-1/caspase-9 and activates caspase-3 [26]. The activation of the caspase cascade decomposes various types of matrix proteins, as well as poly-ADP ribose polymerase (PARP), which resides in the nucleus, to induce apoptosis [27]. Therefore, western blot analysis was performed to detect changes in the expression of Bcl-2 family proteins when DU-145 prostate cancer cells were treated with 500 or 1000 μg/mL fucoidan. Expression of Bax, cleaved caspase-9, and cleaved PARP, all pro-apoptotic proteins, was increased, while that of Bcl-2, an anti-apoptotic protein, was decreased, all in a concentration-dependent manner (Figure 3). A study by Boo et al. [18] also reported a increase in Bax, cleaved caspase-9, and cleaved PARP expression when PC-3 prostate cancer cells were treated with fucoidan.

A

B

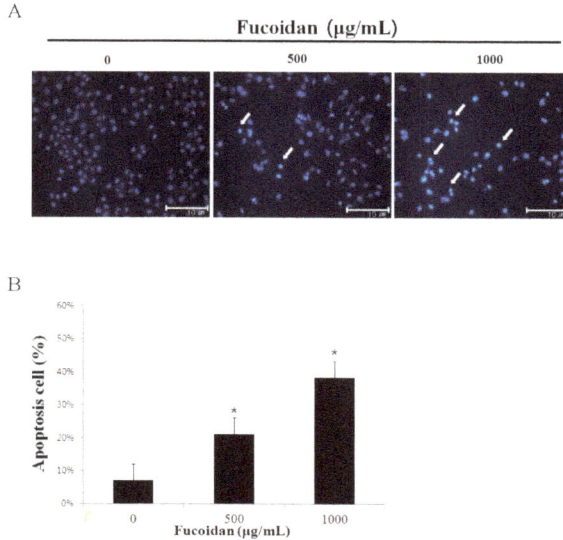

Figure 2. Effect of fucoidan on the chromatin condensation in DU-145 cells. (**A**) DU-145 cells were treated with 0, 500, 1000 μg/mL fucoidan or vehicle in RPMI-1640 medium containing 5% FBS for 24 h, and cell were stained with DAPI. The arrows indicate chromatin condensation in the cancer cell. (**B**) DU-145 cells were treated with fucoidan (0, 500, 1000 μg/mL) for 24 h. Apoptosis cells were counted under a light microscope and expressed as the average of five fields. Each bar represents the mean ± SD calculated from independent experiments. Significance was determined by Dunnett's *t*-test with * *p* < 0.05 compared as statistically significant compared with non-treated controls.

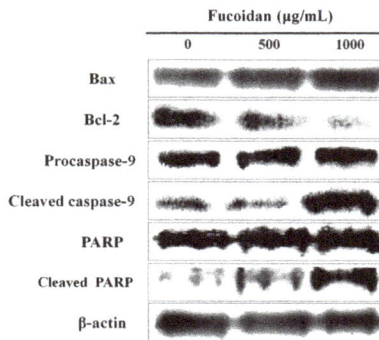

Figure 3. Effect of fucoidan on the apoptotic pathway in DU-145 cells. DU-145 cells were treated with fucoidan 0, 500, and 1000 μg/mL for 24 h and cell were harvested to measure protein levels of Bax, Bcl-2, cspase-9, and PARP by western blotting. The blots were also probed with β-actin antibodies to confirm equal sample loading.

Park et al. [28] demonstrated that, when T24 colon cancer cells were treated with fucoidan, the expression of Bax and cleaved PARP when increased, whereas Bcl-2 and pro-caspase-9 were downregulated. In summary, fucoidan likely induces apoptosis in cancer cells by regulating the expression of Bax and Bcl-2, inducing cleavage of caspase-9 and PARP.

2.4. Effect of Fucoidan on PI3K/Akt Pathways in DU-145 Cancer Cells

Akt is a serine/threonine kinase, also called protein kinase B, is activated by PI3K and regulates many biological responses, including proliferation, differentiation, or the cell cycle-associated survival of cells. When triggered by PI3K, Akt inhibits apoptosis by hindering the expression of BAD (Bcl-2 associated death promoter) or caspase-9, both of which are pro-apoptotic [29]. To investigate the effect of fucoidan on PI3K/Akt signaling pathways, western blotting was performed (Figure 4A). When DU-145 prostate cancer cells were treated with 500 or 1000 µg/mL fucoidan for 24 h, the phosphorylation of Akt and PI3K was decreased in a concentration-dependent manner. In a similar experiment confirmed the apoptosis of androgen-independent PC-3 human prostate cancer cells [18] also reported a decrease in p-Akt dependent on concentration of fucoidan. A study by Lee et al. [29] also reported a decrease in p-Akt and p-PI3K dependent on time and concentration when A549 lung cancer cells were treated with fucoidan. Together, these studies indicate that fucoidan induces apoptosis in DU-145 prostate cancer cells by decreasing activation of Akt and PI3K.

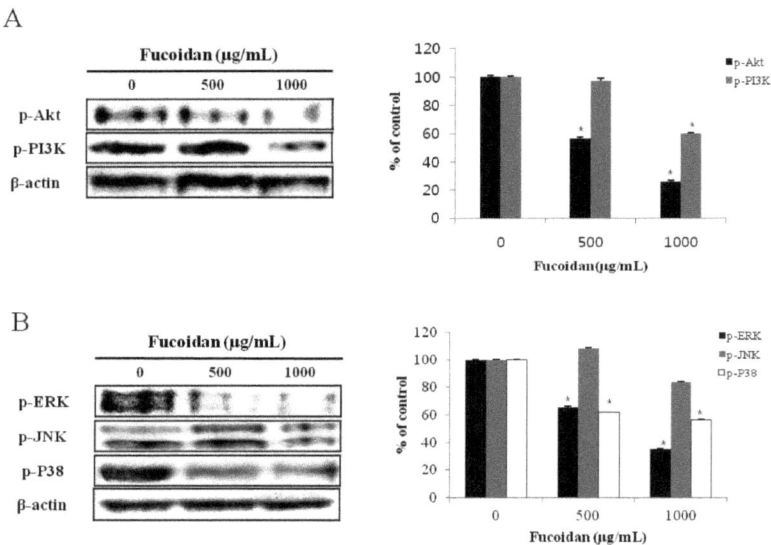

Figure 4. Effect of fucoidan on the activation of PI3K/Akt pathway in DU-145 cells. Cells were treated with fucoidan 0, 500 and 1000 µg/mL for 24 h. Cell lysates were prepared as described in the materials and methods and analyzed by 12% SDS-PAGE followed by western blotting. (**A**) The membranes were incubated with PI3K/AKT pathway antibodies. (**B**) The membranes were incubated with MAPKs pathway antibodies. Each bar represents the mean ± SD calculated from independent experiments. Significance was determined by Dunnett's *t*-test with * p <0.05 compared as statistically significant compared with non-treated controls.

2.5. Effect of Fucoidan on MAPK Pathways in DU-145 Cancer Cells

Various kinases in the MAPK pathways are involved in diverse actions depending on cellular conditions; generally, the ERK signaling pathway is involved in cell proliferation, whereas JNK acts to antagonize cell proliferation [30]. Thus, we investigated how MAPK signaling is affected by fucoidan in DU-145 prostate cancer cells. When DU-145 prostate cancer cells were treated with 500 or 1000 µg/mL fucoidan for 24 h, although there was no change in phosphorylation of JNK, the ERK and p38 was decreased in a concentration-dependent manner (Figure 4B). Boo et al. [18] demonstrated that, when PC-3 prostate cancer cells were treated with fucoidan, the expression of p38 was decreased, whereas p-ERK was upregulated. A study by Aisa et al. [10] also reported a decrease in p-ERK and p-p38 expression when HCT-15 colon cancer cells were treated with fucoidan. These results demonstrate that fucoidan inhibits the growth of DU-145 prostate cancer cells and induces apoptosis by inhibiting the phosphorylation of ERK and p38.

2.6. Effect of Fucoidan on Tumor Growth In Vivo Animal Model

Next, we evaluated the effect of fucoidan on tumors arising from transplantation of DU-145 cells into nude mice. The tumor size was measured twice a week, and fucoidan was diluted with phosphate-buffered saline and intraperitoneally injected at 5 or 10 mg/kg body weight five times a week for three weeks. Tumors were smaller in mice given fucoidan compared with the control group eight days from the commencement of drug administration. At 21 days, compared with the control group, tumors in the low-concentration (5 mg/kg) group were 52.0% smaller, while those in the high-concentration (10 mg/kg) group were 80.0% smaller (Figure 5A). In terms of mass, the mean weight of tumors in mice receiving 5 mg/kg fucoidan was 137 ± 19.0 mg and 89 ± 33.0 mg in those receiving 10 mg/kg; there was a marked trend of decreased tumor weight compared with the control group, in which tumors were 397 ± 15.4 mg (Figure 5B). Han et al. [15] reported that intraperitoneal injection of 5 or 10 mg/kg fucoidan into colon cancer (HT29)-bearing mice led to a decrease in the tumor weight by 39.0% ± 2.6% or 7.5% ± 1.2%, respectively. Such results lead to the reasonable conclusion that fucoidan also inhibits the growth of DU-145 prostate tumors.

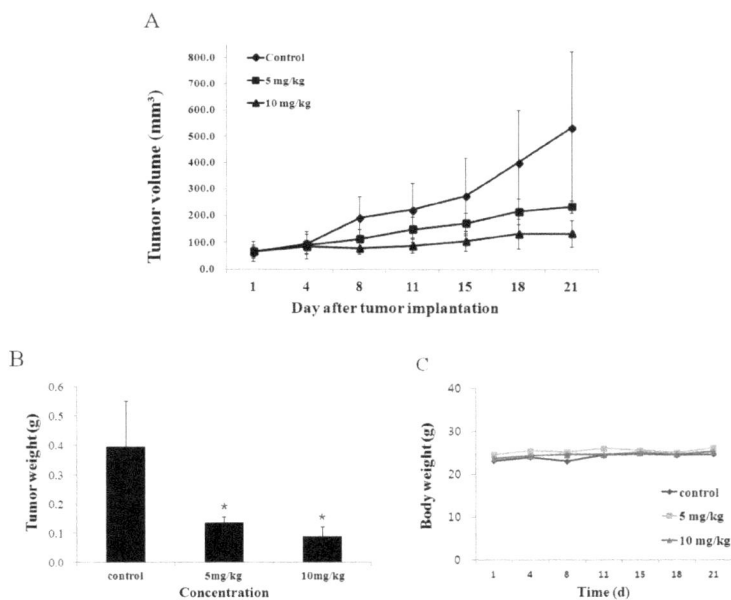

Figure 5. Inhibition of DU-145 prostate tumor growth and enhancement of apoptosis in DU-145 prostate tumors by the fucoidan. (**A**) To identify the effect of fucoidan in DU-145 prostate tumor growth, nude mice were treated with fucoidan (0, 5, 10 mg/kg) for 21 days (*n* = 5). (**B**) The graph expresses final tumor weight. (**C**) The graph is nude mice weight. Each value was expressed as mean ± SE of five mice. Significance was determined by Dunnett's *t*-test with * *p* <0.05 compared as statistically significant compared with non-treated controls.

2.7. Effect of Fucoidan on the Apoptosis Induction of DU-145 Tumor Tissue

To verify the anticancer effect of fucoidan on DU-145 prostate cancer, the drug was administered to mice carrying xenograft tumors. Compared with the control group, tumors from mice given 0 mg/kg or 10 mg/kg fucoidan had more apoptotic cells (4.1% ± 1.0% and 18.6% ± 4.0% more, respectively as measured by the TUNEL (terminal deoxynucleotidyl transferase dUTP nick end labeling) assay (Figure 6). This result implies that DNA fragmentation observed earlier resulted from apoptosis. Xue et al. [31] reported similar effects of 5 or 10 mg/kg fucoidan on 4T1 breast cancer xenografts in mice. Thus, fucoidan likely inhibits the growth of tumors by inducing apoptosis in DU-145 prostate cancer cells.

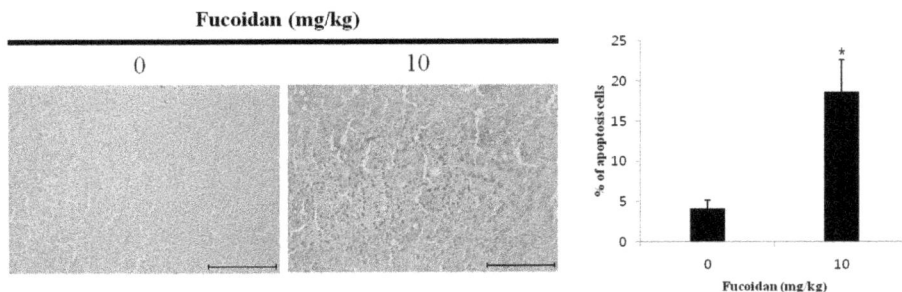

Figure 6. Induction of apoptosis by fucoidan in DU-145 cells. Nude mice were treated with fucoidan for 21 days and apoptosis was assessed by terminal deoxynucleotidyltransferase-mediated Dutp nick-ned labeling (TUNEL) assay. Tumor tissues were observed under a microscope and photographed at a ×200 magnification. The percentage of labeled with TUNEL-positive apoptotic cells was calculated from 1,000 scored cells. Paraffin-embedded tumors were cut into 5 μm sections. Each bar represents the mean ± SD calculated from independent experiments. Significance was determined by Dunnett's *t*-test with * $p < 0.05$ compared as statistically significant compared with non-treated controls. Scale bar, 10 μm.

2.8. Effect of Fucoidan on Akt and ERK Expression in DU-145 Tumor Tissue

Akt and ERK cooperate to maintain cell viability, and are known to be involved in proliferation and differentiation of cells and to regulate a wide spectrum of biological activity [32]. Thus, we employed immunohistochemical assays to measure the activation (phosphorylation) of Akt and ERK in tumor tissues collected from human tumor-xenografted mice after intraperitoneal injection of 5 or 10 mg/kg fucoidan (Figure 7). We observed that fucoidan at either dose decreased phosphorylation of Akt and ERK compared with the control group, similar to the results of western blotting in vitro. Fucoidan thus appears to inhibit the growth and migration of tumors by regulating the activity of Akt and ERK.

2.9. The Histopathological Changes in DU-145 Tumor Tissues by the Fucoidan

Next, to assess organ toxicity due to fucoidan administration, liver, and kidney tissues from tumor-xenografted mice were histologically examined by hematoxylin and eosin staining followed by fluorescence microscopy (original magnification, ×200). No histopathological abnormality was detected, indicating that fucoidan causes no detectable toxic effects (Figure 8).

Fucoidan (mg/kg)

0	5	10

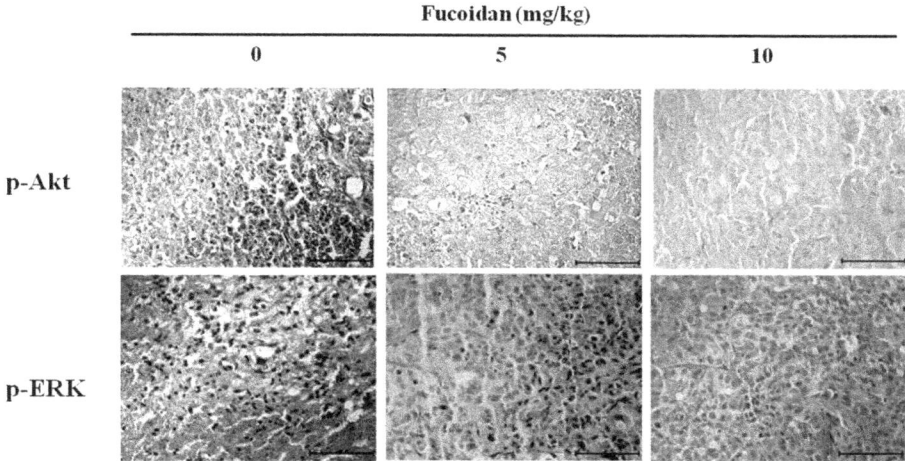

Figure 7. Effect of fucoidan on p-Akt and p-ERK expression in DU-145 prostate tumors. Nude mice were administered fucoidan (0, 5 and 10 mg/kg) for three weeks and assayed by immunohistochemistry using p-Akt and p-ERK antibodes. Tumor tissues were observed under a microscope and photographed at a ×400 magnification. Paraffin-embedded tumors were sectioned to a thickness of 5 μm. Scale bar, 5 μm.

Fucoidan (mg/kg)

0	5	10

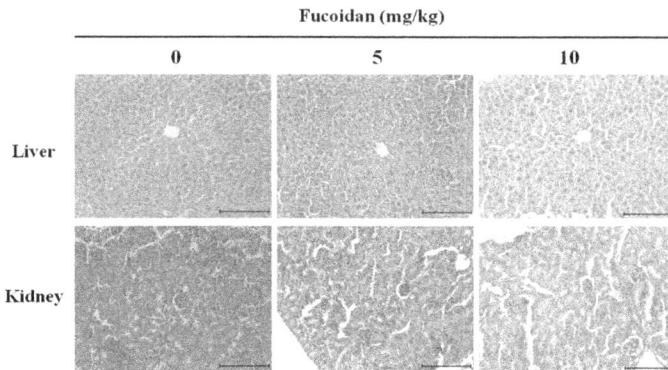

Figure 8. Histological observation of nude mice treated intraperitoneally with fucoidan. Fucoidan was administered at a dose of 5 or 10 mg/kg five times per week, for a total 21 injections. On day 21, mice were sacrificed, and tumors excised and evaluated by hematoxylin & eosin (H & E) staining (×200). The dose of fucoidan had no detectable toxicological effect on nude mice. Scale bar, 10 μm.

3. Materials and Methods

3.1. Chemicals, Drugs, and Antibodies

Fucoidan *(Undaria pinnatifida)* was purchased from Sigma-Aldrich (St. Louis, MO, USA). RPMI-1640 medium, penicillin-streptomycin, trypsin-EDTA and fetal bovine serum (FBS) were purchased from HyClone Laboratories Inc. (Logan, UT, USA). 3-(4,5-Dimethythiazol-2-yl)-2,5-diphenyl tetrazolium bromide (MTT) and dimethylsulfoxide (DMSO) were obtained from Sigma-Aldrich. Antibodies against Bax, Bcl-2, β-actin, Akt, phospho-Akt (Ser473), caspase-9, phospho-PARP, phosphoinositide 3-kinase (PI3K), extracellular signal regulated kinase (ERK) 1/2, c-Jun N-terminal kinase (JNK), P38 and rabbit lgG were purchased from Cell Signaling Technology (Beverly, MA,

USA). Cell lysis buffer and 4',6-diamidino-2-phenylindole (DAPI) were purchased from Invitrogen Life Technologies (Carlsbad, CA, USA). The DeadEnd™ fluorometric terminal deoxyribonucleotide transferase-mediated dUTP nick end-labeling (TUNEL) assay kit was purchased from Promega (Madison, WI, USA).

3.2. Cell Lines and Culture

The human prostate carcinoma cell line, DU-145, was purchased from the Korean Cell Line Bank (Seoul, Korea) and maintained in RPMI-1640 medium supplemented with 5% FBS and 1% penicillin-streptomycin at 37 °C in a humidified 5% CO_2 atmosphere. Culture medium was renewed every 2–3 days. For fucoidan treatment, DU-145 cells were seeded at a density of approximately 3×10^4 cells/cm^2 in a 175 cm^2 flask and were allowed to adhere overnight.

3.3. Cell Viability Assay

The anticancer effects of fucoidan were assessed by MTT assay. DU-145 cells were seeded in a 96-well plate at a density of 2×10^4 cells/mL and a volume of 200 μL/well. After 24 h of incubation, the cells were treated with 250, 500, 750, and 1000 μg/mL fucoidan for either 24 h in triplicate. Following treatment, the medium was discarded, followed by the addition of 40 μL of a 5 mg/mL MTT solution and incubation for a further 2 h. The medium was then aspirated and the formazan product generated by viable cells was solubilized with the addition of 100 μL of DMSO. The absorbance of the solutions at 595 nm was determined using a microplate reader (Bio-Rad, Hercules, CA, USA). The percentage of viable cells was estimated in comparison to the untreated control cells.

3.4. 4',6-diamidino-2-phenylindole (DAPI) Staining

Apoptotic cell death was determined morphologically using a fluorescent nuclear dye, DAPI. DAPI staining showed the number of apoptotic cells with chromatin condensation and nuclear fragmentation. DU-145 cells were incubated with PBS or various concentrations of fucoidan (500 and 1000 μg/mL) for 24 h, then harvested by trypsinization, and fixed in 70% ethanol overnight at 4 °C. The next day, the cells were stained with DAPI, deposited onto the slides, and finally viewed to detect apoptotic characteristics with a fluorescent microscope.

3.5. Western Blot Analysis

Cells were treated with various concentrations of fucoidan for 24 h, and then protein concentrations were determined using the Bradford protein assay (Bio-Rad Laboratories, Hercules, CA). Total proteins in each cell lysate were resolved on various concentrations (6%–14%) of sodium dodecyl sulfate-polyacrylamide gel electrophoresis (SDS PAGE) gels, and then were electro-transferred onto nitrocellulose membranes. The membranes were incubated with blocking buffer (5% non-fat dry milk in Tris-buffered saline with Tween 20 (TBS-T)) for 1 h at room temperature, and then were further incubated with specific antibodies diluted in blocking solution overnight at 4 °C. After washing with TBS-T, membranes were incubated with horseradish peroxidase (HRP)-conjugated secondary antibodies for 1 h at room temperature. After washing, bands were visualized using enhanced chemiluminescence (ECL) detection reagents (Pierce Biotechnology, Rockford, IL, USA) according to the manufacturer's instructions.

3.6. Antitumor Activity In Vivo

Five-week-old male BALB/c nude mice (nu/nu) were purchased from Orient Bio Inc. (Gyeonggi-do, Korea). Experiments on animals were performed in accordance with the Guidelines for the Care and Use of Animals of the Kongju National University Animals Care Committee (Chungcheongnam-do, Korea). Mice were maintained under a 12 h light/dark cycle, and housed under controlled temperature (23 ± 3 °C) and humidity (40% ± 10%) conditions. Mice were allowed access to laboratory pelleted food and water ad libitum. DU-145 cells were maintained in RPMI-1640 supplemented with 10% FBS and 1% penicillin-streptomycin at 37 °C in a humidified 5% CO_2 atmosphere. DU-145 cells were harvested from cultures by exposure to 0.25% trypsin. Trypsinization was stopped with a solution containing 10% FBS, and cells were then washed twice and resuspended in RPMI-1640 medium. A total of 2×10^7 cells in 0.2 mL of medium were injected subcutaneously into the right flank of donor nude mice. Seven days after the subcutaneous injection, DU-145 cells growing under the skin of nude mice established tumors. All animal experiments were performed following the approval of the Institutional Animal Care and Use Committee according to the guidelines of Kongju National University (KNU_2015-06).

3.7. Histological Examination

The excised livers and kidneys were immediately fixed in 10% neutral-buffered formalin and, after embedding in paraffin, cut into 5-μm-thick sections. Following hematoxylin and eosin (H & E) staining, the sections were examined under a light microscope ($\times$200).

3.8. TUNEL Assay

Paraffin-embedded tumor tissues were used for TUNEL staining, which was performed using the Dead End Colorimetric TUNEL system (Promega). Paraffin-embedded sections (5 μm thick) were processed according to the manufacturer's protocol. Briefly, sections were deparaffinized in xylene, and then treated with a graded series of alcohol (100%, 95%, 85%, 70%, and 50% ethanol (*v/v*) in double-distilled H_2O) and rehydrated in PBS (pH 7.5). Then the tissues were treated with proteinase K solution for permeabilization and refixed with 4% paraformaldehyde solution. Slides were treated with the rTdT reaction mix and incubated at 37 for 1 h; reactions were terminated by immersing the slides in 2$\times$ SSC solution for 15 min at room temperature. After blocking endogenous peroxidase activity (with 0.3% hydrogen peroxide), slides were washed with PBS, and then incubated with streptavidin horseradish peroxidase solution for 30 min at room temperature. After washing, slides were incubated with 3,3-diaminobenzidine (substrate) solution until a light brown background appeared (10 min), and then rinsed several times in deionized water. After mounting, slides were observed using a light microscope.

3.9. Immunohistochemistry

To detect p-Akt and p-ERK, 5-μm-thick sections were cut from paraffin-embedded tissue blocks. The sections were deparaffinized and hydrated by sequential immersion in xylene and graded alcohol solutions. The endogenous peroxidase activity was quenched by treatment with 3% hydrogen peroxide for 5 min at room temperature. The sections were incubated with primary antibodies for 1 h at 37 °C and then with the secondary antibody for 30 min at room temperature. Staining was performed using diaminobenzidine (DAB) and counterstaining was performed using methyl green. For the negative control, the incubated antibody diluent was used as a substitute for the primary antibody

3.10. Statistical Analysis

The results are expressed as the means $\pm$ standard deviation (SD). Differences between the mean values for the groups were assessed by a one-way analysis of variance (ANOVA) and Dunnett's *t*-tests. $p < 0.05$ was considered to indicate a statistically significant difference.

4. Conclusions

In this study, we confirmed the effects of fucoidan on androgen-independent prostate cancer via in vitro and in vivo. Fucoidan inhibited the proliferation of and induced apoptosis in DU-145 prostate cancer cells and modulated protein expression associated with apoptosis through the PI3K/Akt and MAPK signaling pathways. Administration of 5 or 10 mg/kg fucoidan to DU-145 prostate-bearing nude mice significantly reduced tumor volume and tumor weight. TUNEL assay results suggest that this results from fucoidan's induction of cancer cell apoptosis. Finally, immunohistochemical analysis of tumor tissue revealed that fucoidan treatment decreased p-Akt and p-ERK levels, indicating that apoptosis of DU-145 prostate cancer cells results from regulation of the PI3K/Akt and MAPK signaling pathways. Thus, the present study provides a molecular basis for the use of fucoidan as a cancer chemopreventive and chemotherapeutic agent.

Acknowledgments: This research was supported by Basic Science Research Program through the National Research Foundation of Korea (NRF) funded by the Ministry of Education, Science and Technology (NRF-2013R1A1A4A01012315). Also, this work was supported by the research grant of the Kongju National University in 2012.

Author Contributions: Ji-Youn Jung conceived and designed the experiments. Gang-Sik Choo, Hae-Nim Lee, Seong-Ah Shin and Hyeong-Jin Kim performed the experiments. Gang-Sik Choo, Hae-Nim Lee and Ji-Youn Jung carried out statistical analysis of the data. All authors contributed to the writing of the manuscript.

Conflicts of Interest: The authors declare no conflict of interest.

References

1. Doll, S.R. The lessons of life: keynote address to the nutrition and cancer conference. *J. Cancer Res.* **1992**, *52*, 2024–2029.
2. Oh, C.M.; Won, Y.J.; Jung, K.W.; Kong, H.J.; Cho, H.; Lee, J.K.; Lee, D.H.; Lee, K.H. Cancer statistics in Korea: Incidence, mortality, survival, and prevalence in 2013. *J. Cancer Res. Ther.* **2014**, *46*, 109–123. [CrossRef] [PubMed]
3. Hwang, E.S.; Bowen, P.E. Effects of tomatoes and lycopene on prostate cancer prevention and treatment. *J. Korean Soc. Food Sci. Nutr.* **2004**, *33*, 455–462.
4. Walsh, P.C.; Partin, A.W.; Epstein, J.I. Cancer control and quality of life following anatomical radical retropubic prostatectomy: Results at 10 years. *J. Urol.* **1944**, *152*, 1831–1836.
5. Isaacs, J.T.; Lundmo, P.I.; Berges, R.; Martikainen, P.; Kyprianou, N. Androgen regulation of programmed death of normal and malignant prostatic cells. *J. Androl.* **1992**, *13*, 457–464. [PubMed]
6. Kwon, M.J.; Nam, T.J. A polysaccharide of the marine alga *Capsosiphon fulvescens* induces apoptosis in AGS gastric cancer cells via an IGF-IR-mediated PI3K/Akt pathway. *Cell Biol. Int.* **2007**, *31*, 768–775. [CrossRef] [PubMed]
7. Li, B.; Lu, F.; Wei, X.; Zhao, R. Fucoidan: Structure and bioactivity. *Molecules* **2008**, *13*, 1671–1695. [CrossRef] [PubMed]
8. Lee, J.B.; Hayashi, K.; Hashimoto, M.; Nakano, T.; Hayashi, T. Novel antiviral fucoidan from sporophyll of *Undaria pinnatifida* (Mekabu). *Chem. Pharm. Bull.* **2004**, *52*, 1091–1094. [CrossRef] [PubMed]
9. Gideon, T.P.; Rengasamy, R. Toxicological evaluation of fucoidan from *Cladosiphon okamuranus*. *J. Med. Food* **2008**, *11*, 638–642. [CrossRef] [PubMed]
10. Aisa, Y.; Miyakawa, Y.; Nakazato, T.; Shibata, H.; Saito, K.; Ikeda, Y.; Kizaki, M. Fucoidan induces apoptosis of human HS-sultan cells accompanied by activation of caspase-3 and down-regulation of ERK pathways. *Am. J. Hematol.* **2005**, *78*, 7–14. [CrossRef] [PubMed]
11. Yamasaki-Miyamoto, Y.; Yamasaki, M.; Tachibana, H.; Yamada, K. Fucoidan induces apoptosis through activation of caspase-8 on human breast cancer MCF-7 cells. *J. Agric. Food Chem.* **2009**, *57*, 8677–8682. [CrossRef] [PubMed]
12. Yang, L.; Wang, P.; Wang, H.; Li, Q.; Teng, H.; Liu, Z.; Yang, W.; Hou, L.; Zou, X. Fucoidan derived from *Undaria pinnatifida* induces apoptosis in human hepatocellular carcinoma SMMC-7721 cells via the ROS-mediated mitochondrial pathway. *Mar. Drugs* **2013**, *11*, 1961–1976. [CrossRef] [PubMed]
13. Park, H.Y.; Han, M.H.; Park, C.; Jin, C.Y.; Kim, G.Y.; Chol, L.W.; Kim, N.D.; Nam, T.J.; Kwon, T.K.; Chol, Y.H. Anti-inflammatory effects of fucoidan through inhibition of NF-κB, MAPK and Akt activation in lipopolysaccharide-induced BV2 microglia cells. *Food Chem. Toxicol.* **2011**, *49*, 1745–1752. [CrossRef] [PubMed]
14. Sharmistha, S.; Akram, A.; Tuhin, G.; Paul, S.; Bimalendu, R. Polysaccharides from *Sargassum tenerrimum*: Structural features, chemical modification and anti-viral activity. *Phytochemistry* **2010**, *71*, 235–242.

15. Han, Y.S.; Lee, J.H.; Lee, S.H. Antitumor effects of fucoidan on human colon cancer cells via activation of AKT signaling. *Biomol. Ther.* **2015**, *23*, 225–232. [CrossRef] [PubMed]
16. Carnero, A. The PKB/AKT pathway in cancer. *Curr. Pharm. Des.* **2010**, *16*, 34–44. [CrossRef] [PubMed]
17. Osaki, M.; Oshimura, M.; Ito, H. PI3K-Akt pathway: its functions and alterations in human cancer. *Apoptosis* **2004**, *9*, 667–676. [CrossRef] [PubMed]
18. Boo, H.J.; Hong, J.Y.; Kim, S.C.; Kang, J.I.; Kim, M.K.; Kim, E.J.; Hyun, J.W.; Koh, Y.S.; Yoo, E.S.; Kwon, J.M.; et al. The Anticancer Effect of Ficoidan in PC-3 Prostate Cancer cells. *Mar. Drugs.* **2013**, *11*, 2982–2999. [CrossRef] [PubMed]
19. Seth, A.; Gonzalez, F.A.; Gupta, S.; Raden, D.L.; Davis, R.J. Signal transduction within the nucleus by mitogen-activated protein kinase. *J. Biol. Chem.* **1992**, *267*, 24796–24804. [PubMed]
20. Zhuang, Z.Y.; Gerner, P.; Woolf, C.J.; Ji, R.R. ERK is sequentially activated in neurons, microglia, and astrocytes by spinal nerve ligation and contributes to mechanical allodynia in this neuropathic pain model. *Pain* **2005**, *114*, 149–159. [CrossRef] [PubMed]
21. Song, G.; Ouyang, G.; Bao, S. The activation of Akt/PKB signaling pathway and cell survival. *J. Cell. Mol. Med.* **2005**, *9*, 59–71. [CrossRef] [PubMed]
22. Lee, Y.K.; Park, S.Y.; Kim, Y.M.; Kim, D.C.; Lee, W.S.; Surh, Y.J.; Park, O.J. Suppression of mTOR via Akt-dependent and -independent mechanisms in selenium-treated colon cancer cells: Involvement of AMPKα_1. *Carcinogenesis* **2010**, *31*, 1092–1099. [CrossRef] [PubMed]
23. Park, H.S.; Kim, G.Y.; Nam, T.J.; Kim, D.N.; Choi, Y.H. Antiproliferative activity of fucoidan was associated with the induction of apoptosis and autophagy in AGS human gastric cancer cells. *J. Food Sci.* **2011**, *76*, 77–83. [CrossRef] [PubMed]
24. Donovan, M.; Cotter, T.G. Control of mitochondrial integrity by Bcl-2 family members and caspase-independent cell death. *Biochim. Biophys. Acta* **2004**, *1644*, 133–147. [CrossRef] [PubMed]
25. Adams, J.M.; Cory, S. The Bcl-2 protein family: Arbiters of cell survival. *Science* **1998**, *281*, 1322–1326. [CrossRef] [PubMed]
26. Wei, C.; Xiao, Q.; Kuang, X.; Zhang, T.; Yang, Z.; Wang, L. Fucoidan inhibits proliferation of the SKM-1 acute myeloid leukaemia cell line via the activation of apoptotic pathways and production of reactive oxygen species. *Mol. Med. Rep.* **2015**, *12*, 6649–6655. [CrossRef] [PubMed]
27. Jin, S.; Yun, S.G.; Oh, Y.N.; Lee, J.Y.; Park, H.J.; Jin, K.S.; Kwon, H.J.; Kim, B.W. Induction of G2/M arrest and apoptosis by methanol extract of *Typha orientalis* in human colon adenocarcinoma HT29 cells. *Microbiol. Biotechnol. Lett.* **2013**, *41*, 425–432. [CrossRef]
28. Park, H.Y.; Kim, G.Y.; Moon, S.K.; Kim, W.J.; Yoo, Y.H.; Choi, Y.H. Fucoidan inhibits the proliferation of human urinary bladder cancer T24 cells by blocking cell cycle progression and inducing apoptosis. *Molecules* **2014**, *19*, 5981–5998. [CrossRef] [PubMed]
29. Lee, H.; Kim, J.S.; Kim, E. Fucoidan from seaweed Fucus vesiculosus inhibits migration and invasion of human lung cancer cell via PI3K-Akt-mTOR pathways. *PLoS ONE* **2012**, *7*, e50624. [CrossRef] [PubMed]
30. Yang, Y.; Zhu, X.; Chen, Y.; Wang, X.; Chen, R. P38 and JNK MAPK, but not ERK1/2 MAPK, play important role in colchicine-induced cortical neurons apoptosis. *Eur. J. Pharmacol.* **2007**, *576*, 26–33. [CrossRef] [PubMed]
31. Xue, M.; Ge, Y.; Zhang, J.; Wang, Q.; Hou, L.; Liu, Y.; Sun, L.; Li, Q. Anticancer properties and mechanisms of fucoidan on mouse breast cancer in vitro and in vivo. *PLoS ONE* **2012**, *7*, e43483. [CrossRef] [PubMed]
32. Zhang, Y.; Wang, L.; Zhang, M.; Jin, M.; Bai, C.; Wang, X. Potential mechanism of interleukin-8 production from lung cancer cells: An involvement of EGF-EGFR-PI3K-Akt-Erk pathway. *J. Cell. Physiol.* **2012**, *227*, 35–43. [CrossRef] [PubMed]

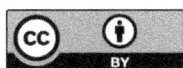

marine drugs

MDPI

Article

Heparanase and Syndecan-4 Are Involved in Low Molecular Weight Fucoidan-Induced Angiogenesis

Oualid Haddad [1], Erwan Guyot [1,2], Nicolas Marinval [1], Fabien Chevalier [3], Loïc Maillard [1], Latifa Gadi [1], Christelle Laguillier-Morizot [1,2], Olivier Oudar [1], Angela Sutton [1,2], Nathalie Charnaux [1,2,†] and Hanna Hlawaty [1,†,*]

[1] Inserm U1148, Laboratory for Vascular Translational Science, UFR SMBH, Université Paris 13, Sorbonne Paris Cité, Groupe Biothérapies et Glycoconjugués, 93000 Bobigny, France; haddad.oualid@univ-paris13.fr (O.H.); erwan.guyot@jvr.aphp.fr (E.G.); nmarinval@yahoo.fr (N.M.); loic_maillard95@hotmail.fr (L.M.); latifa.gadi@yahoo.fr (L.G.); christelle.laguillier@jvr.aphp.fr (C.L.-M.); olivier.oudar@univ-paris13.fr (O.O.); angela.sutton@jvr.aphp.fr (A.S.); nathalie.charnaux@jvr.aphp.fr (N.C.)

[2] Laboratoire de Biochimie, Hôpital Jean Verdier, Assistance Publique-Hôpitaux de Paris, 93140 Bondy, France

[3] ERL CNRS 9215, CRRET Laboratory, Université Paris Est Créteil, 94010 Créteil, France; fabien.che@gmail.com

* Author to whom correspondence should be addressed; hanna.hlawaty@univ-paris13.fr; Tel.: +33-1-48-38-76-97 or +33-1-48-38-77-52; Fax: +33-1-48-38-13-22.

† These authors contributed equally to this work.

Academic Editor: Paola Laurienzo
Received: 29 July 2015; Accepted: 19 October 2015; Published: 28 October 2015

Abstract: Induction of angiogenesis is a potential treatment for chronic ischemia. Low molecular weight fucoidan (LMWF), the sulfated polysaccharide from brown seaweeds, has been shown to promote revascularization in a rat limb ischemia, increasing angiogenesis _in vivo_. We investigated the potential role of two heparan sulfate (HS) metabolism enzymes, exostosin-2 (EXT2) and heparanase (HPSE), and of two HS-membrane proteoglycans, syndecan-1 and -4 (SDC-1 and SDC-4), in LMWF induced angiogenesis. Our results showed that LMWF increases human vascular endothelial cell (HUVEC) migration and angiogenesis _in vitro_. We report that the expression and activity of the HS-degrading HPSE was increased after LMWF treatment. The phenotypic tests of LMWF-treated and _EXT2_- or _HPSE_-siRNA-transfected cells indicated that EXT2 or HPSE expression significantly affect the proangiogenic potential of LMWF. In addition, LMWF increased SDC-1, but decreased SDC-4 expressions. The effect of LMWF depends on SDC-4 expression. Silencing _EXT2_ or _HPSE_ leads to an increased expression of SDC-4, providing the evidence that EXT2 and HPSE regulate the SDC-4 expression. Altogether, these data indicate that EXT2, HPSE, and SDC-4 are involved in the proangiogenic effects of LMWF, suggesting that the HS metabolism changes linked to LMWF-induced angiogenesis offer the opportunity for new therapeutic strategies of ischemic diseases.

Keywords: fucoidan; angiogenesis; human endothelial cell; glycosaminoglycan; syndecan; heparanase

1. Introduction

Heparan sulfate proteoglycans (HSPG) are integral components of the cell surface and extracellular matrix (ECM) of animal cells. These complex molecules consist of sulfated carbohydrate chains of glycosaminoglycans (GAGs) covalently bound to a protein core. The GAGs are composed of disaccharide units composed of galactose or glucuronic/iduronic acid and N-acetyl-glucosamine/-galactosamine. Heparan sulfate (HS) chain compositions are cell-specific and can evolve during the development or tissue regeneration. All HS chains are synthesized _de novo_, and it is still unclear what determines their structures. The enzymes involved in the biosynthesis of a carbohydrate chain have been identified. Two main categories have been described: the enzymes responsible for chain polymerization, mainly exostosin-1 and -2 (EXT1, EXT2), and the enzymes responsible for chain modifications (*N*-deacetylase/*N*-sulfotransferases (NDST), 2-*O*-sulfotransferases (2OST), 3-*O*-sulfotransferases (3OST), 6-*O*-sulfotransferases (6OST), and heparanase (HPSE). Syndecans (SDCs) are heparan-sulfate containing transmembrane proteoglycans [1]. They bind various components of the ECM and are important regulators of cell-cell and cell-ECM interactions. Syndecans are involved in cell migration and angiogenesis [2,3]. Syndecan-4 (SDC-4) is a component of the focal contacts and its activation is associated with cell cytoskeletal rearrangement leading to cell migration [4]. Syndecan-1 (SDC-1) modulates β-integrin- and interleukin-6-dependent breast cancer cell adhesion and migration, and its overexpression in human fibrosarcoma cells leads to increased proliferation and migratory ability [5,6]. Low molecular weight fucoidan (LMWF), a sulfated polysaccharide from brown seaweeds that mimics some biological activities of heparin, has been shown to promote revascularization in a rat critical hindlimb ischemia [7]. It increases human vascular endothelial growth factor (VEGF$_{165}$)-induced endothelial cell migration by enhancing VEGF$_{165}$ binding to VEGFR-2 and neuropilin 1 (NRP1) [8]. Furthermore, fucoidan induces the adoption by endothelial colony-forming cells (ECFC) of an angiogenic phenotype *in vitro* and greatly increases ECFC-mediated angiogenesis *in vivo* [9]. We have previously demonstrated that LMWF, injected in rats, prevented intimal hyperplasia in the thoracic aorta by increasing human vascular endothelial cell (HUVEC) migration, but decreasing vascular smooth muscle cell migration through the modulation of matrix metalloproteinase-2 (MMP-2) expression [10]. Nevertheless, the effects of fucoidan on angiogenesis are somehow controversial. Indeed, depending on the seaweed origin, the sulfatation level, or the size, fucoidan may have antiangiogenic effects. Soeda *et al.* reported that oversulfated fucoidan (100 kDa) from *Fucus vesiculosus* significantly inhibited the fibroblast growth factor-2 (FGF-2) induced HUVEC migration and tube formation by increasing the release of plasminogen activator inhibitor-1 (PAI-1) [11]. In contrast, Kim *et al.* reported that fucoidan acts synergistically with FGF-2 in promoting HUVEC proliferation and agiogenesis by AKT and MMP-2 signalling via activation of the p38 and JNK signalling pathways [12]. In this study, we hypothesized that LMWF (8 kDa) from *Fucus vesiculosus* can also modify the amount and the distribution of heparan sulfate (HS) chains exposed at the endothelial cell surface and of two major heparan sulfate membrane proteoglycans, SDC-1 and SDC-4, causing modifications of cell properties related to proangiogenic abilities.

2. Results and Discussion

2.1. Effects of LMWF on Endothelial Cell Abilities (Migration and 2D-Angiogenesis)

LMWF at 10 µg/mL, but not high molecular weight fucoidan (HMWF) (600 kDa) increased HUVEC migration through fibronectin-coated 8 µm-porous membranes by 36% ± 8% (Figure 1A and data not shown). Confocal microscopy confirmed that LMWF induced the formation of lamellipodia and ruffles, which characterize a migration phenotype and reorganized actin cytoskeleton (Figure 1B). Using a 2D-angiogenesis assay, we demonstrated that LMWF induced the formation of capillary tubes in Matrigel by increasing their length by 4 fold and their area up to 84% ± 8%, as compared to untreated (UT) control cells (Figure 1C).

2.2. LMWF and Level of Glycosaminoglycan Chains Expressed in HUVECs

We first investigated whether LMWF could modify the GAG chain level expressed by HUVECs. For that purpose, the level of total GAGs, HS chains, and chondroitin sulfate (CS) chains were determined by DMMB assays in the lysate of endothelial cells after 24 h of 10 µg/mL LMWF treatment and compared to UT control cells. There was no significant difference in the level of GAGs, HS, and CS after LMWF incubation (Figure S1). Following LMWF treatment, the amount of total GAGs in the conditioned medium of LMWF-treated cells decreased by 28% ± 8% at 24 h, as compared to untreated control cells ($p < 0.05$, $n = 3$, Figure 2A). Further analysis revealed that HS amounts decreased by 25% ± 5% in the conditioned medium of the LMWF-treated cells, whereas there was no variation of CS chain amount (Figure 2A). These data suggests that LMWF may modify the HS and HSPG turnover (HS synthesis or cleavage and HSPG shedding).

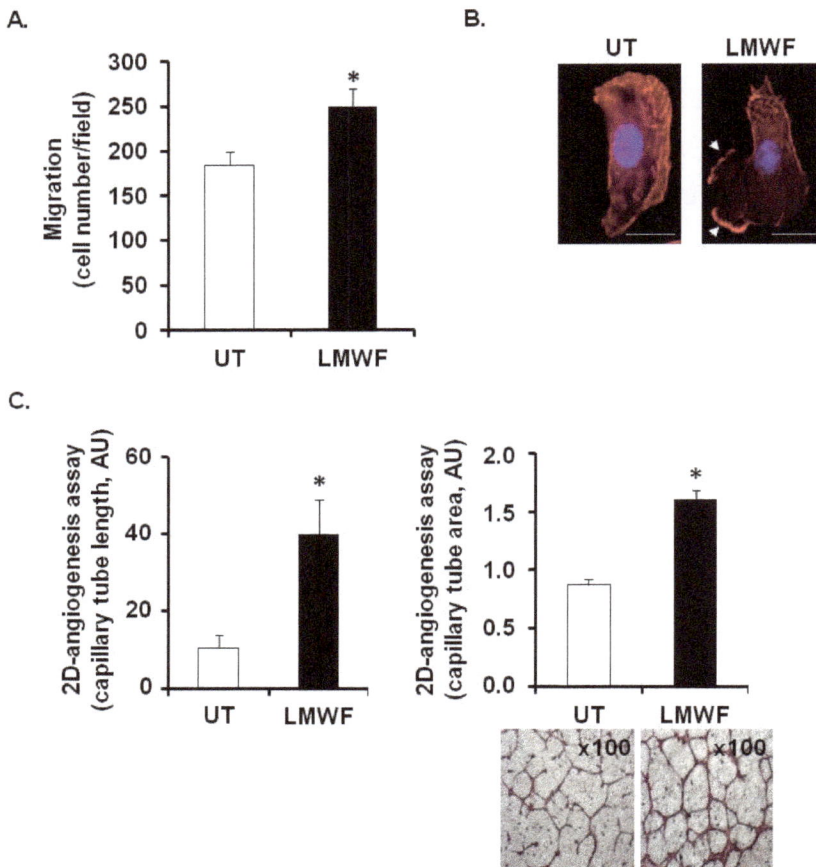

Figure 1. Effects of Low molecular weight fucoidan (LMWF) on endothelial cell abilities: migration and 2D-angiogenesis. Human vascular endothelial cells (HUVEC) were incubated with 10 µg/mL LMWF for 24 h and the migration (**A**), the lamellipodia formation (**B**) and the capillary tube formation (length and area) (**C**) were determined. (**A**) Migration chamber assay. HUVECs incubated with or without 10 µg/mL LMWF, were allowed to migrate through the porous fibronectin-coated membrane. They were stained with Mayer's hemalum and counted. The results are expressed as cell number per field; (**B**) Lamellipodia formation. LMWF induced the formation of lamellipodia and ruffles (white arrows indicate lamellipodia/ruffle formation, DAPI-nucleus (blue), Phalloidin-F-actin (red)). Bar = 10 µm; (**C**) Capillary tube formation (2D-angiogenesis assay) on Matrigel. Left and right panels show the length (**left**) and area (**right**) of endothelial capillaries formed by HUVECs treated with or without 10 µg/mL LMWF. Lower right panel shows a representative image of capillary network, as photographed with phase contrast microscopy (magnification ×100). * $p < 0.05$ *versus* control untreated (UT) cells. A.U.: arbitrary unit.

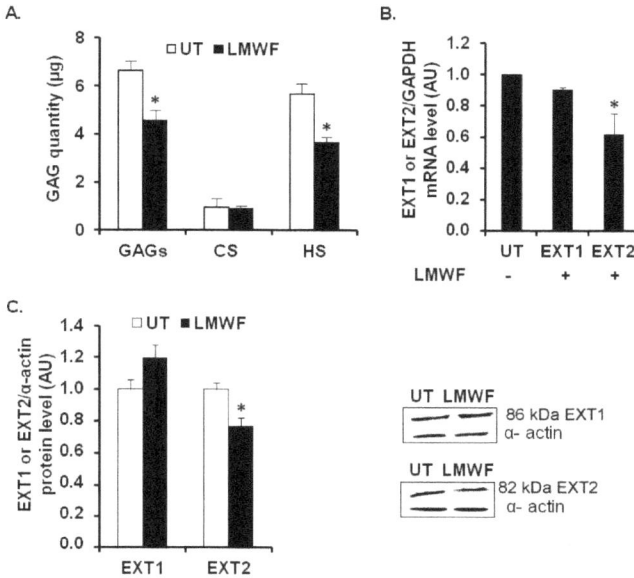

Figure 2. LMWF and glycosaminoglycan chain level in HUVECs. (**A**) Glycosaminoglycan quantification. HUVECs were incubated with 10 μg/mL LMWF for 24 h and the amount of total GAGs, CS and HS chains were determined in the supernatant according to a dimethyl-methylene blue (DMMB) assay; (**B**) Exostosin-1 and -2 (EXT1 or EXT2) mRNA levels were determined by real-time RT-PCR in cells treated with or without 10 μg/mL LMWF. (**C**) EXT1 or EXT2 protein levels were determined by western blot in cells treated with or without 10 μg/mL LMWF. Right panel shows a representative image of the western blot assay. * $p < 0.05$ *versus* control untreated (UT) cells. A.U.: arbitrary unit.

2.3. LMWF and Heparan Sulfate Biosynthesis and Degradation Enzymes in HUVECs

We have first studied the effects of LMWF on enzymes involved in HS biosynthesis (EXT1, EXT2) or degradation (heparanase). These glycosyltransferases EXT1 and EXT2 are responsible for the elongation of HS by catalyzing the addition of alternating β-D-glucuronate (GlcA) and α-D-N-acetylglucosamine (GlcNAc) units to the tetrasaccharide linker of GAGs. We assessed the glycosaminoglycan polymerization (*EXT1* and *EXT2*) mRNA levels by quantitative RT-PCR. The mRNA expression level of *EXT2* in LMWF-treated cells was decreased by 36% ± 13%, as compared to untreated cells at 24 h ($p < 0.05$), whereas the level of mRNA encoding for *EXT1* was unaffected (Figure 2B). The EXT1 and EXT2 protein levels were measured by western blot analysis in HUVEC lysates. A slightly decreased EXT2 level by 23% ± 5% was observed in the LMWF-treated cells ($p < 0.05$). No significant difference was observed for EXT1 (Figure 2C).

The HS-degrading enzyme heparanase (HPSE) is an endo-β-D-glucuronidase, which plays an important role in remodeling of the basement membrane and extracellular matrix during process of inflammation [13–15]. HPSE is synthesized as an inactive 65 kDa pro-form enzyme (pro-HPSE), can be transformed into active heterodimer consisting of 50 and 8 kDa subunits (active HPSE), and cleaves HS chains attached to proteoglycans, such as syndecans and perlecan [15,16]. *HPSE* mRNA expression, as assessed by quantitative RT-PCR, was increased by 2.4 fold in LMWF-treated cells, as compared to untreated control cells (Figure 3A). Active HPSE form (50 kDa) expression, as assessed by western blot, was significantly increased up to 2 fold in the supernatant or by 20% ± 5% in the lysate of the LMWF-treated cells (Figure 4B). HPSE activity was slightly but significantly increased up to 20% ± 3% in the lysate of LMWF-treated cells (Figure 3C), whereas it was not detected in the respective conditioned medium.

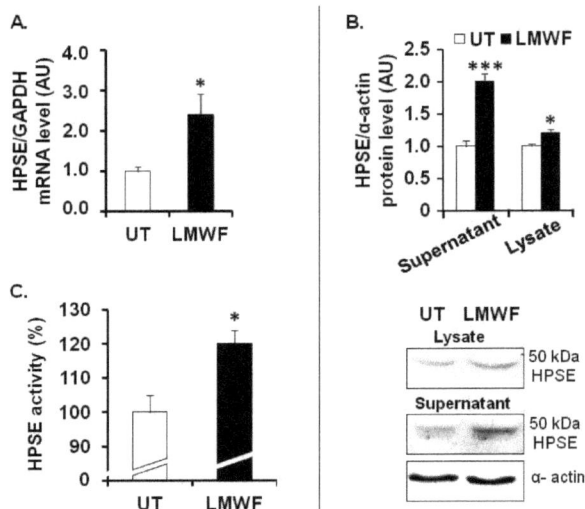

Figure 3. LMWF and heparanase in HUVECs. (**A**) *HPSE* mRNA levels were determined by real-time RT-PCR in cells treated with or without 10 µg/mL LMWF; (**B**) HPSE protein levels were determined by western blot in the supernatant or in the lysate of cells treated with or without 10 µg/mL LMWF. Lower panel shows a representative image of the western blot assay. (**C**) Heparanase activity was checked in the lysate of LMWF-treated cells. HPSE activity in untreated cells was arbitrary set to 100%. * $p < 0.05$, *** $p < 0.0005$, LMWF-treated cells *versus* LMWF-untreated cells (UT). A.U.: arbitrary unit.

2.4. Effects of LMWF on the Syndecan Expression

We therefore focused on the effect of LMWF on the expression of the heparan sulfate transmembrane proteoglycans belonging to the syndecan family, SDC-1 and SDC-4.

In HUVECs, we demonstrated that LMWF increased the level of mRNA encoding for SDC-1 by 48% ± 12% ($p < 0.005$), whereas it decreased that of SDC-4 by 38% ± 9% ($p < 0.05$) (Figure 4A). We then analyzed SDC-1 and SDC-4 levels by western blot. The SDCs contains the core protein (ectodomain, transmembrane, and cytoplasmic domains) and the GAG, which are attached in the ectodomain part of SDCs. As shown previously, it is well known that the western blot expression pattern is heterogeneous (many bands from 20 kDa to 250 kDa) and show many forms of SDC-1 and SDC-4 in the cell lysate [17]. Our results of SDC protein expression showed the presence of 3 different forms for SDC-1 and SDC-4 (Figure 4B,C). Upon LMWF treatment, protein level was significantly increased by 22% ± 2% (33 kDa), 13% ± 5% (75 kDa) and 18% ± 4% (250 kDa) for SDC-1 or decreased by 28% ± 5% (22 kDa), 41% ± 9% (75 kDa), and 48% ± 5% (150 kDa) for SDC-4, respectively (Figure 4B,C). As assessed by dot blot, the shedded ectodomain level of SDC-1 in the supernatant of LMWF-treated cells was increased by 2 fold, as compared to untreated control cells, whereas that of SDC-4 was decreased by 35% ± 8% ($p < 0.05$) (Figure 4D).

Taken together, LMWF modulate SDC-1 and SDC-4 gene expression and ectodomain shedding in HUVEC *in vitro* culture.

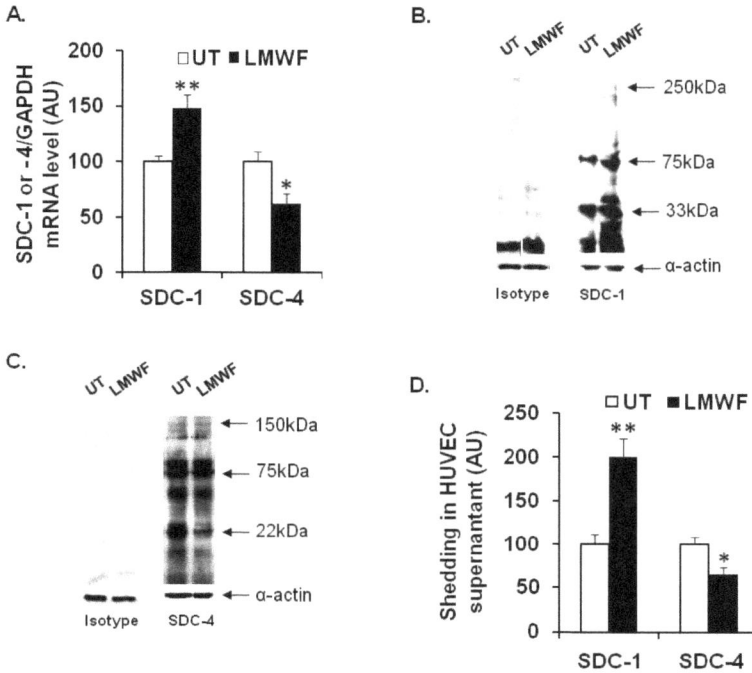

Figure 4. Effects of LMWF on the SDC expression in HUVECs. *SDC-1* and *SDC-4* mRNA or protein levels in endothelial cells treated or not with 10 µg/mL LMWF were analyzed respectively by real time RT-PCR (**A**) or western blot (**B,C**). SDC-1 and SDC-4 ectodomains in the supernatant of cells treated with or without 10 µg/mL LMWF were analyzed by dot blot (**D**). $* p < 0.05$, $** p < 0.005$, significantly different to LMWF-untreated cells (UT). A.U.: arbitrary unit.

In vivo, the influence of LMWF on SDCs expression was assessed in a Sprague Dawley Rat model of intimal hyperplasia. We have already used this model to show the pro-angiogenic effect of LMWF treatment [10]. In addition, SDC-1 and SDC-4 have been shown to play an important role in the pathological response of a balloon-injured wall artery [18]. Briefly, rats were subjected to balloon injury into the thoracic artery to create local destruction of endothelial layer leading to inflammation and intimal hyperplasia development. Two weeks after LMWF-intramuscular injection the level of SDC-1 and SDC-4 in the balloon-injured artery was analyzed.

Our results demonstrated that the expression of SDC-1 and SDC-4 was very low in healthy arteries in the media (M) and adventitia (A) layers, whereas it increased in the neointima (N), media and adventitia layers in balloon-injured, and NaCl-treated arteries (vehicle), leading to development of intimal hyperplasia (Figure 5A–E). The LMWF treatment of injured artery increased SDC-1 expression in the neointima and in the adventitia layers, as compared to vehicle (Figure 5C). Furthermore, upon LMWF treatment, the SDC-4 expression was decreased in the neointima and media, but largely increased in the adventitia layer, as compared to vehicle (Figure 5F). These *in vivo* results were in concordance with our previously described observation obtained in the HUVECs *in vitro* culture [10].

All these results suggest that LMWF has an important influence on the proteoglycan distribution in the endothelial cells and can increase SDC-1 and decrease SDC-4 expression *in vitro* and *in vivo*.

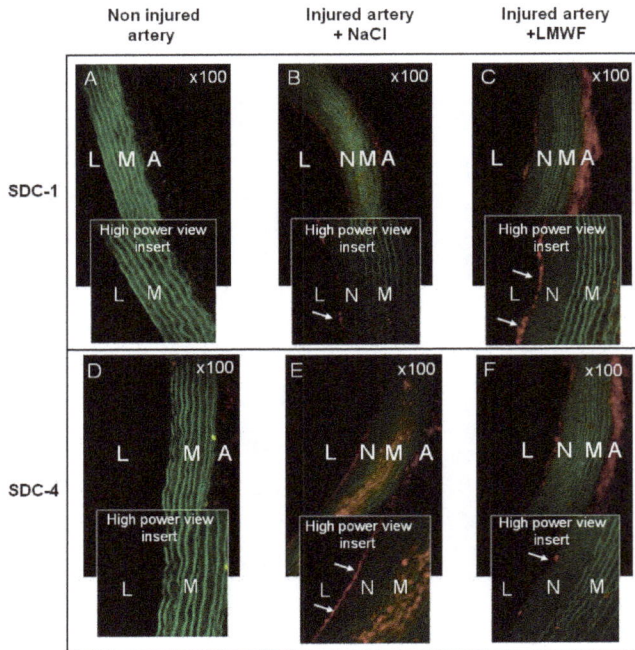

Figure 5. Effects of LMWF on the SDC distribution in rat balloon injured artery. SDC-1 and SDC-4 expressions were assessed using immunohistochemistry in rat model of intimal hyperplasia. (**A**) SDC-1 or (**D**) SDC-4 expressions in non injured arteries; (**B**) SDC-1 or (**E**) SDC-4 expressions in injured arteries treated with NaCl; (**C**) SDC-1 or (**F**) SDC-4 expressions in injured arteries treated with LMWF. White arrows indicate SDC expressions in the neointima layer in high power view inserts (red). Green: autofluorescence of the elastic fibers of the lamina. Magnification ×100, L: lumen, N: neointima, M: media, A: adventitia.

2.5. Assessment of EXT-, HPSE- or SDC Involvement in Biological Effects of LMWF

To assess the potential role of EXT1/EXT2, HPSE or SDC-1/SDC-4 in the biological effects induced by LMWF, specific siRNAs were carried out.

Quantitative RT-PCR showed that the expression of the mRNAs and proteins of EXT2 in *EXT2*-siRNA- and EXT1 in *EXT1*-siRNA-transfected cells was reduced up to 72% ± 16% and 71% ± 15%, respectively, as compared to the *SNC*-siRNA-transfected control cells (Figure 6A). The flow cytometry assay showed that the binding of 10E4 anti-HS antibodies to *EXT2*-siRNA- or *EXT1*-siRNA-transfected cells was respectively reduced by 75% ± 8% or by 80% ± 9%, as compared to *SNC*-siRNA-transfected control cells (Figure 6B).

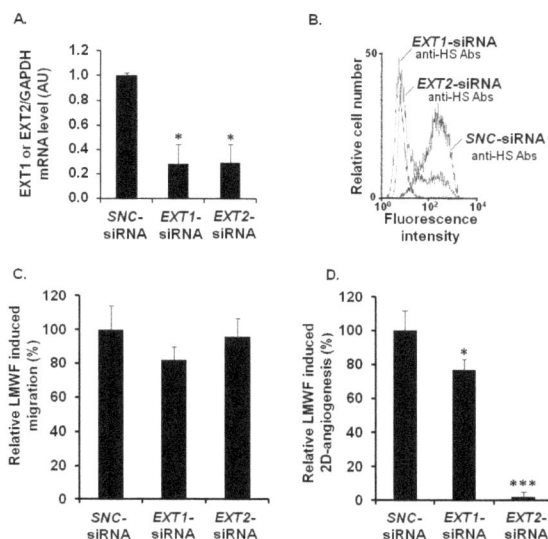

Figure 6. Assessment of EXT involvement in biological effects of LMWF in HUVECs. HUVECs were transfected with *EXT1*-siRNA or *EXT2*-siRNA or with *SNC*-siRNA control. (**A**) *EXT1* or *EXT2* mRNA levels were determined in *EXT1*-siRNA- or *EXT2*-siRNA- or *SNC*-siRNA-transfected control cell by real-time RT PCR. *EXT1*- or *EXT2* mRNA level normalized to *GAPDH* mRNA level in *SNC*-siRNA-transfected control cells was arbitrarily set to 1; (**B**) The binding of 10E4 anti-HS antibodies to *EXT2*- or *EXT1*-siRNA transfected cells was compared to that of *SNC*-siRNA-transfected cells; (**C**) Migration was assayed in cells treated with or without 10 μg/mL LMWF; (**D**) 2D-angiogenesis was assayed in cells treated with or without 10 μg/mL LMWF. The difference in the capillary network length between LMWF-treated and untreated cells in each RNA interference condition (*EXT1 or EXT2* silencing) was compared to that in *SNC*-siRNA-transfected cells. Control LMWF induction was arbitrary set at 100% for *SNC*-siRNA-transfected cells. * $p < 0.05$, *** $p < 0.0005$ *versus* *SNC*-siRNA-transfected control cells. A.U.: arbitrary unit.

There were no significant difference in cell migration after LMWF treatment in *EXT1*-siRNA- or *EXT2*-siRNA-transfected cells, as compared to *SNC*-siRNA-transfected cells (Figure 6C). In contrast, the LMWF induction of 2D-angiogenesis was abolished in LMWF-treated *EXT2*-siRNA-transfected cells by 98% ± 5%, or decreased in LMWF-treated *EXT1*-siRNA-transfected cells by 33% ± 5% ($p < 0.05$), as compared to *SNC*-siRNA-transfected control cells (Figure 6D). These latter data suggest that EXT2 and, to a lesser extent EXT1, affect the pro-angiogenic effect of LMWF.

HPSE-siRNA-transfected cells were used for 2D-angiogenesis or migration assays. Quantitative RT-PCR showed that the expression of the mRNAs encoding for heparanase in *HPSE*-siRNA-transfected cells was reduced up to 74% ± 8%, as compared to the *SNC*-siRNA-transfected control cells (Figure 7A). Under basal conditions (in the absence of LMWF), *HPSE*-siRNA transfection decreased endothelial cell migration by 37% ± 5% ($p < 0.05$), but had no effect on 2D-angiogenesis (Figure S2A,B). However, upon LMWF stimulation and *HPSE*-siRNA transfection, the ability of HUVECs to form capillary network in Matrigel 2D-angiogenesis assay was altered. The capillary network length induced by LMWF treatment was largely decreased by 51% ± 11% in *HPSE*-siRNA-transfected cells, as compared to *SNC*-siRNA-transfected control cells (Figure 7B). In contrast, the cell migration induced by LMWF was significantly increased by 56% ± 9% ($p < 0.05$) in *HPSE*-siRNA-transfected, as compared to *SNC*-siRNA-transfected cells (Figure 7C).

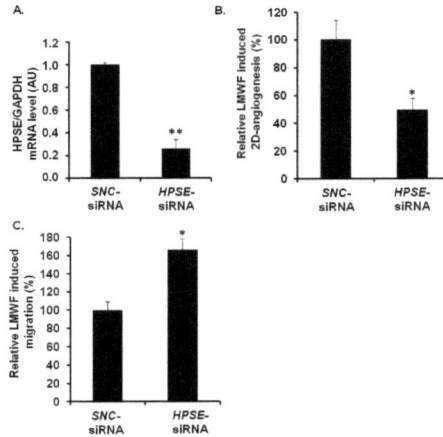

Figure 7. Assessment of HPSE involvement in biological effects of LMWF in HUVECs. HUVECs were transfected with *HPSE*-siRNA or *SNC*-siRNA control. (**A**) *HPSE* mRNA levels were determined in *HPSE*-siRNA- or *SNC*-siRNA-transfected cells by real-time RT-PCR. *HPSE* mRNA level normalized to *GAPDH* mRNA level in *SNC*-siRNA-transfected control cells was arbitrary set to 1; (**B**) 2D-angiogenesis was assayed in cells treated with or without 10 µg/mL LMWF. The difference in the capillary network length between LMWF-treated and untreated cells in *HPSE* RNA interference condition was compared to that in *SNC*-siRNA-transfected cells; (**C**) Migration was assayed in cells treated with or without 10 µg/mL LMWF. Control LMWF induction was arbitrary set at 100% for *SNC*-siRNA-transfected cells. * $p < 0.05$, ** $p < 0.005$ *versus* *SNC*-siRNA-transfected control cells. A.U.: arbitrary unit.

LMWF biological effects have been checked in *SDC-1*-siRNA- or *SDC-4*-siRNA-transfected cells or in cells treated with specific anti-SDC-1 or anti-SDC-4 antibodies. As described [19,20], quantitative RT-PCR showed that the expression of the mRNAs encoding for SDC-1 in *SDC1*-siRNA- or SDC-4 in *SDC4*-siRNA-transfected cells was reduced up to 69% ± 14% and 73% ± 17% respectively, as compared to *SNC*- siRNA-transfected control cells.

Under basal conditions, the 2D-angiogenenis assays showed a significant decrease in cell capillary network length by 23% ± 4% in *SDC-1*- and by 54% ± 7% in *SDC-4*-siRNA-transfected cells, as compared to *SNC*-siRNA-transfected control cells (Figure S3A). Upon LMWF cell treatment, the LMWF-induction of 2D-angiogenenis was unchanged in *SDC-1*-siRNA-transfected cells, whereas it was significantly increased in *SDC-4*-siRNA-transfected cells by 62% ± 5% ($p < 0.005$), as compared to *SNC*-siRNA-transfected control cells (Figure 8A).

Under basal conditions, endothelial cell migration assayed in modified Boyden chambers was decreased by 43% ± 5% and by 40% ± 8% in *SDC-1*-siRNA-transfected and anti-SDC-1 antibody-incubated cells, respectively (Figure S3B). LMWF induction of endothelial cell migration was decreased in *SDC-1*-siRNA-transfected cells by 20% ± 5% and in anti-SDC-1 antibody-incubated cells by 47% ± 3%, as compared to respective control cells (Figure 8B). These data were confirmed by a wound healing assay (Figure S3C). Regarding RNA silencing experiments, these data suggest that SDC-1 does not play a crucial role in LMWF-induced effects.

Basal endothelial cell migration was decreased by 68% ± 5% and by 67% ± 9% in *SDC-4*-siRNA-transfected and anti-SDC-4 antibody-incubated cells, respectively (Figure S3B). However, LMWF-induction of endothelial cell migration was largely increased by 87% ± 5% in *SDC-4*-siRNA-transfected cells or by 2 fold in anti-SDC-4-antibody incubated cells, as compared to respective control cells (Figure 8B). These data were confirmed by a wound healing assay (Figure S3C). These results demonstrated that SDC-4 expression limits the LMWF effect on the cells.

Altogether, we have demonstrated that on the one hand EXT2 (and EXT1 to a lesser extent) and HPSE expression, and on the other hand SDC-4, play critical roles in LMWF pro-angiogenic effects. We have then addressed the question whether silencing of endothelial HPSE or EXT2 could affect SDC-4 level. In *HPSE-* or *EXT2*-siRNA-transfected cells, *SDC-4* mRNA level was up-regulated respectively by 64% ± 19% or 35% ± 10%, as compared to *SNC*-siRNA-transfected control cells (Figure 8C). In addition, there was no effect on *SDC-1* mRNA level in *HPSE-* or *EXT2* silenced cells (Figure 8C).

2.6. Discussion

Fucoidan exhibits various biological effects, among them anti-inflammatory, low anti-coagulant and anti-thrombotic activities. We have previously shown the therapeutic potential of low molecular weight fucoidan (LMWF) in reduction of in-stent restenosis in a rabbit model, vascular tissue repair [21], and in critical hind limb ischemia in a rat model [7].

In this study, we hypothesized that LMWF could modify the amount and the distribution of heparan sulfate chains expressed in endothelial cells and of syndecan-1 (SDC-1) and syndecan-4 (SDC-4), two major heparan sulfate (HS) membrane proteoglycans.

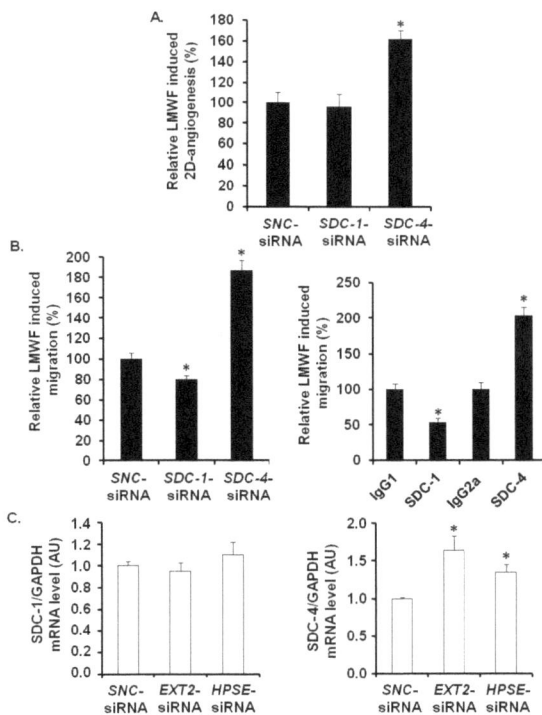

Figure 8. Assessment of SDC involvement in biological effects of LMWF in HUVECs. 2D-angiogenesis (**A**) and migration (**B**) assays were performed in *SDC-1*-siRNA- or *SDC-4*-siRNA- or *SNC*-siRNA-transfected control cells (**B, left panel**), or in cells treated with specific anti-SDC-1 or anti-SDC-4 antibodies (**B, right panel**). Control LMWF induction was arbitrary set at 100% for *SNC*-siRNA-transfected cells or isotypes. (**C**) *SDC-1* and *SDC-4* mRNA expression was analyzed in *EXT2*- or *HPSE*-siRNA-transfected cells. * $p < 0.05$ *versus* *SNC*-siRNA-transfected control cells or isotypes. A.U.: arbitrary unit.

Our results could be summarized as follows: 1/LMWF increased endothelial cell migration and vascular tube formation; 2/LMWF modified HS- and SDC metabolism (increased heparanase (HPSE) level and activity, change in SDC-1/-4 expression and shedding); 3/EXT2, HPSE and SDC-4 are involved in LMWF cellular effects since silencing *EXT2*, *HPSE*, or *SDC-4* affect LMWF-induced angiogenesis; 4/Our data also evidenced a link between EXT2, HPSE, and SDC-4 level since silencing *EXT2* or *HPSE* led to increased translational expression of SDC-4.

Fucoidan as a heparin-like molecule can physically interact with several heparin-binding growth factors and chemokines. Fucoidan may promote or inhibit growth factor effects by trapping endogenously-released growth factors, or by displacing its ligands from their storage sites, increasing their bioavailability. Thus, LMWF has been shown to release the glycosaminoglycan-bound stromal cell-derived factor-1 (SDF-1)/CXCL12, which mobilizes progenitor cells [22]. (SDF-1)/CXCL12 may participate in angiogenesis together with vascular endothelial growth factor (VEGF) and fibroblast growth factor (FGF) [23]. In this context, one could suppose that the modification in HS chain synthesis or degradation would affect LMWF activities. For example, it has been demonstrated that the overall size of HS chains, as well as the specific features of HS chains, including the sulfated patterns, can affect FGF signaling activation [24]. Our data suggest that LMWF effects depend on HS, since LMWF-mediated angiogenesis is decreased either in *EXT2* (involved in HS biosynthesis) or *HPSE* (involved in HS degradation) silencing conditions. Furthermore, our data also demonstrated that LMWF increased HPSE expression and activity, and does not really affect EXT1 and EXT2 expression in endothelial cells. It is of note that LMWF treatment only slightly affects the HS level in our *in vitro* condition of HUVEC culture. This could be related to the law sensitivity of the dimethyl-methylene blue (DMMB) assay.

Interestingly, the inverse relations among HS, EXT1, and HPSE expressions are observed in cancer cell models. Cancer cells with higher EXT1 expression exhibited lower HPSE expression, whereas cancer cells with lower EXT1 expression exhibited higher HPSE expression [25]. In addition, the *EXT1* knockdown with siRNA led to up-regulation of HPSE expression and potentiation of metastatic capacity [25]. Similarly, Huegel *et al.* recently demonstrated that interfering with HS function, both with the chemical antagonist Surfen or treatment with bacterial heparitinase, up-regulated endogenous HPSE gene expression, suggesting a feedback mechanism that would result in further HS reduction and increased signaling [26]. With our data, it suggests that a coordinated regulation of key features of HS expression (EXT enzymes and HPSE) does exist even no mechanism has been brought out yet.

Our results also highlight a more important role of EXT2 than EXT1 in LMWF-inducted angiogenesis. This could be related to the fact that these enzymes can act differently on HS biosynthesis as demonstrated by Busse *et al.* [27].

Besides, HPSE overexpression has already been involved in *in vivo* angiogenesis in mice models. Homozygous transgenic mice that overexpress HPSE demonstrate both a deep reduction in the size of HS chains, as well as enhanced neovascularization of mammary ducts [28], some conclusions that seem consonant with our observations. The overexpression of HPSE by tumors may activate tumor angiogenesis through various mechanisms in addition to promoting the release of growth factor-decorated HS fragments. HPSE has been demonstrated to be a mediator of angiogenesis by different mechanisms [29]. HPSE promotes: 1/endothelial cell migration and degradation of the subendothelial basal lamina; 2/release of active HS-bound FGF and VEGF; 3/release of HS degradation fragments that promote FGF receptor binding, dimerization and signaling. In addition, HPSE has been demonstrated to be related to changes in the distribution of SDC-1, in particular by acting on SDC-1 ectodomain shedding [30]. We have investigated effects of LMWF on SDC-1 and SDC-4. Both heparan sulfate proteoglycans are involved in cell migration through cell cytoskeletal rearrangement, spreading, and 2D-angiogenesis. We have demonstrated that LMWF increases endothelial cell SDC-1 expression and shedding, and has an opposite effect on the same SDC-4 features. In rat injured thoracic aorta, our recent *in vivo* results demonstrate that LMWF treatment increased SDC-1 expression in the neointima layer of the injured artery, but decreased the SDC-4 expression in the neointima and media layers, therefore strengthening the *in vitro* data [10]. *SDC-4*, but not *SDC-1* silencing in HUVECs increases the LMWF-induced angiogenesis and cell migration, suggesting that SDC-4 expression partially counteracts LMWF effects.

Furthermore, our data also evidenced an unknown link between EXT2, HPSE, and SDC-4 level since silencing *EXT2* or *HPSE* led to increased translational expression of SDC-4. In these conditions, SDC-1 expression remains unchanged. These data suggested that the amount of HS present on SDC-4 core proteins could regulate the rate of SDC-4 core protein synthesis. Similarly, Ramani *et al.* recently demonstrated that HS-chains of SDC-1 regulate ectodomain shedding accompanied by a very high increase in core protein synthesis [31].

Altogether, we hypothesize that LMWF affects SDCs shedding and expression by acting through both enzymes HPSE and matrix metalloproteinase-2 [10], leading to change in the binding and the signaling and/or the bioavailability of heparin-binding proteins in the process of angiogenesis.

3. Experimental Section

3.1. Cell Culture

Human umbilical vein endothelial cells (HUVEC, N°CRL-1730, ATCC) were cultured in Endothelial Cell Basal Media 2 (PromoCell, Heidelberg, Germany) supplemented with 10% of fetal calf serum (Lonza, Levallois-Perret, France), and a mix from PromoCell containing EGF (5.0 ng/mL), Hydrocortisone (0.2 µg/mL), VEGF (0.5 ng/mL), bFGF (10 ng/mL), R3 IGF-1 (20 ng/mL), Ascorbic Acid (1 µg/mL), Heparin (22.5 µg/mL), 1% Penicillin Streptomycin (PAA Laboratories, Pasching, Austria). Cells were divided two times per week at a sub cultivation ratio of 1:3.

3.2. Low Molecular Weight Fucoidan

Low molecular weight fucoidan (LMWF) was isolated and hydrolyzed by a radical depolymerization process [32] from high molecular weight (HMW) extracts from *Fucus vesiculosus*, a brown seaweed (Kraeber & Co GmbH, Ellerbek, Germany). The characteristics of LMWF according to previously reported analytical methods [33] are: weight average molecular mass 8 ± 1 kDa; fucose content 35% (wt/wt); uronic acid content 3% (wt/wt); and sulfate content 34% (wt/wt). The structural model of fucoidan prepared from *Fucus vesiculosus* was determined previously by others [34,35].

3.3. Glycosaminoglycan Extraction

Frozen supernatant from HUVEC cell culture were freeze-dried and suspended in the extraction buffer (50 mM Tris pH 7.9, 10 mM NaCl, 2 mM $MgCl_2$ and 1% of Triton X-100). Samples were digested by proteinase K (PK) (50 µg/mL final sample concentration; Merck, Molsheim, France) at 56 °C for 24 h. After PK inactivation (90 °C, 30 min), samples were treated by DNase (10 U/mL final sample concentration; Qiagen, Courtaboeuf, France) at 37 °C, overnight. Then, samples were centrifuged ($13,000 \times g$, 10 min) through a 0.22 µm filter unit (Pall, Saint-Germain-en-Laye, France). NaCl was added to a final concentration of 4 M and the filtered samples were vigorously agitated for 30 min. Proteins were precipitated with TCA (10% final sample concentration; Sigma-Aldrich, Saint-Quentin Fallavier, France) at 4 °C. Pellets were discarded and supernatants were cleared by chloroform washing. Finally, aqueous phases were immediately dialysis (Spectrum, 3500 MWCO) against buffer (50 mM Tris pH 7.5, 50 mM CH_3COONa, 2 mM $CaCl_2$) and then pure water before freeze-drying. Identities of the extracted GAGs were analyzed by specific digestion with chondroitinase ABC (Sigma-Aldrich, Saint-Quentin Fallavier, France), or by nitrous acid treatment as previously described [36].

3.4. Glycosaminoglycan Quantification

Sulfated GAGs were quantified according to the 1–9 dimethyl-methylene blue (DMMB) assay as previously described [35]. Briefly, an aliquot of each sample was pipetted and completed up to 100 µL with pure water, 1 mL of DMMB solution was added and then vigorously agitated. Then samples were centrifuged (13,000× *g*, 10 min) to sediment the GAG/DMMB complex and supernatants were discarded. The pellet was then dissolved in 250 μL of the decomplexating solution by shaking and the absorbance of the resulting solution was measured at 656 nm. A calibration curve constructed with known amounts of chondroitin sulfate (CS) A or HS standard was included in each assay.

3.5. Flow Cytometry Analysis

To identify the level of heparan sulfate on HUVEC cell surface, cells were preincubated for 1 h at 4 °C with anti-HS Abs (10 μg/mL, Clone 10E4; Seikagaku COGER, Paris, France) or with isotypes. After washing, cells were labeled for 30 min at 4 °C with anti-mouse Ig-FITC (1:50; Becton Dickinson, Le Pont de-Claix, France). Cells were fixed in 1% paraformaldehyde (PFA) and analyzed with a FACScan (Becton Dickinson, Le Pont de-Claix, France).

3.6. Real-Time RT-PCR

Real-time RT-PCR were performed using an Applied Step-One device with EXT1 (Hs00609162_m1), EXT2 (Hs00925442_m1), SDC-1 (Hs Hs00896423_m1), SDC-4 (Hs Hs01120909_m1) and Heparanase (Hs00180737_m1) TaqMan Inventoried Assay and TaqMan Gene Expression Master Mix kit (Life Technlologies, Saint Aubin, France). The mRNA levels were normalized with *GAPDH* housekeeping gene levels as described in the manufacturer's instructions (Hs02758991_g1, TaqMan Inventoried Assay; Life Technologies, Saint Aubin, France).

3.7. RNA Interference

EXT1 and *EXT2* gene-specific sense and antisense 21-nt single stranded RNAs with symmetric 2 nt 3′(2′-deoxy) thymidine overhangs validated by Life Technologies (s4891 and s4894, Silencer Select siRNA, Life Thecnologies, Saint Aubin, France). *EXT1*, *EXT2*, *SDC-1*, *SDC-4*, *Heparanase* (*HPSE*) and scramble *SNC* silencing were carried out as previously described [18,19]. HUVEC cells were transfected with 50 nM siRNA in serum-free medium using INTERFERIN transfectant reagent (Polyplus, Ozyme, Saint Quentin en Yvelines, France) following the manufacturer's instructions. In each experiment, a negative siRNA control *SNC* (Eurogentec, Angers, France) was used as a negative control. Cells transfected with specific siRNA or *SNC*-siRNA were used 48 h post transfection for RNA analysis.

3.8. Migration

Cell migration was measured from 6×10^4 HUVECs with Bio-coat cell migration chambers (Becton-Dickinson, Le Pont de Claix, France) [37]. Briefly, inserts of Bio-coat cell migration chamber were coated with fibronectin (100 μg/mL; Beckton Dickinson, Le Pont de-Claix, France). 6×10^4 HUVECs treated with *SDC-1-*, *SDC-4-*, *EXT1-*, *EXT2-*siRNA or *SNC*-siRNA for 48 h were resuspended in basal media supplemented or not with 10 μg/mL LMWF. Cells were added in the upper chamber and complete media was added in the lower chamber. After 24 h, cells migrated through the porous membrane were stained with Mayer's hemalum (Sigma-Aldrich, Saint-Quentin Fallavier, France) and counted manually by two different observers who performed the blind data acquisition. The cell migration rate was $[(D1 - D2)/D1] \times 100$; D1 was the difference between the number of migrated *SNC*-siRNA-transfected cells stimulated by LMWF and that of unstimulated migrated *SNC*-siRNA-transfected cells; D2 was the difference between the number of migrated specific siRNA-transfected cells stimulated with LMWF and that of unstimulated specific siRNA-transfected cells. Alternatively, 6×10^4 cells were pre-incubated or not for 2 h with the following antibodies: anti-SDC-1 (Clone DL101, IgG1; Santa Cruz Biotechnology, Heidelberg, Germany), anti-SDC-4 (Clone 5G9, IgG2a; Santa Cruz, Heidelberg, Germany) or their isotype (Becton–Dickinson, Le Pont de-Claix, France) at 5 μg/mL. The cell migration rate was $[(D3 - D4)/D3] \times 100$; D3 was the difference between the number of migrated isotype-preincubated cells stimulated with LMWF and that of migrated unstimulated isotype-preincubated cells. D4 was the difference between the number of migrated antibodies-preincubated cells stimulated with LMWF and that of migrated unstimulated antibodies-preincubated cells.

3.9. Immunocytochemistry

HUVECs were harvested and put into the labtek chamber (10×10^4 per well), than incubated with 10 µg/mL of LMWF for 2 h and lead to spread. Then the cells were permeabilized in 0.05% Triton X-100 (Sigma-Aldrich), stained with Alexa Fluor 546 phalloidin (F-actin, dilution 1/100; Life Technlologies, Saint Aubin, France) and lamellipodia formation were observed with a confocal microscopy (LSM 510; Carl Zeiss, Marly le Roi, France).

3.10. In Vitro Angiogenesis Assay

2D-angiogenesis assay (capillary tube formation in Matrigel) was performed with 9×10^4 cells/well seeded on Matrigel-coated 24-well plate (Beckton Dickinson, Le Pont de-Claix, France) and treated for 24 h with 10 µg/mL LMWF. Endothelial cells were pre-treated with *EXT1-*, *EXT2*-siRNA or *SNC*-siRNA (control) 48 h before. The capillary tubes were fixed with 4% PFA and stained with 1% Hematoxylin (Sigma-Aldrich, Saint-Quentin Fallavier, France) and photographed in phase contrast microscopy (CK40; Olympus, Rungis, France) after 24 h. The average length of vascular capillary tubes was evaluated using the open source ImageJ Software (Open Source, ImageJ ver 1.47r, National Institutes of Health, Bethesda, MD, USA).

3.11. Western Blot

HUVECs were incubated with 10 µg/mL of LMWF for 24 h and assayed for western blot as previously described [38]. The supernatant was collected and cell lysate protein concentration was determined by bicinchoninic acid (BCA) assay (Pierce Biotechnology, Rockford, IL, USA). Total protein was probed using anti-SDC-1 and anti-SDC-4 (respectively: mouse monoclonal IgG1, clone DL101 and rabbit polyclonal IgG, H-140, for both dilution 1/500; Santa Cruz Biotechnology, Heidelberg, Germany), anti-EXT1 and anti-EXT2 (respectively: rabbit polyclonal IgG, H-114 and goat polyclonal IgG, C-17, for both dilution 1/500; Santa Cruz Biotechnology, Heidelberg, Germany), anti-HPSE (rabbit polyclonal IgG, H-80, 1/500; Santa Cruz Biotechnology, Heidelberg, Germany), or using their isotypes (all at 1/200) and revealed with horseradish peroxidase (HRP) conjugated anti-mouse, anti-rabbit, or anti-goat IgG (dilution 1/2500; Jackson ImmunoResearch, Suffolk, UK). For comparison α- actin (rabbit polyclonal IgG, I-19-R, dilution 1/500; Santa Cruz Biotechnology, Heidelberg, Germany) was used as relevant standard house-keeping protein and revealed with horseradish peroxidase (HRP) conjugated anti-rabbit IgG (dilution 1/2500; Jackson ImmunoResearch, Suffolk, UK). Proteins were detected using Enhanced chemiluminescence detection reagents (GE Healthcare, Orsay, France). The statistical analysis was done after the protein bands quantification by Scion Image Software (Scion Corporation, Frederick, MD, USA).

3.12. Heparanase Activity Assay

HUVEC cell lysate or supernatant was used to determine heparanase activity using Cisbio Heparanase assay (Cisbio, Codolet, France). HepOne (InSight, Rehovot, Israel) was used for heparanase standard range. Briefly, cells lysate, supernatant, or HepOne was mixed with HS labeled with biotin and Eu3+ in reaction buffer (20 mM citrate phosphate buffer pH 5.4, 50 mM NaCl, 1 mM $CaCl_2$, 0.1% BSA, 0.1% Chaps) for 3 h at 37 °C. Then for the detection step we add streptavidin-d2 (300 mM phosphate buffer pH 7, 800 mM potassium fluoride, 0.1% BSA, 2 mg/mL heparin) for 15 min at ambient temperature. Then the fluorescence was read using the following setup: excitation 337 nm, emissions 620 nm and 665 nm on M200 Pro reader (Tecan, Lyon, France).

179

3.13. Experimental Model of Intimal Hyperplasia

The experimental design was approved by the Bichat University Institutional Animal Care and use Committee (N°2011-14/698-0038). Adult male Wistar rats (*n* = 12, purchased from Janvier, CERJ, Laval, France), weighing 280 to 300 g and aged 8 weeks, were anesthetized with intraperitoneal pentobarbital (0.1 mL/kg) (CEVA Santé Animal, Libourne, France). 2F Fogerty balloon catheter (Baxter Healthcare, Maurepas, France) was inserted through an incision made in the external carotid artery and advanced along the length of the common carotid artery to the thoracic aorta [39]. The balloon was then inflated and passed three times along the length of the aortas. The balloon catheter was removed, the external carotid artery was permanently ligated and the skin wound was repaired. Then, the animals were divided into two groups: the first one received the LMWF solution (5 mg/kg/day, *n* = 6) and the second one received the saline solution (control animals, *n* = 6) via intramuscularly injection in the right leg for 14 days. Two weeks after balloon injury, rats were sacrificed by pentobarbital overdose. The thoracic aortas were harvested and divided into two groups. The first one (*n* = 6) was fixed in 4% paraformaldehyde (PFA), embedded in paraffin, and cut in 9-μm-thick cross sections for histology study. The second one (*n* = 6) was embedded in Tissue-Tek OCT Compound (Tissue-Tek, Hatfield, PA, USA), frozen in liquid nitrogen and cut in 9-μm-thick cross sections with a cryostat (Leica CM 1900, Rueil-Malmaison, France) for immunohistochemistry study.

After fixation in 4% PFA, rat aortas were stained with hematoxylin and eosin solution. Digital-slide were acquired and analyzed with a NanoZoomer (Hamamatsu, Massy, France). At least 3 sections of each stained samples were used for analysis representing different levels of the arterial segment.

Adjacent 9-μm-thick fresh arterial cross sections were immunostained with mouse anti-human endothelium CD31 (rat cross-reactive, clone RECA-1, MCA970, dilution 1/20; Abcam, Paris, France) and mouse anti-human smooth-muscle α-actin (α-SMA) (rat cross-reactive, clone 1A4, M0851, dilution 1/100; Dako, Trappes, France) as previously described [40]. Afterwards, slides were co-incubated with the appropriate secondary antibodies (5 μg/mL; Life Technologies, Saint Aubin, France). Negative control sections were incubated only with the secondary antibodies. Representative immunofluorescence photomicrographs were taken using a Leica DMRXA. Specific software (HistoLab Software, Microvision Instruments, Evry, France) allowed the tissue analysis.

3.14. Statistical Analysis

For the determination of statistical significance, ANOVA tests were performed with the StatView software (StatView 4.5 Abacus Concepts, Berkeley, CA, USA). All results are expressed as mean ± SEM for minimum three independent experiments (*n* = 3). A *p*-value of 0.05 was used as the criterion of statistical significance.

Acknowledgments: This work was supported by the Direction de la Recherche et des Enseignements Doctoraux (Ministère de l'Enseignement Supérieur et de la Recherche), the University Paris 13 and INSERM. N. Marinval and L. Maillard were supported by a fellowship from the Ministère de l'Enseignement Supérieur et de la Recherche. The authors would like to thank Liliane Louedec (INSERM U1148, LVTS) for her technical assistance with the animal experiments. This work was supported by Region Ile-de-France doctoral fellowship for F. Chevalier (STEMP-RVT- UNIVPARISEST-AD-P10).
The authors would like to thank Julien Trébaux and Fabienne Chevallier from Cisbio Assays Company for their technical assistance with the analysis of heparanase activity.

Author Contributions: O.H., H.H. and N.C. conceived and designed the experiments; O.H., H.H., N.M., F.C., L.G. and L.M. performed the experiments; H.H., N.C., O.H., A.S. and O.O. analyzed the data; E.G., O.H., N.M. and C.L.M. contributed reagents/materials/analysis tools; N.C., H.H. and O.H. wrote the paper.

Conflicts of Interest: The authors have no conflict of interest to declare.

References

1. Nikolova, V.; Koo, C.Y.; Ibrahim, S.A.; Wangs, Z.; Spillmann, D.; Dreier, R.; Kelsch, R.; Fischgräbe, J.; Smollich, M.; Rossi, L.H.; *et al.* Differential roles for membrane-bound and soluble syndecan-1 (CD138) in breast cancer progression. *Carcinogenesis* **2009**, *30*, 397–407. [CrossRef] [PubMed]

2. Zong, F.; Fthenou, E.; Mundt, F.; Szatmári, T.; Kovalszky, I.; Szilák, L.; Brodin, D.; Tzanakakis, G.; Hjerpe, A.; Dobra, K. Specific syndecan-1 domains regulate mesenchymal tumor cell adhesion, motility and migration. *PLoS ONE* **2011**, *6*. [CrossRef] [PubMed]
3. Corti, F.; Finetti, F.; Ziche, M.; Simons, M. The syndecan-4/protein kinase Cα pathway mediates prostaglandin E2-induced extracellular regulated kinase (ERK) activation in endothelial cells and angiogenesis *in vivo*. *J. Biol. Chem.* **2013**, *288*, 12712–12721. [CrossRef] [PubMed]
4. Longley, R.L.; Woods, A.; Fleetwood, A.; Cowling, G.J.; Gallagher, J.T.; Couchman, J.R. Control of morphology, cytoskeleton and migration by syndecan-4. *J. Cell Sci.* **1999**, *112*, 3421–3431. [PubMed]
5. Hassan, H.; Greve, B.; Pavao, M.S.; Kiesel, L.; Ibrahim, S.A.; Götte, M. Syndecan-1 modulates β-integrin-dependent and interleukin-6-dependent functions in breast cancer cell adhesion, migration, and resistance to irradiation. *FEBS J.* **2013**, *280*, 2216–2227. [CrossRef] [PubMed]
6. Péterfia, B.; Füle, T.; Baghy, K.; Szabadkai, K.; Fullár, A.; Dobos, K.; Zong, F.; Dobra, K.; Hollósi, P.; Jeney, A.; *et al.* Syndecan-1 Enhances Proliferation, Migration and Metastasis of HT-1080 Cells in Cooperation with Syndecan-2. *PLoS ONE* **2012**, *7*. [CrossRef]
7. Luyt, C.E.; Meddahi-Pellé, A.; Ho-Tin-Noe, B.; Colliec-Jouault, S.; Guezennec, J.; Louedec, L.; Prats, H.; Jacob, M.P.; Osborne-Pellegrin, M.; Letourneur, D.; *et al.* Low-molecular-weight fucoidan promotes therapeutic revascularization in a rat model of critical hindlimb ischemia. *J. Pharmacol. Exp. Ther.* **2003**, *305*, 24–30. [CrossRef] [PubMed]
8. Lake, A.C.; Vassy, R.; di Benedetto, M.; Lavigne, D.; le Visage, C.; Perret, G.Y.; Letourneur, D. Low molecular weight fucoidan increases VEGF165-induced endothelial cell migration by enhancing VEGF165 binding to VEGFR-2 and NRP1. *J. Biol. Chem.* **2006**, *281*, 37844–37852. [CrossRef] [PubMed]
9. Sarlon, G.; Zemani, F.; David, L.; Duong van Huyen, J.P.; Dizier, B.; Grelac, F.; Colliec-Jouault, S.; Galy-Fauroux, I.; Bruneval, P.; Fischer, A.M.; *et al.* Therapeutic effect of fucoidan-stimulated endothelial colony-forming cells in peripheral ischemia. *J. Thromb. Haemost.* **2012**, *10*, 38–48. [CrossRef] [PubMed]
10. Hlawaty, H.; Suffee, N.; Sutton, A.; Oudar, O.; Haddad, O.; Ollivier, V.; Laguillier-Morizot, C.; Gattegno, L.; Letourneur, D.; Charnaux, N. Low molecular weight fucoidan prevents intimal hyperplasia in rat injured thoracic aorta through the modulation of matrix metalloproteinase-2 expression. *Biochem. Pharmacol.* **2011**, *81*, 233–243. [CrossRef] [PubMed]
11. Soeda, S.; Kozako, T.; Iwata, K.; Shimeno, H. Oversulfated fucoidan inhibits the basic fibroblast growth factor-induced tube formation by human umbilical vein endothelial cells: Its possible mechanism of action. *Biochim. Biophys. Acta* **2000**, *1497*, 127–134. [CrossRef]
12. Kim, B.S.; Park, J.Y.; Kang, H.J.; Kim, H.J.; Lee, J. Fucoidan/FGF-2 induces angiogenesis through JNK- and p38-mediated activation of AKT/MMP-2 signalling. *Biochem. Biophys. Res. Commun.* **2014**, *450*, 1333–1338. [CrossRef] [PubMed]
13. Vlodavsky, I.; Friedmann, Y. Molecular properties and involvement of heparanase in cancer metastasis and angiogenesis. *J. Clin. Investig.* **2001**, *108*, 341–347. [CrossRef] [PubMed]
14. Levy-Adam, F.; Abboud-Jarrous, G.; Guerrini, M.; Beccati, D.; Vlodavsky, I.; Ilan, N. Identification and characterization of heparin/heparan sulfate binding domains of the endoglycosidase heparanase. *J. Biol. Chem.* **2005**, *280*, 20457–20466. [CrossRef] [PubMed]
15. Levy-Adam, F.; Miao, H.Q.; Heinrikson, R.L.; Vlodavsky, I.; Ilan, N. Heterodimer formation is essential for heparanase enzymatic activity. *Biochem. Biophys. Res. Commun.* **2003**, *308*, 885–891. [CrossRef]
16. Parish, C.R.; Freeman, C.; Hulett, M.D. Heparanase: A key enzyme involved in cell invasion. *Biochim. Biophys. Acta* **2001**, *1471*, 99–108. [CrossRef]
17. Crescimanno, C.; Marzioni, D.; Paradinas, F.J.; Schrurs, B.; Mühlhauser, J.; Todros, T.; Newlands, E.; David, G.; Castellucci, M. Expression pattern alterations of syndecans and glypican-1 in normal and pathological trophoblast. *J. Pathol.* **1999**, *189*, 600–608. [CrossRef]
18. Adhikari, N.; Carlson, M.; Lerman, B.; Hall, J.L. Changes in Expression of Proteoglycan Core Proteins and Heparan Sulfate Enzymes in the Developing and Adult Murine Aorta. *J. Cardiovasc. Transl. Res.* **2011**, *4*, 313–320. [CrossRef] [PubMed]
19. Friand, V.; Haddad, O.; Papy-Garcia, D.; Hlawaty, H.; Vassy, R.; Hamma-Kourbali, Y.; Perret, G.Y.; Courty, J.; Baleux, F.; Oudar, O.; *et al.* Glycosaminoglycan mimetics inhibit SDF-1/CXCL12-mediated migration and invasion of human hepatoma cells. *Glycobiology* **2009**, *19*, 1511–1524. [CrossRef] [PubMed]

20. Charni, F.; Friand, V.; Haddad, O.; Hlawaty, H.; Martin, L.; Vassy, R.; Oudar, O.; Gattegno, L.; Charnaux, N.; Sutton, A. Syndecan-1 and syndecan-4 are involved in RANTES/CCL5-induced migration and invasion of human hepatoma cells. *Biochim. Biophys. Acta* **2009**, *1790*, 1314–1326. [CrossRef] [PubMed]

21. Deux, J.F.; Meddahi-Pelle, A.; Le Blanche, A.F.; Feldman, L.J.; Colliec-Jouault, S.; Brée, F.; Boudghène, F.; Michel, J.B.; Letourneur, D. Low molecular weight fucoidan prevents neointimal hyperplasia in rabbit iliac artery in-stent restenosis model. *Arterioscler. Thromb. Vasc. Biol.* **2002**, *22*, 1604–1609. [CrossRef] [PubMed]

22. Sweeney, E.A.; Lortat-Jacob, H.; Priestley, G.V.; Nakamoto, B.; Papayannopoulou, T. Sulfated polysaccharides increase plasma levels of SDF-1 in monkeys and mice: Involvement in mobilization of stem/progenitor cells. *Blood* **2002**, *99*, 44–51. [CrossRef] [PubMed]

23. Salvucci, O.; Yao, L.; Villalba, S.; Sajewicz, A.; Pittaluga, S.; Tosato, G. Regulation of endothelial cell branching morphogenesis by endogenous chemokine stromal-derived factor-1. *Blood* **2002**, *99*, 2703–2711. [CrossRef] [PubMed]

24. Ferreras, C.; Rushton, G.; Cole, C.L.; Babur, M.; Telfer, B.A.; van Kuppevelt, T.H.; Gardiner, J.M.; Williams, K.J.; Jayson, G.C.; Avizienyte, E. Endothelial heparan sulfate 6-*O*-sulfation levels regulate angiogenic responses of endothelial cells to fibroblast growth factor 2 and vascular endothelial growth factor. *J. Biol. Chem.* **2012**, *287*, 36132–36146. [CrossRef] [PubMed]

25. Wang, Y.; Yang, X.; Yamagata, S.; Yamagata, T.; Sato, T. Involvement of Ext1 and heparanase in migration of mouse FBJ osteosarcoma cells. *Mol. Cell. Biochem.* **2013**, *373*, 63–72. [CrossRef] [PubMed]

26. Huegel, J.; Enomoto-Iwamoto, M.; Sgariglia, F.; Koyama, E.; Pacifici, M. Heparanase stimulates chondrogenesis and is up-regulated in human ectopic cartilage: a mechanism possibly involved in hereditary multiple exostoses. *Am J Pathol.* **2015**, *185*, 1676–1685. [CrossRef] [PubMed]

27. Busse, M.; Feta, A.; Presto, J.; Wilén, M.; Gronning, M.; Kjellén, L.; Kusche-Gullberg, M. Contribution of EXT1, EXT2, and EXTL3 to heparan sulfate chain elongation. *J. Biol. Chem.* **2007**, *282*, 32802–32810. [CrossRef] [PubMed]

28. Zcharia, E.; Metzger, S.; Chajek-Shaul, T.; Aingorn, H.; Elkin, M.; Friedmann, Y.; Weinstein, T.; Li, J.P.; Lindahl, U.; Vlodavsky, I. Transgenic expression of mammalian heparanase uncovers physiological functions of heparan sulfate in tissue morphogenesis, vascularization and feeding behavior. *FASEB J.* **2004**, *18*, 252–263. [CrossRef] [PubMed]

29. Vlodavsky, I.; Blich, M.; Li, J.P.; Sanderson, R.D.; Ilan, N. Involvement of heparanase in atherosclerosis and other vessel wall pathologies. *Matrix Biol.* **2013**, *32*, 241–251. [CrossRef] [PubMed]

30. Purushothaman, A.; Uyama, T.; Kobayashi, F.; Yamada, S.; Sugahara, K.; Rapraeger, A.C.; Sanderson, R.D. Heparanase-enhanced shedding of syndecan-1 by myeloma cells promotes endothelial invasion and angiogenesis. *Blood* **2010**, *115*, 2449–2457. [CrossRef] [PubMed]

31. Ramani, V.C.; Pruett, P.S.; Thompson, C.A.; DeLucas, L.D.; Sanderson, R.D. Heparan sulfate chains of syndecan-1 regulate ectodomain shedding. *J. Biol. Chem.* **2012**, *287*, 9952–9961. [CrossRef] [PubMed]

32. Nardella, A.; Chaubet, F.; Boisson-Vidal, C.; Blondin, C.; Durand, P.; Jozefonvicz, J. Anticoagulant low molecular weight fucans produced by radical process and ion exchange chromatography of high molecular weight fucans extracted from the brown seaweed *Ascophyllum nodosum*. *Carbohydr. Res.* **1996**, *289*, 201–208. [CrossRef]

33. Chevolot, L.; Foucault, A.; Chaubet, F.; Kervarec, N.; Sinquin, C.; Fisher, A.M.; Boisson-Vidal, C. Further data on the structure of brown seaweed fucans: Relationships with anticoagulant activity. *Carbohydr. Res.* **1999**, *319*, 154–165. [CrossRef]

34. Li, B.; Lu, F.; Wei, X.; Zhao, R. Fucoidan: Structure and bioactivity. *Molecules* **2008**, *13*, 1671–1695. [CrossRef] [PubMed]

35. Patankar, M.S.; Oehninger, S.; Barnett, T.; Williams, R.L.; Clark, G.F. A revised structure for fucoidan may explain some of its biological activities. *J. Biol. Chem.* **1993**, *268*, 21770–21776. [PubMed]

36. Barbosa, I.; Garcia, S.; Barbier-Chassefière, V.; Caruelle, J.P.; Martelly, I.; Papy-García, D. Improved and simple micro assay for sulfated glycosaminoglycans quantification in biological extracts and its use in skin and muscle tissue studies. *Glycobiology* **2003**, *13*, 647–653. [CrossRef] [PubMed]

37. Sutton, A.; Friand, V.; Brulé-Donneger, S.; Chaigneau, T.; Ziol, M.; Sainte-Catherine, O.; Poiré, A.; Saffar, L.; Kraemer, M.; Vassy, J.; *et al.* Stromal cell-derived factor-1/chemokine (C-X-C motif) ligand 12 stimulates human hepatoma cell growth, migration, and invasion. *Mol. Cancer Res.* **2007**, *5*, 21–33. [CrossRef] [PubMed]

38. Charnaux, N.; Brule, S.; Hamon, M.; Chaigneau, T.; Saffar, L.; Prost, C.; Lievre, N.; Gattegno, L. Syndecan-4 is a signaling molecule for stromal cell-derived factor-1 (SDF-1)/CXCL12. *FEBS J.* **2005**, *272*, 1937–1951. [CrossRef] [PubMed]

39. Mao, C.; Malek, O.T.; Pueyo, M.E.; Steg, P.G.; Soubrier, F. Differential expression of rat frizzled-related *frzb-1* and frizzled receptor *fz1* and *fz2* genes in the rat aorta after balloon injury. *Arterioscler. Thromb. Vasc. Biol.* **2000**, *20*, 43–51. [CrossRef] [PubMed]

40. Suffee, N.; Hlawaty, H.; Meddahi-Pelle, A.; Maillard, L.; Louedec, L.; Haddad, O.; Martin, L.; Laguillier, C.; Richard, B.; Oudar, O.; *et al.* RANTES/CCL5-induced pro-angiogenic effects depend on CCR1, CCR5 and glycosaminoglycans. *Angiogenesis* **2012**, *15*, 727–744. [CrossRef] [PubMed]

marine drugs

MDPI

Article

Fucoidan Stimulates Monocyte Migration via ERK/p38 Signaling Pathways and MMP9 Secretion

Elene Sapharikas [1,*], Anna Lokajczyk [1], Anne-Marie Fischer [2] and Catherine Boisson-Vidal [1]

[1] Inserm UMR_S 1140, Faculté de Pharmacie, Université Paris Descartes, Sorbonne Paris Cité, 4 Avenue de l'observatoire Paris 75006, France; anna.lokajczyk@parisdescartes.fr (A.L.); catherine.boisson-vidal@parisdescartes.fr (C.B.-V.)

[2] Inserm UMR-S 970, AP-HP, Hôpital Européen Georges Pompidou, 20 rue Leblanc Paris 75015, France; anne-marie.fischer@egp.aphp.fr

* Author to whom correspondence should be addressed; elene.sapharikas@parisdescartes.fr; Tel.: +33-1-5373-9717; Fax: +33-1-4407-1772.

Academic Editor: Paola Laurienzo

Received: 26 May 2015; Accepted: 23 June 2015; Published: 30 June 2015

Abstract: Critical limb ischemia (CLI) induces the secretion of paracrine signals, leading to monocyte recruitment and thereby contributing to the initiation of angiogenesis and tissue healing. We have previously demonstrated that fucoidan, an antithrombotic polysaccharide, promotes the formation of new blood vessels in a mouse model of hindlimb ischemia. We examined the effect of fucoidan on the capacity of peripheral blood monocytes to adhere and migrate. Monocytes negatively isolated with magnetic beads from peripheral blood of healthy donors were treated with fucoidan. Fucoidan induced a 1.5-fold increase in monocyte adhesion to gelatin ($p < 0.05$) and a five-fold increase in chemotaxis in Boyden chambers ($p < 0.05$). Fucoidan also enhanced migration 2.5-fold in a transmigration assay ($p < 0.05$). MMP9 activity in monocyte supernatants was significantly enhanced by fucoidan ($p < 0.05$). Finally, Western blot analysis of fucoidan-treated monocytes showed upregulation of ERK/p38 phosphorylation. Inhibition of ERK/p38 phosphorylation abrogated fucoidan enhancement of migration ($p < 0.01$). Fucoidan displays striking biological effects, notably promoting monocyte adhesion and migration. These effects involve the ERK and p38 pathways, and increased MMP9 activity. Fucoidan could improve critical limb ischemia by promoting monocyte recruitment.

Keywords: fucoidan; monocytes; critical limb ischemia; migration

---

1. Introduction

Cardiovascular disease is the leading cause of death worldwide. Peripheral arterial disease (PAD) is linked to a three- to six-fold increase in cardiovascular mortality compared to the general population [1–3]. With population aging, PAD has become a major public health problem [4]. Revascularization currently relies on bypass surgery or endovascular therapy (balloon angioplasty or stents) [2,5,6]. Conservative surgery is not always possible, and the affected limb must sometimes be amputated to avoid necrosis [7]. PAD is initially asymptomatic, and its diagnosis is based mainly on the ankle brachial pressure index. However, media sclerosis can interfere with this index [8], especially in older people and patients with diabetes, further delaying diagnosis and treatment in some cases [9]. Current treatments do not always avoid limb amputation or death [10–12]. Great hopes are being placed in gene and cell therapies. However, a large randomized placebo-controlled phase III trial in critical limb ischemia, the TAMARIS study, showed no reduction in the amputation rate in patients treated with a plasmid encoding acidic FGF (fibroblast growth factor) [13], thus failing to confirm benefits seen in phase II trials [14,15]. Protective effects have been observed with other angiogenic growth factors (FGF2 and VEGF) [16–18]. Several studies have shown an improvement in patients' health status after intramuscular injection of bone marrow- or peripheral blood-derived mononuclear cells [19–21]. However, none of these trials showed efficient revascularization [22,23]. Endothelial progenitor cells are mononuclear cells involved in vascular and tissue remodeling. Several studies have shown the direct beneficial involvement of monocytes in PAD [24,25]. In particular, the early presence of monocytes at ischemic sites resulted in increased reperfusion in a murine model of lower limb ischemia [26]. Mobilization and recruitment of circulating monocytes from bone marrow to sites of active revascularization, where they differentiate into macrophages, is crucial for tissue regeneration after an ischemic event. The first step of monocyte recruitment involves tethering and rolling along the vessel endothelium, followed by strong adhesion and tissue entry. Several studies have shown an important role for monocyte chemoattractant protein-1 (MCP1) and its receptor CCR2 in monocyte mobilization at ischemic sites. Inhibition of this recruitment negatively affects the angiogenic process, as demonstrated in the CCR2 knock out mouse model [27,28]. During PAD, increased MCP-1 secretion leads to monocyte recruitment and is involved in the angiogenic process. Voskuil *et al.* showed that MCP-1 injection after femoral artery ligation in pigs stimulated collateral vessel formation [29].

Our laboratory studies a low-molecular-weight (LMW) sulfated polysaccharide extracted from brown seaweeds. Fucoidan exhibits exceptional enhancement of new blood vessel formation in animal models [30–33]. LMW fucoidan enhances the proangiogenic properties of endothelial colony-forming cells (ECFC) *in vitro*, by modifying both early events (proliferation and migration) and late events (differentiation into vascular cords) [31]. In a previous study, we showed that fucoidan significantly improved the beneficial effects of ECFC transplantation in a mouse model of hind limb ischemia, preventing tissue necrosis [30]. This tissue protection was associated with enhanced neoangiogenesis and a reduction in rhabdomyolysis. Fucoidan prestimulation enhanced each step of the angiogenic processes, namely cell recruitment to ischemic tissue *via* enhanced ECFC adhesion to activated endothelium, MMP-9 secretion, extravasation, and differentiation into a vascular network. In the present study, we investigated the mechanism of action of fucoidan on peripheral blood monocyte cells (PBMC) adhesion to gelatin and migration through an activated endothelium, as well as adhesion molecule expression and the MMP2/MMP9 secretion. We also explored the signaling pathway involved in fucoidan-induced monocyte migration.

2. Results and Discussion

2.1. Fucoidan Pretreatment Enhances Monocyte Adhesion, Migration and Transmigration

The first step of monocyte recruitment is their adhesion to the endothelium, followed by migration and transmigration through the endothelium. We first investigated the effect of fucoidan on monocyte adhesion to gelatin (Figure 1A). Fucoidan treatment for 24 h enhanced monocyte adhesion by 1.5-fold (Figure 1A,B, $p < 0.05$). As shown in Figure 1C, fucoidan enhanced PBMC migration in a concentration-dependent manner (data not shown). Monocytes pretreated with fucoidan were 5-fold more motile than control cells towards 100 ng/mL MCP-1 ($p < 0.05$, Figure 1D). As shown in Figure 1E, pretreatment of PBMC with fucoidan led to a 2.5-fold increase in transmigration across an activated monolayer of HUVEC (Figure 1F, $p < 0.01$). These results showed that, *ex vivo*, fucoidan enhanced all the major steps of monocyte recruitment to ischemic sites.

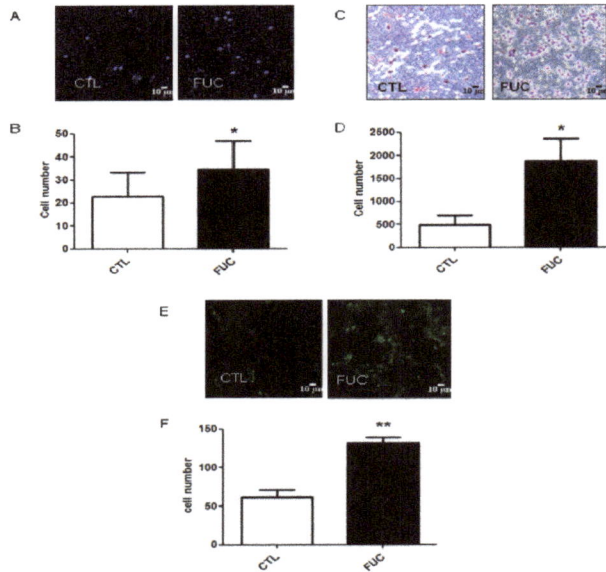

Figure 1. Fucoidan enhances monocyte adhesion to gelatin, and their migration. (**A**) Representative results obtained with PBMC after 30 min, with or without 24 h of fucoidan pretreatment; (**B**) Monocyte adhesion (in white, control monocytes, in black, monocytes incubated with 10 μg/mL fucoidan; (**C**) Representative results for migration of isolated PBMC treated with or without fucoidan (4 h) towards 100 ng/mL MCP-1; (**D**) Migratory cell numbers in five independent fields; (**E**) Representative monocyte transmigration (18 h) with or without fucoidan pretreatment (30 min); (**F**) Transmigratory cell numbers in five independent fields. Three to five independent donors. * $p < 0.05$; ** $p < 0.01$.

2.2. Fucoidan Stimulation of Monocyte Adhesion and Migration Is not Due to Modulation of Integrin Expression or CCR2 Receptor Expression

As fucoidan-treated PBMC showed a striking increase in adhesion and migration, we examined whether fucoidan modulated the expression of integrins involved in these processes. As engagement of monocyte integrins αMβ2 (VLA4) and α4β1 (MAC-1) by endothelial ICAM-1 and VCAM, respectively, is critical for monocyte extravasation, we examined the effect of fucoidan on the expression levels of these integrins after 30 min or 24 h of fucoidan exposure. As shown in Figure 2, neither exposure time affected PBMC integrin expression (Figure 2A–D). MCP-1 receptor (CCR2) expression was not modulated by fucoidan after 20 min of incubation (Figure 2E). Surprisingly, however, CCR2 expression was downregulated after 24 h, in the presence or absence of fucoidan (Figure 2E), possibly because CCR2 is involved in the early phase of recruitment of monocytes, whereas CXCR1 takes over during the second phase [34,35]. Finally, fucoidan did not affect the expression of CD44 or CD87, two receptors involved in monocyte migration and actin cytoskeleton rearrangement involved in cell motility (data not shown).

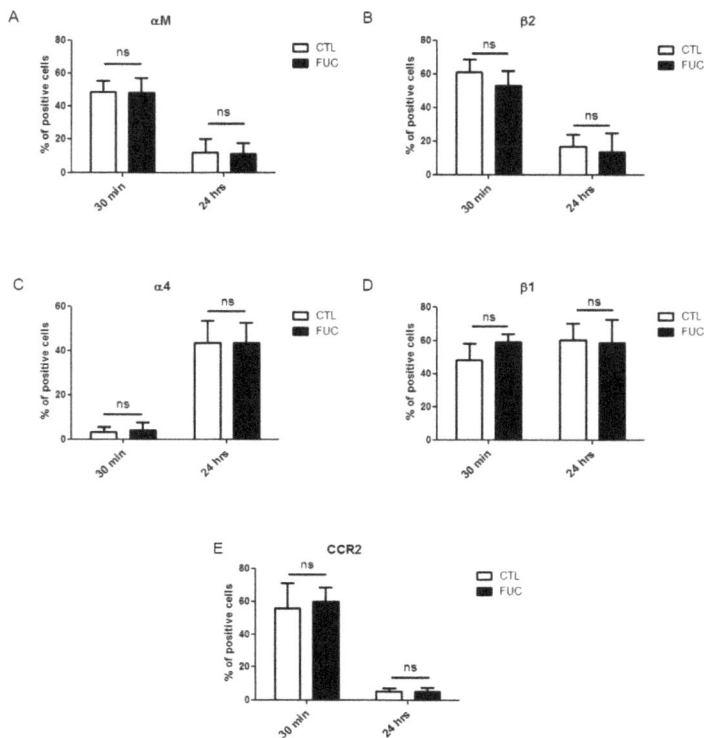

Figure 2. Impact of fucoidan on adhesion molecule and CCR2 receptor expression: PBMC were treated for 30 min or 24 h with (black bars) or without fucoidan (white bars). (**A**) Percentage of monocytes positive for alpha M expression; (**B**) Percentage of beta 2-positive cells; (**C**) Percentage of alpha 4-positive cells; (**D**) Percentage of beta 1-positive cells; (**E**) Percentage of CCR2-positive cells (4 independent donors).

2.3. Fucoidan Enhances PBMC MMP9 Activity

As fucoidan-treated monocytes showed no change in integrin or CCR2 receptor expression, we explored the possible role of matrix metalloproteinases in fucoidan-enhanced migration and adhesion. Extracellular MMPs are involved in monocyte migration: macrophage adhesion to fibronectin via $\alpha 5 \beta 1$ integrin *in vitro* is associated with increased MMP9 secretion [36]. Furthermore, we have shown that fucoidan increases MMP9 activity in HUVEC and ECFC cells [30,31]. Here, MMP9 and MMP2 activities were quantified by gelatin zymography (Figure 3A). We observed a significant increase in MMP9 activity in conditioned media of fucoidan-treated PBMC (Figure 3B, $p < 0.05$). MMP2 activity was unaffected (Figure 3C). This effect of fucoidan on MMP9 secretion is unlikely to be sole mechanism underlying the observed effect of fucoidan on monocyte migration and adhesion.

A

CTL FUC

Pro-MMP9 ⟶

MMP9 ⟶

Pro-MMP2 ⟶
MMP2 ⟶

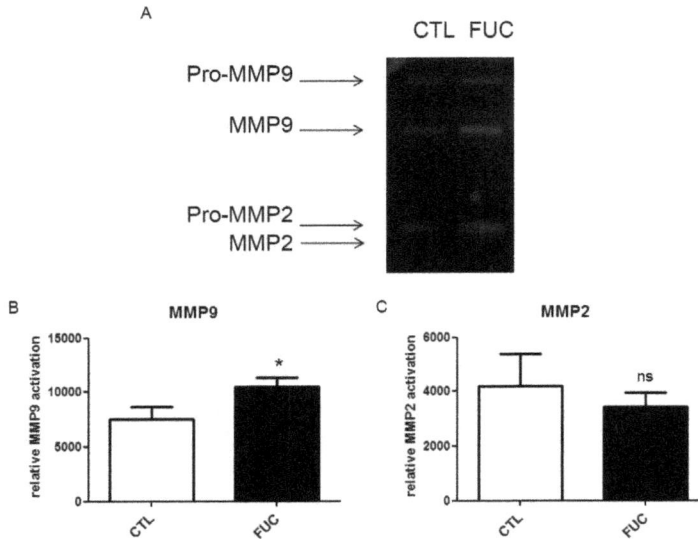

B MMP9

C MMP2

Figure 3. Impact of fucoidan on monocyte MMP9 expression (gelatinolytic activity): (**A**) Representative gelatin zymography of culture supernatant of monocytes treated with or without fucoidan for 30 min; (**B**) MMP9 gelanitolytic activity; (**C**) MMP2 gelatinolytic activity. Three independent donors; * $p < 0.05$

2.4. Fucoidan Enhancement of PBMC Migration Is Countered by ERK and p38 Pathway Inhibition

The MAPK ERK and p38 pathways have been shown to be involved in monocyte migration. We used Western blot to analyze the phosphorylation levels of ERK1/2 and p38 in starved and re-stimulated monocytes, treated with or without fucoidan, in the presence of specific inhibitors of these kinases (Figure 4A). Fucoidan-treated monocytes showed a two-fold increase in ERK phosphorylation, and this increase was inhibited by the ERK inhibitor PD98059 (Figure 4B). Fucoidan treatment also increased p38 phosphorylation to a lesser extent, an effect also inhibited by the p38-specific inhibitor SB203580 (Figure 4C). Finally, we explored the role of the ERK and p38 pathways in PBMC migration towards MCP-1 (Figure 4D). As expected, ERK and p38 inhibition abrogated the ability of fucoidan to enhance monocyte migration. Although neither pathway seemed to be involved in monocyte migration nor in control conditions, ERK and p38 inhibition reduced the migration of fucoidan-treated monocytes by 2.5-fold (Figure 4E), highlighting the prominent role of these pathways in fucoidan-enhanced monocyte migration.

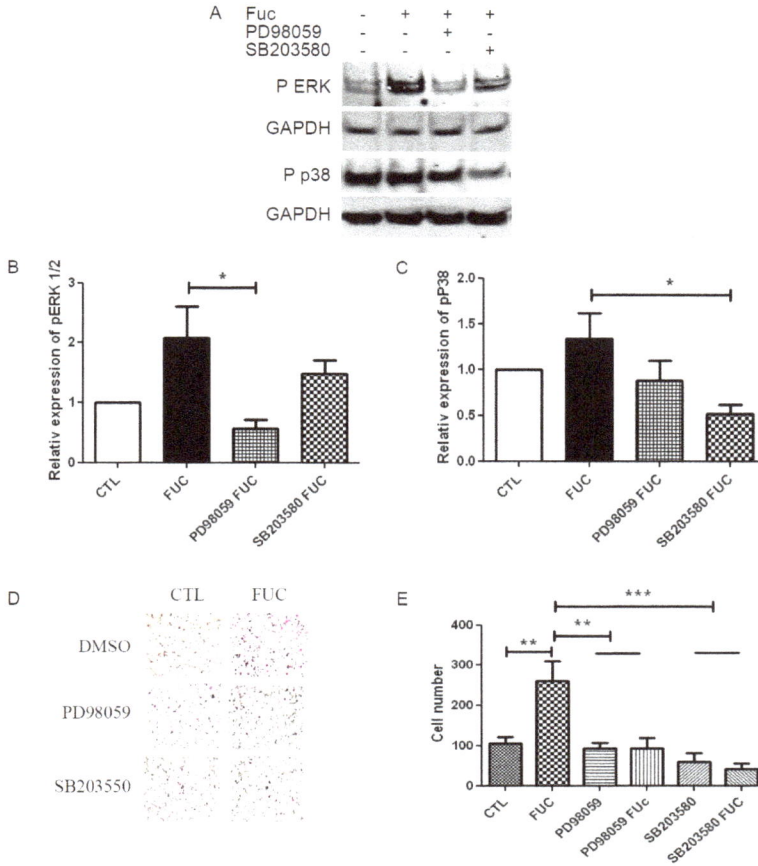

Figure 4. ERK and p38 signaling pathway involvement in fucoidan-treated monocyte migration: (**A**) Representative Western blot illustrating phosphorylation of ERK1/2 and P38 when PBMC were treated with or without fucoidan (in the presence or absence of PD98059 or SB203580) for 30 min; (**B**) Quantitative analysis of ERK phosphorylation; (**C**) Quantitative analysis of p38 phosphorylation. Results are represented relative to the corresponding control, with with independent donors; (**D**) Representative fields showing migratory cells treated as in A; (**E**) Migratory cell numbers in five independent fields. * $p < 0.05$; ** $p < 0.01$; *** $p < 0.001$ compared to control. Four independent donors.

3. Discussion

We provide new evidence for a major effect on fucoidan on monocyte migration. We found that fucoidan did not modulate integrin or receptor expression on the monocyte cell membrane. However, fucoidan enhanced monocyte migration towards MCP-1, an effect associated with ERK and p38 signaling pathway activation and with MMP9 secretion (Figure 5).

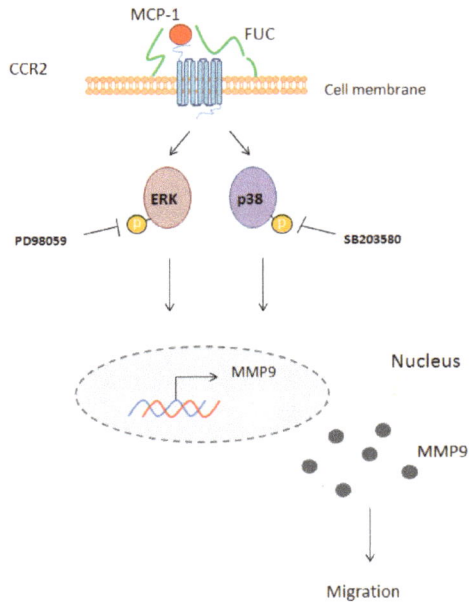

Figure 5. Schematic overview of the effect of fucoidan on monocyte migration. Fucoidan bound to the cell membrane enhances MCP-1 interaction with its receptor CCR2. This interaction leads to phosphorylation of ERK1/2 and p38 and activates MM9 secretion. PD98059 and SB203580 inhibit this phosphorylation, leading to reduced monocyte migration.

In response to diverse pro-inflammatory signals released from damaged tissue, circulating blood monocytes attach transiently to the activated vascular endothelium and resist shear stress before crossing the vessel wall [37]. Several studies have highlighted the importance of monocyte recruitment for tissue and vessel repair [28,38,39]. Here we show that PBMC pretreatment with fucoidan enhanced their adhesion to gelatin. Elsewhere, fucoidan-treated ECFC have been found to adhere more efficiently to activated endothelium in flow conditions [30]. We also found that fucoidan enhanced monocyte migration towards MCP-1 as chemoattractant, and also favored monocyte transmigration on a monolayer of activated endothelial cells. This increased response of PMBC to MCP-1 may have therapeutic relevance, as this chemoattractant has been shown to be involved in monocyte recruitment, particularly during neovessel formation. Vein graft intimal hyperplasia is associated with MCP-1 upregulation, leading to monocyte recruitment. Furthermore, macrophage depletion with liposome clodronate diminishes MCP-1 and TGF beta 1 expression, an effect associated with reduced vein graft healing in rats [40]. Schepers and collaborators confirmed these results with anti-MCP-1 in mice, as did Tatewaki *et al.* using adenoviral gene transfer to block MCP-1 expression in dogs [41,42]. Our results indicate that fucoidan promotes the early phase of monocyte recruitment to activated endothelium and, subsequently, new vessel formation.

The precise mechanism of action of fucoidan on PBMC is not fully understood. We have previously demonstrated that GAG abrasion on the cell surface hinders ECFC migration, and that fucoidan treatment restores this migration [30]. Like glycosaminoglycans, fucoidan, by its ionic structure, is able to bind adhesion proteins [43], growth factors [44] and cytokines [45]. The activity of fucoidan is due mainly to its sulfatation: desulfated fucoidan loses its proangiogenic properties *in vitro* and *in vivo*, and is unable to recruit hematopoietic stem cells [46]. As fucoidan interacts with adhesion proteins, we examined whether fucoidan treatment enhanced PBMC expression of integrins involved in monocyte migration. Fucoidan had no effect on the expression of integrins or CCR2, the main MCP-1 receptor. Interestingly, $\alpha M/\beta 2$ integrin expression was reduced after 24 h of culture, while $\alpha 4$ integrin expression was increased, but these changes occurred irrespective of fucoidan treatment.

Fucoidan treatment increased the phosphorylation of ERK 1/2 and p38, two signaling pathways involved in monocyte migration and transmigration [47,48]. Surprisingly, we found that these two signaling pathways were not involved in monocyte chemoattraction *ex vivo*, as their inhibition did not inhibit the migration of monocytes not treated with fucoidan. This discrepancy with previous reports may be explained by the use of different models, as most published studies used monocytic cell lines such as THP1. Ashida *et al.* reported that the ERK pathway is involved in monocyte adhesion, while the p38 pathway would be involved in cell migration [49]. In contrast, and in accordance with our findings, it has been shown that the ERK and p38 pathways are not involved in the migration of fresh PBMC [50]. Our results support a direct role of ERK and p38 in fucoidan-enhanced monocyte migration. Indeed, inhibition of either pathway abolished the effect of fucoidan. Finally, we found that fucoidan enhancement of *ex vivo* monocyte migration was associated with MMP9 secretion. It has been shown that monocyte migration is specifically associated with MMP9 activity, through ERK activation [48,51]. Fucoidan was also reported to be an antitumor compound inhibiting migration, invasion and MMP-2/-9 activities in human fibrosarcoma cells (HT1080), human lung cancer cells (A549) and mouse hepatocarcinoma cells lines (Hca-F) [52–54]. This biological effect varies with species and fucoidan's molecular weight [55]. Indeed, fucoidan of over 30 kDa or high concentration of LMWF may deplete the medium from growth factors and thus interfere with their activities [56,57]. This sequestration by fucoidan on growth factor could explain the inhibition of MMP-2 and -9 secretions.

Interestingly, in the absence of growth factors, cytokines or serum in the culture medium, fucoidan had no effect on the activation of the ERK 1/2 or p38 signaling pathways (data not shown). Being a glycosaminoglycan, fucoidan behaves as a heparin sulfate and binds to the cell surface. Fucoidan would appear to facilitate the interaction between MCP-1 and its receptor CCR2. We have previously demonstrated that fucoidan potentiates the activity of specific factors like FGF-2 on blood vessel formation *in vitro* [58] and *in vivo* [30]. Overall, our results help to explain the effects of fucoidan on monocyte adhesion and migration and support the therapeutic potential of fucoidan in chronic limb ischemia.

4. Experimental

4.1. Reagents

Fetal bovine serum, PBS $-/-$, HBSS $+/+$ and RPMI 1640 culture medium were from Gibco (Life Technologies, Saint-Aubin, France). Calcein-AM and PD98059 were from Calbiochem (Merck KGaA, Darmstadt, Germany). Giemsa, bovine serum albumin, gelatin and saponin were from Sigma Aldrich (Saint-Quentin-en-Yvelines, France). SB203580 was a kind gift from Bachelot-Loza (Inserm UMR_S 1140, Faculty of Pharmacy, Paris Descartes University, France). pERK was from Cell Signaling (Ozyme, Saint-Quentin-en-Yvelines, France), pP38 was from Promega (Lyon, France), αM-PE, $\alpha 4$-PE and CCR2-APC were from BD Biosciences (Le Pont de Claix, France), $\beta 1$-FITC, ERK and GAPDH were from Santa Cruz (Heidelberg, Germany), $\beta 2$ was from Chemicon-Europe (Merck KGaA, Darmstadt, Germany), and MCP-1 was from R&D systems (Bio Techn Lille, Lilie, France). LMW fucoidan was obtained by radical depolymerization of high-molecular-weight fucoidan extracted from *Ascophylum nodosum*, using procedures adapted from Nardella *et al.* [59]. The molecular weight average mass was 4 ± 1 kDa and characterized by high-performance steric chromatography (HPSEC) in 0.15 M NaCl, 0.005 M NaH2PO4 at pH 7.0, using two columns connected in series (Licrospher Si300 diol and Hema Sec Bio 40 columns) (Merck S.A., Molsheim, France) calibrated using narrow cut heparin fractions as described in Mulloy *et al.* [60]. The chemical composition was as follows: 34% fucose, 4% galactose, 3% xylose, 3% uronic acid and 32.2% sulfate. The human monocyte isolation kit II was from Miltenyi Biotec (Paris, France) and Histopaque solution from Sigma (Saint Quentin Fallavier, France).

4.2. Monocyte and HUVEC Isolation

Monocytes were isolated from healthy donor blood purchased from Etablissement Français du Sang (EFS, convention number: 13/EFS/064). Mononuclear cells were isolated by density-gradient centrifugation using 1.077 g/mL Histopaque solution and then negatively purified following the manufacturer's procedure. Human umbilical vein endothelial cells (HUVEC) were isolated from cord blood with the mothers' consent, as described by Zemani *et al.* [31].

4.3. Cell Adhesion Assay

Ten thousand monocytes were treated with fucoidan 10 μg/mL for 24 h and seeded on Millicell EZ slides (from Millipore, Merck KGaA, Darmstadt, Germany) coated with 0.2% gelatin. They were allowed to adhere for 30 min and then washed with PBS to detach non-adherent cells. Adherent cells were fixed with paraformaldehyde for 10 min at room temperature, then washed with PBS and permeabilized with 0.5% saponin. Cell nuclei were stained with TOPRO for 10 min. The slides were then coverslipped with Ibidi mounting medium and examined with a confocal fluorescence microscope.

4.4. Cell Migration Assay

Boyden chambers were used for migration assays with 8-μm pore-size inserts (BD Biosciences, Le Pont de Claix, France) in 24-well plates. Six hundred microliters of RPMI 1640 medium-1% FBS with 100 ng/mL MCP-1 was placed in the lower chamber. Seventy-five thousand monocytes treated with 10 μg/mL fucoidan were placed in the upper chamber in RPMI 1640 medium-0.1% BSA. After 4 h of migration, the inserts were fixed and stained with Giemsa (Sigma-Aldrich, Saint-Quentin-en-Yvelines, France). Migratory cells were counted in 10 randomly selected fields (200× magnification).

4.5. Transmigration Assay

HUVEC were seeded at 60,000 cells per Transwell chamber coated with 0.5% gelatin for 2 days. They were then activated for 4 h with 10 ng/mL TNFα, and 75,000 monocytes treated with 10 μg/mL of fucoidan were stained with 5 M calcein-AM at 37 °C for 20 min before being added to HUVEC. After 18 h of transmigration, the upper part of the insert was cotton-swabbed to remove non-migrated cells. The remaining cells were fixed, then the Transwell inserts were cut out, placed on slides and coverslipped with Ibidi mounting medium. The lower side of the insert was examined with a confocal fluorescence microscope. Labeled monocytes were counted in 10 randomly selected fields (200× magnification).

4.6. Western Blot

Total protein was prepared from monocytes treated with lysis buffer (Tris 50 mM, NaCl 150 mM, 1% Triton X100, PMSF 1 mM, Na3VO4 1 mM) supplemented with a protease and phosphatase inhibitor cocktail (Sigma Aldrich, Saint-Quentin-en-Yvelines, France) for 20 min on ice, then centrifuged for 10 min at 14,000× *g*. Supernatants were fractionated by SDS-PAGE 4%–12% (NuPAGE® Bis-Tris Pre-Cast gels, Life Technologies, Saint-Aubin, France), transferred to nitrocellulose membranes, and incubated with the following primary antibodies: phosphor ERK, phosphor p38 and GAPDH (all at 1/300 in 0.1% milk/TTBS 1×) and then incubated for 10 min with SNAP i.d.® (Millipore, Merck KGaA, Darmstadt, Germany). Secondary antibodies were either anti-mouse or anti-rabbit Dylight fluor 680 or 800 conjugated antibodies (Thermo Fisher Scientific, Villebon-sur-Yvette, France) (1/3000). Images of the blots were scanned with the Odyssey Infra-Red Imaging System (Li-Cor Biotechnology Eurobio, Courtaboeuf, France). Phosporylation was quantified with ImageJ software (National Institutes of Health, Bethesda, MD, USA).

4.7. Flow Cytometry

Monocytes treated with fucoidan for 30 min or 24 h were collected in HBSS containing 10% FBS. Cells were then labeled for 30 min at 4 °C with the following antibodies: αM-PE, α4-PE, CCR2-APC or β1-FITC. For β2 staining, cells were incubated for 30 min with anti-β2 then washed with HBSS–10% FBS and incubated with FITC-conjugated secondary antibodies for 30 min. Fluorescence was quantified in a BD Accuri C6 flow cytometer (BD Biosciences, Le Pont de Claix, France).

4.8. Zymography

One hundred five monocytes were seeded in 22.6-mm-diameter culture dishes starved overnight before being treated with fucoidan for 30 min. The culture supernatant was collected and 20 µL was analyzed as described by Sarlon *et al.* [30].

4.9. Statistical Analysis

Data are expressed as mean and S.E.M. Data were analyzed by one-way ANOVA followed by Turkey's multiple comparisons test or Student's *t* test. A *p* value < 0.05 was considered to denote statistical significance. GraphPad Prism software version Prism 5 (GraphPad, Sandiego, CA, USA) was used for all analyses.

Acknowledgments: We thank the nursing services of Hôpital St Louis for providing umbilical cord blood samples. E. Sapharikas received grants from Fondation pour la Recherche Médicale and Ministère de l'enseignement Supérieur et de la Recherche. CNRS pays the salary of C. Boisson-Vidal.

Author Contributions: E.S. conceived, designed and performed the experiment, analyzed the data and wrote the paper; A.L. performed the experiments; A.-M.F. contributed to finding funding; and C.B.-V. found funding, supervised the work and wrote the paper.

Conflicts of Interest: The authors declare no conflict of interest.

References

1. Golomb, B.A.; Dang, T.T.; Criqui, M.H. Peripheral arterial disease: Morbidity and mortality implications. *Circulation* **2006**, *114*, 688–699. [CrossRef] [PubMed]
2. Norgren, L.; Hiatt, W.R.; Dormandy, J.A.; Nehler, M.R.; Harris, K.A.; Fowkes, F.G.R.; Rutherford, R.B. TASC II Working Group Inter-society consensus for the management of peripheral arterial disease. *Int. Angiol. J. Int. Union Angiol.* **2007**, *26*, 81–157.
3. Shanmugasundaram, M.; Ram, V.K.; Luft, U.C.; Szerlip, M.; Alpert, J.S. Peripheral arterial disease—What do we need to know? *Clin. Cardiol.* **2011**, *34*, 478–482. [CrossRef] [PubMed]
4. Fowkes, F.G.R.; Rudan, D.; Rudan, I.; Aboyans, V.; Denenberg, J.O.; McDermott, M.M.; Norman, P.E.; Sampson, U.K.A.; Williams, L.J.; Mensah, G.A.; *et al.* Comparison of global estimates of prevalence and risk factors for peripheral artery disease in 2000 and 2010: A systematic review and analysis. *Lancet* **2013**, *382*, 1329–1340. [CrossRef]
5. Rastan, A.; Krankenberg, H.; Baumgartner, I.; Blessing, E.; Müller-Hülsbeck, S.; Pilger, E.; Scheinert, D.; Lammer, J.; Beschorner, U.; Noory, E.; *et al.* Stent Placement *vs.* Balloon Angioplasty for Popliteal Artery Treatment: Two-Year Results of a Prospective, Multicenter, Randomized Trial. *J. Endovasc. Ther. Off. J. Int. Soc. Endovasc. Spec.* **2015**, *22*, 22–27. [CrossRef] [PubMed]
6. Varol, C.; Mildner, A.; Jung, S. Macrophages: Development and tissue specialization. *Annu. Rev. Immunol.* **2015**, *33*, 643–675. [CrossRef] [PubMed]
7. McGinigle, K.L.; Kalbaugh, C.A.; Marston, W.A. Living in a medically underserved county is an independent risk factor for major limb amputation. *J. Vasc. Surg.* **2014**, *59*, 737–741. [CrossRef] [PubMed]
8. Lau, J.F.; Weinberg, M.D.; Olin, J.W. Peripheral artery disease. Part 1: Clinical evaluation and noninvasive diagnosis. *Nat. Rev. Cardiol.* **2011**, *8*, 405–418. [CrossRef] [PubMed]
9. Aerden, D.; Massaad, D.; von Kemp, K.; van Tussenbroek, F.; Debing, E.; Keymeulen, B.; van den Brande, P. The ankle-brachial index and the diabetic foot: A troublesome marriage. *Ann. Vasc. Surg.* **2011**, *25*, 770–777. [CrossRef] [PubMed]
10. Weinberg, M.D.; Lau, J.F.; Rosenfield, K.; Olin, J.W. Peripheral artery disease. Part 2: Medical and endovascular treatment. *Nat. Rev. Cardiol.* **2011**, *8*, 429–441. [CrossRef] [PubMed]
11. Novo, S.; Coppola, G.; Milio, G. Critical limb ischemia: Definition and natural history. *Curr. Drug Targets Cardiovasc. Haematol. Disord.* **2004**, *4*, 219–225. [CrossRef] [PubMed]

12. Bertelè, V.; Roncaglioni, M.C.; Pangrazzi, J.; Terzian, E.; Tognoni, E.G. Clinical outcome and its predictors in 1560 patients with critical leg ischaemia. Chronic Critical Leg Ischaemia Group. *Eur. J. Vasc. Endovasc. Surg. Off. J. Eur. Soc. Vasc. Surg.* **1999**, *18*, 401–410. [CrossRef] [PubMed]

13. Baumgartner, I.; Chronos, N.; Comerota, A.; Henry, T.; Pasquet, J.-P.; Finiels, F.; Caron, A.; Dedieu, J.-F.; Pilsudski, R.; Delaère, P. Local gene transfer and expression following intramuscular administration of FGF-1 plasmid DNA in patients with critical limb ischemia. *Mol. Ther. J. Am. Soc. Gene Ther.* **2009**, *17*, 914–921. [CrossRef] [PubMed]

14. Hiatt, W.R.; Hirsch, A.T.; Creager, M.A.; Rajagopalan, S.; Mohler, E.R.; Ballantyne, C.M.; Regensteiner, J.G.; Treat-Jacobson, D.; Dale, R.A.; Rooke, T. Effect of niacin ER/lovastatin on claudication symptoms in patients with peripheral artery disease. *Vasc. Med. Lond. Engl.* **2010**, *15*, 171–179. [CrossRef] [PubMed]

15. Nikol, S.; Baumgartner, I.; van Belle, E.; Diehm, C.; Visoná, A.; Capogrossi, M.C.; Ferreira-Maldent, N.; Gallino, A.; Wyatt, M.G.; Wijesinghe, L.D.; et al. TALISMAN 201 investigators Therapeutic angiogenesis with intramuscular NV1FGF improves amputation-free survival in patients with critical limb ischemia. *Mol. Ther. J. Am. Soc. Gene Ther.* **2008**, *16*, 972–978. [CrossRef] [PubMed]

16. Belch, J.; Hiatt, W.R.; Baumgartner, I.; Driver, I.V.; Nikol, S.; Norgren, L.; van Belle, E. TAMARIS Committees and Investigators Effect of fibroblast growth factor NV1FGF on amputation and death: A randomised placebo-controlled trial of gene therapy in critical limb ischaemia. *Lancet* **2011**, *377*, 1929–1937. [CrossRef]

17. Lederman, R.J.; Mendelsohn, F.O.; Anderson, R.D.; Saucedo, J.F.; Tenaglia, A.N.; Hermiller, J.B.; Hillegass, W.B.; Rocha-Singh, K.; Moon, T.E.; Whitehouse, M.J.; et al. TRAFFIC Investigators Therapeutic angiogenesis with recombinant fibroblast growth factor-2 for intermittent claudication (the TRAFFIC study): A randomised trial. *Lancet* **2002**, *359*, 2053–2058. [CrossRef]

18. Rajagopalan, S.; Mohler, E.R.; Lederman, R.J.; Mendelsohn, F.O.; Saucedo, J.F.; Goldman, C.K.; Blebea, J.; Macko, J.; Kessler, P.D.; Rasmussen, H.S.; et al. Regional angiogenesis with vascular endothelial growth factor in peripheral arterial disease: A phase II randomized, double-blind, controlled study of adenoviral delivery of vascular endothelial growth factor 121 in patients with disabling intermittent claudication. *Circulation* **2003**, *108*, 1933–1938. [PubMed]

19. Tateishi-Yuyama, E.; Matsubara, H.; Murohara, T.; Ikeda, U.; Shintani, S.; Masaki, H.; Amano, K.; Kishimoto, Y.; Yoshimoto, K.; Akashi, H.; et al. Therapeutic Angiogenesis using Cell Transplantation (TACT) Study Investigators Therapeutic angiogenesis for patients with limb ischaemia by autologous transplantation of bone-marrow cells: A pilot study and a randomised controlled trial. *Lancet* **2002**, *360*, 427–435. [CrossRef]

20. Ishida, A.; Ohya, Y.; Sakuda, H.; Ohshiro, K.; Higashiuesato, Y.; Nakaema, M.; Matsubara, S.; Yakabi, S.; Kakihana, A.; Ueda, M.; et al. Autologous peripheral blood mononuclear cell implantation for patients with peripheral arterial disease improves limb ischemia. *Circ. J. Off. J. Jpn. Circ. Soc.* **2005**, *69*, 1260–1265. [CrossRef]

21. Huang, P.; Li, S.; Han, M.; Xiao, Z.; Yang, R.; Han, Z.C. Autologous transplantation of granulocyte colony-stimulating factor-mobilized peripheral blood mononuclear cells improves critical limb ischemia in diabetes. *Diabetes Care* **2005**, *28*, 2155–2160. [CrossRef] [PubMed]

22. Fadini, G.P.; Agostini, C.; Avogaro, A. Autologous stem cell therapy for peripheral arterial disease meta-analysis and systematic review of the literature. *Atherosclerosis* **2010**, *209*, 10–17. [CrossRef] [PubMed]

23. Moazzami, K.; Majdzadeh, R.; Nedjat, S. Local intramuscular transplantation of autologous mononuclear cells for critical lower limb ischaemia. *Cochrane Database Syst. Rev.* **2011**, *12*, CD008347. [PubMed]

24. Silvestre, J.-S.; Smadja, D.M.; Lévy, B.I. Postischemic revascularization: From cellular and molecular mechanisms to clinical applications. *Physiol. Rev.* **2013**, *93*, 1743–1802. [CrossRef] [PubMed]

25. Magri, D.; Vasilas, P.; Muto, A.; Fitzgerald, T.N.; Fancher, T.T.; Feinstein, A.J.; Nishibe, T.; Dardik, A. Elevated monocytes in patients with critical limb ischemia diminish after bypass surgery. *J. Surg. Res.* **2011**, *167*, 140–150. [CrossRef] [PubMed]

26. Capoccia, B.J.; Shepherd, R.M.; Link, D.C. G-CSF and AMD3100 mobilize monocytes into the blood that stimulate angiogenesis *in vivo* through a paracrine mechanism. *Blood* **2006**, *108*, 2438–2445. [CrossRef] [PubMed]

27. Heil, M.; Ziegelhoeffer, T.; Pipp, F.; Kostin, S.; Martin, S.; Clauss, M.; Schaper, W. Blood monocyte concentration is critical for enhancement of collateral artery growth. *Am. J. Physiol. Heart Circ. Physiol.* **2002**, *283*, H2411–H2419. [CrossRef] [PubMed]

28. Heil, M.; Ziegelhoeffer, T.; Wagner, S.; Fernández, B.; Helisch, A.; Martin, S.; Tribulova, S.; Kuziel, W.A.; Bachmann, G.; Schaper, W. Collateral artery growth (arteriogenesis) after experimental arterial occlusion is impaired in mice lacking CC-chemokine receptor-2. *Circ. Res.* **2004**, *94*, 671–677. [CrossRef] [PubMed]

29. Voskuil, M.; van Royen, N.; Hoefer, I.E.; Seidler, R.; Guth, B.D.; Bode, C.; Schaper, W.; Piek, J.J.; Buschmann, I.R. Modulation of collateral artery growth in a porcine hindlimb ligation model using MCP-1. *Am. J. Physiol. Heart Circ. Physiol.* **2003**, *284*, H1422–H1428. [CrossRef] [PubMed]

30. Sarlon, G.; Zemani, F.; David, L.; Duong van Huyen, J.P.; Dizier, B.; Grelac, F.; Colliec-Jouault, S.; Galy-Fauroux, I.; Bruneval, P.; Fischer, A.M.; *et al.* Therapeutic effect of fucoidan-stimulated endothelial colony-forming cells in peripheral ischemia. *J. Thromb. Haemost. JTH* **2012**, *10*, 38–48. [CrossRef] [PubMed]

31. Zemani, F.; Silvestre, J.-S.; Fauvel-Lafeve, F.; Bruel, A.; Vilar, J.; Bieche, I.; Laurendeau, I.; Galy-Fauroux, I.; Fischer, A.M.; Boisson-Vidal, C. *Ex vivo* priming of endothelial progenitor cells with SDF-1 before transplantation could increase their proangiogenic potential. *Arterioscler. Thromb. Vasc. Biol.* **2008**, *28*, 644–650. [CrossRef] [PubMed]

32. Boisson-Vidal, C.; Zemani, F.; Caligiuri, G.; Galy-Fauroux, I.; Colliec-Jouault, S.; Helley, D.; Fischer, A.-M. Neoangiogenesis induced by progenitor endothelial cells: Effect of fucoidan from marine algae. *Cardiovasc. Hematol. Agents Med. Chem.* **2007**, *5*, 67–77. [CrossRef] [PubMed]

33. Luyt, C.-E.; Meddahi-Pellé, A.; Ho-Tin-Noe, B.; Colliec-Jouault, S.; Guezennec, J.; Louedec, L.; Prats, H.; Jacob, M.-P.; Osborne-Pellegrin, M.; Letourneur, D.; *et al.* Low-molecular-weight fucoidan promotes therapeutic revascularization in a rat model of critical hindlimb ischemia. *J. Pharmacol. Exp. Ther.* **2003**, *305*, 24–30. [CrossRef] [PubMed]

34. Nahrendorf, M.; Swirski, F.K.; Aikawa, E.; Stangenberg, L.; Wurdinger, T.; Figueiredo, J.-L.; Libby, P.; Weissleder, R.; Pittet, M.J. The healing myocardium sequentially mobilizes two monocyte subsets with divergent and complementary functions. *J. Exp. Med.* **2007**, *204*, 3037–3047. [CrossRef] [PubMed]

35. Geissmann, F.; Jung, S.; Littman, D.R. Blood monocytes consist of two principal subsets with distinct migratory properties. *Immunity* **2003**, *19*, 71–82. [CrossRef]

36. Hartney, J.M.; Brown, J.; Chu, H.W.; Chang, L.Y.; Pelanda, R.; Torres, R.M. Arhgef1 regulates alpha5beta1 integrin-mediated matrix metalloproteinase expression and is required for homeostatic lung immunity. *Am. J. Pathol.* **2010**, *176*, 1157–1168. [CrossRef] [PubMed]

37. Nourshargh, S.; Alon, R. Leukocyte migration into inflamed tissues. *Immunity* **2014**, *41*, 694–707. [CrossRef] [PubMed]

38. Bergmann, C.E.; Hoefer, I.E.; Meder, B.; Roth, H.; van Royen, N.; Breit, S.M.; Jost, M.M.; Aharinejad, S.; Hartmann, S.; Buschmann, I.R. Arteriogenesis depends on circulating monocytes and macrophage accumulation and is severely depressed in op/op mice. *J. Leukoc. Biol.* **2006**, *80*, 59–65. [CrossRef] [PubMed]

39. Arras, M.; Ito, W.D.; Scholz, D.; Winkler, B.; Schaper, J.; Schaper, W. Monocyte activation in angiogenesis and collateral growth in the rabbit hindlimb. *J. Clin. Invest.* **1998**, *101*, 40–50. [CrossRef] [PubMed]

40. Wolff, R.A.; Tomas, J.J.; Hullett, D.A.; Stark, V.E.; van Rooijen, N.; Hoch, J.R. Macrophage depletion reduces monocyte chemotactic protein-1 and transforming growth factor-beta1 in healing rat vein grafts. *J. Vasc. Surg.* **2004**, *39*, 878–888. [CrossRef] [PubMed]

41. Schepers, A.; Eefting, D.; Bonta, P.I.; Grimbergen, J.M.; de Vries, M.R.; van Weel, V.; de Vries, C.J.; Egashira, K.; van Bockel, J.H.; Quax, P.H.A. Anti-MCP-1 gene therapy inhibits vascular smooth muscle cells proliferation and attenuates vein graft thickening both *in vitro* and *in vivo*. *Arterioscler. Thromb. Vasc. Biol.* **2006**, *26*, 2063–2069. [CrossRef] [PubMed]

42. Tatewaki, H.; Egashira, K.; Kimura, S.; Nishida, T.; Morita, S.; Tominaga, R. Blockade of monocyte chemoattractant protein-1 by adenoviral gene transfer inhibits experimental vein graft neointimal formation. *J. Vasc. Surg.* **2007**, *45*, 1236–1243. [CrossRef] [PubMed]

43. Haroun-Bouhedja, F.; Lindenmeyer, F.; Lu, H.; Soria, C.; Jozefonvicz, J.; Boisson-Vidal, C. *In vitro* effects of fucans on MDA-MB231 tumor cell adhesion and invasion. *Anticancer Res.* **2002**, *22*, 2285–2292. [PubMed]

44. Sadir, R.; Baleux, F.; Grosdidier, A.; Imberty, A.; Lortat-Jacob, H. Characterization of the stromal cell-derived factor-1alpha-heparin complex. *J. Biol. Chem.* **2001**, *276*, 8288–8296. [CrossRef] [PubMed]

45. Thorlacius, H.; Vollmar, B.; Seyfert, U.T.; Vestweber, D.; Menger, M.D. The polysaccharide fucoidan inhibits microvascular thrombus formation independently from P- and L-selectin function *in vivo*. *Eur. J. Clin. Invest.* **2000**, *30*, 804–810. [CrossRef] [PubMed]

46. Frenette, P.S.; Weiss, L. Sulfated glycans induce rapid hematopoietic progenitor cell mobilization: Evidence for selectin-dependent and independent mechanisms. *Blood* **2000**, *96*, 2460–2468. [PubMed]

47. Cambien, B.; Pomeranz, M.; Millet, M.A.; Rossi, B.; Schmid-Alliana, A. Signal transduction involved in MCP-1-mediated monocytic transendothelial migration. *Blood* **2001**, *97*, 359–366. [CrossRef] [PubMed]

48. Ge, H.; Yuan, W.; Liu, J.; He, Q.; Ding, S.; Pu, J.; He, B. Functional Relevance of Protein Glycosylation to the Pro-Inflammatory Effects of Extracellular Matrix Metalloproteinase Inducer (EMMPRIN) on Monocytes/Macrophages. *PLoS ONE* **2015**, *10*, e0117463. [CrossRef] [PubMed]

49. Ashida, N.; Arai, H.; Yamasaki, M.; Kita, T. Distinct signaling pathways for MCP-1-dependent integrin activation and chemotaxis. *J. Biol. Chem.* **2001**, *276*, 16555–16560. [CrossRef] [PubMed]

50. McGilvray, I.D.; Tsai, V.; Marshall, J.C.; Dackiw, A.P.B.; Rotstein, O.D. Monocyte adhesion and transmigration induce tissue factor expression: Role of the mitogen-activated protein kinases. *Shock* **2002**, *18*, 51–57. [CrossRef] [PubMed]

51. Liao, C.-C.; Ho, M.-Y.; Liang, S.-M.; Liang, C.-M. Recombinant protein rVP1 upregulates BECN1-independent autophagy, MAPK1/3 phosphorylation and MMP9 activity via WIPI1/WIPI2 to promote macrophage migration. *Autophagy* **2013**, *9*, 5–19. [CrossRef] [PubMed]

52. Ye, J.; Li, Y.; Teruya, K.; Katakura, Y.; Ichikawa, A.; Eto, H.; Hosoi, M.; Hosoi, M.; Nishimoto, S.; Shirahata, S. Enzyme-digested Fucoidan Extracts Derived from Seaweed Mozuku of Cladosiphon novae-caledoniae kylin Inhibit Invasion and Angiogenesis of Tumor Cells. *Cytotechnology* **2005**, *47*, 117–126. [CrossRef] [PubMed]

53. Lee, H.; Kim, J.-S.; Kim, E. Fucoidan from Seaweed Fucus vesiculosus Inhibits Migration and Invasion of Human Lung Cancer Cell via PI3K-Akt-mTOR Pathways. *PLoS ONE* **2012**, *7*, e50624. [CrossRef] [PubMed]

54. Teng, H.; Yang, Y.; Wei, H.; Liu, Z.; Liu, Z.; Ma, Y.; Gao, Z.; Hou, L.; Zou, X. Fucoidan Suppresses Hypoxia-Induced Lymphangiogenesis and Lymphatic Metastasis in Mouse Hepatocarcinoma. *Mar. Drugs* **2015**, *13*, 3514–3530. [CrossRef] [PubMed]

55. Fitton, J.H. Therapies from fucoidan; Multifunctional marine polymers. *Mar. Drugs* **2011**, *9*, 1731–1760. [CrossRef] [PubMed]

56. Ustyuzhanina, N.E.; Bilan, M.I.; Ushakova, N.A.; Usov, A.I.; Kiselevskiy, M.V.; Nifantiev, N.E. Fucoidans: Pro- or antiangiogenic agents? *Glycobiology* **2014**, *24*, 1265–1274. [CrossRef] [PubMed]

57. Matsubara, K.; Xue, C.; Zhao, X.; Mori, M.; Sugawara, T.; Hirata, T. Effects of middle molecular weight fucoidans on *in vitro* and *ex vivo* angiogenesis of endothelial cells. *Int. J. Mol. Med.* **2005**, *15*, 695–699. [CrossRef] [PubMed]

58. Zemani, F.; Benisvy, D.; Galy-Fauroux, I.; Lokajczyk, A.; Colliec-Jouault, S.; Uzan, G.; Fischer, A.M.; Boisson-Vidal, C. Low-molecular-weight fucoidan enhances the proangiogenic phenotype of endothelial progenitor cells. *Biochem. Pharmacol.* **2005**, *70*, 1167–1175. [CrossRef] [PubMed]

59. Nardella, A.; Chaubet, F.; Boisson-Vidal, C.; Blondin, C.; Durand, P.; Jozefonvicz, J. Anticoagulant low molecular weight fucans produced by radical process and ion exchange chromatography of high molecular weight fucans extracted from the brown seaweed *Ascophyllum nodosum*. *Carbohydr. Res.* **1996**, *289*, 201–208. [CrossRef]

60. Mulloy, B.; Gee, C.; Wheeler, S.F.; Wait, R.; Gray, E.; Barrowcliffe, T.W. Molecular weight measurements of low molecular weight heparins by gel permeation chromatography. *Thromb. Haemost.* **1997**, *77*, 668–674. [PubMed]

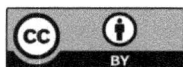

marine drugs

MDPI

Article

Prophylactic Administration of Fucoidan Represses Cancer Metastasis by Inhibiting Vascular Endothelial Growth Factor (VEGF) and Matrix Metalloproteinases (MMPs) in Lewis Tumor-Bearing Mice

Tse-Hung Huang [1,2,†], Yi-Han Chiu [3,†], Yi-Lin Chan [4], Ya-Huang Chiu [3,5], Hang Wang [3,6], Kuo-Chin Huang [7], Tsung-Lin Li [8], Kuang-Hung Hsu [2,9,*] and Chang-Jer Wu [3,10,*]

[1] Department of Traditional Chinese Medicine, Chang Gung Memorial Hospital, Keelung 20401, Taiwan; huangtsehung@gmail.com
[2] Graduate Institute of Clinical Medicine Sciences, Chang Gung University, Taoyuan 33302, Taiwan
[3] Department of Food Science, National Taiwan Ocean University, Keelung 20224, Taiwan; chiuyiham@hotmail.com (Y.-H.C.); p19810222@yahoo.com.tw (Y.-H.C.); sandy72066@hotmail.com (H.W.)
[4] Department of Life Science, Chinese Culture University, Taipei 11114, Taiwan; phd.elainechan@gmail.com
[5] Aquatic Technology Laboratories, Agricultural Technology Research Institute, Hsinchu 30093, Taiwan
[6] Institute of Biomedical Nutrition, Hung Kuang University, Taichung 43302, Taiwan
[7] Holistic Education Center, Mackay Medical College, New Taipei City 25245, Taiwan; kchsports@mmc.edu.tw
[8] Genomics Research Center, Academia Sinica, Taipei 11529, Taiwan; tlli@gate.sinica.edu.tw
[9] Laboratory for Epidemiology, Department and graduate institute of health care management, Chang Gung University, Taoyuan 33302, Taiwan
[10] Center of Excellence for the Oceans, National Taiwan Ocean University, Keelung 20224, Taiwan
* Authors to whom correspondence should be addressed; khsu@mail.cgu.edu.tw (K.-H.H.); wuchangjer@yahoo.com.tw (C.-J.W.); Tel.: +886-3-2118800 (ext.5473) (K.-H.H.); +886-2-24622192 (ext. 5137) (C.-J.W.).
† These authors contributed equally to this work.

Academic Editor: Paola Laurienzo
Received: 12 February 2015; Accepted: 27 March 2015; Published: 3 April 2015

Abstract: Fucoidan, a heparin-like sulfated polysaccharide, is rich in brown algae. It has a wide assortment of protective activities against cancer, for example, induction of hepatocellular carcinoma senescence, induction of human breast and colon carcinoma apoptosis, and impediment of lung cancer cells migration and invasion. However, the anti-metastatic mechanism that fucoidan exploits remains elusive. In this report, we explored the effects of fucoidan on cachectic symptoms, tumor development, lung carcinoma cell spreading and proliferation, as well as expression of metastasis-associated proteins in the Lewis lung carcinoma (LLC) cells-inoculated mice model. We discovered that administration of fucoidan has prophylactic effects on mitigation of cachectic body weight loss and improvement of lung masses in tumor-inoculated mice. These desired effects are attributed to inhibition of LLC spreading and proliferation in lung tissues. Fucoidan also down-regulates expression of matrix metalloproteinases (MMPs), nuclear factor kappa-light-chain-enhancer of activated B cells (NF-κB) and vascular endothelial growth factor (VEGF). Moreover, the tumor-bearing mice supplemented with fucoidan indeed benefit from an ensemble of the chemo-phylacticity. The fact is that fucoidan significantly decreases viability, migration, invasion, and MMPs activities of LLC cells. In summary, fucoidan is suitable to act as a chemo-preventative agent for minimizing cachectic symptoms as well as inhibiting lung carcinoma metastasis through down-regulating metastatic factors VEGF and MMPs.

Keywords: fucoidan; sulfated polysaccharide; lung carcinoma; metastasis; cachexia; chemo-preventative agent

1. Introduction

The international agency for research on cancer (IARC) estimates in 2012 that >14.1 million people were diagnosed with cancer and >8.2 million people died of cancer or cancer-related diseases [1]. Lung cancer accounts for 19.5% of all cancer deaths, the leading cause of cancer death. The non-small-cell lung cancer (NSCLC) takes up approximately 85% out of all lung cancer cases [2]. The five-year survival rate for patients receiving surgical resection, radiation ablation or systemic chemotherapy is as incredibly low as 10%–15%. Recent studies suggested that the primary neoplasm of lung cancer is prone to invade surrounding tissues and then metastasize to distant organs [3]. Metastasis often determines the survival time and the life quality of lung cancer patients [4].

Tumor metastasis of primary tumor cells to distant organs is a multistep process that follows a typical tumor metastatic cascade, such as uncontrolled cell proliferation, tissue remodeling, angiogenesis and invasion [5]. The colonization of tumor cells in secondary organs generally recruits specific sets of proteins at a given time point. Matrix metalloproteinases (MMPs) are known to be closely related to integrity of extracellular matrix (ECM) and basal membrane, of which their disruption is thus correlated to tumor invasiveness. Husmann *et al.* reported that an increase of MMPs in the human osteosarcoma cell model destructs ECM, thus correlating the level of MMPs to tumor metastasis [6]. In NSCLC, tissue inhibitors of metalloproteinases (TIMPs) reported regulate the NSCLC tumor invasion and metastasis [7]. Generally, high expression of MMPs in lung tissues signals a bad prognosis in NSCLC [8].

It has been known that MMPs promote migration of endothelial cells and facilitate formation of new blood vessels. The density of microvessels of tumorigenesis thus reflects patient's prognosis. The vascular endothelial growth factor (VEGF) is one of major proangiogenic factors [9]. VEGF promotes vascular endothelial growth and mediates vessel permeability, thus facilitating tumor progression and metastatic spread [10]. Chen *et al.* reported that over-expression of VEGF in small-cell lung cancer patients has to do with lymph node metastasis [11]. Liu *et al.* also reported that the levels of VEGF-B and MMP9 in the NSCLC metastatic patients are significantly elevated [12]. High expression of VEGF-A but low expression of both VEGF-B and VEGF-D manifests both poor time to progression (TTP) and overall survival (OS) in NSCLC [13].

The ocean is a gigantic pool of biologically active substances [14–17]. Fucoidan, a heparin-like sulfated polysaccharide, is abundant in brown seaweeds. Fucoidan is composed of L-fucose as well as other sugars, such as D-xylose, D-galactose, D-mannose, and glucuronic acid [18]. Several studies have reported that fucoidan carries many desired biological effects, such as anticoagulation/antithrombosis [19], anti-inflammation [20], antioxidation [21], anticancer activity [22], and antiviral activity [23]. Specifically, fucoidan is able to induce senescence against hepatocellular carcinoma [24], induce apoptosis of human breast and colon carcinoma [25], as well as prevent migration and invasion of human lung cancer cells [26]. Additionally, fucoidan is able to suppress tumor growth in NSCLC-bearing nude mice [27], prevent tumor-induced angiogenesis in sarcoma 180-bearing mice [28] and induce apoptosis against 4T1 mouse breast cancer cells [29].

The anticancer mechanism of fucoidan remains far from clear. In this report, we wanted to evaluate the inhibition effects of fucoidan on cachectic symptoms, tumor development, lung carcinoma cell spreading/proliferation, as well as expression of metastasis-associated proteins in an LLC cells-inoculated mice model in order to know whether fucoidan is suitable to serve as a prophylactic agent in the prevention of cancer-cell invasion and metastasis. We also wanted to explore the effect of fucoidan on tumor cell viability, wound healing, invasiveness and MMPs activities. Finally, we summarize that fucoidan is an excellent agent capable of improving cachectic symptoms, inhibiting colonization of lung metastasis, and decreasing tumor cell viability by inhibition of MMPs activities and reduction of VEGF expression.

2. Results

2.1. Fucoidan Mitigates Cachectic Symptoms in LLC-Inoculated C57BL/6 Mice

We set out to establish the prophylactic effect of fucoidan by observing cancer cachectic symptoms and tumor development/metastasis, for which the body weight, and Lewis lung carcinoma cell spreading/proliferation were monitored. The alterations of body weight in testing animals are summarized in Figure 1. The body weights are increased by $16.51\% \pm 3.05\%$ in control mice, while the body weights are slightly increased by $3.34\% \pm 2.75\%$ in tumor bearing control (TB-Con) mice (Figure 1A), indicating that inoculation of tumor cells results in body weight loss ($p < 0.05$). In contrast, the body weights are significantly increased by $19.35\% \pm 3.12\%$ and $19.47\% \pm 6.51\%$ in TB-Lfu and TB-Hfu groups, respectively ($p < 0.001$, Figure 1A).

Table 1 summarizes hematological and spleen immunological parameters. In the TB-Con group, the total red cell (RBC) count is low when compared with those of other groups. The total RBC counts in the mice receiving either a low or high dose of fucoidan are similar to that of control ($p < 0.05$), suggesting that fucoidan can keep tumor-induced RBC steady. In terms of total white cell (WCB) count (including absolute neutrophil, monocyte and lymphocyte), they are all similar. After inoculation of LLC cells, the cell counts of absolute neutrophils, monocytes and lymphocytes were determined to be 6.9 ± 0.8, 2.1 ± 0.6, 0.6 ± 0.1, and $4.4 \pm 0.7 \times 10^9$/L, respectively; significantly lower than those in control. After administration of fucoidan, the leukopenia effects (including neutropenia and lymphopenia) were considerably reduced ($p < 0.05$; Table 1A), indicating that fucoidan alleviates cachectic leukopenia in tumor-bearing mice. However, the subpopulation distributions of spleenocytes did not change in the group subject to tumor inoculation and fucoidan administration (Table 1B).

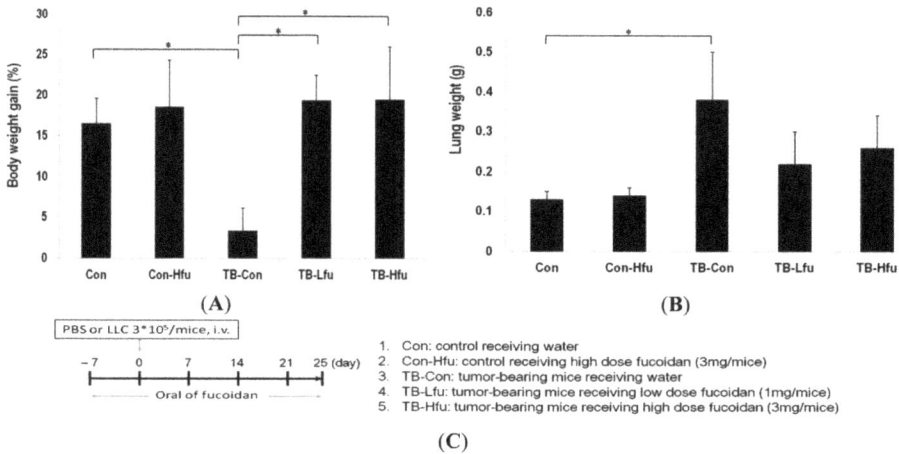

Figure 1. Effects of fucoidan on body weight and lung mass in the LLC xenografted mouse model. At the 25th day, mice were sacrificed and examined for final gains of body weights (**A**) and lung masses (**B**); (**C**) The treatment protocol of fucoidan in tumor-bearing mice. Mice were fed orally with water or low- or high-dose of fucoidan (1 or 3 mg/mice) seven days before tumor implantation. Data are expressed as means $\pm$ SD (n = 6 mice per group; two independent experiments). Asterisk (*) stands for a significant difference when compared with the control group ($p < 0.05$).

The changes of lung masses are relatively minor, which are 0.13 ± 0.02 and 0.14 ± 0.02 g for the control and Con-Hfu mice, respectively, (Figure 1B) as opposed to 0.38 ± 0.12 g for the TB-con mice. These results indicate that fucoidan does not considerably influence the masses of lungs, but LLCs significantly increase lung masses. The increase of lung masses is likely as result of LLCs spreading and proliferation in lung. The lung masses of the TB-Lfu and TB-Hfu groups are 0.22 ± 0.08 and 0.26 ± 0.08 g, respectively, which are significantly smaller than those of the TB-con group ($p < 0.001$, Figure 1B). As a result, the administration of fucoidan does have an effect on reduction of tumor size (Figure 1B).

Table 1. Effects of fucoidan on hematological and spleen immunological parameters in the Lewis lung carcinoma (LLC) xenografted mouse model.

Parameter	Con	Con-Hfu	TB-Con	TB-Lfu	TB-Hfu
		(A) Hematology parameter			
Total red cell count (10^{12}/L)	9.7 ± 0.2	9.4 ± 0.2	6.5 ± 0.2	9.2 ± 0.4 [b]	9.1 ± 0.8 [b]
Total white cell count (10^9/L)	18.9 ± 1.4	23 ± 1.0 [a]	6.9 ± 0.8	14.2 ± 2.0 [b]	14.2 ± 2.2 [b]
Absolute neutrophil count (10^9/L)	3.8 ± 0.7	4.9 ± 0.4 [a]	2.1 ± 0.6	4.1 ± 0.9 [b]	3.4 ± 0.1 [b]
Absolute monocyte count (10^9/L)	1.1 ± 0.2	1.3 ± 0.1	0.6 ± 0.1	0.9 ± 0.3 [b]	0.9 ± 0.3 [b]
Absolute lymphocyte count (10^9/L)	14.1 ± 0.5	16.8 ± 1.3 [a]	4.4 ± 0.7	10.7 ± 1.7 [b]	10.6 ± 1.6 [b]
		(B) Spleenocyte parameter			
CD3[+] (%)	37.6 ± 4.2	35.8 ± 5.6	31.2 ± 2.7	35.5 ± 2.5 [b]	33.5 ± 1.5
CD4[+] (%)	19.4 ± 1.8	15.8 ± 0.8 [a]	16.28 ± 2.6	15.1 ± 2.0	15.4 ± 1.9
CD8[+] (%)	16.8 ± 3.7	17.3 ± 1.5	14.5 ± 1.7	17.1 ± 3.0	15.4 ± 1.4
CD19[+] (%)	45.7 ± 5.0	43.4 ± 4.4	47.5 ± 4.4	47.2 ± 3.9	45.4 ± 3.5

Data are expressed as means $\pm$ S.E. ($n = 6$). [a] $p < 0.05$ *versus* the control group; [b] $p < 0.05$ *versus* the LLC cell-inoculated group.

2.2. Fucoidan Inhibits Lung Metastatic Colonization of LLC Cells in C57BL/6 Mice

Whether fucoidan is able to inhibit lung metastatic colonization of LLC cells was examined. The LLC cells were injected into C57BL/6 mice via tail vein, and observed tumor formation in lung for 25 days. Pulmonary metastasis of the mice treated with/without fucoidan was assessed by counting the number of tumor nodules on the surface of lungs and pleura under macroscopic or microscopic observation at the 25th day (Figure 2A). Multiple metastatic nodules (with a characteristic opaque tumor spot) appeared in lungs for all TB-Con mice (100%), most of which had tumors across pleural and bronchus surfaces. Interestingly, addition with a low or high dose of fucoidan reduced both the number of metastasis in lungs and impeded the dissemination of tumor cells to adjacent areas (Figure 2A). Histological examination using H&E staining identified LLC colonies in lungs of mice intravenously inoculated with LLC cells (Figure 2B). It is worth noting that the tumor sections of TB-Con mice show noticeable increases of metastatic colonies and tumor cells with mitotic nuclei, which agree with macroscopic observations. The histological analysis confirmed that fucoidan significantly suppresses cancer metastasis to lungs. The low dose treatment of fucoidan reduced the number of lung metastatic foci; the high dose treatment had an even stronger effect (Figure 2B), thus concluding that fucoidan possesses anti-metastatic activity.

(A)

(B)

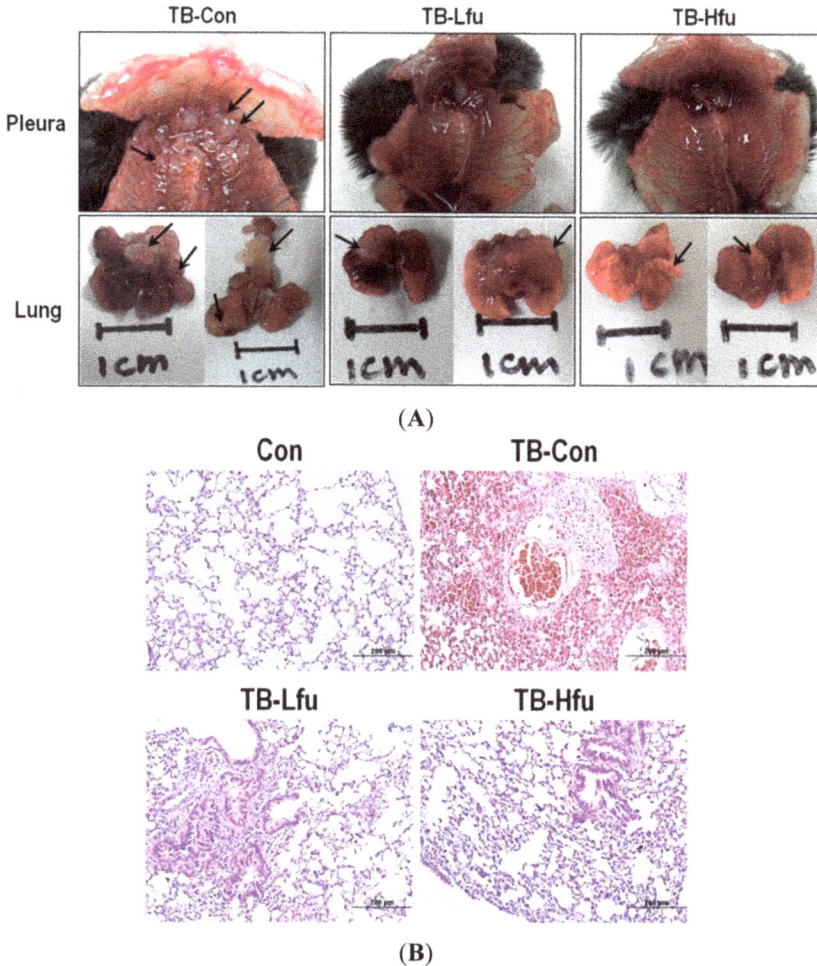

Figure 2. Fucoidan reduces growth of lung tumor in mice. (**A**) Lung, pleural and bronchus tissues. 3×10^5 LLC cells were injected by tail vein in mice. Mice were sacrificed at the 25th day. The solid tumors (indicated by arrows) were spotted on multiple sites in mice; (**B**) Lungs were subjected to histological analysis (H&E stain) for determining metastasis. Six representative samples are shown.

2.3. Fucoidan Restrains LLCs Metastasis by Suppressing Expression of VEGF and MMPs

To determine the mechanism that fucoidan alleviates lung angiogenesis and metastasis of LLCs, we examined protein expression of VEGF, NF-kB and MMPs in lungs and/or sera. The expression of VEGF in sera and lung tissues are summarized in Figures 3 and 4. The level of VEGF in serum was significantly elevated in the LLCs inoculated mice (Figure 3), which is positively correlated with both the expression level of VEGF in lung tissues (Figure 4) and the severity of tumor metastasis. As shown in the immunohistochemical staining, the VEGF immunoreactivity occurs mainly in the cytoplasm of the lung tissues in TB-Con mice (Figure 4C). Upon the fucoidan treatment (1 mg), the expression of VEGF reduced in sera and cytoplasmas in lung tissues as compared to those in TB-Con. This effect is

Mar. Drugs **2015**, *13*, 1882–1990

enhanced when a higher dose (3 mg) of fucoidan was supplemented (Figure 4A,B). MMP-2 and MMP-9 are extracellular metalloproteinases, which play an important role in the degradation of extracellular matrix, thus facilitating cancer cell invasion and migration. It is not surprising that the protein levels of MMP-2 and -9 were increased in mice inoculated with LLCs (Figure 4). Administration of a low or high dose of fucoidan, however, showed declines of MMP-2 and -9. Since the redox-sensitive transcription factor is in charge of sensing oxidative stresses [30], the level of NF-κB is used to index lung cancer progression. The expression of NF-κB in lung tissues is shown in Figure 4, where NF-κB increases significantly upon inoculation with LLCs as compared to that of controls. On receiving either a low or high dose of fucoidan, the expression of NF-κB decreases when compared to that in TB-Con mice. The effect of the high dose is higher than that of the low dose (Figure 4A,B). Fucoidan is thus concluded to carry an anti-metastasis activity.

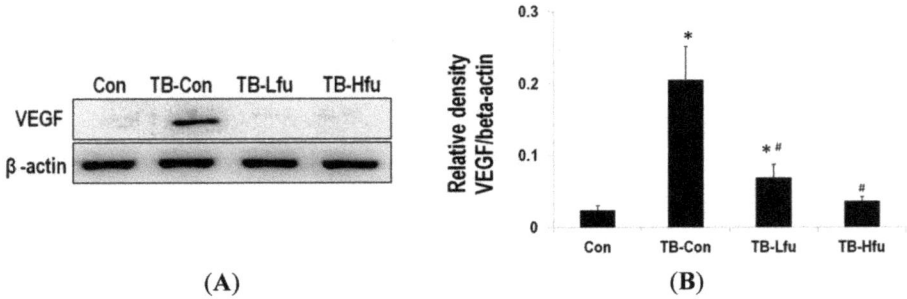

(A) (B)

Figure 3. Expression of metastatic proteins in sera of tumor bearing mice treated with fucoidan. (**A**) Western blot analyses of VEGF from representative mice. Expression levels of VEGF normalized to β-actin (**B**). Asterisk (*) indicates a significant difference (*p* value < 0.05) when compared to the con group. Pound (#) indicates a significant difference (*p* value < 0.05) when compared to TB-Con.

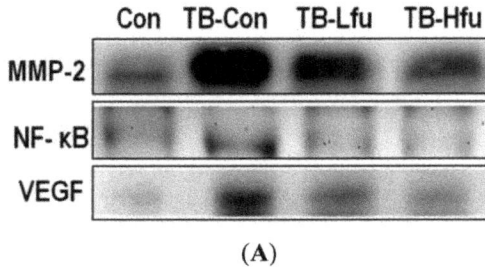

(A)

Figure 4. *Cont.*

(B)

(C)

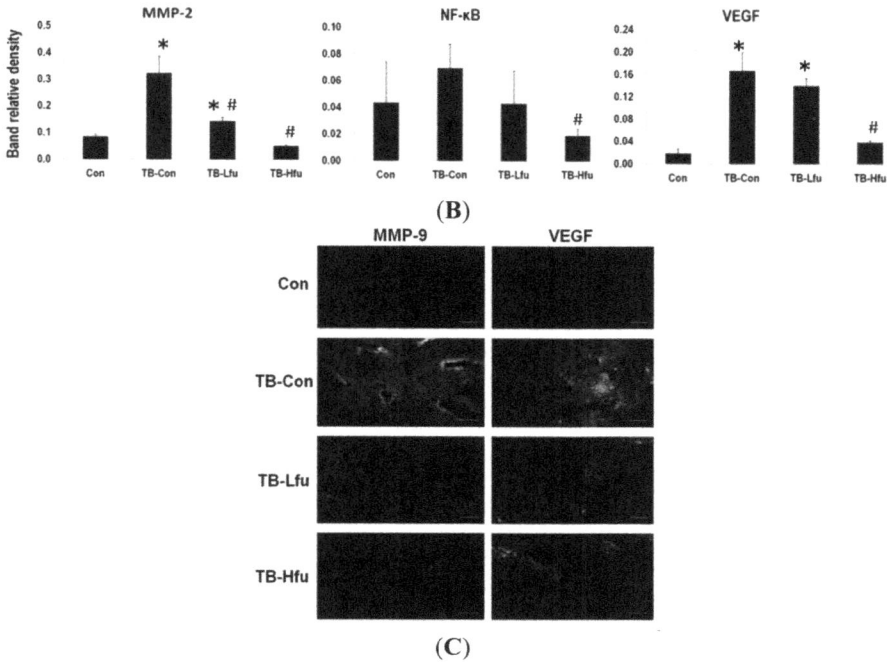

Figure 4. Expression of metastatic proteins in lung tissues of tumor bearing mice treated with fucoidan. (**A**) Western blot analyses of MMP-2, NF-κB and VEGF (from representative samples); (**B**) Protein expression levels that are quantified and expressed as a fold-change relative to the control. Asterisk (*) indicates a significant difference (p value < 0.05) when compared to the con group. Pound (#) indicates a significant difference (p value < 0.05) when compared to TB-Con; (**C**) Immunofluorescence analysis for lung tumors treated and untreated (TB-Con) with fucoidan. Images are shown at 200× magnification.

2.4. Fucoidan Has a Cytotoxic Effect on the LLC Cell Line

Having learned that fucoidan is able to inhibit tumor growth and metastasis in the Lewis lung carcinoma transplantation model, we were keen to know its molecular/cellular mechanism. For this, the Vero normal kidney epithelial cells and Lewis lung carcinoma cells were incubated for 24 h in the presence of various concentrations of fucoidan. The MTS assay showed that fucoidan damages cell viability of LLCs in a concentration-dependent manner. As shown in Figure 5, the cell viabilities are 92.86% ± 3.97%, 94.57% ± 6.77%, 85.99% ± 7.51% and 82.43% ± 5.08% in the presence of 0.05, 0.1, 0.2 and 0.4 mg/mL fucoidan, respectively. LLCs decline significantly in the presence of 0.4 mg/mL fucoidan when compared to the one with no added fucoidan ($p < 0.05$). In contrast, the Vero normal kidney epithelial cells increase (Figure 5); hence fucoidan sensitizes LLC cancer cells but not Vero normal cells.

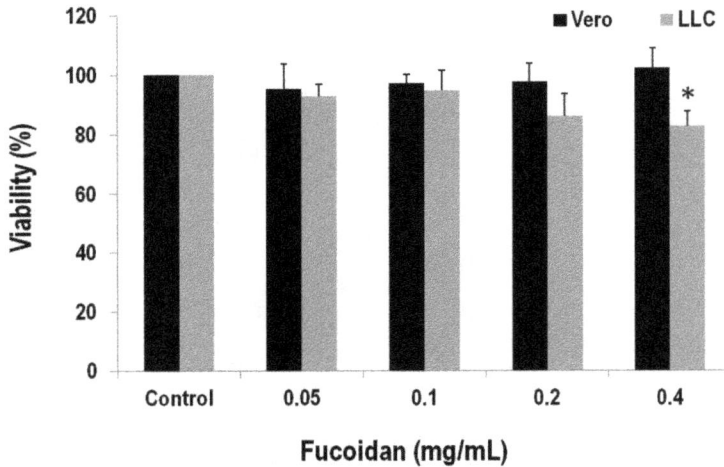

Figure 5. Effects of fucoidan on cell viability in African green monkey kidney Vero and mouse Lewis lung carcinoma cells. Cells were incubated in a culture medium containing various concentrations of fucoidan for 24 h. After the treatment, cell viability was determined by the MTS assay. Values relative to that of vehicle control were determined, in which the cell viability of control is set as 100%. Data (each value is an average of at least three independent experiments (six tests)) are presented as mean ± SEM. Asterisk (*) indicates a significant difference (p value < 0.05) relative to the vehicle-treated cells.

2.5. Fucoidan Prevents Metastasis of Lung Adenocarcinoma Cells

To verify the *in vivo* inhibitory effect of fucoidan on LLC metastasis, we tested various concentrations of fucoidan on the migration and invasion of the LLC cells by the wound healing and chamber assays. In the wound-healing assay, the control cells migrated to a wound area where the wound edges became undistinguishable, whereas the cells with addition of fucoidan displayed slower wound closure (Figure 6A). To correlate the cell movement with the quantity of fucoidan, the migration inhibition was determined to be 24.76% ± 2.04%, 29.97% ± 8.15%, 49.03% ± 7.55% and 68.70% ± 7.94% *versus* 0.05, 0.1, 0.2 and 0.4 mg/mL fucoidan, respectively (Figure 6B).

In the invasion chamber assay, matrigel-coated membranes were used to investigate the invasive properties of the cells treated with/without fucoidan. After LLC cells were incubated for 24 h in a transwell assay system, the number of cells for those that had moved through the membrane of the chamber declined as 33.50% ± 7.63%, 45.92% ± 9.35%, 59.61% ± 9.44% and 70.83% ± 6.61% against the number of the control (p < 0.01, Figure 6C,D) for the cells added with 0.05, 0.1, 0.2 and 0.4 mg/mL fucoidan, respectively. Fucoidan is thus concluded able to prevent metastasis of lung adenocarcinoma cells.

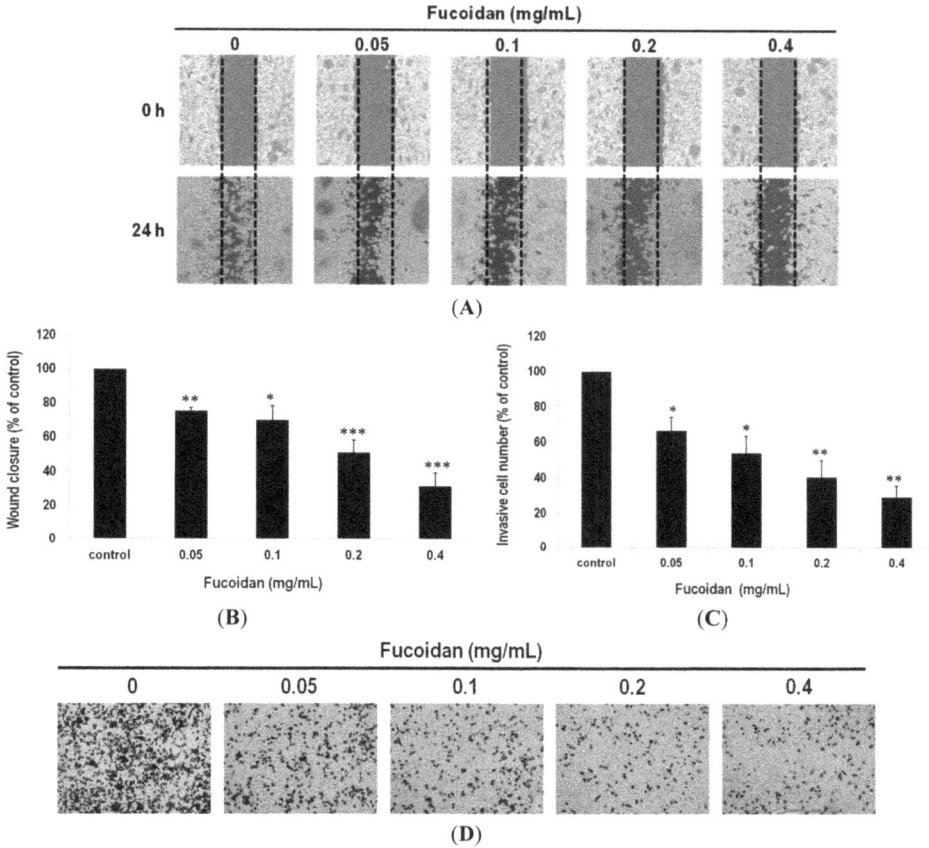

Figure 6. Suppression of migration and invasion of lung adenocarcinoma cells by fucoidan. (**A**) Representative photographs of three independent experiments, showing a dose-dependent inhibition of migration after treatment of fucoidan (24 h). Images of wound closures (10× magnification); (**B**) Black dotted lines indicate the wound edge. The cell-free areas invaded by cells (across the black dotted lines) were quantified by three random fields as shown in the lower panels; (**C**) The invasiveness of the LLC cells were quantified by counting the stained cells that invade into the porous polycarbonate membrane; (**D**) Invasiveness of the LLC cells treated with fucoidan. The LLC cells were pretreated with fucoidan for 24 h and then seeded onto the transwell chamber. Photographs were taken by an inverted microscope with 10× magnification. Data were derived from three independent experiments and presented as mean ± SEM. * $p < 0.05$, ** $p < 0.001$, *** $p < 0.0001$ when compared to the vehicle-treated cells.

2.6. Effects of Fucoidan on Expression and Activity of MMPs

Whether the reduced invasion/migration upon addition of fucoidan is related to MMP proteins in LLC cells was examined. As shown in Figure 7A, the enzyme activities of both MMP-2 and MMP-9 declined significantly in the gelatin zymography assays. Namely, the MMP-2 activities dropped to 36.44% ± 14.74%, 22.22% ± 7.30%, 13.07% ± 4.49% and 2.89% ± 2.50% for the samples with 0.05, 0.1, 0.2 and 0.4 mg/mL fucoidan added, respectively (Figure 7B). MMP-9 behaved similarly when exposed to fucoidan. Likewise, the MMP-9 activities dropped to 6.44% ± 5.68%, 5.04% ± 4.59% and 0.12% ± 0.20% for the samples with 0.05, 0.1 and 0.2 mg/mL fucoidan added, respectively (Figure 7B).

Interestingly, the MMP-9 activity was not detected when the concentration of fucoidan was raised to 0.4 mg/mL.

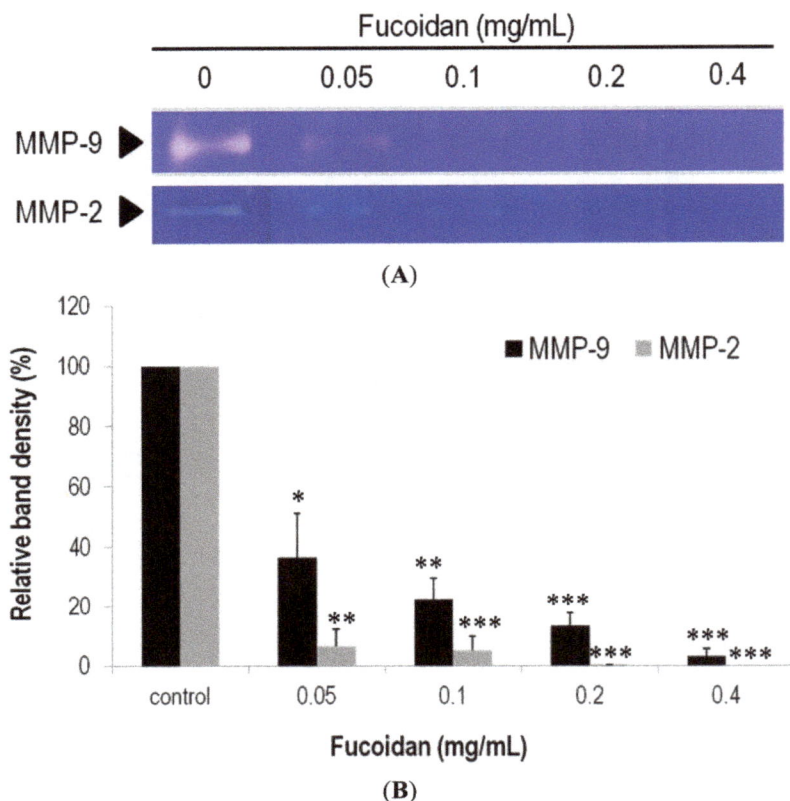

Figure 7. Enzymatic activities of MMP-2 and MMP-9 in the LLC cell lines treated with fucoidan. (**A**) The activity of MMPs was determined by the gelatinase zymography, in which the bright zones stand for gelatin digested; (**B**) The MMPs activity was quantified by measuring the band intensity in the zymography. Data were derived from three independent experiments and presented as mean ± SEM. * $p < 0.05$, ** $p < 0.001$, *** $p < 0.0001$ when compared to the vehicle-treated cells.

3. Discussion

Fucoidan was reported with anticancer activity [24–29]. It was also reported that the people that consume higher fucoidan-containing seaweeds have low incidences of certain tumors. Given that Lewis lung carcinoma cells (LLCs) specifically invade lungs and that removal of the primary tumor facilitates tumor metastasis, we herein verified that administration of fucoidan considerably reduces the metastatic load in a dose-dependent manner. The fact is partially due to that administration of fucoidan reduces cachectic body weight loss, hematological anemia/leukopenia, and the tumor-induced mass increase of lungs. In all TB-Con animals multiple metastatic nodules located in lungs, where they showed as opaque spots invading bilaterally throughout the pleural and bronchus surfaces. When pretreated with a low or high dose of fucoidan, metastatic nodules declined significantly, strongly supporting that fucoidan has a high anti-metastatic activity.

Metastasis impairs quality of life and results in a poor prognosis [4]. Current mainstay treatments, such as chemotherapy, radiation therapy and target therapy, all come along with severe side-effects. The prophylactic treatment now emerges as a new way to control or prevent micrometastases. An effective anti-VEGF agent ideally is able to block formation of new tumor vessels or even to prune away existing ones. One sad example is that bevacizumab seemed able to wither tumor vessels and reduce tumor microvascular density by 40%–50% in the phase I trial for rectal cancer patients [31], while it failed in the phase III trial as result of increased expression of some angiogenic factors [32]. Prophylactic cranial irradiation has shown a promising outcome, where brain metastases in NSCLC patients were prevented [33]. In our study, fucoidan was shown to prophylactically inhibit lung metastasis colonization of LLC cells in C57BL/6 mice. Fucoidan acts likely to down-regulate the expression of MMPs, NF-κB and VEGF. VEGF was described as a multifunctional angiogenic regulator that stimulates epithelial cell proliferation, blood vessel formation and endothelial cell survival [34]. High levels of VEGF were detected in sera and tumor tissues in mice, well correlating VEGF overexpression with tumor metastasis as well as poor survival rate. Interestingly, fucoidan can reduce the tumor-induced VEGF expression as well as the expression of MMP-2, MMP-9 and NF-κB in lung tissues, suggesting fucoidan restrains cancer cells from invasion and metastasis through suppressing epithelial cell proliferation and blood vessel formation.

To further explore the mechanism underlying fucoidan's protective effect, we evaluated the effects of fucoidan on cell viability of normal and cancer cells. LLC mouse lung cancer cells are more susceptible to fucoidan than Vero kidney normal cells, as fucoidan significantly reduced viability of LLC cells at the level of 0.4 mg/mL. In contrast, fucoidan does not have cytotoxicity to Vero cells. Our result agrees with previous studies, where fucoidan inhibited the growth of skin and lung cancer cells but enhanced normal cell immune activity [35].

The motility factors, such as MMP-2 and MMP-9, which govern metastasis, have been well documented. On the basis of our results, fucoidan is able to mediate the activities of MMP-2 and MMP-9, also in line with the report that fucoidan suppressed migration and invasion of A549 lung cancer cells by suppressing secretion and/or expression of MMP-2 [26]. Although both LLC and A549 cells are highly invasive and metastatic [36,37], the LLC cells are more susceptible to MMPs under the mediation of fucoidan on the basis of our results.

4. Materials and Method

4.1. Cells and Cell Culture

Lewis lung carcinoma cells (LLC, C57BL/6 strain mice lung cancer cell line, ATCC CRL-1642) were obtained from the Bioresource Collection and Research Center (Hsinchu, Taiwan). LLC cells were maintained in Dulbecco's modified Eagle's medium (DMEM) supplemented with 10% fetal bovine serum. Cells were cultured at 37 °C in a humidified incubator with an atmosphere of 5% CO_2.

4.2. Preparation of Fucoidan Extract

Commercially available fucoidan purified from *F. vesiculosus* (F5631) was purchased from Sigma-Aldrich, Inc. (St. Louis, MO, USA). Due to a substantial difficulty (the fact is that the structures of fucoidan polysaccharides have not yet been determined in detail), the purchased fucoidan was not subjected to further purification. The purchased fucoidan was used to examine its *in vitro* effects on anti-migration and -invasion in a simulated gastric fluid (SGF) or intestinal fluid (SIF) system. The fucoidan powders were dissolved in PBS and the simulated gastric (pH 1.2) and intestinal fluids (pH 7.5) with continuous mixing at 200 rpm for 3 h. The mixture was then placed in an 80 °C water bath (Julabo, Germany) to denature the enzymes in the gastric and intestinal fluids. It was sterilized using a 0.45 mm pore filter (Merck KGaA, Darmstadt, Germany) and stored as "fucoidan extract (20 mg/mL)" at 4 °C until use.

4.3. Ethical Approval and Animals

Male C57BL/6 mice (6–8 weeks) were obtained from the National Laboratory Animal Center (Taipei, Taiwan, ROC) and housed in a climate controlled room (12:12 dark-light cycle with a constant room temperature of 21 ± 1 °C). Mice underwent at least 4-day adjustment to new environment and diet before treatments were performed. Food and water were given *ad libitum*. All methods were performed with approval from the Animal Care and Use Committee of National Taiwan Ocean University.

4.4. Experimental Design

To examine the effects of fucoidan on the cancer metastasis, mice were divided into five weight-matched groups in the preventive model: (1) control receiving water (Con); (2) control receiving high dose (3 mg/mice) fucoidan (Con-Hfu); (3) tumor-bearing mice receiving water (TB-Con); (4) tumor-bearing mice receiving low dose (1 mg/mice) fucoidan (TB-Lfu); and (5) tumor-bearing mice receiving high dose (3 mg/mice) fucoidan (TB-Hfu). Commercially available fucoidan without further process was used in animal study. One milligram or three milligram fucoidan were diluted in 500 μL water and feed to mice once a day by intragastric gavage 7 days prior to tumor inoculation. At the 7th day post oral administration, 3×10^5 live LLC cells in 100 μL PBS were injected into mice through tail vein. Mice were kept to receive fucoidan or water orally until the due course of the experiment. In all experiments, animals were anaesthetized by CO_2 inhalation method and weighted at the termination of the experiment on day 25. Following sacrifice, the lung tissues were fixed in 4% paraformaldehyde and stained with hematoxylin and eosin. Final body weight gain was calculated as the difference between the carcass and initial weight.

4.5. Blood Sample Analysis

Blood samples (0.5 mL) for measurements of red blood cells (RBC), white blood cells (WBC), lymphocyte, monocyte and neutrophil counts were determined by a blood cell analyzer (Symex K-1000, Sysmex American, Mundelein, IL, USA).

4.6. Flow Cytometry

During flow cytometry, at least 5×10^5 spleenocytes were analyzed by Becton–Dickinson FACSan flow cytometer (Franklin Lakes, NJ, USA) with CellQuest software (Becton–Dickinson, Oxford, UK). Lymphocytes were gated based on the expression of CD3 and CD4 or CD8. B cells were gated based on the expression of $CD19^+$.

4.7. Lewis Lung Carcinoma Cells Metastasis Models

For the passive metastasis model, Lewis lung carcinoma cells (3×10^5 cells in 100 μL PBS) were injected via the tail vein into mice as described previously. At the end of the experiments, the lungs were harvested and the surface nodules were counted to evaluate the metastatic spread of the tumor. Tissues with metastases were either photographed for gross morphology or further analyzed by histology. For pulmonary nodule enumeration, the number of metastatic foci in H&E stained lung sections was counted in a blinded fashion.

4.8. Western Blot Analysis

Confluent cell lines cultures were washed with buffered salt solution and treated with fucoidan in the serum-free medium for 24 h. At the end of the experiments, medium was removed and 500 mL was concentrated using Microcon concentrators (Millipore, Bedford, MA, USA) for 30 min at 25 °C. Concentrated samples with equal amounts of protein (25 mg) were mixed with 2 mL reducing sample buffer and resolved by SDS/PAGE, transferred to nitrocellulose membrane (Bio-Rad, Hercules, CA, USA), and the blot was probed with polyclonal goat anti-mice MMP-2, NF-κB, VEGF and β-actin antibodies (Santa Cruz Biotechnology, Santa Cruz, CA, USA). Immunoreactive proteins were visualized by Immobilon™ Western chemiluminescent HRP Substrate kit (Millipore, Bedford, MA, USA). Images were captured and the intensities of the protein bands were analyzed using the Lab works® software (V4.5, UVP Inc., Upland, CA, USA) are expressed as arbitrary optical density unit.

4.9. Histopathological Analysis

Tumor and lung tissues were collected from mice, washed carefully by cold normal saline 3 times, then fixed in 10% formalin solution, processed, and embedded in a paraffin film. Sections of 5-μm thick slices of tissues were prepared. The sections were stained with H&E. Microscopic observations were carried out at 200× magnifications.

4.10. Immunofluorescence Assay

Sections were blocked by blocking buffer for 1 h at room temperature then stained with primary antibody at 1:200 dilution for 24 h. The primary antibody was washed by phosphate buffered saline (PBS). Sections were stained with secondary antibody at 1:100 dilution for 24 h at room temperature then washed with PBS. The primary antibodies that were used are as follows: rabbit anti-mouse VEGF (Santa Cruz Biotechnology, Santa Cruz, CA, USA) and rabbit anti-mouse MMP-9 (Santa Cruz Biotechnology, Santa Cruz, CA, USA). The secondary antibodies were FITC-conjugates goat anti-rabbit IgG (Sigma, Sanint Louis, MO, USA).

4.11. Cell Viability Assay

(3-(4,5-dimethylthiazol-2-yl)-5-(3-carboxymethoxyphenyl)-2-(4-sulfophenyl)-2H-tetrazolium) (MTS) assay is a colorimetric assay based on the ability of viable cells to change from soluble yellow tetrazolium salt to blue formazan crystals. LLC cells (0.5×10^4 cells/mL) were first pretreated with varying concentrations of fucoidan for 24 h. After drugs treatment, cells were washed with incubation buffer, collected by centrifugation, and then suspended in the incubation buffer, containing 0.5 mg/mL MTS for 4 h. After MTS treatment, cells were collected by centrifugation, and then suspended in DMSO for 10 min to thoroughly dissolve the dark blue crystals. The absorbency at a wavelength of 490 nm was measured by spectrophotometer. The cell viability was determined by comparing the results with the absorbency of the untreated cells.

4.12. Cell Migration and Invasion Assays

LLC cells migration and invasion were determined using the wound healing assays and transwell plate as previously described. Briefly, for wound healing assays, LLC cells (5×10^5/well) were seeded and grown overnight to 90%–95% confluence in 12-well plates before wounds of similar size were introduced into the monolayer by a sterile pipette tip. The monolayers were rinsed with phosphate buffer saline (PBS) to remove detached cells and then cultured in medium containing varying concentration of fucoidan. The speed of wound closure was documented 24 h post-wounding using the Nikon Eclipse TE2000U microscope (Melville, NY, USA).

Cell invasion assays were performed using transwell cell culture inserts (Becton Dickinson, Franklin Lakes, NJ, USA). As many as 3.5×10^5 cells were placed in the top part of the chamber. The top part of the chamber was filled with DMEM or with medium supplemented with varying concentration of fucoidan, while DMEM supplemented with 10% FBS was added in the bottom part of the chamber. Incubation was carried out at 37 °C for 24 h. The filters were removed and fixed with 100% methanol for 8–10 min at room temperature. Cells on the upper filter surface were removed with a cotton swab. The filters were stained with 0.2% w/v crystal violet, washed with PBS (pH 7.4), and observed under a light microscope operating at 200× magnification. The invasion index was defined as the ratio of the percent invasion obtained with invaded cells (LLC cells) to the percent invaded obtained with non-invaded cells.

4.13. Gelatin Zymography

LLC cell lines were starved for 24 h with medium containing no FBS. Subsequently, the cells in media containing 0.5% FBS were stimulated with varying concentration of fucoidan for different time periods, and then the supernatants were collected. The samples were analyzed with gelatin zymography, (0.1% w/v) gelatin (Sigma, Sanint Louis, MO, USA) as the substrate. Each lane was loaded with a total protein concentration of 3 μg and subjected to SDS-PAGE electrophoresis at 48 °C. Gels were washed twice in 50 mM Tris (pH 7.4) containing 2.5% (v/v) Triton X-100 for 1 h, followed by two 10-min rinses in 50 mM Tris (pH 7.4). After SDS removal, the gels were incubated overnight in 50 mM Tris (pH 7.5) containing 10 mM $CaCl_2$, 0.15 M NaCl, 0.1% (v/v) Triton X-100, and 0.02% sodium azide at 37 °C under constant gentle shaking. After incubation, the gels were stained with 0.25% Coomassie brilliant blue R-250 (Sigma, Sanint Louis, MO, USA) and destained in 7.5% acetic acid with 20% methanol. The gelatinase bands appeared white on a blue background.

4.14. Statistical Analysis

All experiments were performed at least 3 times, each time in triplicate. Data were analyzed by multivariate ANOVA test. If a significant difference was found, a least significant differences (LSD) multiple comparison test was used to identify significant groups. Statistical analyses used The Statistical Software Package for the Social Sciences, version 12.0.1 for Windows (SPSS Inc., Chicago, IL, USA). A p value < 0.05 was considered statistically significant.

5. Conclusions

Fucoidan exhibits an anti-metastasis activity, which could ensure traditional therapeutic efficacy. The beneficial effects of fucoidan are largely attributed to down-regulation of MMPs, NF-κB and VEGF.

Acknowledgments: This study was partially supported by the Ministry of Science and Technology (NSC102-2628-B-019-001-MY3), Technology Development Program for Academia, Ministry of Economic Affairs (101, 102, 103-EC-17-A17-S1-210) and Chang-Gung Memorial Hospital Research Foundation (CMRPG2C0441-2 and CMRPG2C0491-2), Taiwan.

Author Contributions: T.-H.H., Y.H.-C., K.-H.H. and C.-J.W. conceived and designed the experiments. T.-H.H., Y.H.-C., Y.-L.C., Y.-H.C. and H.W. performed the experiments and analyzed the data. K.-C.H. and T.-L.L. helped acquired data and statistical analysis. T.-H.H., Y.H.-C., Y.-L.C., T.-L.L., K.-H.H. and C.-J.W. wrote the paper.

Conflicts of Interest: The authors disclose no potential conflicts of interest.

References

1. Ferlay, J.; Soerjomataram, I.I.; Dikshit, R.; Eser, S.; Mathers, C.; Rebelo, M.; Parkin, D.M.; Forman, D.D.; Bray, F. Cancer incidence and mortality worldwide: Sources, methods and major patterns in GLOBOCAN 2012. *Int. J. Cancer* **2014**. [CrossRef]
2. Meoni, G.; Cecere, F.L.; Lucherini, E.; di Costanzo, F. Medical treatment of advanced non-small cell lung cancer in elderly patients: A review of the role of chemotherapy and targeted agents. *J. Geriatr. Oncol.* **2013**, *4*, 282–290. [CrossRef] [PubMed]
3. Bremnes, R.M.; Camps, C.; Sirera, R. Angiogenesis in non-small cell lung cancer: The prognostic impact of neoangiogenesis and the cytokines VEGF and bFGF in tumours and blood. *Lung Cancer* **2006**, *51*, 143–158. [CrossRef] [PubMed]
4. Juhász, E.; Kim, J.H.; Klingelschmitt, G.; Walzer, S. Effects of erlotinib first-line maintenance therapy versus placebo on the health-related quality of life of patients with metastatic non-small-cell lung cancer. *Eur. J. Cancer* **2013**, *49*, 1205–1215. [CrossRef] [PubMed]
5. Folkman, J. Role of angiogenesis in tumor growth and metastasis. *Semin. Oncol.* **2002**, *29*, 15–18. [CrossRef] [PubMed]
6. Husmann, K.; Arlt, M.J.; Muff, R.; Langsam, B.; Bertz, J.; Born, W.; Fuchs, B. Matrix Metalloproteinase 1 promotes tumor formation and lung metastasis in an intratibial injectionosteosarcoma mouse model. *Biochim. Biophys. Acta* **2013**, *1832*, 347–354. [CrossRef] [PubMed]

7. Safranek, J.; Pesta, M.; Holubec, L.; Kulda, V.; Dreslerova, J.; Vrzalova, J.; Topolcan, O.; Pesek, M.; Finek, J.; Treska, V. Expression of MMP-7, MMP-9, TIMP-1 and TIMP-2 mRNA in lung tissue of patients with non-small cell lung cancer (NSCLC) and benign pulmonary disease. *Anticancer Res.* **2009**, *29*, 2513–2517. [PubMed]

8. Zhou, H.; Wu, A.; Fu, W.; Lv, Z.; Zhang, Z. Significance of semaphorin-3A and MMP-14 protein expression in non-small cell lung cancer. *Oncol. Lett.* **2014**, *7*, 1395–1400. [PubMed]

9. Wimberger, P.; Chebouti, I.; Kasimir-Bauer, S.; Lachmann, R.; Kuhlisch, E.; Kimmig, R.; Süleyman, E.; Kuhlmann, J.D. Explorative investigation of vascular endothelial growth factor receptor expression in primary ovarian cancer and its clinical relevance. *Gynecol. Oncol.* **2014**, *133*, 467–472. [CrossRef] [PubMed]

10. Shinkaruk, S.; Bayle, M.; Laïn, G.; Déléris, G. Vascular endothelial cell growth factor (VEGF), an emerging target for cancer chemotherapy. *Curr. Med. Chem. Anticancer Agents* **2003**, *3*, 95–117. [CrossRef] [PubMed]

11. Chen, P.; Zhu, J.; Liu, D.Y.; Li, H.Y.; Xu, N.; Hou, M. Over-expression of survivin and VEGF in small-cell lung cancer may predict the poorer prognosis. *Med. Oncol.* **2014**, *31*, 775. [CrossRef] [PubMed]

12. Liu, G.; Xu, S.; Jiao, F.; Ren, T.; Li, Q. Vascular endothelial growth factor B coordinates metastasis of non-small cell lung cancer. *Tumour. Biol.* **2014**. [CrossRef]

13. Sanmartín, E.; Sirera, R.; Usó, M.; Blasco, A.; Gallach, S.; Figueroa, S.; Martínez, N.; Hernando, C.; Honguero, A.; Martorell, M.; *et al.* A gene signature combining the tissue expression of three angiogenic factors is a prognostic marker in early-stage non-small cell lung cancer. *Ann. Surg. Oncol.* **2014**, *21*, 612–620. [CrossRef] [PubMed]

14. Chen, J.; Wu, Q.; Rowley, D.C.; Al-Kareef, A.M.; Wang, H. Anticancer agent-based marine natural products and related compounds. *J. Asian Nat. Prod. Res.* **2015**, *3*, 1–18.

15. Nagamine, T.; Nakazato, K.; Tomioka, S.; Iha, M.; Nakajima, K. Intestinal absorption of fucoidan extracted from the brown seaweed, Cladosiphon okamuranus. *Mar. Drugs* **2014**, *13*, 48–64. [CrossRef] [PubMed]

16. Silva, T.H.; Moreira-Silva, J.; Marques, A.L.; Domingues, A.; Bayon, Y.; Reis, R.L. Marine origin collagens and its potential applications. *Mar. Drugs* **2014**, *12*, 5881–5901. [CrossRef] [PubMed]

17. Nair, D.G.; Weiskirchen, R.; Al-Musharafi, S.K. The use of marine-derived bioactive compounds as potential hepatoprotective agents. *Acta Pharmacol. Sin.* **2014**. [CrossRef]

18. Kwak, J.Y. Fucoidan as a marine anticancer agent in preclinical development. *Mar. Drugs* **2014**, *12*, 851–870. [CrossRef] [PubMed]

19. Zhu, Z.; Zhang, Q.; Chen, L.; Ren, S.; Xu, P.; Tang, Y.; Luo, D. Higher specificity of the activity of low molecular weight fucoidan for thrombin-induced platelet aggregation. *Thrombo. Res.* **2010**, *125*, 419–426. [CrossRef]

20. Semenov, A.V.; Mazurov, A.V.; Preobrazhenskaia, M.E.; Ushakova, N.A.; Mikhaĭlov, V.I.; Berman, A.E.; Usov, A.I.; Nifant'ev, N.E.; Bovin, N.V. Sulfated polysaccharides as inhibitors of receptor activity of P-selectin and P-selectin-dependent inflammation. *Vopr. Med. Khim.* **1998**, *44*, 135–144. [PubMed]

21. Wang, J.; Zhang, Q.; Zhang, Z.; Song, H.; Li, P. Potential antioxidant and anticoagulant capacity of low molecular weight fucoidan fractions extracted from Laminaria japonica. *Int. J. Biol. Macromol.* **2010**, *46*, 6–12. [CrossRef] [PubMed]

22. Veena, C.K.; Josephine, A.; Preetha, S.P.; Varalakshmi, P.; Sundarapandiyan, R. Renal peroxidative changes mediated by oxalate: The protective role of fucoidan. *Life Sci.* **2006**, *79*, 1789–1795. [CrossRef] [PubMed]

23. Hayakawa, K.; Nagamine, T. Effect of fucoidan on the biotinidase kinetics in human hepatocellular carcinoma. *Anticancer Res.* **2009**, *29*, 1211–1217. [PubMed]

24. Min, E.Y.; Kim, I.H.; Lee, J.; Kim, E.Y.; Choi, Y.H.; Nam, T.J. The effects of fucodian on senescence are controlled by the p16INK4a-pRb and p14Arf-p53 pathways in hepatocellular carcinoma and hepatic cell lines. *Int. J. Oncol.* **2014**, *45*, 47–56. [PubMed]

25. Chen, S.; Zhao, Y.; Zhang, Y.; Zhang, D. Fucoidan induces cancer cell apoptosis by modulating the endoplasmic reticulum stress cascades. *PLoS ONE* **2014**, *9*, e108157. [CrossRef] [PubMed]

26. Lee, H.; Kim, J.S.; Kim, E. Fucoidan from seaweed fucus vesiculosus inhibits migration and invasion of human lung cancer cell via PI3K-Akt-mTOR pathways. *PLoS ONE* **2012**, *7*, e50624. [CrossRef] [PubMed]

27. Riou, D.; Colliec-Jouault, S.; Pinczon du Sel, D.; Bosch, S.; Siavoshian, S.; le Bert, V.; Tomasoni, C.; Sinquin, C.; Durand, P.; Roussakis, C. Antitumor and antiproliferative effects of a fucan extracted from ascophyllum nodosum against a non-small-cell bronchopulmonary carcinoma line. *Anticancer Res.* **1996**, *16*, 1213–1218. [PubMed]

28. Koyanagi, S.; Tanigawa, N.; Nakagawa, H.; Soeda, S.; Shimeno, H. Oversulfation of fucoidan enhances its anti-angiogenic and antitumor activities. *Biochem. Pharmacol.* **2003**, *65*, 173–179. [CrossRef] [PubMed]

29. Xue, M.; Ge, Y.; Zhang, J.; Wang, Q.; Hou, L.; Liu, Y.; Sun, L.; Li, Q. Anticancer properties and mechanisms of fucoidan on mouse breast cancer *in vitro* and *in vivo*. *PLoS ONE* **2012**, *7*, e43483. [CrossRef] [PubMed]

30. Meng, Q.; Peng, Z.; Chen, L.; Si, J.; Dong, Z.; Xia, Y. Nuclear factor-κB modulates cellular glutathione and prevents oxidative stress in cancer cells. *Cancer Lett.* **2010**, *299*, 45–53. [CrossRef] [PubMed]

31. Willett, C.G.; Boucher, Y.; Duda, D.G.; di Tomaso, E.; Munn, L.L.; Tong, R.T.; Kozin, S.V.; Petit, L.; Jain, R.K.; Chung, D.C.; *et al.* Surrogate markers for antiangiogenic therapy and dose-limiting toxicities for bevacizumab with radiation and chemotherapy: Continued experience of a phase I trial in rectal cancer patients. *J. Clin. Oncol.* **2005**, *23*, 8136–8139. [CrossRef] [PubMed]

32. Miller, K.D.; Chap, L.I.; Holmes, F.A.; Cobleigh, M.A.; Marcom, P.K.; Fehrenbacher, L.; Dickler, M.; Overmoyer, B.A.; Reimann, J.D.; Sing, A.P.; *et al.* Randomized phase III trial of capecitabine compared with bevacizumab plus capecitabine in patients with previously treated metastatic breast cancer. *J. Clin. Oncol.* **2005**, *23*, 792–799. [CrossRef] [PubMed]

33. Lester, J.F.; MacBeth, F.R.; Coles, B. Prophylactic cranial irradiation for preventing brain metastases in patients undergoingradical treatment for non-small- cell lung cancer: A Cochrane Review. *Int. J. Radiat. Oncol. Biol. Phys.* **2005**, *63*, 690–694. [CrossRef] [PubMed]

34. Hicklin, D.J.; Ellis, L.M. Role of the vascular endothelial growth factor pathway in tumor growth and angiogenesis. *J. Clin. Oncol.* **2005**, *23*, 1011–1027. [CrossRef] [PubMed]

35. Ale, M.T.; Maruyama, H.; Tamauchi, H.; Mikkelsen, J.D.; Meyer, A.S. Fucoidan from *Sargassum.* sp. and Fucus. vesiculosus reduces cell viability of lung carcinoma and melanoma cells in vitro and activates natural killer cells in mice *in vivo*. *Int. J. Biol. Macromol.* **2011**, *49*, 331–336. [CrossRef] [PubMed]

36. Lee, K.R.; Lee, J.S.; Song, J.E.; Ha, S.J.; Hong, E.K. Inonotus obliquus-derived polysaccharide inhibits the migration and invasion of human non-small cell lung carcinoma cells via suppression of MMP-2 and MMP-9. *Int. J. Oncol.* **2014**, *45*, 2533–2540. [PubMed]

37. Rask, L.; Fregil, M.; Høgdall, E.; Mitchelmore, C.; Eriksen, J. Development of a metastatic fluorescent Lewis Lung carcinoma mouse model: Identification of mRNAs and microRNAs involved in tumor invasion. *Gene* **2013**, *517*, 72–81. [CrossRef] [PubMed]

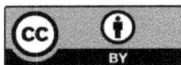

marine drugs

MDPI

Review

Perspective on the Use of Sulfated Polysaccharides from Marine Organisms as a Source of New Antithrombotic Drugs

Paulo A. S. Mourão [1,2]

[1] Connective Tissue Research Laboratory, University Hospital Clementino Fraga Filho,
Rio de Janeiro, RJ 21941-590, Brazil; pmourao@hucff.ufrj.br; Tel./Fax: +55-21-3938-2090

[2] Program of Glycobiology, Institute of Medical Biochemistry, Federal University of Rio de Janeiro,
Caixa Postal 68041, Rio de Janeiro, RJ 21941-590, Brazil

Academic Editor: Paola Laurienzo
Received: 26 February 2015; Accepted: 17 April 2015; Published: 6 May 2015

Abstract: Thromboembolic diseases are increasing worldwide and always require anticoagulant therapy. We still need safer and more secure antithrombotic drugs than those presently available. Sulfated polysaccharides from marine organisms may constitute a new source for the development of such drugs. Investigation of these compounds usually attempts to reproduce the therapeutic effects of heparin. However, we may need to follow different routes, focusing particularly in the following aspects: (1) defining precisely the specific structures required for interaction of these sulfated polysaccharides with proteins of the coagulation system; (2) looking for alternative mechanisms of action, distinct from those of heparin; (3) identifying side effects (mostly pro-coagulant action and hypotension rather than bleeding) and preparing derivatives that retain the desired antithrombotic action but are devoid of side effects; (4) considering that sulfated polysaccharides with low anticoagulant action on *in vitro* assays may display potent effects on animal models of experimental thrombosis; and finally (5) investigating the antithrombotic effect of these sulfated polysaccharides after oral administration or preparing derivatives that may achieve this effect. If these aspects are successfully addressed, sulfated polysaccharides from marine organisms may conquer the frontier of antithrombotic therapy and open new avenues for treatment or prevention of thromboembolic diseases.

Keywords: sulfated fucans; sulfated galactans; anticoagulant drugs; glycosaminoglycan-like polysaccharides; fucosylated chondroitin sulfate; fucoidan; carrageenans

1. We Need New Antithrombotic Drugs

Cardiovascular diseases are the leading cause of mortality worldwide. Among them are the thromboembolic events due to the formation of a thrombus or clot inside the circulatory system. Stasis, changes in blood coagulation, damage of the vascular wall and changes in the concentrations of leukocytes or platelets cause thrombus formation.

The occurrence of thromboembolic processes necessarily requires anticoagulant therapy. Dicumarinic (or warfarin) was the first widely used anticoagulant shortly followed by heparin. Heparin has the highest negative charge density of any known biomolecule described in vertebrate tissues so far. Just behind insulin, heparin is the second-most used naturally occurring drug in medicine. Besides being one of the first biopolymers employed as a medicine, and certainly the principal example of a carbohydrate-based drug, heparin is perhaps one of the oldest natural products still in use [1]. Its clinical use dates back more than 65 years [2]. Although it is primarily destined for treatment and prophylaxis of thromboembolic disorders, extracorporeal circulations during cardiovascular surgeries [3] and hemodialysis [4] also require heparin.

Besides its long-standing and varied clinical applications, heparin long-term therapy causes a number of side effects, such as bleeding, thrombocytopenia, changes in lipid metabolism and osteoporosis [5]. Additionally, heparin originates from animal tissues, and therefore is highly susceptible to contamination by pathogenic particles, such as in the case of spongiform encephalopathy. Furthermore, there is doubt if animal sources of heparin (mostly porcine or bovine intestine) will match the increasing demand for this drug. Nowadays, EUA and European countries obtain heparin exclusively from porcine intestinal mucosa. These countries are now looking for new sources of the drug [6]. However, heparins extracted from different tissues may possess distinct structures and activities, requiring separate monographs in the Pharmacopeia. This is the case of heparins obtained from bovine and porcine intestinal mucosa [7].

Even more serious are the recent reports of contamination of heparin preparations. In late 2007, the microorganism *Serratia marcescens* contaminated unopened heparin syringes, which leaded to a recall in the USA [8]. In early 2008, there were reports of contamination of heparin preparations with oversulfated chondroitin sulfate. This contaminant has a potent hypotensive effect and induces anaphylactic reactions. These side effects were associated with the death of ~200 patients in the United States [9,10]. Another negative example related to the use of mammalian heparin, which took place in Brazil, was the increase of bleeding when porcine intestinal heparin was replaced by bovine intestinal heparin [7,11].

These observations indicate we still need to search for new antithrombotic drugs, and marine organisms may constitute new sources of heparin analogs.

2. A Step Forward in the Study of Sulfated Polysaccharides from Marine Organisms

Marine organisms are a rich source of new substances with potential applications in medicine, though they are not yet well-explored. In particular, sulfated polysaccharides from marine invertebrates and algae possess unique structures and specific biological effects when tested in mammalian systems. The most abundant sulfated polysaccharides found in algae and marine invertebrates are sulfated fucans (also known as fucoidan when isolated from brown algae) and sulfated galactans (also known as carrageenans when isolated from red algae) [12–14]. In general, algal polysaccharides have more complex structures than polymers from marine invertebrates. Figure 1 illustrates this observation by comparing structures of sulfated galactans and sulfated fucans from red or brown algae (highlighted in blue) with those from sea urchins (in red).

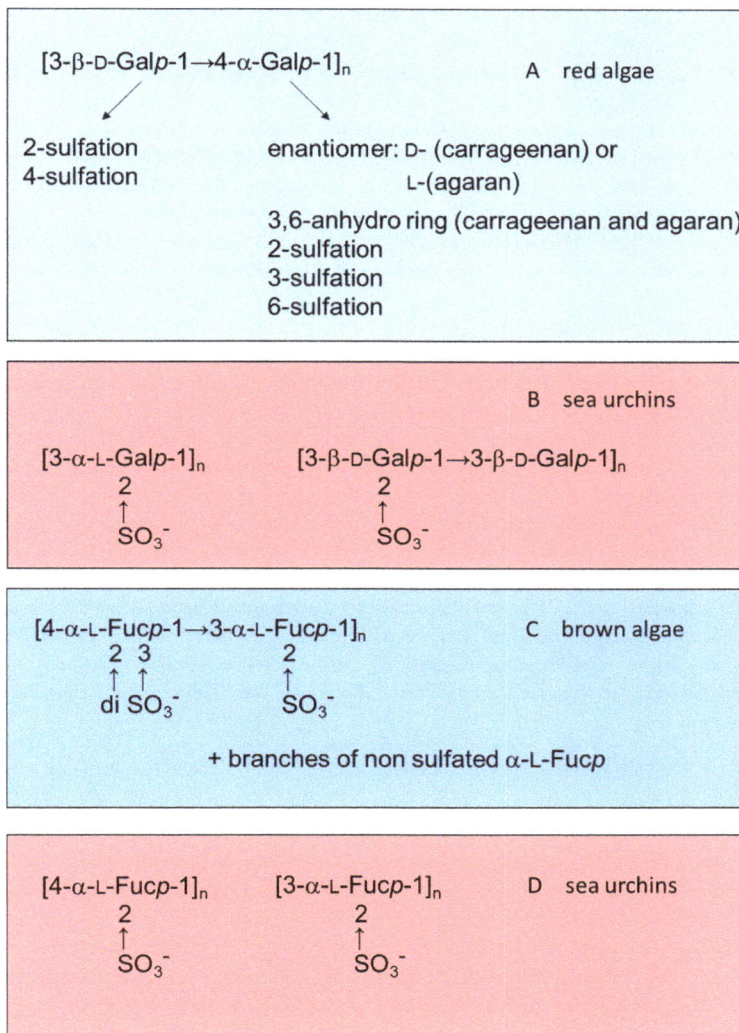

Figure 1. Examples of the structures of sulfated galactans from (**A**) red algae [15–19]; (**B**) sea urchins [20, 21]; (**C**) sulfated fucan from brown algae [22–24]; and (**D**) from sea urchins [25,26]. Structures of the sulfated polysaccharides from marine algae highlighted in blue and those from sea urchins in red.

Most studies on the effects of anticoagulant sulfated polysaccharides aim at selecting the most active native or chemically sulfated derivatives of natural polysaccharides in biological assays. Thus, the anticoagulant activity of the sulfated fucans increases with increasing sulfate content [27,28]. These studies follow an approach seeking to establish similarities between these molecules and heparin, the gold standard. The objective is to select active compounds based on general coagulation tests (mostly clotting assays). Thereafter, the aim is to compare the effects of these polysaccharides with those of heparin in more specific assays looking for similarities between them.

This approach raises skepticism since it is difficult to believe in the possibility of mimicking the effects of heparin on the coagulation system using sulfated polysaccharides with very distinct structures. The mechanism of the anticoagulant action of heparin constitutes a paradigm of interaction between carbohydrate and protein that triggers a potent biological effect [29]. A rare pentasaccharide sequence in the heparin molecule is responsible for the interaction and conformational activation of antithrombin, which is the major plasma serpin. This is the initial step, which determines the inhibition of serpin-dependent proteases of the coagulation system, especially thrombin and factor Xa.

Attempts to simulate the effect of heparin using other sulfated polysaccharides led to criticism that the structures of these compounds cannot simulate the same effect of heparin due to the obvious absence of the specific pentasaccharide sequence with high antithrombin affinity. The observation that a sulfated galactan, with high anticoagulant activity, does not induce the same conformational change on antithrombin as heparin supports this view [30]. The skeptics attributed the anticoagulant activity of the sulfated polysaccharides from marine organisms to non-specific and low-affinity interactions between their highly sulfated carbohydrate chains and basic regions in proteins of the coagulation system.

Another event which discouraged the study of sulfated polysaccharides as anticoagulants was the report that oversulfated chondroitin sulfate has an anticoagulant effect, although with much less potency than heparin and one that is associated with a strong toxic effect. This polysaccharide activates factor XII and releases bradykinin with potent hypotensive effect. Contamination of heparin preparation with oversulfated chondroitin sulfate has been responsible for ~200 deaths in the USA [9, 10]. Sulfated polysaccharides from algae and marine invertebrates may have similar effects, as already reported for a sea cucumber polysaccharide [31]. These observations further increased the disbelief in the possibility of simulating the effects of heparin with other sulfated polysaccharides.

However, it is possible to follow different routes to investigate these sulfated polysaccharides from marine organisms as anticoagulant drugs using a more innovative approach. The essential point is to look for distinct effects of these sulfated polysaccharides in the coagulation system, different from those reported for heparin. Sulfated polysaccharides with new mechanisms of action may open new avenues for therapeutic applications in thromboembolic diseases. This review will focus on some of these possibilities.

3. The Anticoagulant Effect of Sulfated Galactans and Sulfated Fucans Depends on Specific Structures

In a study performed in our laboratory, we tested the anticoagulant effects of sulfated galactans and sulfated fucans obtained from marine invertebrates. More than 20 types of sulfated polysaccharides with well-defined and repetitive structures were tested. The substantial number of results obtained allowed us to ensure that the structure of the sulfated polysaccharide correlates with its specific effects on the coagulation system. Three examples of this type of approach are described below.

Initially we compared the anticoagulant effect of a set of sulfated fucans obtained from sea urchins, all composed of linear chains of 3-linked α-L-fucopyranosyl (Fuc*p*) units with different patterns of 2- and 4-sulfation. We observed that the presence of 2,4-disulfated Fuc*p* units is the major requirement for antithrombin-mediated anticoagulant activity [32].

In another approach we compared the antithrombotic effect of two types of polysaccharides rich in 2,4-disulfated α-L-Fuc*p* units. One of them was a fucosylated chondroitin sulfate isolated from the sea cucumber. This polysaccharide has a backbone like that of vertebrate chondroitin sulfate: [4-β-D-glucuronic acid (GlcA)-1→3-β-D-*N*-acetylgalactosamine (GalNAc)-1]$_n$ but substituted at the 3-position of the β-D-GlcA with branches of 2,4-disulfated α-L-Fuc*p* [33]. Another polysaccharide was a sulfated fucan isolated from the same invertebrate but containing 2,4-disulfated α-Fuc*p* units as part of a linear chain: [α-L-Fuc*p*-2,4(OSO$_3^-$)-1→3-α-L-Fuc*p*-1→3-α-L-Fuc*p*-2(OSO$_3^-$)-1→3-α-L-Fuc*p*-2(OSO$_3^-$)]$_n$ [34] (Figure 2, Panels A and B). The result shown in Figure 2, Panel C, illustrates the effect of these two sulfated polysaccharides in an experimental model of arterial thrombosis. Clearly, occurrence of 2,4-disulfated α-Fuc*p* as branched residues (as in fucosylated chondroitin sulfate) ensures a more potent antithrombotic effect compared to the linear polymer containing the same type of residue [35].

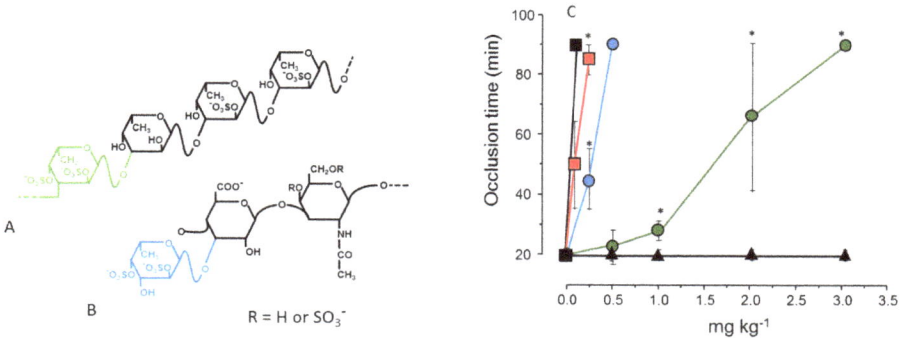

Figure 2. Structures (**A,B**) and antithrombotic effect (**C**) of sulfated polysaccharides rich in 2,4-disulfated α-L-Fucp units. (**A**) The sulfated fucan is composed of [3-α-L-Fucp-2,4(OSO$_3$$^-$)-1→3-α-L-Fucp-1→3-α-L-Fucp-2(OSO$_3$$^-$)-1→3-α-L-Fucp-2(OSO$_3$$^-$)]$_n$ repeating units; (**B**) Fucosylated chondroitin sulfate has a chondroitin sulfate-like backbone, but contains branches of 2,4-disulfated α-L-Fucp units linked to the β-D-GlcA residues on the polysaccharide core. The 2,4-disulfated α-L-Fucp units in these two polysaccharides are highlighted in green or blue; (**C**) Antithrombotic effect of sulfated fucan (●), fucosylated chondroitin sulfate (●), unfractionated heparin (■), low-molecular-weight heparin (■) and vertebrate chondroitin 6-sulfate (▲) on an arterial thrombosis model induced in carotid artery of rats by laser irradiation. See Ref. [35] for further details.

Another example of the stereospecificity of the anticoagulant effect of sulfated polysaccharides arises from comparison between a α-L-fucan and a α-L-galactan, both 2-sulfated and 3-linked (Figure 3, Panels A and B). The sulfated α-galactan is significantly more active than the sulfated α-fucan as an antithrombin-mediated thrombin inhibitor (Figure 3, Panel C) [36].

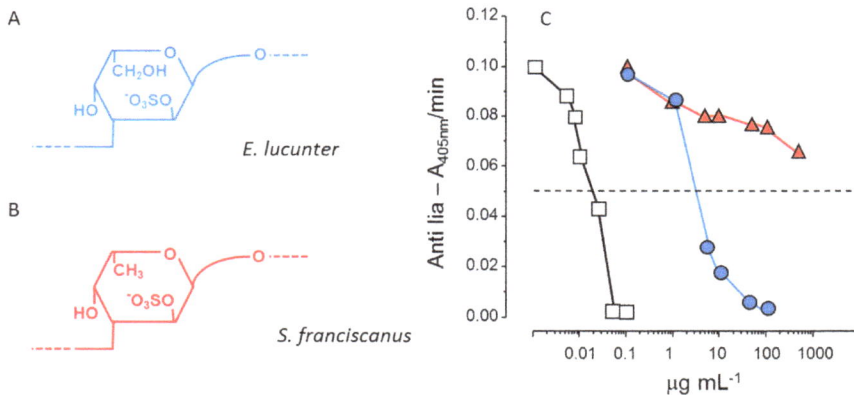

Figure 3. Structures and anticoagulant effect of a sulfated galactan and a sulfated fucan. (**A,B**) Structures of the sulfated α-L-galactan from the sea urchin *E. lucunter* (in blue, Panel A) and sulfated α-L-fucan from *S. franciscanus* (in red, Panel B). Both polysaccharides are 3-linked with a regular sulfation at the 2-position, but differ in their constituent monosaccharides; (**C**) Thrombin inhibition mediated by antithrombin *vs.* concentrations of the sulfated galactan (●), sulfated fucan () and heparin (□). See Ref. [36] for further details.

In conclusion, pattern of sulfation, position of the residue, either internal or non-reducing unit, and type of constituent sugar [α-L-galactopyranosyl (Gal*p*) or α-L-Fuc*p* unit] ensure the anticoagulant and antithrombotic effects. The anticoagulant activity of the polysaccharide is not only a consequence of negative charge density, but of precise structural constituents.

These studies were possible using the sulfated polysaccharides from marine invertebrates that possess well-defined structures. However, these polysaccharides occur in low concentrations, or some of the invertebrate species are scarce. In several cases, we can obtain these polysaccharides only in small amounts, which limits their practical use. A practical alternative to develop antithrombotic drug is to employ sulfated polysaccharides from marine algae, which are abundant. Nevertheless, the invertebrate polymers are model molecules and may reveal a specific structural sequence we need to look for in the algal polysaccharides.

4. Serpin-Independent Anticoagulant Effect

Serpins (as antithrombin and heparin cofactor II) mediate the anticoagulant activity of heparin, resulting in the inhibition of the coagulation proteases. Consequently, the effect of that glycosaminoglycan disappears on serpins-depleted plasmas. Sulfated polysaccharides from marine organisms have a similar serpin-mediated activity, demonstrated on assays using purified reagents (proteases and serpins) [16,32,33,36]. It intrigued us when it was observed that the anticoagulant effect of a fucosylated chondroitin sulfate from the sea cucumber [37] and of a sulfated galactan from red algae [38] remains unchanged when tested in serpin-depleted plasma. This observation is even more striking when tests of thrombin or factor Xa generation in serpin-depleted plasma was employed. Clearly, the inhibitory effect of the blood coagulation proteases disappears in tests using heparin, but persists with fucosylated chondroitin sulfate or sulfated galactan [37,38].

Further examination revealed that fucosylated chondroitin sulfate and sulfated galactan inhibit the intrinsic tenase and prothrombinase complexes that are critical for the generation of factor Xa and thrombin. Assays using purified proteins of the coagulation system assure this conclusion. The sulfated polysaccharides inhibit the interaction between factor Va and factor X [38]. These results reveal an anticoagulant effect with a distinct mechanism of action compared with heparin or any other known antithrombotic drug. Figure 4 summarizes the preponderant target sites for the sulfated polysaccharides from marine organisms on the coagulation system. Blue arrows at right of the Figure indicate the anticoagulant effects.

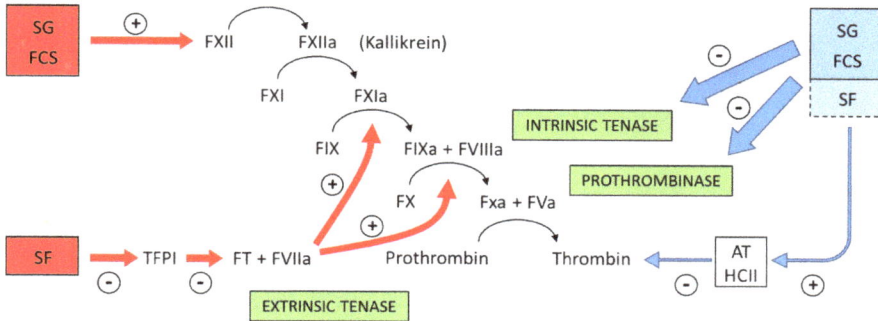

Figure 4. Major target sites for the sulfated polysaccharides from marine organisms on the coagulation system. Blue and red arrows indicate anticoagulant and pro-coagulant effects, respectively. + indicates activation and − indicates inhibitory effects. Anticoagulant effect: sulfated galactans (SG) from marine red algae and fucosylated chondroitin sulfates (FCS) from sea cucumbers inhibit the intrinsic tenase and prothrombinase complexes [37,38]. It is still unclear if sulfated fucans (SF) have similar effects. These polysaccharides also potentiate the inhibitory effect of antithrombin (AT) and/or heparin cofactor II (HCII) on thrombin [16,32,33,36]. Their effects on factor Xa are very modest. The serpin-independent action preponderates on the plasma system. Pro-coagulant effect: SG and FCS activate factor XII [31,39]. This effect may result in severe hypotension (due to bradykinin release) and pro-coagulant (and pro-thrombotic) action. It is unclear if SF activates factor XII. SF inhibits Tissue Factor Protease Inhibitor (TFPI), a specific inhibitor of the extrinsic tenase complex. Consequently, SF has a pro-coagulant effect [40,41].

Of course, further studies are necessary to investigate whether this distinct mechanism of action may confer favorable effects to the marine polysaccharides for the prevention and treatment of thromboembolic events. In particular, it is necessary to clarify which one of the two mechanisms (serpin-dependent or serpin-independent) is more favorable for an antithrombotic therapy.

5. Sulfated Polysaccharides with Low Anticoagulant Activity May Have Potent Antithrombotic Effects

Screening for new anticoagulant polysaccharides usually requires an initial assessment with general coagulation tests. The compound, which is most active, moves to a more detailed stage of evaluation using animal testing. Following this methodological guideline, our laboratory carried out a study of sulfated polysaccharides from 50 species of marine algae. The work leaded to a sulfated galactan from the red alga *Botryocladia occidentalis* with very high anticoagulant activity [16]. This polysaccharide has a relatively simple structure as compared with that of similar compounds obtained from seaweeds. The presence of 2,3-disulfated α-Gal*p* units was associated with the high anticoagulant activity of the sulfated polysaccharide.

However, we can proceed in a different way, looking for sulfated polysaccharides with low anticoagulant activity. We can propose, conceptually, that a polysaccharide with low activity in coagulation tests using *in vitro* assays may exhibit a potent antithrombotic effect when tested in animal models of thrombosis.

We followed this approach and ended up with a sulfated galactan from the red alga *Acanthophora muscoides* with low anticoagulant activity. Despite this data, we continued to go deeper with the coagulation study. The polysaccharide presented a very complex structure. Its backbone consists of alternating units of α- and β-Gal*p* units, as is the characteristic of seaweed galactans. However, we observed a wide variety of structural modifications, such as sulfation in different positions, the presence of methyl ether, and anhydrous sugars. Another unique feature of this sulfated galactan is its low molecular weight (~20 kDa) [19]. Most seaweed-sulfated galactans have extremely high molecular weights.

We reduced the molecular weight of the sulfated galactan from *B. occidentalis* using mild acid hydrolysis and obtained a derivative with the same molecular weight as that of the native polysaccharide from *A. muscoides*. The clotting assay using these two sulfated galactans, with similar molecular weights, revealed that the compound from *B. occidentalis* was more active (Figure 5, Pane A, closed circles in blue *vs.* closed diamond in red). However, more importantly, it turns out that these two sulfated galactans, with low molecular weights, are practically inactive in coagulation assays using purified coagulation proteases and serpins [19]. That is, its anticoagulant effect, albeit modest as compared to heparin, is independent of serpins. The clotting assays using serpin-depleted plasma confirmed this proposition (Figure 5, Panels B and D, compare closed *vs.* open symbols).

The next step was to test these sulfated galactans, with low anticoagulant activity and serpin-free effects, in animal models of experimental thrombosis. Figure 5, Panel C, shows the test using an experimental model of arterial thrombosis. Surprisingly, the sulfated galactan from *A. muscoides* is very active, whereas that obtained from *B. occidentalis* is completely inactive (closed circles in blue *vs.* closed diamond in red).

These results are very important because they reveal a sulfated polysaccharide, with only modest anticoagulant action on *in vitro* assay but potent arterial antithrombotic effect in the experimental animal model. We attribute this effect to the inhibition of the tenase and prothrombinase complexes that generate the coagulation proteases. This approach consolidates the molecular basis of a new antithrombotic mechanism by a sulfated polysaccharide, involving inhibition of factor Xa and thrombin generations by the tenase and prothrombinase systems.

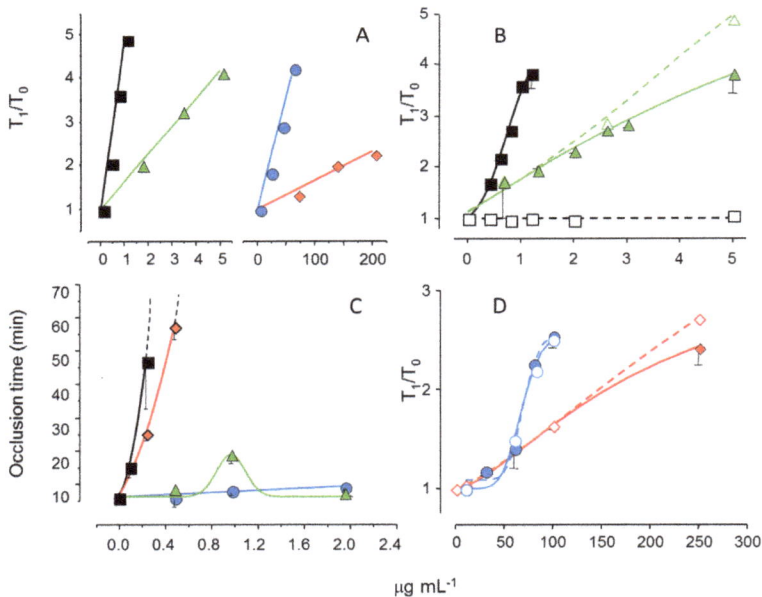

Figure 5. Effect of sulfated galactans on anticoagulant assays (**A,C,D**) and on arterial experimental thrombosis in rats (**B**). Different concentrations or doses of heparin (■,□), native sulfated galactan from *B. occidentalis* (,Δ) or from *A. muscoides* (,◊) or the sulfated galactan from *B. occidentalis* with reduced molecular weight (●,) were tested. In Panels C and D closed and open symbols refer to assays performed using normal or serpin-depleted plasma, respectively. Data from Ref. [19].

6. Balance between Pro- and Anticoagulant Effects

Sulfated galactans have no bleeding tendency [19,39,42], which is the major side effect of heparin and other antithrombotic drugs. Instead, the major side effect of these polysaccharides is activation of factor XII. This action results in the release of bradykinin, leading to severe hypotension [9,10,31]. Conceptually, we expect that activation of factor XII should trigger coagulation, resulting in pro-thrombotic action. In the case of the sulfated galactan from the red alga *B. occidentalis* we observed a dual effect, as a potent anticoagulant and as an activator of factor XII [39]. This observation is very clear with the use of a recalcification time assay, without the addition of phospholipids (Figure 6, Panel A). Heparin has a potent anticoagulant action (open squares), while the sulfated galactan has a dual effect: up to ~8 $\mu g.mL^{-1}$, an anticoagulant effect, and above 8 $\mu g.mL^{-1}$, a pro-coagulant effect (closed triangles in Figure 6, Panel A). A 14 kDa fragment shows the same effect as the native polysaccharide but at different concentrations (open circles). Decrease of the molecular weight to ~5 kDa eliminates this dual effect (closed circles).

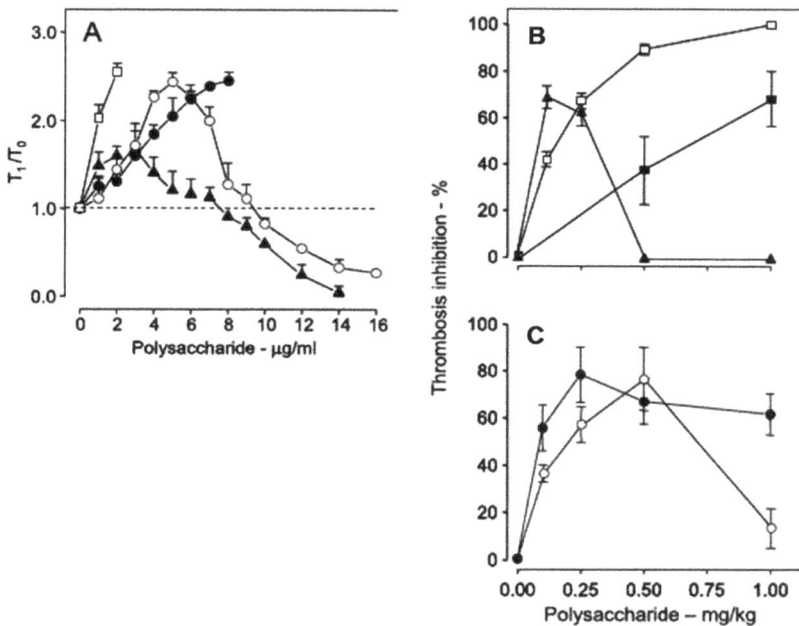

Figure 6. Anticoagulant activity based on recalcification time (**A**) and antithrombotic effect on a stasis thrombosis model in vena cava of rats (**B,C**). Different concentrations (**A**) or doses (**B,C**) of unfractionated heparin (□), low-molecular-weight heparin (■), native sulfated galactan (▲), ~14 kDa (O) and ~5 kDa (●) fragments were tested. In Panel A the anticoagulant activity was expressed as T_1/T_0, which is the ratio between the clotting time in the presence or absence of sulfated polysaccharide. The broken line ($T_1/T_0 = 1$) indicates no effect from the polysaccharide on coagulation. Data from Ref. [39].

Because of the dual effect on coagulation, this sulfated galactan has two distinct effects in the experimental thrombosis model. At lower doses, up to approximately 0.25 $mg.kg^{-1}$ body weight, it is a potent antithrombotic, similar to heparin; at higher doses, above 0.25 $mg.kg^{-1}$ body weight, this effect disappears and is replaced by a pro-coagulant effect (Figure 6, Panel B), due to activation of factor XII.

In order to develop an antithrombotic drug for practical use, it is essential to dissociate the anticoagulant action from the undesirable pro-coagulant effect. We achieved this goal by means of partial acid hydrolysis of the polysaccharide. The sulfated galactan with low molecular weight (~ 5 kDa) proved to be a promising antithrombotic, devoid of pro-coagulant action (Figure 6, Panel C, closed circles) [39].

Curiously, even fucoidan presents the concomitant anti- and pro-coagulant effects [40,41]. Selected modified derivatives from this polysaccharide, devoid of anticoagulant activity, have been used as a therapeutic option in bleeding disorders, such as hemophilia. The pro-coagulant effect of fucoidan is distinct from the activation of factor XII proposed for the sulfated galactans. It involves a blockade of the extrinsic pathway down-regulator, the tissue factor pathway inhibitor, by the non-anticoagulant fucoidan derivatives. Red arrows at left of Figure 4 indicate the pro-coagulant effects of the sulfated polysaccharides from marine organisms.

Protamine neutralizes the effects of sulfated polysaccharides from marine organisms on the coagulation system, as occurs with heparin. It decreases the pro-coagulant effect of a sulfated galactan from red alga [42] and the anticoagulant action of fucosylated chondroitin sulfate from sea cucumber. These observations are relevant to ensure we can antagonize the effects of the polysaccharides if severe side effects occur. Induction of thrombocytopenia with the sulfated polysaccharides from marine organisms is another important aspect that requires future investigation.

7. Sulfated Polysaccharide with Oral Antithrombotic Effects

The use of sulfated polysaccharides as antithrombotic drug requires intravascular or subcutaneous administration, which limits their use. The new oral antithrombotic agents, which directly inhibit thrombin or factor Xa, have overcome this limitation although they may cause bleeding and have unpredicted responses [43,44].

Sulfated polysaccharides are not promising for oral administration due to their high molecular weight. Even attempts to administer heparin orally were also unsuccessful. Possibly, degradation of heparin by bacteria of the intestinal flora or by enzymes produced by the vertebrate also reduced its absorption after oral administration. However, the different chemical nature of the sulfated galactans and sulfated fucans from marine organisms makes them resistant to degradation by most enzymes that normally act on vertebrate glycosaminoglycans.

A number of studies indicate biological effects after oral ingestion of sulfated fucans from brown algae (fucoidan) [45]. Early work on digestion of these polysaccharides suggested that they were not changed by human bacterial flora and were wholly excreted [46,47]. Following oral administration to rats, we observed that fucosylated chondroitin sulfate has anticoagulant and antithrombotic effects, with low hemorrhagic action [48]. This finding allowed us to overcome the main limitation to the development of new antithrombotics based on sulfated polysaccharides. Of course, we need to extend this kind of study to other types of sulfated polysaccharides from marine organisms, especially sulfated galactans and sulfated fucans.

The observation that a sulfated polysaccharide has antithrombotic effect after oral administration raises a challenging question: how extensive is the gastrointestinal absorption of this polysaccharide? Answering this question requires a careful investigation of the metabolism of sulfated polysaccharides from marine organisms after administration to mammals, including their route of absorption and pharmacokinetics. Studies about the intestinal absorption of fucoidan have been reported recently [49].

8. Conclusions

In this review, we discussed possible ways to proceed in order to develop new antithrombotic drugs based on sulfated polysaccharides from marine organisms. These compounds occur in high amounts in marine algae. However, their therapeutic use in humans faces several challenges. We need to look for alternative approaches in order to establish a new paradigm, instead of continuing to look at them as "heparin-like molecules." Possibly, we need to consider the following points:

(1) Precisely define the specific structures required for the interaction of sulfated polysaccharides with the proteins and complexes of the coagulation system.

(2) Look for alternative mechanisms of action distinct from those of heparin, including serpin-independent effects. Clarification of the precise target molecules of these sulfated polysaccharides will help to establish new drugs on a more rational basis.

(3) Identify major side effects in order to design the preparation of derivatives that retain the desirable antithrombotic action but are devoid of toxic ones. Pro-coagulant effect and hypotension, both due to activation of factor XII, instead of bleeding, may be the major obstacle for the therapeutic use of sulfated polysaccharides from marine organisms.

(4) Consider that sulfated polysaccharides with low activity on *in vitro* coagulation tests may exhibit potent activity on animal models of experimental thrombosis.

(5) Investigate the effect of these sulfated polysaccharides after oral administration. If unsuccessful, we may attempt to prepare derivatives that achieve this effect. The discovery of new oral anticoagulants derived from the sulfated polysaccharides of marine organisms will put these compounds on the frontier of antithrombotic therapeutics.

Acknowledgments: The author would like to acknowledge the funding from Conselho Nacional de Desenvolvimento Científico e Tecnológico (CNPq) and Fundação de Amparo à Pesquisa do Estado do Rio de Janeiro (FAPERJ).

Conflicts of Interest: The author declares no conflict of interest.

References

1. Norma, R. 100 years. Looking back. Skill, drive and luck: The discovery and development of heparin. *CMAJ* **2011**, *13*, 2139–2140. [CrossRef]
2. Mulloy, B.; Gray, E.; Barrowcliffe, T.W. Characterization of unfractionated heparin: Comparison of materials from the last 50 years. *Thromb. Haemost.* **2000**, *84*, 1052–1056. [PubMed]
3. Tagarakis, G.; Tsilimingas, N.B. Heparin-coated extracorporeal circulation systems in heart surgery. *Recent Pat. Cardiovasc. Drug Discov.* **2009**, *4*, 177–179. [CrossRef] [PubMed]
4. Molitor, B.; Klingel, R.; Hafner, G. Monitoring of the heparin therapy during acute haemodialysis. *Hamostaseologie* **2005**, *25*, 272–278. [PubMed]
5. Alban, S. Adverse Effects of Heparin. *Handb. Exp. Pharmacol.* **2012**, *207*, 211–264. [PubMed]
6. Introduction of Proposal for Reintroduction of Bovine Heparin to the U.S Market. Available online: http://www.fda.gov/downloads/UCM399418.pdf (accessed on 4 March 2015).
7. Aquino, R.S.; Pereira, M.S.; Vairo, B.C.; Cinelli, L.P.; Santos, G.R.C.; Fonseca, R.J.C.; Mourão, P.A.S. Heparins from porcine and bovine intestinal mucosa: Are they similar drugs? *Thromb. Haemost.* **2010**, *103*, 1005–1015. [CrossRef] [PubMed]
8. Chemaly, R.F.; Rathod, D.B.; Sikka, M.K.; Hayden, M.K.; Hutchins, M.; Tracy Horn, T.; Jeffery Tarrand, J.; Javier Adachi, J.; Kim Nguyen, K.; Trenholme, G.; *et al.* Serratia marcescens bacteremia because of contaminated prefilled heparin and saline syringes: A multi-state report. *Am. J. Infect. Control* **2011**, *39*, 521–524. [CrossRef] [PubMed]
9. Kishimoto, T.K.; Viswanathan, K.; Ganguly, T.; Elankumaran, S.; Smith, S.; Pelzer, K.; Lansing, J.C.; Sriranganathan, N.; Zhao, G.; Galcheva-Gargova, Z.; *et al.* Contaminated heparin associated with adverse clinical events and activation of the contact system. *N. Engl. J. Med.* **2008**, *358*, 2457–2467. [CrossRef] [PubMed]
10. Guerrini, M.; Beccati, D.; Shriver, Z.; Naggi, A.; Viswanathan, K.; Bisio, A.; Capila, I.; Lansing, J.C.; Guglieri, S.; Fraser, B.; *et al.* Oversulfated chondroitin sulfate is a contaminant in heparin associated with adverse clinical events. *Nat. Biotechnol.* **2008**, *26*, 669–675. [CrossRef] [PubMed]
11. Melo, E.I.; Pereira, M.S.; Cunha, R.S.; Sá, M.P.; Mourão, P.A.S. Heparin quality control in the Brazilian market: Implications in the cardiovascular surgery. *Rev. Bras. Cir. Cardiovasc.* **2008**, *23*, 169–174. [CrossRef] [PubMed]
12. Mourão, P.A.S. Use of sulfated fucans as anticoagulant and antithrombotic agents: Future perspectives. *Curr. Pharm. Des.* **2004**, *10*, 967–981. [CrossRef] [PubMed]
13. Pomin, V.H.; Mourão, P.A.S. Structure, biology, evolution, and medical importance of sulfated fucans and galactans. *Glycobiology* **2008**, *18*, 1016–1027. [CrossRef] [PubMed]

14. Mourão, P.A.S. A carbohydrate-based mechanism of species recognition in sea urchin fertilization. *Braz. J. Med. Biol. Res.* **2007**, *40*, 5–17. [CrossRef] [PubMed]

15. Usov, A.I. Structural analysis of red seaweed galactans of agar and carrageenan groups. *Food Hydrocoll.* **1998**, *12*, 301–308. [CrossRef]

16. Farias, W.R.; Valente, A.P.; Pereira, M.S.; Mourão, P.A.S. Structure and anticoagulant activity of sulfated galactans. Isolation of a unique sulfated galactan from the red algae *Botryocladia occidentalis* and comparison of its anticoagulant action with that of sulfated galactans from invertebrates. *J. Biol. Chem.* **2000**, *275*, 29299–29307. [CrossRef] [PubMed]

17. Lahaye, M. Developments on gelling algal galactans, their structure and physico-chemistry. *J. Appl. Phycol.* **2001**, *13*, 173–184. [CrossRef]

18. Pereira, M.G.; Benevides, N.M.; Melo, M.R.; Valente, A.P.; Melo, F.R.; Mourão, P.A.S. Structure and anticoagulant activity of a sulfated galactan from the red alga, *Gelidium crinale*. Is there a specific structural requirement for the anticoagulant action? *Carbohydr. Res.* **2005**, *340*, 2015–2023. [CrossRef] [PubMed]

19. Quinderé, A.L.G.; Santos, G.R.C.; Oliveira, S.N.M.C.G.; Glauser, B.F.; Fontes, B.F.; Queiroz, I.N.L.; Benevides, N.M.B.; Pomin, V.H.; Mourão, P.A.S. Is the antithrombotic effect of sulfated galactans independent of serpin? *J. Thromb. Haemost.* **2014**, *12*, 43–53. [CrossRef] [PubMed]

20. Alves, A.P.; Mulloy, B.; Diniz, J.A.; Mourão, P.A.S. Sulfated polysaccharides from the egg jelly layer are species-specific inducers of acrosomal reaction in sperms of sea urchins. *J. Biol. Chem.* **1997**, *272*, 6965–6971. [CrossRef] [PubMed]

21. Castro, M.O.; Pomin, V.H.; Santos, L.L.; Vilela-Silva, A.C.E.S.; Hirohashi, N.; Pol-Fachin, L.; Verli, H.; Mourão, P.A.S. A unique 2-sulfated β-galactan from the egg jelly of the sea urchin *Glyptocidaris crenularis*: Conformational flexibly *versus* induction of the sperm acrosome reaction. *J. Biol. Chem.* **2009**, *284*, 18790–18800. [CrossRef] [PubMed]

22. Chevolot, L.; Foucault, A.; Kervarec, N.; Sinquin, C.; Fisher, A.M.; Boisson-Vidal, C. Further data on the structure of brown seaweed fucans: Relationships with anticoagulant activity. *Carbohydr. Res.* **1999**, *319*, 154–165. [CrossRef] [PubMed]

23. Chevolot, L.; Mulloy, B.; Ratiskol, J.; Foucault, A.; Colliec-Jouault, S. A disaccharide repeat unit is the major structure in fucoidans from two species of brown algae. *Carbohydr. Res.* **2000**, *330*, 529–535. [CrossRef]

24. Bilan, M.I.; Grachev, A.A.; Ustuzhanina, N.E.; Shashkov, A.S.; Nifantiev, N.E.; Usov, A.I. Structure of a fucoidan from the brown seaweed *Fucus evanescens*. *Carbohydr. Res.* **2002**, *337*, 719–730. [CrossRef] [PubMed]

25. Vilela-Silva, A.C.E.S.; Alves, A.P.; Valente, A.P.; Vacquier, V.D.; Mourão, P.A.S. Structure of the sulfated α-L-fucan from the egg jelly coat of the sea urchin *Strongylocentrotus franciscanus*: Patterns of preferential 2-O- and 4-O-sulfation determine sperm cell recognition. *Glycobiology* **1999**, *9*, 225–232. [CrossRef]

26. Vilela-Silva, A.C.E.S.; Castro, M.O.; Valente, A.P.; Biermann, C.H.; Mourão, P.A.S. Sulfated fucans from the egg jellies of the closely related sea urchins *Strongylocentrotus droebachiensis* and *Strongylocentrotus pallidus* ensure species specific fertilization. *J. Biol. Chem.* **2002**, *277*, 379–387. [CrossRef] [PubMed]

27. Soeda, S.; Ohmagari, Y.; Shimeno, H.; Nagamatsu, A. Preparation of oversulfated fucoidans fragments and evaluation of their antithrombotic activities. *Thromb. Res.* **1993**, *72*, 247–256. [CrossRef] [PubMed]

28. Haroun-Bouhedja, F.; Ellouali, M.; Sinquin, C.; Boisson-Vidal, C. Relationship between sulfate groups and biological activities of fucans. *Thromb. Res.* **2000**, *100*, 453–458. [CrossRef] [PubMed]

29. Gray, E.; Hogwood, J.; Mulloy, B. The anticoagulant and antithrombotic mechanisms of heparin. *Handb. Exp. Pharmacol.* **2012**, *207*, 347–360. [PubMed]

30. Melo, F.R.; Pereira, M.S.; Foguel, D.; Mourão, P.A.S. Antithrombin-mediated anticoagulant activity of sulfated polysaccharides: Different mechanisms for heparin and sulfated galactans. *J. Biol. Chem.* **2004**, *279*, 20824–20835. [CrossRef] [PubMed]

31. Fonseca, R.J.C.; Oliveira, S.N.M.C.G.; Pomin, V.H.; Mecawi, A.S.; Iracema, G.; Araujo, I.G.; Mourão, P.A.S. Effects of oversulfated and fucosylated chondroitin sulfates on coagulation, Challenges for the study of anticoagulant polysaccharides. *Thromb. Haematol.* **2010**, *103*, 994–1004.

32. Pereira, M.S.; Melo, F.R.; Mourão, P.A.S. Is there a correlation between structure and anticoagulant action of sulfated galactans and sulfated fucans? *Glycobiology* **2002**, *12*, 573–580. [CrossRef] [PubMed]

33. Mourão, P.A.S.; Pereira, M.S.; Pavão, M.S.G.; Mulloy, B.; Tollefsen, D.M.; Mowinckel, M.C.; Abildgaard, U. Structure and anticoagulant activity of a fucosylated chondroitin sulfate from echinoderm: Sulfated fucose branches on the polysaccharide account for its high anticoagulant activity. *J. Biol. Chem.* **1996**, *271*, 23973–23984. [CrossRef]

34. Ribeiro, A.C.; Vieira, R.P.; Mourão, P.A.S.; Mulloy, B. A sulfated α-L-fucan from sea cucumber. *Carbohydr. Res.* **1994**, *255*, 225–240. [CrossRef] [PubMed]

35. Fonseca, R.J.C.; Santos, G.R.C.; Mourão, P.A.S. Effects of polysaccharides enriched in 2,4-disulfated fucose units on coagulation, thrombosis and bleeding. Practical and conceptual implications. *Thromb. Haematol.* **2009**, *102*, 829–836.

36. Pereira, M.S.; Vilela-Silva, A.C.E.S.; Valente, A.P.; Mourão, P.A.S. A 2-sulfated, 3-linked α-L-galactan is an anticoagulante polysaccharide. *Carbohydr. Res.* **2002**, *337*, 2231–2238. [CrossRef] [PubMed]

37. Glauser, B.F.; Pereira, M.S.; Monteiro, R.Q.; Mourão, P.A.S. Serpin-independent anticoagulant activity of a fucosylated chondroitin sulfate. *Thromb. Haemost.* **2008**, *100*, 420–428. [PubMed]

38. Glauser, B.F.; Rezende, R.M.; Melo, F.R.; Pereira, M.S.; Francischetti, I.M.B.; Monteiro, R.Q.; Rezaie, A.R.; Mourão, P.A.S. Anticoagulant activity of a sulfated galactan: Serpin-independent effect and specific interaction with factor Xa. *Thromb. Haemost.* **2009**, *102*, 1183–1193. [PubMed]

39. Melo, F.R.; Mourão, P.A.S. Sulfated galactan has an unusual effect on thrombosis due to activation of factor XII and inhibition of the coagulation proteases. *Thromb. Haemost.* **2008**, *99*, 531–538. [PubMed]

40. Liu, T.; Scallan, C.D.; Broze, G.J., Jr.; Patarroyo-White, S.; Pierce, G.F.; Johnson, K.W. Improved coagulation in bleeding disorders by non-anticoagulant sulfated polysaccharides (NASP). *Thromb. Haemostas.* **2006**, *95*, 68–76.

41. Zhang, Z.; Till, S.; Jiang, C.; Knappe, S.; Reutterer, S.; Scheiflinger, F.; Szabo, C.M.; Dockal, M. Structure-activity relationship of the pro- and anticoagulant effects of *Fucus vesiculosus* fucoidan. *Thromb. Haemost.* **2014**, *111*, 429–437. [CrossRef] [PubMed]

42. Farias, W.F.; Nazareth, R.A.; Mourão, P.A.S. Dual effects of sulfated d-galactans from the red algae *Botryocladia occidentalis* preventing thrombosis and inducing platelet aggregation. *Thromb. Haemost.* **2001**, *86*, 1540–1546. [PubMed]

43. Holster, I.L.; Valkhoff, V.E.; Kuipers, E.J.; Tjwa, E.T. New oral anticoagulants increase risk for gastrointestinal bleeding: A systematic review and meta-analysis. *Gastroenterology* **2013**, *145*, 105–112. [CrossRef] [PubMed]

44. Holster, I.L.; Hunfeld, N.G.; Kuipers, E.J.; Kruip, M.J.; Tjwa, E.T. On the treatment of new oral anticoagulant-associated gastrointestinal hemorrhage. *J. Gastrointestin. Liver Dis.* **2013**, *22*, 229–231. [PubMed]

45. Fitton, J.H. Therapies from fucoidan; multifunctional marine polymers. *Mar. Drugs* **2011**, *9*, 1731–1760. [CrossRef] [PubMed]

46. Michel, C.; Lahaye, M.; Bonnet, C.; Mabeau, S.; Barry, J.L. *In vitro* fermentation by human fecal bacteria of total and purified dietary fibers from brown seaweeds. *Br. J. Nutr.* **1996**, *75*, 263–280. [CrossRef] [PubMed]

47. Yamada, Y.; Miyoshi, T.; Tanada, S.; Imaki, M. Digestibility and energy availability of Wakame (*Undaria pinnatifida*) seaweed in Japanese. *Nippon Eiseigaku Zasshi* **1991**, *46*, 788–794. [CrossRef] [PubMed]

48. Fonseca, R.J.C.; Mourão, P.A.S. Fucosylated chondroitin sulfate as a new oral antithrombotic agent. *Thromb. Haemost.* **2006**, *96*, 822–829. [PubMed]

49. Nagamine, T.; Nakazato, K.; Tomioka, S.; Iha, M.; Nakajima, K. Intestinal absorption of fucoidan extracted from the brown seaweed, *Cladosiphono kamuranus*. *Mar. Drugs* **2015**, *13*, 48–64. [CrossRef]

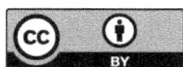

marine drugs

MDPI

Review

Marine Polysaccharides: A Source of Bioactive Molecules for Cell Therapy and Tissue Engineering

Karim Senni [1,†], **Jessica Pereira** [2,†], **Farida Gueniche** [3], **Christine Delbarre-Ladrat** [4], **Corinne Sinquin** [4], **Jacqueline Ratiskol** [4], **Gaston Godeau** [3], **Anne-Marie Fischer** [2,5], **Dominique Helley** [2,5] and **Sylvia Colliec-Jouault** [4,*]

[1] Seadev-FermenSys SAS, Technopole Brest Iroise, 185 rue René Descartes, Plouzané 29280, France; senni@seadev.fr

[2] INSERM U765, Faculté de Pharmacie, UMR-S765, Université Paris Descartes, Sorbonne Paris Cité, 4 avenue de l'Observatoire, Paris 75006, France; jessica.pereira@etu.parisdescartes.fr (J.P.); anne-marie.fischer@egp.aphp.fr (A.-M.F.); dominique.helley@egp.aphp.fr (D.H.)

[3] Biochemistry Department, Faculty of Dental Surgery, Paris Descartes University, Montrouge 92120, France; gueniche_farida@yahoo.fr (F.G.); godeau_g@yahoo.fr (G.G.)

[4] Laboratory of Biotechnology and Marine Molecules, Ifremer, Rue de l'Ile d'Yeu, BP 21105, Nantes Cedex 03 44311, France; Christine.Delbarre.Ladrat@ifremer.fr (C.D.-L.); Corinne.Sinquin@ifremer.fr (C.S.); Jacqueline.Ratiskol@ifremer.fr (J.R.)

[5] AP-HP, Biological Hematology Department, European Hospital Georges Pompidou, 20 rue Leblanc, Paris 75015, France

[*] Author to whom correspondence should be addressed; Sylvia.Colliec.Jouault@ifremer.fr; Tel.: +33-2-4037-4093; Fax: +33-2-4037-4071.

[†] These authors contributed equally to this work.

Received: 22 July 2011; in revised form: 2 September 2011; Accepted: 5 September 2011; Published: 23 September 2011

Abstract: The therapeutic potential of natural bioactive compounds such as polysaccharides, especially glycosaminoglycans, is now well documented, and this activity combined with natural biodiversity will allow the development of a new generation of therapeutics. Advances in our understanding of the biosynthesis, structure and function of complex glycans from mammalian origin have shown the crucial role of this class of molecules to modulate disease processes and the importance of a deeper knowledge of structure-activity relationships. Marine environment offers a tremendous biodiversity and original polysaccharides have been discovered presenting a great chemical diversity that is largely species specific. The study of the biological properties of the polysaccharides from marine eukaryotes and marine prokaryotes revealed that the polysaccharides from the marine environment could provide a valid alternative to traditional polysaccharides such as glycosaminoglycans. Marine polysaccharides present a real potential for natural product drug discovery and for the delivery of new marine derived products for therapeutic applications.

Keywords: marine bacteria; marine algae; exopolysaccharides; sulfated polysaccharides; structure; chemical modification; biological activity; blue biotechnology; cell therapy; tissue engineering

---

1. Introduction

Sulfated polysaccharides have diverse functions in the tissues from which they originate. They are capable of binding with proteins at several levels of specificity and are involved mainly in the development, cell differentiation, cell adhesion, cell signaling and cell matrix interactions. These bioactive molecules present a great potential for medical, pharmaceutical and biotechnological applications such as wound dressings, biomaterials, tissue regeneration and 3D culture scaffolds and even drugs. The most studied for their biological properties are mammalian sulfated polysaccharides or glycoconjugates constituted by glycosaminoglycans (GAGs) composed of negatively charged osidic chains, most of them covalently linked to proteins. The discovery of the biological importance of the mammalian glycoconjugates has been the beginning of a new modern research field focusing on the carbohydrate based recognition phenomena, glycobiology [1,2]. It has been demonstrated that these particular biological properties were due to the chemical diversity of the osidic chains in which the patterns of sulfate substitution can give specific biological functions. It was also noted that the chemical diversity of the sulfated polysaccharides was largely species specific [3].

Marine polysaccharides present an enormous variety of structures; they are still under-exploited and they should therefore be considered as an extraordinary source of chemical diversity for drug discovery [4]. Sulfated polysaccharides, possessing GAG-like biological properties, can be found either in marine eukaryotes or in marine prokaryotes. This marine origin should offer potentially safer compounds than mammalian polysaccharides for drug discovery. In this review, we will present first the biological properties of GAGs from mammalian origin in relation to cell therapy and tissue engineering. Then we will describe different studies made on marine polysaccharides, showing that these polysaccharides could advantageously replace mammalian GAGs in some therapeutic applications.

2. Glycosaminoglycans: Structural Features, Biological Properties and Limitations for Therapeutic Use

Glycosaminoglycans (GAGs) are present in all animals; some of them such as heparin and dermatan-sulfate are extracted from mammalian mucosa for therapeutical uses. GAGs can be located in the extracellular matrix, on the cell surface or within the intracellular compartment. These polysaccharides are composed of disaccharide repeating units including one uronic acid (or neutral sugar for one of them) and one amino sugar. GAGs can be sulfated (chondroitin-sulfate, dermatan-sulfate, heparin/heparan-sulfate, keratan-sulfate) or not (hyaluronic acid). Furthermore, sulfated glycosaminoglycans can be covalently bound to a protein to form proteoglycans. Hyaluronic acid (HA) is very peculiar because it is neither sulfated, nor covalently linked to a protein to form proteoglycan. Moreover this polysaccharide has a very high molecular weight (up to 8×10^6 g/mol in tissue) in contrast to sulfated GAGs (from 10 to 100×10^3 g/mol) [5,6]. GAGs interact with a wide range of proteins involved in physiological and pathological processes. They display many biological activities which can influence tissue repair as well as inflammatory response [1,7,9].

For example, heparan-sulfate chains borne by the cell surface proteoglycans are required to mediate signals of heparin-binding growth factors such as fibroblast growth factors (FGFs), heparin binding-epidermal growth factor (HB-EGF) or vascular endothelial growth factor (VEGF) (Figure 1) [10,12]. Furthermore in extracellular matrix, sulfated glycosaminoglycans are specifically involved in growth factor bioavailability and protection against proteinase degradation [13,14]. Their ability to structure matrix macromolecules has been described on collagens as well as on matrix glycoproteins or elastic fibers [15,17]. Other studies demonstrated that heparin and chondroitin-sulfate directly inhibit serine-proteinase activity and modulate matrix metalloproteinase activity in cell culture [18,19]. Due to specific interactions with chemokines and selectins, heparan-sulfates found on endothelial cell surface are also major actors in leukocyte rolling and chemo-attraction [20,21].

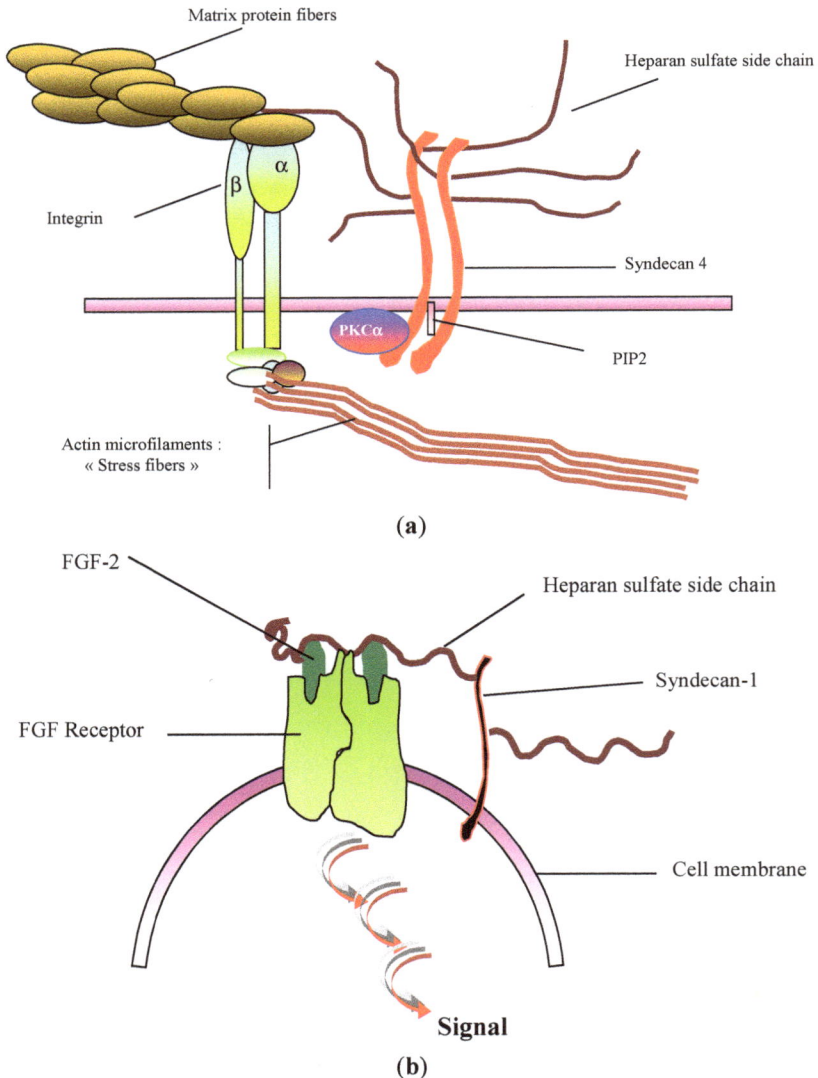

Figure 1. Cell surface GAGs and cell behavior. (**a**) GAGs and cell adhesion; (**b**) GAGs and growth factor promotion.

The HA, a non-sulfated GAG, is also a major actor in tissue structuring and remodeling. The hallmark of this polysaccharide is its ability to form hydrogels allowing joint lubrication and space creation to cell migration during wound healing and embryonic morphogenesis [22]. During cutaneous wound healing, HA prevents fibrosis [23]. Thus, during fetal skin repair, which is characterized by scarless wound healing, high amounts of HA are produced whereas a dramatic downregulation of this GAG synthesis is observed in the keloids [24]. HA stimulates endothelial cell proliferation, migration and differentiation following activation of specific cell receptors (CD44 receptor and hyaluronan-mediated motility receptor or RHAMM). HA is also involved in inflammatory response after injury by stimulation of macrophage cytokine secretion through CD44 signaling pathway [21].

Thus, these polysaccharides could be advantageously proposed as pharmacological agents or biomaterials for tissue repair and engineering. Unfortunately, the strong anti-coagulant activity of some of them (heparin, heparan-sulfate), their animal origin increasing the risk for the presence of infectious agents such as viruses or prions, and an unreliable availability (cost, volume) restrict their use in Human. Marine organisms such as macroalgae, microalgae, bacteria, cyanobacteria, invertebrates and chordata offer a rich source of carbohydrates with original structures largely species specific.

3. GAG-Like Polysaccharides from Marine Eukaryotes

3.1. GAGs

Hyaluronic acid, chondroitin sulfate, dermatan sulfate and heparan sulfate can be found in marine invertebrates; they have been isolated from marine mollusks or echinoderms such as sea urchins or sea cucumbers (ascidians). GAGs can be extracted from marine mollusk such as *Amussium pleuronectus* (Linne). The structural characterization showed that they are sulfated like heparin and contain equivalent amount of uronic acid and hexosamine. They could be an alternative source of heparin [25]. The dermatan sulfates isolated from sea urchin and chondroitin sulfates from ascidians have the same backbone structures as the mammalian GAGs but possess different sulfation patterns [26,27]. In animal models, the fucosylated chondroitin sulfate obtained from sea cucumber was a promising molecule with possible beneficial effects in pathological conditions such as thrombosis and ischemia [27]. Chondroitin/dermatan sulfate hybrid chains extracted from shark skin showed a high affinity for growth factors and neurotrophic factors [28].

3.2. Alginate

Marine alginate is found in all brown seaweeds (Phaeophyceae) in a proportion of 18 to 40% of the total plant. Alginate is both a biopolymer and a polyelectrolyte and is considered to be biocompatible, non-toxic, non-immunogenic and biodegradable. Alginate is a high-molecular weight (in the range $200–500 \times 10^3$ g/mol) polyuronic acid composed of two types of uronic acid distributed as blocks of guluronic acid (GulA or "G") or mannuronic acid (ManA or "M") as well as heteropolymeric mixed sequences (GulA-ManA, usually alternating). Often commercial alginate is characterized by its "M:G" ratio. The alginate is known to form a physical gel by hydrogen bonding at low pH (acid gel) and by ionic interactions with divalent or trivalent ions, which act as crosslinkers between adjacent polymer chains. The alginate and alginate with chemical modifications on carboxyl or hydroxyl groups, present real promise for obtaining new biomaterials useful in cell immobilization, controlled drug delivery and tissue engineering [29,30]. Tailored alginate hydrogels have been studied to transplant cells such as chondrocytes and osteoblasts and improve neo-cartilage or neo-bone formation. The beneficial use of these modified alginate gels as biomaterials has been demonstrated in a number of *in vitro* and *in vivo* studies [31].

3.3. Fucoidans

3.3.1. From Marine Echinoderms

Biological properties of sulfated fucoidans (or fucans) extracted from marine invertebrates such as sea urchins or sea cucumbers have been extensively studied. These polymers of L-fucose are homogeneous and unbranched and bear no substituent other than sulfate. As described for mammalian GAGs, they present anticoagulant and antithrombotic activities. They can act as a ligand for either L- or P-selectins like heparin or heparan sulfate. They also are active on cell growth, migration and adhesion [3].

3.3.2. From Seaweeds

Fucoidans can also be isolated from Phaeophyceae cell wall; algal sulfated fucoidans are more complex than fucoidans found in marine invertebrates. Algal fucoidans are composed of fucosyl disaccharide repeating units substituted by sulfates or uronic acids; they present other substituents such as *O*-acetyl, and branches adding considerably to their heterogeneity (Figure 2) [32,34].

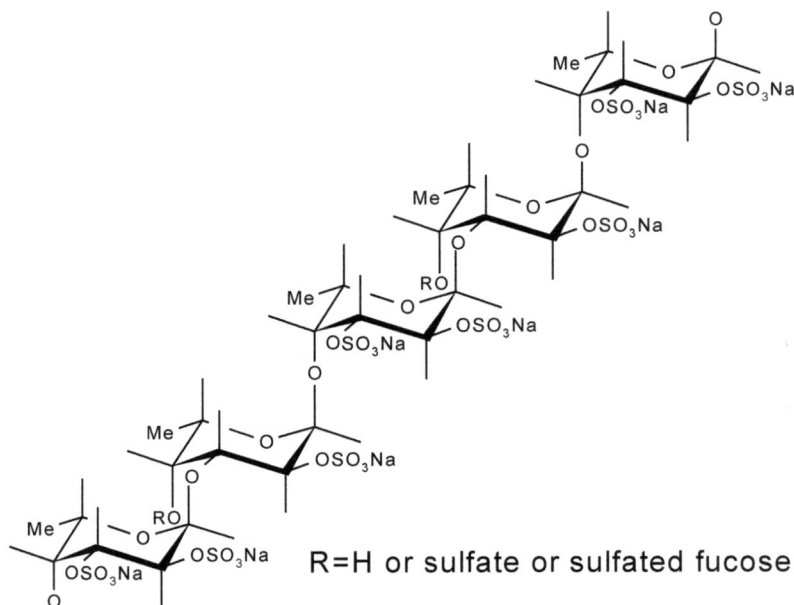

Figure 2. Structure of sulfated oligofucoidan constitutive of algal fucoidan from *Ascophyllum nodosum* [32].

After depolymerization (by acidic hydrolysis or free radical process), low-molecular-weight fractions of fucoidans (LMW fucans, <30 kDa) have been obtained and shown to exhibit some heparin-like properties, with less side effects. Heparin is a sulfated polysaccharide from porcine origin used as an antithrombotic drug; however, its antithrombotic efficacy is limited by its strong anticoagulant properties correlated with a high hemorrhagic risk. The venous antithrombotic activity of LMW fucans (LMWF) has been compared with a low-molecular-weight heparin in the Wessler rabbit model and exhibited a better ratio antithrombotic effect/hemorrhagic risk [35,37]. Moreover LMWF exhibited arterial antithrombotic activity *in vivo* as well. Indeed, LMWF injections improved residual muscle blood flow and increased vessel formation in acute hind limb ischemia model in rat; they prevented arterial thrombosis induced by apoptosis in rabbit with no increase of bleeding risk (Figure 3) [38,39]. This antithrombotic activity may, in part, be explained by the decrease of tissue factor expression in the media of denuded arteries and the significant increase of plasma TFPI (inhibitor of the extrinsic coagulation pathway) released from endothelial cell by fucoidan as previously shown *in vitro* [39,40].

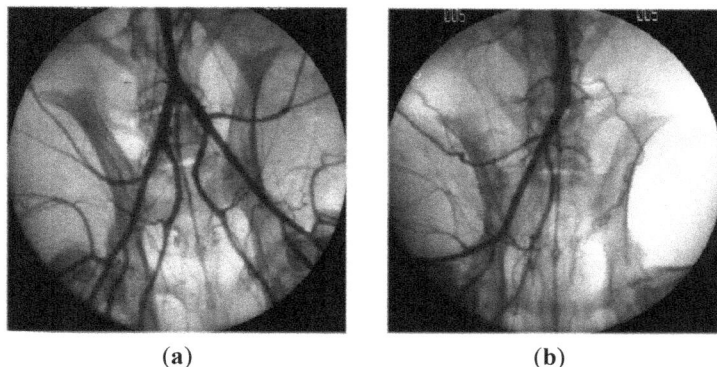

Figure 3. Angiographies of hind limbs from rabbits, 3 days after apoptosis induction. (**a**) Rabbit receiving LMWF; (**b**) Rabbit receiving placebo.

These results led us to further study sulfated polysaccharide-endothelial cell interaction. Owing to their ionic structure, LMWF, like heparin, can bind and modulate the activity of proangiogenic growth factors such as fibroblast growth factors (FGF) [41,42]. Fucoidan enhanced *in vitro* tube formation by mature endothelial cells in the presence of FGF-2 [43]. This effect correlated with a decrease of PAI-1 (plasminogen activator inhibitor) release, and an upregulation of the cell-surface α6 integrin subunit, which could explain the proangiogenic activity [42,44].

Until recently, vessel formation was claimed to be related to *in situ* mature endothelial cell proliferation, migration and differentiation. In 1997, Asahara and Isner demonstrated the presence of endothelial progenitor cells (EPCs) in circulating blood, which play a major role in vasculogenesis in physiological and pathological situations when organ vascularization, and regeneration, is required [45]. Autologous infusion of EPCs would potentially be a promising therapy for revascularizing ischemic tissues. Unfortunately these EPCs are very rare in blood. Moreover further evidence indicates that not only the cell number but also functional properties of transplanted EPCs determine the outcome of autologous stem cell transplantation. The poor graft efficiency seems to be related to unfavorable functional changes during the expansion procedure. We demonstrated that fucoidan induced EPCs to adopt a proangiogenic phenotype. It enhanced their proliferation, migration and differentiation into capillary-like structures on Matrigel [46]. LMWF could act through SDF-1, which when stimulated during EPCs expansion increased their therapeutic potential after cell transplantation in a model of hind limb ischemia [47,48].

LMWF has demonstrated some anti-inflammatory properties such as anti-complementary activities with both inhibition of leukocyte margination and connective tissue proteolysis. LMWF could be used for treating some inflammatory diseases in which uncontrolled extracellular matrix degradation takes place [49]. As described above, LMWF can also promote tissue rebuilding parameters such as signaling by heparin-binding growth factors (FGF-2, VEGF) and collagen processing in fibroblasts, smooth muscle cells or endothelial cells in culture. Recently, a study showed that LMWF can bind fibrillar collagens and provide protection and signal promotion of heparin binding growth factors to improve biocompatibility of purified cancellous bone substitute. Indeed, it was demonstrated that LMWF mimicks and restores the properties of bone non collagenous matrix (proteoglycans, glycoproteins) that were eliminated by drastic purification process during design of the biomaterial, to regulate soluble factors bioavailability [50].

4. GAG-Like Polysaccharides from Marine Prokaryotes

4.1. Extracellular Polymeric Substances (EPS)-Producing Cyanobacteria

Cyanobacteria (blue-green algae) are Gram-negative photosynthetic prokaryotes considered as a rich source of novel molecules of a great importance from a biotechnological and industrial point of view. Many cyanobacteria produce extracellular polymeric substances (EPS) mainly of polysaccharidic nature. These EPS can remain associated to the cell surface as sheaths, capsules and/or slimes, or be liberated into the surrounding environment as released polysaccharides [51].

4.2. Spirulina (Arthrospira)

Spirulina is a microalga which offers a broad range of applications such as a nutritive or pharmaceutical additive with no risk to health. Clinical studies suggest that compounds in the microalgae have therapeutic functions and especially polysaccharides with antiflammatory effects [52]. Spirulan, existing as a ionic form (calcium or sodium), is a sulfated polysaccharide isolated from *Arthrospira platensis* (formely *Spirulina platensis*) and consisting of two types of disaccharide repeating units, [→3)-α-L-Rha(1→2)-α-L-Aco-(1→] where Aco (acofriose) is 3-*O*-methyl-Rha with sulfate groups and *O*-hexuronosyl-rhamnose. It also contains trace amounts of xylose, glucuronic acid and galacturonic acid. Its molecular weight is about 200×10^3 g/mol and it bears from 5 to 20% sulfate depending on the source [53]. Spirulan is reported to inhibit pulmonary metastasis in humans and to prevent the adhesion and proliferation of tumor cells. Highly porous scaffolds have been constructed by electrospining biomass of *Spirulina*. In these conditions, well defined nanofibers were produced to be used as extracellular matrices for stem cell culture and future treatment of spinal cord injury [54].

Other EPS-Producing Cyanobacteria

Cyanobacteria of the genera *Aphanocapsa*, *Cyanothece*, *Gloeothece*, *Synechocystis*, *Phormidium*, *Anabaena* and *Nostoc* are able to produce sulfated polysaccharides containing uronic acids. Applications of cyanobacterial polysaccharides have been poorly investigated in the biomedical field except as antiviral agents. Moreover, the overall negative charge of cyanobacterial EPS may be essential for sequestering metal cations that are essential for cell growth but present at low concentrations in their surroundings, and/or preventing the direct contact between the cells and toxic heavy metals dispersed in the environment [55].

4.3. Bacterial Exopolysaccharides (EPS)

Marine biosphere offers wealthy flora and fauna living in different unusual ecosystems embracing diverse microbial communities: deep-sea hydrothermal vents, Arctic and Antartic sea-ice, Mediterranean shallow vents, microbial mats located in some polynesian atolls [56,63].

Deep-sea microorganisms, bacteria and archaea, or the processes they mediate *in situ*, and the promise of their primary and secondary products present a great interest to biotechnology and a potential for pharmaceutical applications [64,66]. From different oceanographic cruises organised to explore deep-sea hydrothermal vent environments (East Pacific Rise, North Fiji, Guaymas basin and Mid Atlantic Ridge), several polysaccharide-producing bacteria have been discovered. Screenings have been performed mainly on mesophilic bacteria rather than on psychrophilic, thermophilic or hyperthermophilic strains. Up to date, three main genera of polysaccharide-producing bacteria have been identified: *Pseudoalteromonas* sp., *Alteromonas* sp. and *Vibrio* sp. By fermentation, each bacterium can liberate into the culture medium (an aerobic carbohydrate-based medium) one specific polysaccharide with an original structure and with an interesting yield, from 0.5 g to 4 g of polysaccharide/liter of culture broth [59].

4.3.1. HE 800 EPS from *Vibrio diabolicus*

The *Vibrio diabolicus* bacterium was isolated from a Pompei worm tube (polychaete *Alvinella pompejana*); the EPS it secreted was characterized by equal amounts of glucuronic acid and hexosamine (*N*-acetyl glucosamine and *N*-acetyl galactosamine). It is a hyaluronic acid-like polymer (Figure 4) [67, 68] and its commercial name is Hyalurift®.

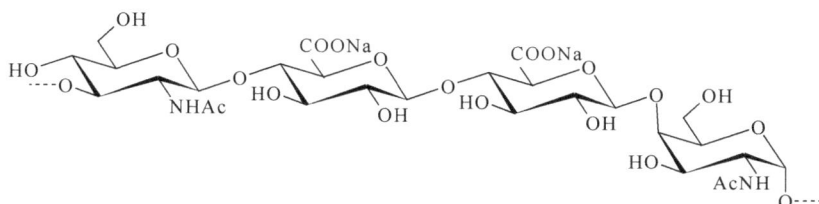

Figure 4. Repeating unit of the marine bacterial polysaccharide (HE800 EPS) produced by *Vibrio diabolicus* [68].

The efficiency of this high-molecular-weight (>10^6 g/mol) linear polysaccharide was evaluated on the restoration of bone integrity for critical size defects (CSD) performed on the calvaria of Wistar male rats. Collagen was used as a control. Briefly, bacterially produced polysaccharide or collagen (as control) was put into a hole made in the right parietal bone while another hole made in the left parietal bone was kept free of any compound. In the presence of EPS secreted by *Vibrio diabolicus*, bone healing was almost complete after 15 days; the anatomy of the defect with trabecular and cortical structure was totally restored. Neovascularization was also observed along with an organized trabecular bone. No abnormal bone growth or conjunctival abnormalities were noticed. Conversely, the collagen-treated animals did not demonstrate significant healing [69].

These results could be explained by the HE800 EPS effects observed subsequently in *in vitro* models of tissue remodeling. Indeed, it was demonstrated that HE800 EPS enhanced collagen structuring in engineering connective tissue model and promoted fibroblast settled in extracellular matrix. Using the capability of acido-soluble collagen I to auto-associate into fibrils after pH neutralizing, a reconstructed extracellular matrix containing human fibroblasts was produced and studied by electron microscopy and classical histology. By electron microscopy, it was observed that addition of HE800 EPS, during collagenous matrix building, increased and accelerated collagen fibrils formation with 67 nm periodic striations.

Study on fibroblasts distribution in different parts of reconstructed connective tissues demonstrated the ability of HE800 EPS to modulate signals mediated by cell-matrix interactions. In this *in vitro* model, proliferating cells were preferentially located at the tissue surface. In order to distinguish between fibroblasts colonizing the extracellular matrix and fibroblasts living and proliferating at the surface of the reconstructed tissue, stained histological sections were studied by image analysis. Observations showed that in reconstructed tissue containing HE800 EPS, cells at the periphery proliferated and massively migrated in the extracellular matrix. We could conclude that this EPS specifically improved cytocompatibility of the engineered tissue. Therefore, the use of HE800 EPS to design collagenic engineered tissue for skin or cartilage grafting can be suggested [70]. These efforts to design innovative medical devices or tissue engineering products demonstrate that HE800 EPS in native form could find application in the future as a new biomaterial for tissue therapy.

With the purpose of preparing a GAG-like compound, this high-molecular-weight EPS was first depolymerized by a free-radical reaction. Then the newly depolymerized EPS was chemically sulfated with pyridine-sulfur trioxyde in dimethylformamide. These chemical modifications can yield a low molecular weight (<20 kDa) and sulfated polysaccharide with new properties. In fact, depolymerization, *N*-deacetylation and sulfation produced a HE800 EPS derivative, referred to as

DRS HE800, which is structurally close to heparan-sulfate. It was also demonstrated that other EPS having no GAG structural features could be modified in order to acquire heparan sulfate properties. The effect of this HE800 EPS derivative was tested in proliferation assays. Thus, in two-dimensional culture this derivative was capable of stimulating the proliferation of dermal and gingival fibroblasts. And moreover, this derivative could inhibit the secretion of matrix metalloproteinases (MMPs) such as gelatinase A (MMP-2) and stromelysin 1 (MMP-3) by fibroblasts after IL-1β induction [71].

Vascularization in tissue engineering is a challenge; indeed tissue repair is possible only in the presence of new vessels contributing to tissue growth. New vessels, contributing to vascular and tissue repair, are formed by two different processes. The first involves proliferation and migration of *in situ* mature endothelial cells. In the second process, the new vessels of proliferating, migrating, and differentiating endothelial progenitor cells (EPCs) from the bone marrow, are incorporated under the influence of proangiogenic factors such as VEGF. *In vitro* studies showed that DRS HE800 exhibited no proangiogenic properties (proliferation, migration, differentiation tested by vascular tube formation on Matrigel) either on mature endothelial cells such as HUVEC (human umbilical vein endothelial cells), or on EPCs [72] (Figure 5).

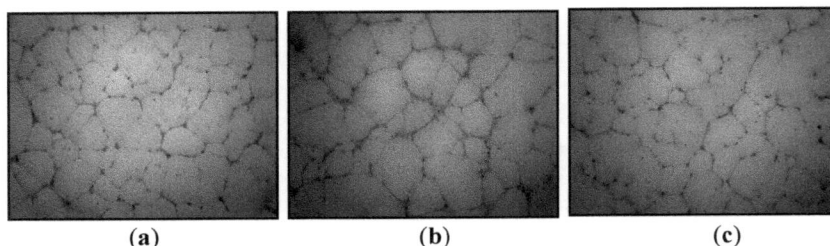

(a)   (b)   (c)

Figure 5. Effect of the DRS HE800 derivative on vascular tube formation on Matrigel from endothelial progenitor cells (EPCs). Photographs show vascular tube formation by EPCs previously treated (a) with 5% of fetal calf serum (control); (b) with proangiogenic factor VEGF (40 ng/mL); and (c) with proangiogenic factor VEGF (40 ng/mL) and DRS HE800 derivative (10 µg/mL).

4.3.2. EPS GY 785 from *Alteromonas infernus*

A bacterium named *Alteromonas infernus* was isolated from a sample of fluid collected among a dense population of *Riftia pachyptila*. The EPS it secretes is a highly branched acidic heteropolysaccharide with a high molecular weight (>1.5 × 10^6 g/mol) and a low sulfate content (≤10%). Its nonasaccharide repeating unit is composed of uronic acid (galacturonic and glucuronic acid) and neutral sugars (galactose and glucose) and substituted with one sulfate group (Figure 6) [73,74].

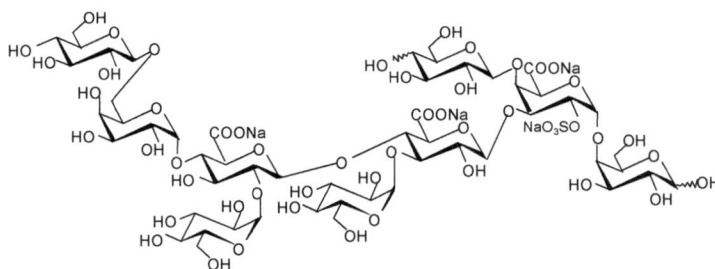

Figure 6. Repeating unit of marine bacterial polysaccharide (GY785 EPS) produced by *Alteromonas infernus* [74,75].

A very recent study demonstrated that the high molecular weight GY785 EPS associated with an injectable silylated hydroxypropylmethylcellulose-based hydrogel (Si-HPMC) could significantly improve the mechanical properties of this new hydrogel construct. The attachment of chondrocytes and osteoblasts was induced when the cells were cultivated in two-dimensional culture on the top of the hydrogel containing 0.67% of GY785 EPS. In three-dimensional culture, GY785 EPS increased viability and proliferation of the chondrocytes. The hydrogel supplemented with 0.67% GY785 EPS presented an interesting feature for cartilage tissue engineering applications [76].

As described above, with the aim of promoting biological activities, preparations of GY785 derivatives have been undertaken to obtain oversulfated low molecular weight polysaccharides. These derivatives demonstrated a weak anticoagulant activity compared to heparin (10 times less). Two types of derivatives (SDR and DRS) were obtained according to the process used. A process with a first step of sulfation (S) and a subsequent second step of free radical depolymerization (DR) gave the SDR derivatives. A process with a first step of free-radical depolymerization (DR) and a subsequent second step of sulfation (S) resulted in DRS derivatives. Surprisingly, the two types of derivatives did not present the same biological properties. The addition of SDR derivative in the culture medium containing FGF-2 increased the proliferation of mature endothelial cells, whereas the DRS derivative had no effect. In the *in vitro* angiogenesis assay, performed to observe the differentiation of mature endothelial cells into vascular tubes on Matrigel, pre-treatment of cells with SDR derivative increased significantly the formation of vascular tubes, whereas DRS derivatives did not have the same effect. In conclusion SDR GY785 EPS derivative has pro-angiogenic effect contrary to DRS GY785 EPS derivative [77]. However, in the same experimental conditions, SDR GY785 EPS derivative had no effect on proliferation, migration and vascular tube formation on Matrigel from endothelial progenitor cells [72]. In summary, SDR GY785 EPS derivative exhibits pro-angiogenic effect contrary to DRS GY785 EPS derivative, but only in the presence of mature endothelial cells.

In other models of study, it was demonstrated that DRS GY785 EPS stimulated some human mesenchymal cells: dermal fibroblasts, gingival fibroblasts, stromal medullar cells. In two-dimensional cultures, this EPS derivative promoted FGF-2 signaling, and thus cell proliferation. This effect was also observed when cells were associated with extracellular collagenous matrix. Furthermore, DRS GY785 EPS derivatives were able to inhibit some processes involved in tissue breakdown and inflammation such as complement cascade, and induction of MMPs by inflammatory cytokines such as IL-1β and TNF-α [71]. Recently, the effect of this derivative on osteogenesis was investigated because it was previously described that the growth and differentiation of bone cells is controlled by several factors, which can be modulated by heparan sulfates [78]. It was shown that this DRS GY785 EPS derivative inhibited osteoclastogenesis. In addition, the DRS GY785 EPS derivative reduced proliferation and accelerated osteoblastic differentiation, leading to strong inhibition of mineralised nodule formation, which would be in favor of an increase of bone resorption. Taken together, these data show different levels of bone resorption regulation by the DRS GY785 EPS derivative, leading to proresorptive effects [79].

5. Conclusions

Marine organisms offer a great diversity of polysaccharides showing interesting biological properties mimicking those described for the mammalian GAGs. Among the different sources of polysaccharides, algal polysaccharides such as fucoidans and especially their LMW derivatives could play an important role in future development of cell therapy and regenerative medicine. Bacterial polysaccharides present also a real potential in cell therapy and tissue engineering with an advantage over the polysaccharides from eukaryotes, since they can be produced totally under controlled conditions in bioreactors. As described for other polysaccharides, some derivatives can be obtained by chemical modifications, to optimize the biological properties and design drugs with improved benefit and low risk for the patient.

References

1. Lindahl, U. Heparan sulfate—a polyanion with multiple messages. *Pure Appl. Chem* **1997**, *69*, 1897–1902.
2. Shriver, Z; Raguram, S; Sasisekharan, R. Glycomics: A pathway to a class of new and improved therapeutics. *Nat. Rev. Drug. Discov* **2004**, *3*, 863–873.
3. Berteau, O; Mulloy, B. Sulfated fucans, fresh perspectives: Structures, functions, biological properties of sulfated fucans and overview of enzymes active towards this class of polysaccharide. *Glycobiology* **2003**, *6*, 29R–40R.
4. Laurienzo, P. Marine polysaccharides in pharmaceutical applications: An overview. *Mar. Drugs* **2010**, *8*, 2435–2465.
5. Jackson, RL; Busch, SJ; Cardin, AD. Glycosaminoglycans—Molecular-properties, proteins interactions, and role in physiological processes. *Physiol. Rev* **1991**, *71*, 481–539.
6. Iozzo, RV. Matrix proteoglycans: From molecular design to cellular function. *Annu. Rev. Biochem* **1998**, *67*, 609–652.
7. Ernst, B; Magnani, JL. From carbohydrate leads to glycomimetic drugs. *Nat. Rev. Drug. Discov* **2009**, *8*, 661–677.
8. Gandhi, NS; Mancera, RL. The structure of glycosaminoglycans and their interactions with proteins. *Chem. Biol. Drug Des* **2008**, *72*, 455–482.
9. Mulloy, B; Linhardt, RJ. Order out of complexity—Protein structures that interact with heparin. *Curr. Opin. Struct. Biol* **2001**, *11*, 623–628.
10. Yayon, A; Klagsbrun, M; Esko, JD; Leder, P; Ornitz, DM. Cell surface, heparin-like molecules are required for binding of basic fibroblast growth factor to its high affinity receptor. *Cell* **1991**, *64*, 841–848.
11. Yu, W-H; Woessner, JF; McNeish, JD; Stamenkovic, I. CD44 anchors the assembly of matrilysin/MMP-7 with heparin-binding epidermal growth factor precursor and ErbB4 and regulates female reproductive organ remodeling. *Genes Dev* **2002**, *16*, 307–323.
12. Stringer, SE. The role of heparan sulphate proteoglycans in angiogenesis. *Biochem. Soc. Trans* **2006**, *34*, 451–453.
13. Penc, SF; Pomahac, B; Winkler, T; Dorschner, RA; Eriksson, E; Herndon, M; Gallo, RL. Dermatan sulfate released after injury is a potent promoter of fibroblast growth factor-2 function. *J. Biol. Chem* **1998**, *273*, 28116–28121.
14. Feige, JJ; Baird, A. Crinopexy: Extracellular regulation of growth factor action. *Kidney Int. Suppl* **1995**, *49*, S15–S18.
15. Chung, CY; Erickson, HP. Glycosaminoglycans modulate fibronectin matrix assembly and are essential for matrix incorporation of tenascin-C. *J. Cell Sci* **1997**, *110*, 1413–1419.
16. Wu, WJ; Vrhovski, B; Weiss, AS. Glycosaminoglycans mediate the coacervation of human tropoelastin through dominant charge interactions involving lysine side chains. *J. Biol. Chem* **1999**, *274*, 21719–21724.
17. Buczek-Thomas, JA; Chu, CL; Rich, CB; Stone, PJ; Foster, JA; Nugent, MA. Heparan sulfate depletion within pulmonary fibroblasts: Implications for elastogenesis and repair. *J. Cell. Physiol* **2002**, *192*, 294–303.
18. Volpi, N. Inhibition of human leukocyte elastase activity by chondroitin sulfates. *Chem. Biol. Interact* **1997**, *105*, 157–167.
19. Gogly, B; Dridi, M; Hornebeck, W; Bonnefoix, M; Godeau, G; Pellat, B. Effect of heparin on the production of matrix metalloproteinases and tissue inhibitors of metalloproteinases by human dermal fibroblasts. *Cell Biol. Int* **1999**, *23*, 203–209.
20. Kawashima, H. Roles of sulfated Glycans in lymphocyte homing. *Biol. Pharm. Bull* **2006**, *29*, 2343–2349.
21. Taylor, KR; Gallo, RL. Glycosaminoglycans and their proteoglycans: Host-associated molecular patterns for initiation and modulation of inflammation. *FASEB J* **2006**, *20*, 9–22.
22. Juhlin, L. Hyaluronan in skin. *J. Int. Med* **1997**, *242*, 61–66.
23. Croce, MA; Dyne, K; Boraldi, F; Quaglino, D; Cetta, G; Tiozzo, R; Ronchetti, IP. Hyaluronan affects protein and collagen synthesis by *in vitro* human skin fibroblasts. *Tissue Cell* **2001**, *33*, 326–331.
24. Meyer, LJM; Russell, SB; Russell, JD; Trupin, JS; Egbert, BM; Shuster, S; Stern, R. Reduced hyaluronan in keloid tissue and cultured keloid fibroblasts. *J. Invest. Dermatol* **2000**, *114*, 953–959.

25. Saravanan, R; Shanmugam, A. Isolation and Characterization of Low Molecular Weight Glycosaminoglycans from Marine Mollusc *Amussium pleuronectus* (Linne) using Chromatography. *Appl. Biochem. Biotechnol* **2010**, *160*, 791–799.
26. Vilela-Silva, AC; Alves, AP; Valente, AP; Vacquier, VD; Mourao, PA. Structure of the sulfated alpha-L-fucan from the egg jelly coat of the sea urchin *Strongylocentrotus franciscanus*: Patterns of preferential 2-*O*- and 4-*O*-sulfation determine sperm cell recognition. *Glycobiology* **1999**, *9*, 927–933.
27. Tapon-Bretaudiere, J; Chabut, D; Zierer, M; Matou, S; Helley, D; Bros, A; Mourao, PA; Fischer, AM. A fucosylated chondroitin sulfate from echinoderm modulates *in vitro* fibroblast growth factor 2-dependent angiogenesis. *Mol. Cancer Res* **2002**, *1*, 96–102.
28. Nandini, CD; Itoh, N; Sugahara, K. Novel 70-kDa chondroitin sulfate/dermatan sulfate hybrid chains with a unique heterogenous sulfation pattern from shark skin, which exhibit neuritogenic activity and binding activities for growth factors and neurotrophic factors. *J. Biol. Chem* **2005**, *280*, 4058–4069.
29. Gomez d'Ayala, G; Malinconico, M; Laurienzo, P. Marine derived polysaccharides for biomedical applications: Chemical modification approaches. *Molecules* **2008**, *13*, 2069–2106.
30. Yang, J-S; Xie, Y-J; He, W. Research progress on chemical modification of alginate: A review. *Carbohydr. Polym* **2011**, *84*, 33–39.
31. Augst, AD; Kong, HJ; Mooney, DJ. Alginate Hydrogels as Biomaterials. *Macromol. Biosci* **2006**, *6*, 623–633.
32. Chevolot, L; Mulloy, B; Ratiskol, J; Foucault, A; Colliec-Jouault, S. A disaccharide repeat unit is the major structure in fucoidans from two species of brown algae. *Carbohydr. Res* **2001**, *330*, 529–535.
33. Bilan, MI; Grachev, AA; Ustuzhanina, NE; Shashkov, AS; Nifantiev, NE; Usov, AI. Structure of a fucoidan from the brown seaweed *Fucus evanescens*. *Carbohydr. Res* **2002**, *337*, 719–730.
34. Nishino, T; Nagumo, T; Kiyohara, H; Yamada, H. Structural characterization of a new anticoagulant fucan sulfate from the brown seaweed *Ecklonia kurome*. *Carbohydr. Res* **1991**, *211*, 77–90.
35. Millet, J; Jouault, SC; Mauray, S; Theveniaux, J; Sternberg, C; Boisson Vidal, C; Fischer, AM. Antithrombotic and anticoagulant activities of a low molecular weight fucoidan by the subcutaneous route. *J. Thromb. Haemost* **1999**, *81*, 391–395.
36. Colliec-Jouault, S; Millet, J; Helley, D; Sinquin, C; Fischer, AM. Effect of low-molecular-weight fucoidan on experimental arterial thrombosis in the rabbit and rat. *J. Thromb. Haemost* **2003**, *1*, 1114–1115.
37. Colliec-Jouault, S; Durand, P; Fischer, A-M; Jozefonvicz, J; Letourneur, D; Millet, J. Low Molecular Weight Sulphated Polysaccharide to Obtain a Medicine with Antithrombotic Activity. US Patent 6,828,307, 7 December 2004.
38. Luyt, CE; Meddahi-Pelle, A; Ho-Tin-Noe, B; Colliec-Jouault, S; Guezennec, J; Louedec, L; Prats, HE; Jacob, MP; Osborne-Pellegrin, M; Letourneur, D; Michel, JB. Low-molecular-weight fucoidan promotes therapeutic revascularization in a rat model of critical hindlimb ischemia. *J. Pharmacol. Exp. Ther* **2003**, *305*, 24–30.
39. Durand, E; Helley, D; Zen, AAH; Dujols, C; Bruneval, P; Colliec-Jouault, S; Fischer, AM; Lafont, A. Effect of low molecular weight fucoidan and low molecular weight heparin in a rabbit model of arterial thrombosis. *J. Vasc. Res* **2008**, *45*, 529–537.
40. Giraux, JL; Tapon-Bretaudiere, J; Matou, S; Fischer, AM. Fucoidan, as heparin, induces tissue factor pathway inhibitor release from cultured human endothelial cells. *J. Thromb. Haemost* **1998**, *80*, 692–695.
41. Matou, S; Helley, D; Chabut, D; Bros, A; Fischer, A-M. Effect of fucoidan on fibroblast growth factor-2-induced angiogenesis *in vitro*. *Thromb. Res* **2002**, *106*, 213–221.
42. Chabut, D; Fischer, AM; Colliec-Jouault, S; Laurendeau, I; Matou, S; Le Bonniec, B; Helley, D. Low molecular weight fucoidan and heparin enhance the basic fibroblast growth factor-induced tube formation of endothelial cells through heparan sulfate-dependent alpha 6 overexpression. *Mol. Pharmacol* **2003**, *64*, 696–702.
43. Matou, S; Colliec-Jouault, S; Galy-Fauroux, I; Ratiskol, J; Sinquin, C; Guezennec, J; Fischer, A-M; Helley, D. Effect of an oversulfated exopolysaccharide on angiogenesis induced by fibroblast growth factor-2 or vascular endothelial growth factor *in vitro*. *Biochem. Pharmacol* **2005**, *69*, 751–759.
44. Chabut, D; Fischer, AM; Helley, D; Colliec, S. Low molecular weight fucoidan promotes FGF-2-induced vascular tube formation by human endothelial cells, with decreased PAI-1 release and ICAM-1 downregulation. *Thromb. Res* **2004**, *113*, 93–95.

45. Asahara, T; Krasinski, KL; Chen, DH; Sullivan, AB; Kearney, M; Silver, M; Li, T; Isner, JM. Circulating endothelial progenitor cells in peripheral blood incorporate into re-endothelialization after vascular injury. *Circulation* **1997**, *96*, 4064–4064.

46. Zemani, F; Benisvy, D; Galy-Fauroux, I; Lokajczyk, A; Colliec-Jouault, S; Uzan, G; Fischer, AM; Boisson-Vidal, C. Low-molecular-weight fucoidan enhances the proangiogenic phenotype of endothelial progenitor cells. *Biochem. Pharmacol* **2005**, *70*, 1167–1175.

47. Sweeney, EA; Priestley, GV; Nakamoto, B; Collins, RG; Beaudet, AL; Papayannopoulou, T. Mobilization of stem/progenitor cells by sulfated polysaccharides does not require selectin presence. *Proc. Natl. Acad. Sci. USA* **2000**, *97*, 6544–6549.

48. Zemani, F; Silvestre, JS; Fauvel-Lafeve, F; Bruel, A; Vilar, J; Bieche, I; Laurendeau, I; Galy-Fauroux, I; Fischer, AM; Boisson-Vidal, C. *Ex vivo* priming of endothelial progenitor cells with SDF-1 before transplantation could increase their proangiogenic potential. *Arterioscler. Thromb. Vasc. Biol* **2008**, *28*, 644–650.

49. Senni, K; Gueniche, F; Foucault-Bertaud, A; Igondjo-Tchen, S; Fioretti, F; Colliec-Jouault, S; Durand, P; Guezennec, J; Godeau, G; Letourneur, D. Fucoidan a sulfated polysaccharide from brown algae is a potent modulator of connective tissue proteolysis. *Arch. Biochem. Biophys* **2006**, *445*, 56–64.

50. Changotade, SI; Korb, G; Bassil, J; Barroukh, B; Willig, C; Colliec-Jouault, S; Durand, P; Godeau, G; Senni, K. Potential effects of a low-molecular-weight fucoidan extracted from brown algae on bone biomaterial osteoconductive properties. *J. Biomed. Mater. Res. A* **2008**, *87*, 666–675.

51. De Philippis, R; Sili, C; Paperi, R; Vincenzini, M. Exopolysaccharide-producing cyanobacteria and their possible exploitation: A review. *J. Appl. Phycol* **2001**, *13*, 293–299.

52. Matsui, MS; Muizzuddin, N; Arad, S; Marenus, K. Sulfated polysaccharides from red microalgae have antiinflammatory properties *in vitro* and *in vivo*. *Appl. Biochem. Biotechnol* **2003**, *104*, 13–22.

53. Lee, JB; Hayashi, T; Hayashi, K; Sankawa, U. Structural Analysis of Calcium Spirulan (Ca-SP)-Derived Oligosaccharides Using Electrospray Ionization Mass Spectrometry. *J. Nat. Prod* **2000**, *63*, 136–138.

54. de Morais, MG; Stillings, C; Dersch, R; Rudisile, M; Pranke, P; Costa, JAV; Wendorff, J. Preparation of nanofibers containing the microalga *Spirulina* (*Arthrospira*). *Bioresour. Technol* **2010**, *101*, 2872–2876.

55. Pereira, S; Micheletti, E; Zille, A; Santos, A; Moradas-Ferreira, P; Tamagnini, P; De Philippis, R. Using extracellular polymeric substances (EPS)-producing cyanobacteria for the bioremediation of heavy metals: Do cations compete for the EPS functional groups and also accumulate inside the cell? *Microbiology* **2011**, *157*, 451–458.

56. Arrieta, JM; Arnaud-Haond, S; Duarte, CM. What lies underneath: Conserving the oceans' genetic resources. *Proc. Natl. Acad. Sci. USA* **2010**, *107*, 18318–18324.

57. Satpute, SK; Banat, IM; Dhakephalkar, PK; Banpurkar, AG; Chopade, BA. Biosurfactants, bioemulsifiers and exopolysaccharides from marine microorganisms. *Biotechnol. Adv* **2010**, *28*, 436–450.

58. Deming, JW. Deep ocean environmental biotechnology. *Curr. Opin. Biotechnol* **1998**, *9*, 283–287.

59. Guezennec, J. Deep-sea hydrothermal vents: A new source of innovative bacterial exopolysaccharides of biotechnological interest? *J. Ind. Microbiol. Biotechnol* **2002**, *29*, 204–208.

60. Nichols Mancuso, CA; Garon, S; Bowman, JP; Raguenes, G; Guezennec, J. Production of exopolysaccharides by Antarctic marine bacterial isolates. *J. Appl. Microbiol* **2004**, *96*, 1057–1066.

61. Nichols Mancuso, CA; Guezennec, J; Bowman, JP. Bacterial exopolysaccharides from extreme marine environments with special consideration of the southern ocean, sea ice, and deep-sea hydrothermal vents: A review. *Mar. Biotechnol* **2005**, *7*, 253–271.

62. Arena, A; Gugliandolo, C; Stassi, G; Pavone, B; Iannello, D; Bisignano, G; Maugeri, TL. An exopolysaccharide produced by Geobacillus thermodenitrificans strain B3-72: Antiviral activity on immunocompetent cells. *Immunol. Lett* **2009**, *123*, 132–137.

63. Guézennec, J; Moppert, X; Raguénès, G; Richert, L; Costa, B; Simon-Colin, C. Microbial mats in French Polynesia and their biotechnological applications. *Process Biochem* **2011**, *46*, 16–22.

64. Pace, NR. Origin of life-facing up to the physical setting. *Cell* **1991**, *65*, 531–533.

65. Desbruyeres, D; Chevaldonne, P; Alayse, AM; Jollivet, D; Lallier, FH; Jouin-Toulmond, C; Zal, F; Sarradin, PM; Cosson, R; Caprais, JC. Biology and ecology of the "Pompeii worm" (*Alvinella pompejana*), a normal dweller of an extreme deep-sea environment: A synthesis of current knowledge and recent developments. *Deep Sea Res. Part II* **1998**, *45*, 383–422.

66. Vincent, P; Pignet, P; Talmont, F; Bozzi, L; Fournet, B; Guezennec, J. Production and characterization of an exopolysaccharide excreted by a deep-sea hydrothermal vent bacterium isolated from the polychaete annelid *Alvinella pompejana*. *Appl. Environ. Microbiol* **1994**, *60*, 4134–4141.

67. Raguenes, G; Christen, R; Guezennec, J; Pignet, P; Barbier, G. *Vibrio diabolicus* sp. nov., a new polysaccharide-secreting organism isolated from a deep-sea hydrothermal vent polychaete annelid, *Alvinella pompejana*. *Int. J. Syst. Bacteriol* **1997**, *47*, 989–995.

68. Rougeaux, H; Kervarec, N; Pichon, R; Guezennec, J. Structure of the exopolysaccharide of Vibrio diabolicus isolated from a deep-sea hydrothermal vent. *Carbohydr. Res* **1999**, *322*, 40–45.

69. Zanchetta, P; Lagarde, N; Guezennec, J. A new bone-healing material: A hyaluronic Acid-like bacterial exopolysaccharide. *Calcif. Tissue Int* **2003**, *72*, 74–79.

70. Senni, K; Sinquin, C; Colliec-Jouault, S; Godeau, G; Guezennec, J. Use of a polysaccharide wich is excreted by the *Vibrio diabolicus* species for the engineering of non-mineralized connective-tissue. US Patent 0,317,860, 25 December 2008.

71. Senni, K; Gueniche, F; Yousfi, M; Fioretti, F; Godeau, G; Colliec-Jouault, S; Ratiskol, J; Sinquin, C; Raguenes, G; Courtois, A; Guezennec, J. Sulfated depolymerized derivatives of exopolysaccharides (EPS) from mesophilic marine bacteria, method for preparing same, and use thereof in tissue regeneration. US Patent 0,131,472, 5 June 2008.

72. Pereira, J. *The bacterial exopolysaccharides DRS HE800 and SDR GY785 have no effect on proangiogenic properties of human endothelial progenitors cells* in vitro; Université Paris Descartes: Sorbonne Paris Cité, UMR-S765, Paris, France, Unpublished work; 2008.

73. Raguenes, GH; Peres, A; Ruimy, R; Pignet, P; Christen, R; Loaec, M; Rougeaux, H; Barbier, G; Guezennec, JG. *Alteromonas infernus* sp. nov., a new polysaccharide-producing bacterium isolated from a deep-sea hydrothermal vent. *J. Appl. Microbiol* **1997**, *82*, 422–430.

74. Roger, O; Kervarec, N; Ratiskol, J; Colliec-Jouault, S; Chevolot, L. Structural studies of the main exopolysaccharide produced by the deep-sea bacterium *Alteromonas infernus*. *Carbohydr. Res* **2004**, *339*, 2371–2380.

75. Rederstorff, E; Fatimi, A; Sinquin, C; Ratiskol, J; Merceron, C; Vinatier, C; Weiss, P; Colliec-Jouault, S. Sterilization of Exopolysaccharides Produced by Deep-Sea Bacteria: Impact on Their Stability and Degradation. *Mar. Drugs* **2011**, *9*, 224–241.

76. Rederstorff, E; Weiss, P; Source, S; Pilet, P; Xie, F; Sinquin, C; Colliec-Jouault, S; Guicheux, J; Laïb, S. An *in vitro* study of two GAG-like marine polysaccharides incorporated into injectable hydrogels for bone and cartilage tissue engineering. *Acta Biomater* **2011**, *7*, 2119–2130.

77. Matou, S; Colliec-Jouault, S; Helley, D; Ratiskol, J; Sinquin, C; Boisset, C; Guezennec, J; Fischer, A-M. Use of low-molecular weight highly sulfated polysaccharide derivatives for modulating angiogenesis. US Patent 0,259,833, 8 November 2007.

78. Velasco, CR; Colliec-Jouault, S; Redini, F; Heymann, D; Padrines, M. Proteoglycans on bone tumor development. *Drug Discov. Today* **2010**, *15*, 553–560.

79. Ruiz Velasco, C; Baud'huin, M; Sinquin, C; Maillasson, M; Heymann, D; Colliec-Jouault, S; Padrines, M. Effects of a sulfated exopolysaccharide produced by *Altermonas infernus* on bone biology. *Glycobiology* **2011**, *21*, 781–795.

Samples Availability: Available from the authors.

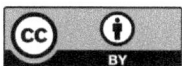

Article

The Anti-Inflammatory Effect and Structure of EPCP1-2 from *Crypthecodinium cohnii* via Modulation of TLR4-NF-κB Pathways in LPS-Induced RAW 264.7 Cells

Xiaolei Ma *, Baolong Xie, Jin Du, Aijun Zhang, Jianan Hao, Shuxun Wang, Jing Wang and Junrui Cao *

The Institute of Seawater Desalination and Multipurpose Utilization, SOA, Tianjin 300192, China;
xiebaolong@tju.edu.cn (B.X.); dujin111@126.com (J.D.); meimei842858@163.com (A.Z.);
phoenix328@163.com (J.H.); w_shuxun@126.com (S.W.); wangjing@126.com (J.W.)
* Correspondence: huandaoyu@126.com or 13929001@mail.tust.edu.cn (X.M.); 13602057810@163.com (J.C.);
  Tel.: +86-022-8755-1825 (X.M.)

Received: 3 November 2017; Accepted: 17 November 2017; Published: 1 December 2017

Abstract: Exopolysaccharide from *Crypthecodinium cohnii* (EPCP1-2) is a marine exopolysaccharide that evidences a variety of biological activities. We isolated a neutral polysaccharide from the fermentation liquid of *Crypthecodinium cohnii* (CP). In this study, a polysaccharide that is derived from *Crypthecodinium cohnii* were analyzed and its anti-inflammatory effect was evaluated on protein expression of toll-like receptor 4 and nuclear factor κB pathways in macrophages. The structural characteristics of EPCP1-2 were characterized by GC (gas chromatography) and GC-MS (gas Chromatography-Mass Spectrometer) analyses. The molecular weight was about 82.5 kDa. The main chain of EPCP1-2 consisted of $(1{\rightarrow}6)$-linked mannopyranosyl, $(1{\rightarrow}6)$-linked glucopyranosyl, branched-chain consisted of $(1{\rightarrow}3,6)$-linked galactopyranosyl and terminal consisted of t-L-Rhapyranosyl. The in vitro anti-inflammatory activity was represented through assay of proliferation rate, pro-inflammatory factor (NO) and expressions of proteins on RAW 264.7, the macrophage cell line. The results revealed that EPCP1-2 exhibited significant anti-inflammatory activity by regulating the expression of toll-like receptor 4, mitogen-activated protein kinases, and Nuclear Factor-κB protein.

Keywords: *Crypthecodinium cohnii*; exo-polysaccharide; anti-inflammatory; TLR4-MAPKs/NF-κB pathways

1. Introduction

Inflammatory response is the process of the human body that attempts to counteract potential injurious agents, including invading viruses, bacteria, and other pathogens [1–3]. Inflammation can also have harmful effects on the host, which is caused by multistage biochemistry, pharmacology, and molecular control of various cells and various soluble medium, including cytokines [4,5]. Pro-inflammatory factor (NO) has been identified as a molecular that involved in the regulation process in nerves and immune system [6]. NO that is generated by activated macrophages can mediate host defense functions, such as antimicrobial and anti-tumor activities, but excess NO production induces tissue damage associated with acute and chronic inflammation. NO secreted by activated macrophages has shown antibacterial and antitumor activities, but the overproduction NO induces acute and chronic inflammation, which causes tissue damage [7]. NO is enzymatically catalyzed by nitric oxide synthases (NOSs) and formed by iNOS in macrophages. In the inflammatory response, NO plays a role by stimulating a variety of proteins of inflammatory reactions pathway, including the NF-κB and MAPKs pathways [8]. Furthermore, such specific anti-inflammatory properties are associated with certain characteristic structures, such as a main backbone of $(1\rightarrow6)$-linked Manp and $(1\rightarrow6)$-linked Glcp residues [9].

Naturally occurring polysaccharides are usually found in marine microorganism, marine invertebrates, such as sea cucumbers and some seaweed [10,11]. Polysaccharide structure and composition of the nature of different marine vary from species to species, but they mainly consist of fucose and sulfate with various monosaccharide and uronic acids [12–15]. *Crypthecodinium cohnii* is oleaginous heterotrophic marine dinoflagellate, in which DHA can account for more than 30% of the total fatty acids (TFA) [16,17]. It is an ideal candidate for DHA production [18]. EPA (Eicosapentaenoic acid) and DHA (Docosahexaenoic Acid) from *Crypthecodinium cohnii* have been extensively studied because of their diverse biological activities, such as antitumor, anti-inflammatory, and immunomodulatory [19]. However, the effects of immunomodulatory activity of water-soluble exopolysaccharides from *Crypthecodinium cohnii* on RAW 264.7 cell line have not been reported. The polysaccharides extracted from plants, fungi, and terrestrial microorganisms have recently attracted to researchers and consumers, due to their bioactivities and relatively low toxicity. Therefore, the detection and evaluation of polysaccharides with antitumor, anti-inflammatory, and immunostimulating bioactivities has become one of the important researches in the field of chemistry and biology [20]. This study was designed to assess the in vitro anti-inflammatory effect of exopolysaccharides extracted from *Crypthecodinium cohnii* on lipopolysaccharide-stimulated RAW 264.7 cell line.

2. Materials and Methods

2.1. Materials and Reagents

Crypthecodinium cohnii was supply by Third Insititude Oceanography, State Oceanic Administration. L-rhamnose, D-glucuronic, D-arabinose, dxylose, D-fructose, D-galactose, and D-mannose were purchased from Solarbio Co. (Beijing, China), while HiTrap Capto Q (16/25) and Superose 6B (10/300) were purchased from GE Co. (Fairfield, CT, USA). T-series dextrans (T-10, T-40, T-70, T-500, T-2000) as standard samples with different molecular weights were purchased from Solarbio Co. (Beijing, China). Methyl iodide (CH_3I) was purchased from Sigma Co., Ltd. (Shanghai, China). Trifluoroacetic acid (TFA) and sodium periodate ($NaIO_4$) were purchased from BLOT Co., Ltd. (Tianjin, China). 3-(4,5-Dimethylthiazol-2-y1)-2,5-diphenyltetrazolium bromide, dimethylsulphoxide (DMSO) was purchased from Sigma Co., Ltd. (Shanghai, China). RPMI-1640 medium and fetal bovine serum (FBS) was purchased from Gibco Invitrogen Co. (New York, NY, USA). Primary antibodies were purchased from CST Co. (Cell Signaling Technology, Danvers, MA, USA), secondary antibodies (HRP-IgG) were purchased from Beyotime Co. (Zhengzhou, China). NC (nitrocellulose) membrane for transfering was purchased from PALL Co. (New York, NY, USA). Other chemicals and reagents were of analytical grade.

2.2. Preparation, Extraction and Purification of Polysaccrides

The fermentation procedures of *Crypthecodinium cohnii* (CP) were based on previous work with some modifications [21]. Crude exopolysaccharide isolated from *Crypthecodinium cohnii* (EPCP) fermentation broth, according to a previous method in reported work [22]. Briefly, fermentation broth of *Crypthecodinium cohnii* was centrifuged ($10,000\times g$, 20 min), and then the supernatant was filtered with 0.22 µm Millipore membrane. After being filtered, the deproteinization of supernatant according to Sevage method [23]. The resulting aqueous fractions without organic solvent were extensively dialyzed by distilled water for two days. The polysaccharides were precipitated by the addition of ethanol to a final concentration of 75% (v/v), after centrifugation ($4000\times g$, 10 min) the precipitates were collected, the precipitates were solubilized in deionized water, and were lyophilized for 48 h. The yield of crude polysaccharides was 58.06%.

The crude polysaccharides were (10 mg) dissolved in 1 mL distilled water, centrifuged ($10,000\times g$, 10 min), and then the supernatant was loaded with a column of Superose 6B (10/300) chromatography and the fraction (EPCP1) was collected. Then, the fraction (EPCP1) was purified by a column HiTrap Capto Q (16/25) [15]. After loading with EPCP1 1 mL, the column was eluted with distilled water, followed by stepwise elution with increased concentration of NaCl (0.1, 0.5, 1.0, and 1.5 M), respectively, at 1 mL/min/tube. The polysaccharide fractions were collected, dialyzed by distilled water for two days, and finally lyophilized to get the polysaccharide fraction named EPCP1-1, EPCP1-2, EPCP1-3, and EPCP1-4. The resulting elute was collected automatically and the soluble sugar content of polysaccharides were detected at 490 nm by the phenol–sulfuric acid method [24]. Finally, the fractions EPCP1-2 were lyophilized for further investigation.

2.3. Characterizations Analysis of EPCP1-2

The carbohydrate content was measured according to phenol-sulfuric acid colorimetric method, using glucose as a standard [24]. Protein content was measured by Bradford's method, using bovine serum albumin (BSA) as the standard [25]. Sulfate group and the uronic acid content were determined according to the reported methods [26,27].

Gas chromatography (GC) is an efficient method to determine polysaccharides. Monosaccharide composition was analyzed based on previous researches [9,28]. For monosaccharide analysis, 5 mg EPCP1-2 was hydrolyzed with 5 mL TFA (2 M) in polytetrafluoroethylene reactor with protection of nitrogen at 110 °C for 3 h. Mole ratio calculation method was as the formula follows:

$$\text{Relative molar number} = CB/AD, \tag{1}$$

(A = Peak area of standard, B = quality of standard, C = Peak area of sample, D = Mw (molecular weight)).

The molecular weight of EPCP1-2 was determined by using a SHIMADZU High Performance Liquid Chromatography (HPLC) analysis system (Tokyo, Japan) with a Shodex SB-804 column ($L \times D$: 8.0 mm × 300 mm, Showa Denko K.K, Tokyo, Japan), according to our previous method [9]. Briefly, NaNO$_3$ solution (0.1 mol/L) was used as the eluent at 0.8 mL·min^{-1} for 30 °C. The molecular weight was calibrated with T-series dextran standard (T-10, T-40, T-70, T-500, T-2000). The injection concentration was 2 mg/mL and volume was 15 μL.

To determine glycosyl linkages, 10–15 mg EPCP1-2 was methylated for seven times according to Needs' method [29]. Briefly, EPCP1-2 was methylated with CH$_3$I (1 mL) in distilled NaOH/DMSO. After reaction, the mixture was extracted with CCl$_4$, and the organic phase was washed by distilled water. Complete methylation was confirmed by FTIR spectrum analysis, in which the disappearance or significantly decreased of the –OH band (3200–3700 cm^{-1}). The per-methylated EPCP1-2 was hydrolyzed, reduced, and acetylated, as described above.

2.4. Cell Culture and Cell Viability Assay

Macrophage cell line, RAW 264.7 cells were maintained and cultured in RPMI 1640 (Gibco Invitrogen Co., Grand Island, NY, USA), supplemented with 10% fetal bovine serum (FBS) at 37 °C under 5% CO$_2$ atmosphere. The cells were seeded into 96-well plates with the density of 5×10^4 cells/well, cultured for 12 h. After being treated with EPCP (100, 200, 400, 800 μg/mL) in the presence or absence of LPS (1 μg/mL) for 36 h, MTT solution (5 mg/mL) was added to each well and incubated for another 4 h. After incubation, culture medium was removed and DMSO was added to dissolve purple precipitates. Then, plates were read at 570 nm using a Microplate spectrophotometer (Thermo Fisher, Co., Waltham, MA, USA).

2.5. NO Assay

Cells were plated at 5×10^4 cell/well in 96-well plates, then it were incubated with or without LPS (1 μg/mL) in the presence or absence of various concentrations EPCP1-2 (50, 100, 200, 400, 800 μg/mL) for 36 h. In brief, 50 μL of cell culture medium was mixed with 50 μL of Griess reagent, the mixture was incubated at room temperature for 15 min, the absorbance at 540 nm was measured in a microplate reader. Fresh culture media were used as blanks for all of the experiments. Nitrite levels in samples were calculated with a standard sodium nitrite curve.

2.6. ELISA Assay of Cytokines

Cells were plated at 5×10^4 cell/well in 96-well plates and then incubated with or without LPS (1 μg/mL) in the presence various concentrations EPCP1-2 (0, 50, 100, 200, 400, 800 μg/mL) of sample for 36 h. In brief, culture medium was collected for detection according to the specification in ELISA kit (Jiancheng, Nanjing, China), the absorbance was measured in a microplate reader. Fresh culture media was used as blanks for all of the experiments. *Cytokines* levels in samples were calculated with standard curves (Supplement Data S2).

2.7. Protein Extraction and Western Blotting

Cells were plated at 5×10^4 cells/well in T-25 culture flask and then incubated with or without LPS (1 μg/mL) in the presence of various concentrations EPCP1-2 (0, 100, 200, 400, 800 μg/mL). After incubation, the cells were collected by centrifugation and washed twice with cold PBS. The cells were lysed in RIPA buffer with 1 mM PMSF (phenylmethylsulfonyl fluoride) on ice for 15 min. The cell lysates were determined as the previous research reported [29]. Finally, the immune-active proteins were separated by Western blot.

2.8. Statistical Analysis

All data were expressed as means ± S.D. $n = 6$. Significant differences among the groups were determined using the unpaired t-test. A value of * $p < 0.05$ and ** $p < 0.01$ were considered to be statistically significant.

3. Result

The EPCP were purified by Superose 6B (10/300) chromatography and HiTrap Capto Q (16/25). Four major fractions were isolated with 0.1 mol/L, 0.5 mol/L, 1.0 mol/L, 1.5 mol/L NaCl. All of these fractions possess anti-inflammatory properties in a range of tests, but one of these fractions possesses the most potent.

3.1. Purification of Hydrolysates of Exopolysaccharide of Crypthecodinium Cohnii (EPCP)

EPCP was firstly separated through a gel chromatography of Superose 6B (10/300) column and anion-exchange column of HiTrap Capto Q (16/25). Two fractions were clearly separated, coded as EPCP1, EPCP2. The proportion of EPCP1 was 98%. EPCP1 was eluted consecutively by 0.1, 0.5, 1.0 and 1.5 mol/L NaCl, coded as EPCP1-1, EPCP1-2, EPCP1-3 and EPCP1-4, respectively. As shown in the profile of gel filtration chromatograms (Figure 1a), two fractions were clearly separated. The anion-exchange chromatogram of the four fractions is shown in (Figure 1b). As Figure 2 showed, only EPCP1-2 had strong activity of anti-inflammatory. In order to explore the cytotoxicity of EPCP1-2 on RAW 264.7 cell line, MTT assay was conducted to test the cell proliferation. As shown by Figure 3, EPCP1-2 promoted proliferation of RAW 264.7 at low concentrations (50, 100, 200 μg/mL). With increase of EPCP1-2 concentration the proliferation showed decrease gradually. But generally, when compared with the control group (0 μg/mL EPCP1-2), the treatment group with EPCP1-2 (400, 800 μg/mL) showed no significant decrease. The results indicated EPCP1-2 exhibited anti-inflammatory effect without cytotoxicity on RAW 264.7 cell line.

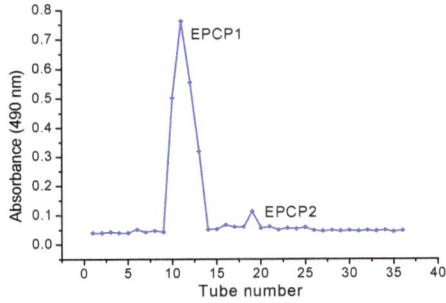

(a)

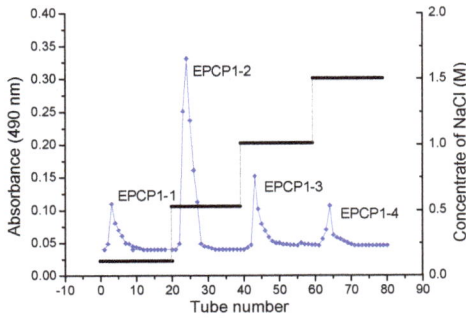

(b)

Figure 1. (a) Stepwise elution curve of crude *Crypthecodinium cohnii* (EPCP) on size-exclusion chromatography column of Superose 6B (10/300) and (b) elution curve of polysaccharide fractions from Superose 6B on anion-exchange chromatography column of HiTrap Capto Q (16/25).

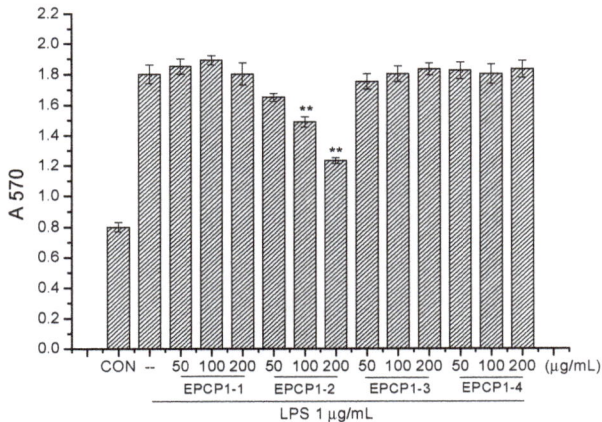

Figure 2. Anti-inflammatory effect of EPCP1 (EPCP1-1, EPCP1-2, EPCP1-3, EPCP1-4) on RAW 264.7 induced by LPS. (Results are expressed as the mean ± S.D. of three separate experiments). Statistical significance was tested using a Student's *t*-test. EPCP group ** $p < 0.01$.

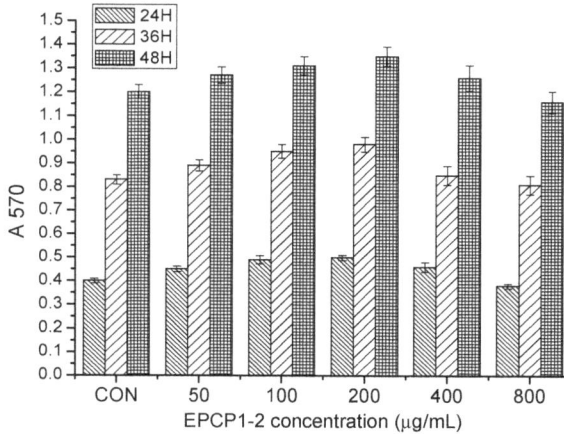

Figure 3. Cytotoxicity assay of EPCP1-2 (50, 100, 200, 400, 800 μg/mL) on RAW 264.7. (Results are expressed as the mean ± S.D. of three separate experiments). Statistical significance was tested using a Student's *t*-test.

3.2. Basic Properties of EPCP1-2

The ratio of the peak area was 99.5% (Figure 4). The extraction process had a relatively high reproducibility, thus the EPCP1-2 molecular weight was estimated to be 82.5 kDa (Mw = 82.52, Mn = 74.86), which was calibrated by the dextran calibration curve (T-series dextran). (Mw: weight-average molecular weight, Mn: number average molecular weight).

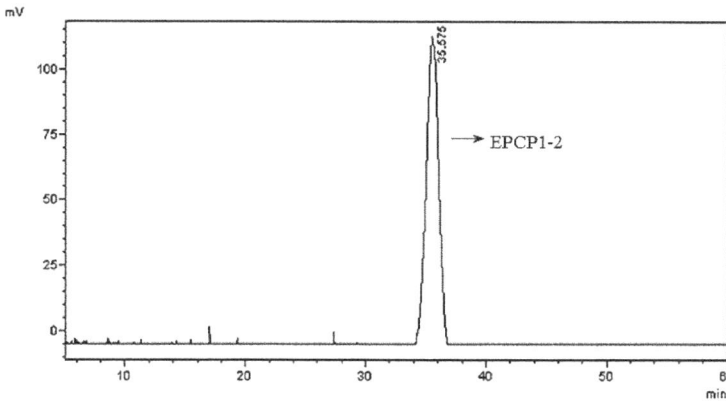

Figure 4. High Performance Liquid Chromatography (HPLC) analysis of EPCP1-2.

No absorption at 280 nm and 260 nm was detected indicated the EPCP1-2 did not contain proteins or nucleic acids. EPCP1-2 was free of proteins, which was detected by Lowry assay. No uronic acid was detected using the m-hydroxydiphenol method with D-glucuronic acid as the standard. The phenol sulfuric acid assay suggests that total sugar content of EPCP1-2 is 92%. These results demonstrate that EPCP1-2 is a neutral polysaccharide.

From monosaccharide and absolute configuration analyses, EPCP1-2 was hydrolyzed, reduced, and acetylated. GC spectrum indicated that EPCP1-2 was composed of rhamnose, mannose, glucose, and galactose with a molar ratio of 1, 17.13, 3.45 and 7.43 (Supplement Data S1).

Methylation analysis by GC-MS was used to investigate the glycosyl linkages of EPCP1-2. Figure 5 and Table 1 showed the three types of linkages, were, namely, 2,4-Me2-Galap, 2,3,4-Me3-Manp, 2,3,4-Me3-Glcp, 2,3,4,6-Me3-Rha, at a percentage of 23.21%, 60.56%, 11.11%, 3.02%. The molar ratio of monosaccharide agrees with the percentages of methylated sugar residues in EPCP1-2. These findings indicated that the repeating unit of EPCP1-2 consists of 1,6-linked-Mannose, 1,3,6-linked-Galactose, 1,6-linked-glucose, and t-L-Rhap.

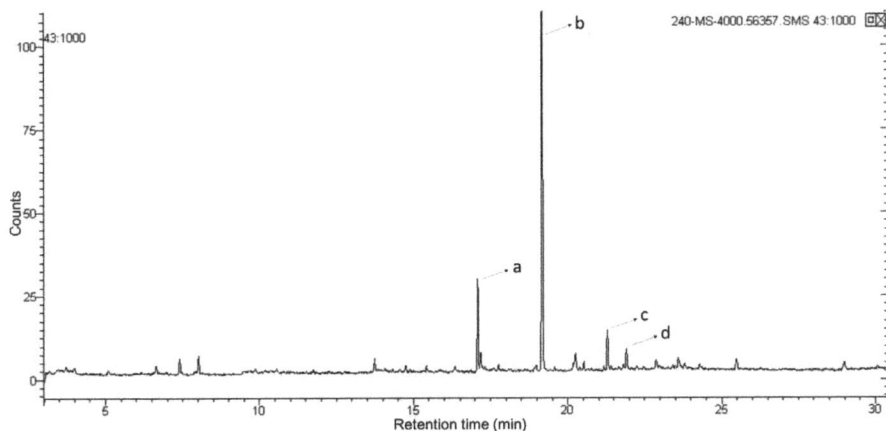

Figure 5. Total ion gas chromatogram of methylation patterns of EPCP1-2 using GC-MS. Note: signals a–d represent 2,4-Me2-Galap, 2,3,4-Me3-Manp, 2,3,4-Me3-Glcp, respectively. The x-axis represents retention time in minutes; the y-axis represents signal intensity by counts.

Table 1. Gas chromatography (GC)/MS data on methylated sugar residues in EPCP1-2.

Peak No.	Methylated Sugar Residue	Retention Time (min)	Linkage Type
a	2,4-Me2-Gala	17.085	1,3-6-D-Galacp
b	2,3,4-Me3-Man	19.175	1,6-D-Manp
c	2,3,4-Me3-Glc	21.294	1,6-D-Glcp
d	2,3,4,6-Me3-Rha	21.911	t-L-Rhap

3.3. Effect of EPCP1-2 on LPS Induced NO Production from RAW 264.7

In order to identify the anti-inflammatory effects of EPCP1-2, we investigated the inhibitory effects of EPCP1-2 on NO production. As Figure 6 showed, when RAW 264.7 cells were stimulated with LPS, nitrite was produced as a biomarker of NO. Various concentration of EPCP1-2 (50, 100, 200, 400, 800 μg/mL) were tested on RAW 264.7 cells with or without stimulation of LPS. Treatment with EPCP1-2 and without LPS stimulation had a mild inhibitory effect on NO production, the inhibition only happened at the highest concentration (800 μg/mL). EPCP1-2 reduced NO production in a concentration-dependent manner after treated for 36 h (Figure 6), with a maximum effects of 64% NO reduction with 800 μg/mL of EPCP1-2, and exhibited the strong inhibitory properties and the lack of any cytotoxic effects. In addition, there was no significant difference between the negative control group and the control group, so the treatment of 800 μg/mL dose EPCP1-2 did not inhibited NO reduction of the cells.

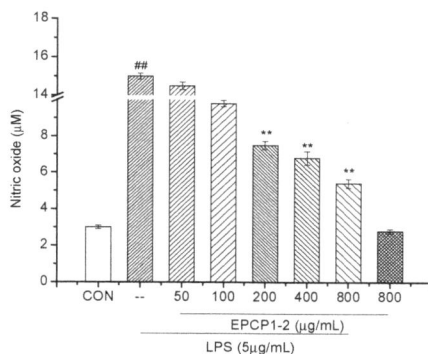

Figure 6. Effects of EPCP1-2 on pro-inflammatory factor (NO) production in RAW 264.7. (Results are expressed as the mean ± S.D. of three separate experiments). Statistical significance was tested using a Student's *t*-test. EPCP1-2 group ** $p < 0.01$; LPS group (positive control) ## $p < 0.01$.

3.4. Effect of EPCP1-2 on LPS Induced Cytokines Production from RAW 264.7

IL-1β is produced by activated monocytes and macrophages, which can promote the proliferation and secretion of B lymphocytes in the immune response. Tumor necrosis factor (TNF-α) is produced by monocytes, macrophages, and T lymphocytes, playing an important role in the immune defense and immune stability of the body. The physiological function of IFN-γ is macrophage activation, immune response, and host defensive immunity, is an important factor that mediates cellular immunity and humoral immunity. In order to investigate the effect of EPCP1-2 on the secretion of inflammatory cytokines in RAW 264.7, the level of cytokines in the cell culture medium was measured by ELISA assay. As Table 2 showed, a certain concentration (200, 400, 800 μg/mL) of EPCP1-2 could inhibit the secretion of inflammatory cytokines and showed a certain dose-dependent. In addition, there was no significant difference between the negative control group and the control group, so that the treatment of 800 μg/mL dose EPCP1-2 did not cause excitation or inhibition to the cells.

Table 2. Effect of EPCP1-2 on the protein expression of cytokines (IL-1β, IFN-γ, TNF-α) in RAW 264.7 cells. (Results are expressed as the mean ± S.D. of three separate experiments). Statistical significance was tested using a Student's *t*-test. EPCP1-2 group ** $p < 0.01$, LPS group (positive control) ## $p < 0.01$.

Group	EPCP1-2 (μg/mL)	LPS (μg/mL)	IL-1β (ng/L)	IFN-γ (ng/L)	TNF-α (ng/L)
Control	-	-	175.5 ± 5.8	200.3 ± 5.1	187.8 ± 3.5
Positive control	-	5	365.3 ± 9.1 ##	445.6 ± 3.5 ##	315.3 ± 6.4 ##
	200	5	320.3 ± 5.3 **	395.4 ± 5.6 **	300.5 ± 9.2 **
Treatment group	400	5	284.7 ± 6.2 **	318.6 ± 8.1 **	281.3 ± 7.4 **
	800	5	214.1 ± 4.4	245.4 ± 6.7	226.4 ± 7.3
Negative control	800	-	180.5 ± 7.5	204.9 ± 4.3	195.2 ± 6.3

3.5. Effect of EPCP1-2 on Expression of Phosphorylation and Total TLR4

TLRs are recognized as a wide variety of pathogen-associated molecular patterns (PAMP) in viruses, bacteria, fungi, and cell, they play an important role in immune-regulatory functions [30]. Previous research reported that TLRs are related to NF-κB, JNK, and p38 MAPK. Their downstream signaling pathways are related to induction and secretion of cytokines, chemokines, and other inflammatory mediators [31]. RAW 264.7 culture were treated with different concentrations of EPCP1-2 (200, 400, 800 μg/mL) and stimulated with 5 μg/mL of LPS for 6 h. Western blotting showed that 5 μg/mL LPS induced strong activation of TLR4, and treated with EPCP1-2 (200, 400, 800 μg/mL) showed a reduced of TLR4 expression with dose dependent. Moreover, we investigated the effect of EPCP1-2 (200, 400, 800 µg/mL) on the interaction of TLR4 with adapter molecule TAK1 in LPS-induced RAW 264.7. As shown in Figure 7A, LPS stimulation of RAW 264.7 caused an increase in TAK1 expression, which was significantly inhibited by EPCP1-2. In a conclusion, the formation of TLR4/TAK1 complex significantly increased after LPS stimulation. Cells that were treated with different concentrations EPCP1-2 showed a reduction in the expression of the TAK1 protein.

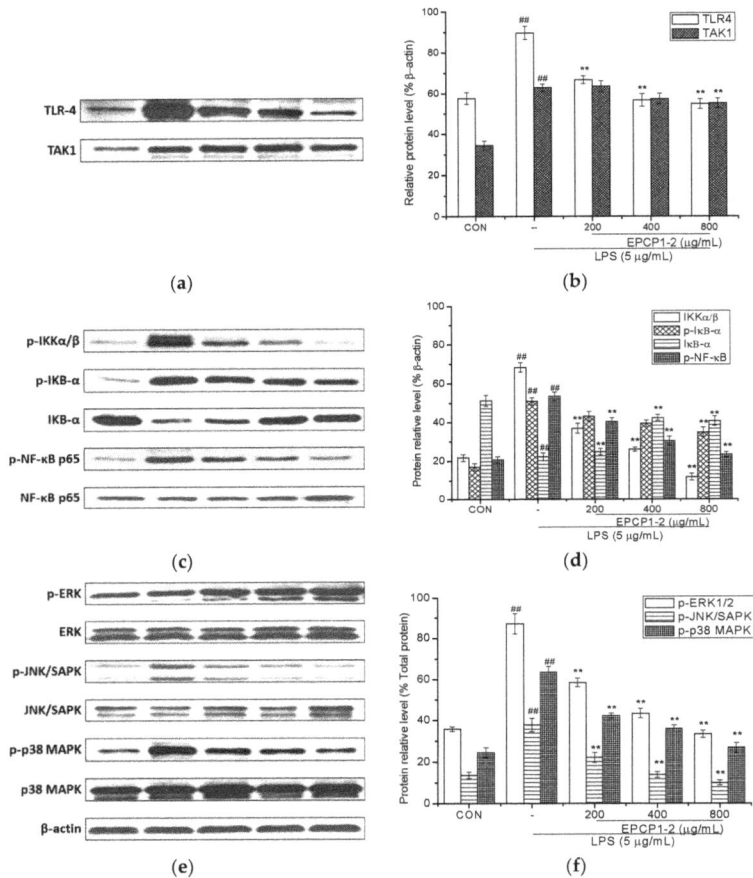

Figure 7. Inhibitory effect of EPCP1-2 isolated from *Crypthecodinium cohnii* on the NF-κB protein activation in LPS-induced RAW 264.7 cells. Cells were stimulated by LPS (5 µg/mL) for 1 h with or without the presence of EPCP1-2 (200, 400, 800 µg/mL). The protein levels of IκB-α and NF-κB were determined using ECL (electrochemiluminescence) immunoblotting method. (**a**) TLR4 protein and TAK1 protein expression were examined by Western blotting analysis. (**b**) Densitometric analysis showed the effects of EPCP1-2 on LPS-induced expressions of TLR4 and TAK1 proteins. (**c**) NF-κB p65 signal relative proteins expression was examined by Western blotting analysis. (**d**) Densitometric analysis showed the effects of EPCP1-2 on LPS-induced expressions of NF-κB p65 signal relative proteins. (**e**) Densitometric analysis showed the effects of EPCP1-2 on LPS-induced expressions of IKKα/β, IκB-α and NF-κB proteins. (**f**) Densitometric analysis showed the effects of EPCP1-2 on LPS-induced expressions of ERK1/2, JNK/SAPK, p38 MAPK proteins. (Results are expressed as the mean ± S.D. of three separate experiments). Statistical significance was tested using a Student's *t*-test. EPCP1-2 group ** $p < 0.01$; LPS group (positive control) ## $p < 0.01$.

3.6. Effect of EPCP1-2 on Expression of Phosphorylation and Total NF-κB

To further examine the effects of EPCP1-2 on the up-stream regulators of immune signaling, the effects were determined on IκB-α phosphorylation by Western blot. As shown in Figure 7c, LPS induced the phosphorylation of IκB-α, which was inhibited by the treatment of EPCP1-2. These results were consistent with the anti-inflammatory effect of EPCP1-2 that is mediated by the inhibition of IκB-α phosphorylation. Therefore, there was dose-dependent effect found. NF-κB is an important transcription factor complex that controls the expression of pro-inflammatory mediators, such as iNOS and NO [32]. To investigate the molecular mechanism underlying the mediated inhibition of iNOS and NO expression, western blot analysis was performed to quantify the presence of NF-κB in its phosphorylated states as an indirect measure for NF-κB transcriptional activity. As shown in Figure 7c, treatment with LPS increased the phosphorylation of NF-κB p65, and EPCP1-2 inhibited these LPS-induced phosphorylations.

3.7. Effect of EPCP1-2 on Expression of MAPKS Phosphoorylation and JNK/SAPK Phosphoorylation Induced by LPS

LPS induction of cytokine expression occurs via activation of MAPK and ERK phosphorylation following binding to TLR4 [33]. The MAPK signaling pathways have been shown to modulate the synthesis and release of pro-inflammatory mediators and cytokines in macrophages that are stimulated by LPS [34]. To understand whether the anti-inflammatory activities of EPCP1-2 are mediated through the MAPK pathway, the effects of EPCP1-2 on LPS-induced phosphorylations of p38 MAPK and ERK1/2 were examined by Western blot. The effect of EPCP1-2 on the activation of MAPK pathways was examined by quantitating MAPK in the phosphorylated form using specific antibodies. RAW 264.7 cells were treated with different concentrations of EPCP1-2 and stimulated with 1 μg/mL of LPS for 6 h. As shown in Figure 7e, the activation of MAPK (p38 MAPKand ERK1/2) and JNK signaling did occur in RAW 264.7 cells compared with the control group. LPS induced p38 ERK and JNK phosphorylation was attenuated by EPCP1-2. Co-treatment with increasing concentrations of EPCP1-2 suppressed LPS-induced phosphorylation of p38, ERK 1/2, and JNK in dose-dependent manner. The amounts of non-phosphorylated p38 ERK 1/2 and JNK were treated with or without LPS and EPCP1-2. As the results shown in Figure 7e, the anti-inflammatory activity of EPCP1-2 was mediated by inhibition of the phosphorylation of p38, ERK1/2, JNK induced by LPS.

4. Discussion

Macrophages play a key role in inflammation and immune responses by secreting chemokines and cytokines, recognizing and phagocytizing pathogens, processing antigens, and repairing tissue damage [35]. LPS can activate macrophages and initiate inflammatory and immune responses, which induces the production of inflammatory cytokines, including TNF-α and IL-8 [36,37]. During inflammation, LPS induces the production of pro-inflammatory mediators, such as NO and PGE2 by modulating iNOS and COX-2 expression, respectively [38]. NO is a key inflammatory mediator, and excessive NO production occurs in both chronic and acute inflammation [39]. Furthermore, NO and iNOS production levels significantly correlate with the degree of inflammation [40]. To further investigate the mechanisms that are underlying EPCP1-2 activity, the expression levels of TLR4, TAK1, and NF-κB were examined by Western Blot. Our present studies showed that EPCP1-2 exerted potent inhibition effects of NF-κB pathway via mediating TLR4-TAK1 complex signaling pathway.

Toll like receptors (TLRs) have been generally considered as therapeutic targets of autoimmune diseases [41]. TLR4 is involved in inflammation and injury of renal. As previous research showed, TLR4-deficient lupus prone mice demonstrated a more global decrease in immune responses, cytokine production, autoantibody production, and attenuation in renal damage [42,43]. In this research, we identified the potent pro-inflammatory effects on LPS-induced RAW 264.7, confirming the correlation to the inflammation of LPS induced in previous findings RAW 264.7. According to our research, the protein expression of TLR4 was upregulated with LPS induction, treatment with EPCP1-2 showed inhibiting effect on expression of TLR4 in LPS-induced RAW 264.7. Moreover, treatment with EPCP1-2 showed inhibiting effect on TLR4 expression with a dose-dependent manner. EPCP1-2 may competitive suppress the binding of LPS and receptor protein TLR4, which might be a mechanism of anti-inflammatory activity of EPCP1-2 on LPS-induced RAW 264.7. In this research, TLR4 has been identified as the cellular receptor that transduces LPS signaling. The binding of LPS and receptor protein TLR4 triggers intracellular signaling, including the NF-κB pathway. NF-κB was involved in initiating the transcription of genes that are involved in mediating the fibrotic and inflammatory process in RAW 264.7 [44,45]. The results in our study indicated that EPCP1-2 inhibited LPS-activated NF-κB pathway through downregulating IκB expression and NF-κB-P65 nuclear translocation, as shown in Figure 8. These results (Figure 7c,d) showed that EPCP1-2 suppresses LPS-stimulated NF-κB activation by preventing the degradation of IκB-α.

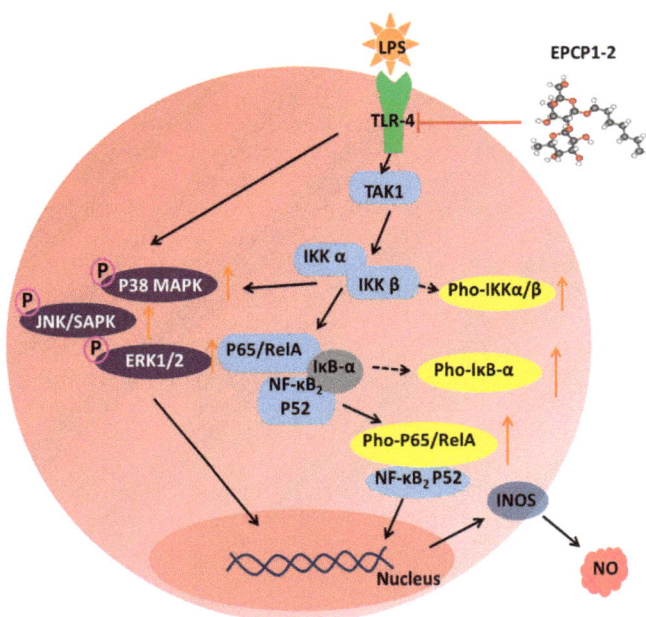

Figure 8. Schematic diagram of the propose target for the anti-inflammatory effects of EPCP1-2 in the RAW 264.7 cells stimulated by LPS, potentially leading to the inhibition of the pro-inflammatory cytokines and related mediators.

The results in our research suggested that EPCP1-2 contains a long main backbone of (1→6)-linked Man*p* and (1→6)-linked Gal*p* residues and (1,3→6)-linked Man*p* as the branch, which inhibited the activation of RAW 264.7 through the IκB-NF-κB signal transduction pathway, thus elucidating the relationship between its chain conformation and anti-inflammation activity. The EPCP1-2 fractions with molecular weights about 82.5 kDa showed significant immunomodulatory effects, which agreed with the previous research, in which the water-soluble polysaccharide fraction showed immunomodulatory effects with molecular weight was ≈100 kDa [46]. The bioactivity of EPCP1-2 may depend on the composition of main backbone (1→6)-linked Man*p*, which serves as the main backbone of a neutral heteropolysaccharide extracted from *Auricularia polytricha* [47].

5. Conclusions

EPCP1-2 was an extracellular polysaccharide extracted from *Crypthecodinium cohnii* which contained a long main backbone of (1→6)-linked Man*p* and (1→6)-linked Gal*p* residues and (1,3→6)-linked Man*p* as the branch. EPCP1-2 had a high capacity to inhibit macrophage proliferation, downregulation of the expression of TRL4, TAK1, MAPKs, and NF-κB protein, and acted as an anti-inflammatory agent through macrophage suppression. In conclusion, our findings demonstrated that the EPCP1-2 extracted from *Crypthecodinium cohnii* against inflammation was considered to be a potent regulatory element in TLR4-TAK1 complex mediated MAPK and NF-κB signaling pathways, as Figure 8 showed.

Supplementary Materials: The following are available online at www.mdpi.com/1660-3397/15/12/376/s1, Supplement Data S1: GC spectrum of monosaccharide composition of EPCP1-2; Supplement Data S2: Standard curve of cytokines protein expression by Elisa (**a**) IL-1β (**b**) IFN-γ (**c**) TNF-α.

Acknowledgments: This work was financially supported by the Central research institutes project (K-JBYWF-2017-G11, K-JBYWF-2017-G12, K-JBYWF-2015-T11, K-JBYWF-2016-G9) and Marine public welfare project (No. 201505032-2).

Author Contributions: Xiaolei Ma, Jing Wang conceived and designed the experiments; Xiaolei Ma performed the experiments; Baolong Xie, Jin Du and Aijun Zhang analyzed the data; Jianan Hao, Shuxun Wang contributed reagents/materials/analysis tools; Xiaolei Ma wrote the paper; Junrui Cao revised and modified the paper.

Conflicts of Interest: The authors declare no conflict of interest. The founding sponsors had no role in the design of the study; in the collection, analyses, or interpretation of data; in the writing of the manuscript, and in the decision to publish the results.

References

1. Henderson, B.; Poole, S.; Wilson, M. Bacterial modulins: A novel class of virulence factors which cause host tissue pathology by including cytokine synthesis. *Microbiol. Rev.* **1996**, *60*, 316–341. [PubMed]
2. Hersh, D.; Weiss, J.; Zychlinsky, A. How bacteria initiate inflammation: Aspects of the emerging story. *Curr. Opin. Microbiol.* **1998**, *1*, 43–48. [CrossRef]
3. Ulevitch, R.J.; Tobias, P.S. Receptor-dependent mechanisms of cell stimulation by bacterial endotoxin. *Annu. Rev. Immunol.* **1995**, *13*, 437–457. [CrossRef] [PubMed]
4. Dinarello, C.A. Proinflammatory cytokines. *Chest* **2000**, *188*, 503–508. [CrossRef]
5. Turcanu, V.; Williams, N.A. Cell identification and isolation on the basis of cytokine secretion: A novel tool for investigating immune responses. *Nat. Med.* **2001**, *7*, 373–376. [CrossRef] [PubMed]
6. Moncada, S.; Palmer, R.M.; Higgs, E.A. Nitric oxide: Physiology, pathophysiology. *Pharmacol. Rev.* **1992**, *43*, 109–142.
7. MacMiking, J.; Xie, Q.W.; Nathan, C. Nitric oxide and macrophage function. *Annu. Rev. Immunol.* **1997**, *15*, 323–350. [CrossRef] [PubMed]
8. Nijkamp, F.P.; Parnham, M.J. *Principles of Immunopharacology*, 2nd ed.; Birkhauser: Basel, Switzerland, 2005; p. 188.
9. Ma, X.; Meng, M.; Han, L.; Cheng, D.; Cao, X.; Wang, C. Structural characterization and immunomodulatory activity of Grifola frondosa polysaccharide via toll-like receptor 4-mitogen-activated protein-kinases-nuclear factor κB pathways. *Food Funct.* **2016**, *7*, 2763–2772. [CrossRef] [PubMed]
10. Chevolot, L.; Foucault, A.; Chaubet, F.; Kervarec, N.; Sinquin, C.; Fisher, A.M. Further data on the structure of brown seaweed fucans: Relationships with anticoagulant activity. *Carbohydr. Res.* **1999**, *319*, 154–165. [CrossRef]
11. Vieira, R.P.; Mourao, P.A. Occurrence of a unique fucose-branched chondroitin sulfate in the body wall of a sea cucumber. *J. Biol. Chem.* **1988**, *263*, 18176–18183. [PubMed]
12. Bilan, M.I.; Grachev, A.A.; Ustuzhanina, N.E.; Shashkov, A.S.; Nifantiev, N.E.; Usov, A.I. Structure of a fucoidan from the brown seaweed Fucus evanescens C.Ag. *Carbohydr. Res.* **2002**, *337*, 719–730. [CrossRef]
13. Chizhov, A.O.; Dell, A.; Morris, H.R.; Haslam, S.M.; McDowell, A. A study of fucoidan from the brown seaweed Chorda filum. *Carbohydr. Res.* **1999**, *320*, 108–119. [CrossRef]

14. Partankar, M.S.; Oehninger, S.; Barnett, T.; Williams, R.L.; Clark, G.F. A revised structure for fucoidan may explain some of its biological activities. *J. Biol. Chem.* **1993**, *268*, 21770–21776.

15. Xu, J.; Xu, L.; Zhou, Q.; Hao, S.; Zhou, T.; Xie, H. Isolation, purification, and antioxidant activities of degraded polysaccharides from Enteromorpha prolifera. *Int. J. Biol. Macromol.* **2015**, *81*, 1026–1030. [CrossRef] [PubMed]

16. Da Silva, T.L.; Reis, A. The use of multi-parameter flow cytometry to study the impact of *n*-dodecane additions to marine dinoflagellate microalga *Crypthecodinium cohnii* batch fermentations and DHA production. *J. Ind. Microbiol. Biotechnol.* **2008**, *35*, 875–887. [CrossRef] [PubMed]

17. De Swaaf, M.E.; de Rijk, T.C.; Eggink, G.; Sijtsma, L. Optimisation of docosahexaenoic acid production in batch cultivations by *Crypthecodinium cohnii*. *J. Biotechnol.* **1999**, *70*, 185–192. [CrossRef]

18. Seung-Hong, L.; Chang-Ik, K.; Youngheun, J.; Yoonhwa, J.; Misook, K.; Jin-Soo, K.; You-Jin, J. Anti-inflammatory effect of fucoidan extracted from Ecklonia cava in zebrafish model. *Carbohydr. Polym.* **2013**, *92*, 84–89.

19. Li, B.; Lu, F.; Wei, X.; Zhao, R. Fucoidan: Structure and bioactivity. *Molecules* **2008**, *13*, 1671–1695. [CrossRef] [PubMed]

20. Xiao-Lei, M.; Meng, M.; Li-Rong, H.; Zheng, L.; Xiao-Hong, C.; Chun-Ling, W. Immunomodulatory activity of macromolecular polysaccharide isolated from Grifola frondosa. *Chin. J. Nat. Med.* **2015**, *13*, 906–914.

21. Liu, B.; Sun, Z.; Ma, X.; Yang, B.; Jiang, Y.; Wei, D.; Chen, F. Mutation breeding of extracellular polysacchride-producing microalga *Crypthecodinium cohnii* by novel mutagenesis with atmospheric and room temperature plasma. *Int. J. Mol. Sci.* **2015**, *16*, 8201–8212. [CrossRef] [PubMed]

22. Qiao, D.; Hu, B.; Gan, D.; Sun, Y.; Ye, H.; Zeng, X. Extraction optimized by using response surface methodology, purification and preliminary characterization of polysaccharides from *Hyriopsis cumingii*. *Carbonhydr. Polym.* **2009**, *76*, 422–429. [CrossRef]

23. Staub, A.M. Removal of protein: Sevag method. *Methods Carbohydr. Chem.* **1965**, *5*, 5–7.

24. Dubois, M.; Gilles, K.A.; Hamilton, J.K.; Rebers, P.A.; Smith, F. Colorimetric method for determination of sugars and related substances. *Anal. Chem.* **1956**, *28*, 350–356. [CrossRef]

25. Bradford, M.M. A rapid and sensitive method for the quantitation of microgram quantities of protein utilizing the principle of protein-dye binding. *Anal. Biochem.* **1976**, *78*, 248–254. [CrossRef]

26. Dodgson, K.S.; Price, R.G. A note on the determination of theester sulphate content of sulphated polysaccharides. *Biochem. J.* **1962**, *84*, 106–110. [CrossRef] [PubMed]

27. Blumencrantz, N.; Asboe-Hansen, G. New methods for quantitative determination of uronic acids. *Anal. Biochem.* **1973**, *54*, 484–489. [CrossRef]

28. Cheong, J.Y.; Jung, W.T.; Park, W.B. Characterization of an alkaliextracted peptidoglycan from Korean *Ganoderma lucidum*. *Arch. Pharm. Res.* **1999**, *22*, 515–519. [CrossRef] [PubMed]

29. Ma, X.; Zhou, F.; Chen, Y.; Zhang, Y.; Hou, L.; Cao, X.; Wang, C. A polysaccharide from Grifola frondosa relieves insulin resistance of HepG2 cell by Akt-GSK-3 pathway. *Glycoconj. J.* **2014**, *31*, 355–363. [CrossRef] [PubMed]

30. Beutler, B. Inferences, questions and possibilities in Toll-like receptor signalling. *Nature* **2004**, *430*, 257–263. [CrossRef] [PubMed]

31. Yan, H.; Wua, M.; Yuan, Y.; Wang, Z.Z.; Jiang, H.; Chen, T. Priming of Toll-like receptor 4 pathway in mesenchymal stem cells increases expression of B cell activating factor. *Biochem. Biophys. Res. Commun.* **2014**, *448*, 212–217. [CrossRef] [PubMed]

32. Gloire, G.; Legrand-Poels, S.; Piette, J. NF-κB activation by reactive oxygen species: Fifteen years later. *Biochem. Pharmacol.* **2006**, *72*, 1493–1505. [CrossRef] [PubMed]

33. Guo, Y.M.; Zhang, X.T.; Meng, J.; Wang, Z.Y. An anticancer agent icaritin induces sustained activation of the extracellular signal-regulated kinase (ERK) pathway and inhibits growth of breast cancer cells. *Eur. J. Pharmacol.* **2011**, *658*, 114–122. [CrossRef] [PubMed]

34. Coskun, M.; Olsen, J.; Seidelin, J.B.; Nielsen, O.H. MAP kinases in inflammatory bowel disease. *Clin. Chim. Acta* **2011**, *412*, 513–520. [CrossRef] [PubMed]

35. Herrero, C.; Sebastian, C.; Marques, L.; Comalada, M.; Xaus, J.; Valledor, A.F.; Lloberas, J.; Celada, A. Immunosenescence of macrophages: Reduced MHC class II gene expression. *Exp. Gerontol.* **2002**, *37*, 389–394. [CrossRef]

36. Dziarski, R.; Gupta, D. Role of MD-2 in TLR2- and TLR4-mediated recognition of Gram-negative and Gram-positive bacteria and activation of chemokine genes. *J. Endotoxin Res.* **2000**, *6*, 401–405. [CrossRef] [PubMed]

37. Wang, Z.; Jiang, W.; Zhang, Z.; Qian, M.; Du, B. Nitidine chloride inhibits LPS-induced inflammatory cytokines production via MAPK and NF-kappaB pathway in RAW 264.7 cells. *J. Ethnopharmacol.* **2012**, *144*, 145–150. [CrossRef] [PubMed]

38. Li, X.; Xu, W. TLR4-mediated activation of macrophages by the polysaccharide fraction from *Polyporus umbellatus (pers.) Fries*. *J. Ethnopharmacol.* **2011**, *135*, 1–6. [CrossRef] [PubMed]

39. Janeway, C.A.; Medzhitov, R. Innate immune recognition. *Annu. Rev. Immunol.* **2002**, *20*, 197–216. [CrossRef] [PubMed]

40. Kimura, H.; Hokari, R.; Miura, S.; Shigematsu, T.; Hirokawa, M.; Akiba, Y.; Kurose, I.; Higuchi, H.; Fujimori, H.; Tsuzuki, Y.; et al. Increased expression of an inducible isoform of nitric oxide synthase and the formation of peroxynitrite in colonic mucosa of patients with active ulcerative colitis. *Gut* **1998**, *42*, 180–187. [CrossRef] [PubMed]

41. Hang, L.; Slack, J.H.; Amundson, C.; Izui, S.; Theofilopoulos, A.N.; Dixon, F.J. Induction of murine autoimmune disease by chronic polyclonal B cell activation. *J. Exp. Med.* **1983**, *157*, 874–883. [CrossRef] [PubMed]

42. Summers, S.A.; Hoi, A.; Steinmetz, O.M.; O'Sullivan, K.M.; Ooi, J.D.; Odobasic, D.; Akira, S.; Kitching, A.R.; Holdsworth, S.R. TLR9 and TLR4 are required for the development of autoimmunity and lupus nephritis in pristane nephropathy. *J. Autoimmun.* **2010**, *35*, 291–298. [CrossRef] [PubMed]

43. Lartigue, A.; Colliou, N.; Calbo, S.; Francois, A.; Jacquot, S.; Arnoult, C.; Tron, F.; Gilbert, D.; Musette, P. Critical role of TLR2 and TLR4 in autoantibody production and glomerulonephritis in lpr mutation-induced mouse lupus. *J. Immunol.* **2009**, *183*, 6207–6216. [CrossRef] [PubMed]

44. Andreucci, M.; Lucisano, G.; Faga, T.; Bertucci, B.; Tamburrini, O.; Pisani, A.; Sabbatini, M.; Salzano, S.; Vitale, M.; Fuiano, G.; et al. Differential activation of signaling pathways involved in cell death, survival and inflammation by radiocontrast media in human renal proximal tubular cells. *Toxicol. Sci.* **2011**, 408–416. [CrossRef] [PubMed]

45. Guo, Y.; Yuan, W.; Wang, L.; Shang, M.; Peng, Y. Parathyroid hormonepotentiated connective tissue growth factor expression in human renal proximal tubular cells through activating the MAPK and NF-kappaB signalling pathways. *Nephrol. Dial. Transplant.* **2011**, *26*, 839–847. [CrossRef] [PubMed]

46. Lee, J.S.; Synytsya, A.; Kim, H.B.; Choi, D.J.; Lee, S.; Lee, J.; Kim, W.J.; Jang, S.; Park, Y.I. Purification, characterization and immunomodulating activity of a pectic polysaccharide isolated from Korean mulberry fruit Oddi (*Morus alba* L.). *Int. Immunopharmacol.* **2013**, *17*, 858–866. [CrossRef] [PubMed]

47. Song, G.; Du, Q. Structure characterization and antitumor activity of an α β-glucan polysaccharide from *Auricularia polytricha*. *Food Res. Int.* **2012**, *45*, 381–387. [CrossRef]

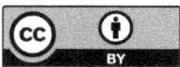

marine drugs

Review

The Structural Diversity of Carbohydrate Antigens of Selected Gram-Negative Marine Bacteria

Evgeny L. Nazarenko [1], Russell J. Crawford [2] and Elena P. Ivanova [2,*]

[1] Pacific Institute of Bioorganic Chemistry, Far East Branch of the Russian Academy of Sciences, Vladivostok 690022, Russia; elnaz@piboc.dvo.ru

[2] Faculty of Life and Social Sciences, Swinburne University of Technology, PO Box 218, Hawthorn, Victoria 3122, Australia; rcrawford@swin.edu.au

* Author to whom correspondence should be addressed; eivanova@swin.edu.au; Tel.: +61-3-9214-5237; Fax: +61-3-9819-0834.

Received: 3 August 2011; in revised form: 7 September 2011; Accepted: 13 September 2011; Published: 14 October 2011

Abstract: Marine microorganisms have evolved for millions of years to survive in the environments characterized by one or more extreme physical or chemical parameters, e.g., high pressure, low temperature or high salinity. Marine bacteria have the ability to produce a range of biologically active molecules, such as antibiotics, toxins and antitoxins, antitumor and antimicrobial agents, and as a result, they have been a topic of research interest for many years. Among these biologically active molecules, the carbohydrate antigens, lipopolysaccharides (LPSs, O-antigens) found in cell walls of Gram-negative marine bacteria, show great potential as candidates in the development of drugs to prevent septic shock due to their low virulence. The structural diversity of LPSs is thought to be a reflection of the ability for these bacteria to adapt to an array of habitats, protecting the cell from being compromised by exposure to harsh environmental stress factors. Over the last few years, the variety of structures of core oligosaccharides and O-specific polysaccharides from LPSs of marine microrganisms has been discovered. In this review, we discuss the most recently encountered structures that have been identified from bacteria belonging to the genera *Aeromonas*, *Alteromonas*, *Idiomarina*, *Microbulbifer*, *Pseudoalteromonas*, *Plesiomonas* and *Shewanella* of the *Gammaproteobacteria* phylum; *Sulfitobacter* and *Loktanella* of the *Alphaproteobactera* phylum and to the genera *Arenibacter*, *Cellulophaga*, *Chryseobacterium*, *Flavobacterium*, *Flexibacter* of the *Cytophaga-Flavobacterium-Bacteroides* phylum. Particular attention is paid to the particular chemical features of the LPSs, such as the monosaccharide type, non-sugar substituents and phosphate groups, together with some of the typifying traits of LPSs obtained from marine bacteria. A possible correlation is then made between such features and the environmental adaptations undertaken by marine bacteria.

Keywords: carbohydrate antigens; O-specific polysaccharides; marine microorganisms

1. Introduction

Gram-negative bacteria are ubiquitous in marine environments. As with other microorganisms present in sea habitats, they represent an interesting taxonomic lineage, and are a valuable source of natural biologically active substances [1,4]. These substances comprise a wide range of antibiotics, toxins and antitoxins, antitumor and antimicrobial agents and enzymes with a wide activity spectrum. Recently, the peculiar metabolic pathways of marine bacteria have been the subject of intensive research due to their possible employment in the biological decontamination of polluted sites. Head *et al.* [1] reviewed the processes underlying the degradation of hydrocarbons by marine microorganisms in light of current bioremediation strategies. For example, several species belonging to the genus *Shewanella* have been considered for their great biotechnological potential, due to their capabilty of dissimilatory reduction of a wide range of electron acceptors, including metal oxides (e.g., those of Fe(III) and Mn(IV)) and organic pollutants [2].

The lipopolysaccharides (LPSs) from non-pathogenic bacteria have also been the focus of intensive medical and veterinary research because in many cases bacteria that were not previously considered to be human pathogens were found in infected, immuno-compromised patients. In other cases, bacteria that were pathogenic for other mammals, became pathogens for humans, whether they were immuno-compromised or not, and *vice versa* [3]. At present, considerable attention is being given to the elucidation of the chemical structures of LPSs of Gram-negative marine bacteria.

The most complete form of LPS (*S*-type) has a tripartite structure, in which the *O*-antigenic side-chain (normally consisting of polymerized oligosaccharide units) is attached to the hydrophobic anchor, lipid A, via a connecting (core) oligosaccharide, the inner region of which is typically constructed from 3-deoxy-D-*manno*-oct-2-ulosonic acid (Kdo) and L-*glycero*-D-*manno*-heptose (L,D-Hep). In classical LPS, the backbone of lipid A is a β-1′,6-linked disaccharide of 2-amino-2-deoxy-D-glucose (D-glucosamine, D-GlcN) to which fatty acids, typically 3-hydroxyalkanoic acids, are attached by ester or amide linkages. Both the inner core region and lipid A are commonly carried ionizing groups. Anionic functions are contributed by Kdo, phosphate and, sometimes, hexuronic or other acid residues. The phosphate groups often serve as bridges to an amino alcohol (ethanolamine, Et_3N) or 4-amino-4-deoxy-L-arabinose (L-Ara4N), while glycosidically-linked amino sugar residues sometimes have a free amino group. It seems clear that the charged groups in LPS, like the polar head groups of phospholipids, are important to the molecular organization and functions of the bacterial outer membrane [4].

All regions of LPS display heterogeneity. For example, products described as *S*-type LPS normally consist of the populations of molecular species with different degrees of polymerization of the *O*-specific side chain, including species with few and/or single repeating unit (also called as semi-rough antigen, *SR*-type), and also contain the species without a side chain, *R*-type) and perhaps even species with an incomplete core oligosaccharide (core-defective *R*-types). In many bacteria, the *O*-specific side chains of the LPS vary widely in structure and composition, giving biological identity to individual strains (serotypes or serovars).

In non-encapsulated Gram-negative bacteria producing *S*-type LPS, the side chains are the dominant, heat-stable surface antigen. Biological specificity is achieved through chemical diversity, by means of the variations in composition and structure for which carbohydrates are pre-eminently suited. In addition to the enormous potential for complexity and diversity already being available, even with common hexoses, the scope of variation in *O*-antigens is often further enhanced by the utilization of less common enantiomers and other stereoisomers, monosaccharides of different chain length (C_5 to C_{10}), ketoses as well as aldoses, structural modifications (e.g., positional and cumulative permutations of deoxy, amino and carboxyl functions; esterification, etherification and amidation), branched monosaccharides and non-carbohydrate residues (e.g., polyols, carboxylic and amino acids) [5].

Bacterial *O*-specific heteropolysaccharides are generally composed of oligosaccharide repeating units. In the biosynthesis of polysaccharides, the so-called "biological" repeating unit is first assembled and then polymerised. In most structural studies, only the "chemical" repeating unit has been determined, whereas the "biological" repeating unit may be any cyclic permutation (rearrangement) of that structure. A number of reviews have dealt with the structures of bacterial carbohydrate antigens e.g., those by Kenne and Lindberg [6], Knirel and Kochetkov [7], Jansson [8], Knirel [9].

The *O*-specific polysaccharides (OPSs) obtained from marine bacteria are often anionic in nature. This has been related to their process of adaptation to the marine environment, since the availability of negatively charged sites on the polysaccharide chains creates a suitable site for the formation of ionic interactions mediated by divalent cations. These bridges strengthen the overall packing of the membrane, thus providing further stability towards external stressors as high pressure. Polysaccharides obtained from marine bacteria have been previously reviewed [10,12].

The OPS is covalently attached to the core oligosaccharide. This region of the LPS shows lower intra-species variability, and is characterized by the presence, in the inner region, of typical monosaccharides, namely 3-deoxy-D-*manno*-oct-2-ulosonic acid (Kdo) and L-*glycero*-D-*manno*-heptose (L,D-Hep) [13]. In the outer core region, neutral or acidic monosaccharides, as well as 2-deoxy-2-aminosugars, are typically encountered. In marine bacteria, archetypal chemical features of the core region have also been encountered, such as the replacement of Kdo by its 8-deoxy-8-amino analogue (Kdo8N) in *Shewanella* [14,16], the occurrence of the D-*glycero*-D-*manno*-heptose (D,D-Hep) [15, 16], and the occurrence of monosaccharides connected via phosphodiester bonds to the linear backbone of the oligosaccharide, as observed in the core region of the LPS from *Arenibacter certesii* [17] and *Alteromonas addita* [18]. Furthermore, as for the OPSs, core oligosaccharides from marine bacteria often show a remarkable negative charge density, inferred by the presence of a great number of phosphate substituents and/or acidic monosaccharides.

The methods leading to the structural characterization of LPSs and lipooligosaccharides (LOSs) include a complex series of extraction, purification and degradation steps. These are obviously supported by an extensive succession of chemical analyses, mainly based on chemical derivatization and gas chromatography-mass spectrometry (GC-MS) analyses, in order to achieve the complete definition of the monosaccharide and lipid content, and completed by matrix-assisted laser desorption/ionization mass spectrometry (MALDI-MS) and high resolution nuclear magnetic resonance spectroscopy (NMR), both of which allow the full structural description of the sub-domains composing the LPS structure.

The chemical structures are determined using mainly sugar and methylation analyses, ^{1}H and ^{13}C NMR spectroscopy, including 2D NMR experiments, homo- and heteronuclear correlation spectroscopy such as homonuclear ^{1}H,^{1}H correlation spectroscopy (COSY), total correlation spectroscopy (TOCSY), heteronuclear H-detected multuquantum and multi bond correlation (^{1}H,^{13}C HMQC and HMBC), nuclear Overhauser effect (NOE) spectroscopy (one- and two-dimensional 1D NOE, 2D nuclear Overhauser effect spectroscopy NOESY and rotational Overhauser effect spectroscopy ROESY), and by the attached proton test (APT).

In this review, we consider the chemical composition and structure of *O*-antigens, as well as LPS core oligosaccharides that are integral components of the cell wall surfaces of some Gram-negative marine bacteria. These bacteria are abundant in the marine environment inhabiting coastal, deep-sea and high sea areas, hydrothermal vents and bottom sediments, marine invertebrates and animals.

2. Structure of Carbohydrate Antigens of *Gammaproteobacteria*

2.1. Genus Alteromonas

This genus belongs to Alteromonadaceae family and comprises 13 validly described species [19,20]. To date, the structural investigation of the LPS of three species of the genus *Alteromonas* have been completed. Two structures of the R-LPSs from *Alteromonas addita* KMM 3600^T, *Alteromonas macleodii* ATCC 27126^T have been reviewed by Leone *et al.* [12], and were found to be an extremely short oligosaccharide chain with a high negative charge density due to the occurrence of 3-deoxy-D-*manno*-oct-2-ulosonic acid (Kdo) and phosphate groups.

The *O*-specific polysaccharide from the *S*-type LPS of *Alteromonas addita* KMM 3600^T [21,22] is comprised of trisaccharide repeating units containing L-rhamnose, D-glucose, and D-galactose residues. It was established that the *O*-specific polysaccharide consists of linear trisaccharide repeating units having the following structure (1) [23]:

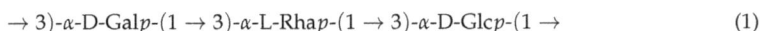

$$\rightarrow 3)\text{-}\alpha\text{-D-Gal}p\text{-}(1 \rightarrow 3)\text{-}\alpha\text{-L-Rha}p\text{-}(1 \rightarrow 3)\text{-}\alpha\text{-D-Glc}p\text{-}(1 \rightarrow \qquad (1)$$

The structure of the highly acidic extracellular polysaccharide produced by the mesophilic species, "*Alteromonas infernus*" [24], found in deep-sea hydrothermal vents and grown under laboratory conditions, has been investigated using partial depolymerization, methylation analysis, mass spectrometry and NMR spectroscopy. The repeating unit of this polysaccharide is a nonasaccharide with the following structure (2) [25]:

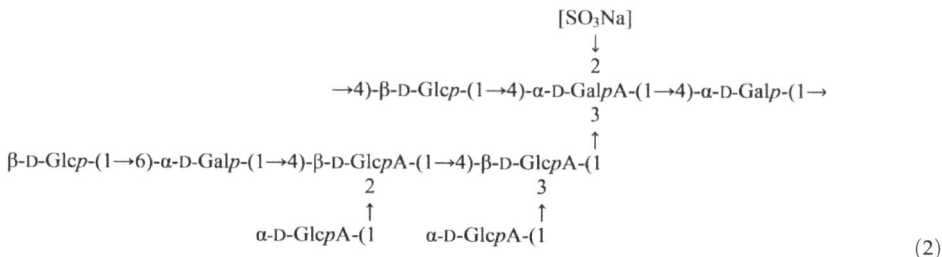

$$
\begin{array}{c}
[SO_3Na] \\
\downarrow \\
2 \\
\rightarrow 4)\text{-}\beta\text{-}D\text{-}Glc}p\text{-}(1\rightarrow4)\text{-}\alpha\text{-}D\text{-}Gal}pA\text{-}(1\rightarrow4)\text{-}\alpha\text{-}D\text{-}Gal}p\text{-}(1\rightarrow \\
3 \\
\uparrow \\
\beta\text{-}D\text{-}Glc}p\text{-}(1\rightarrow6)\text{-}\alpha\text{-}D\text{-}Gal}p\text{-}(1\rightarrow4)\text{-}\beta\text{-}D\text{-}Glc}pA\text{-}(1\rightarrow4)\text{-}\beta\text{-}D\text{-}Glc}pA\text{-}(1 \\
2 \qquad\qquad\qquad 3 \\
\uparrow \qquad\qquad\qquad \uparrow \\
\alpha\text{-}D\text{-}Glc}pA\text{-}(1 \qquad \alpha\text{-}D\text{-}Glc}pA\text{-}(1
\end{array}
$$

(2)

2.2. Genus Microbulbifer

The genus *Microbulbifer* was proposed by González *et al.* (1997) to accommodate a novel rod-shaped and strictly aerobic marine bacterium belonging to the *Gammaproteobacteria*. Isolates belonging to this genus have been isolated from a marine enrichment community growing on pulp-mill effluent, and the original inoculum was obtained from a salt marsh on the coast of Georgia, USA [26]. At present the genus consists of 14 validly described species isolated from various marine sources [19]. The composition and structure of carbohydrate-containing biopolymers from the cell membrane of this genus species have not been studied.

The capsular polysaccharide (CPS) containing D-galactosamine uronic acid and D-alanine residues were isolated from the culture of *Microbulbifer* sp. KMM 6242 [27]. The combined chemical and NMR analyses showed that the CPS is a homopolymer of 2-acetamido-2-deoxy-N-(D-galacturonyl)-D-alanine of the following structure (3):

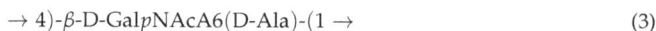

$$\rightarrow 4)\text{-}\beta\text{-}D\text{-}Gal}pNAcA6(D\text{-}Ala)\text{-}(1 \rightarrow \tag{3}$$

Such an amide of D-galactosamine uronic acid was found in bacterial exopolysaccharides for the first time.

An *O*-specific polysaccharide containing D-ribose and D-galactose residues was isolated from the cell-membrane lipopolysaccharide. On the basis of sugar analysis and NMR spectroscopy data the following structure of the disaccharide repeating unit of the polysaccharide was established (4):

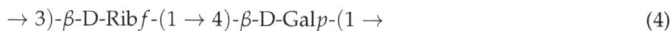

$$\rightarrow 3)\text{-}\beta\text{-}D\text{-}Rib}f\text{-}(1 \rightarrow 4)\text{-}\beta\text{-}D\text{-}Gal}p\text{-}(1 \rightarrow \tag{4}$$

2.3. Genus Pseudoalteromonas

Gram-negative bacteria of the genus *Pseudoalteromonas* are aerobic non-fermentative prokaryotes. They are widespread obligatory marine microorganisms and require seawater based culture media for their growth. The bacteria produce a wide range of biologically active compounds, such as antibiotics, toxins and antitoxins, antitumor and antimicrobial agents, as well as enzymes with a wide spectrum of action.

Common features of most polysaccharides of the genus *Pseudoalteromonas* are their acidic character and the presence of unusual sugars and non-sugar substituents with the absence of any structural similarity of the repeating units. For example, L-iduronic acid [28], 2-acetamido-2-deoxyhexuronic acids with the D-*galacto* [29,30], L-*galacto* [29,31] and L-*gulo* [32] configurations, 3-deoxy-D-*mannooct*-2-ulosonic acid [33,34], 5-acetamido-3,5,7,9-tetradeoxy-7-formamido-L-*glycero*-L-*manno*-non-2- ulosonic acid [30], 2,3-diacetamido-2,3-dideoxy-D-mannuronoyl-L-alanine [35], *R*-lactic acid [36], sulfate [37,38] and glycerophosphate [39] have been found among uncommon acidic components of the polysaccharides of *Pseudoalteromonas*.

The typical components include various *N*-acyl derivatives of 6-deoxyamino sugars, such as *N*-acetylated 2-amino-2,6-dideoxy-D-glucose (D-quinovosamine) [30], L-galactose (L-fucosamine) [33] and L-talose [33], 3-(*N*-acetyl-D-alanyl)amino-3,6-dideoxy-D-glucose [29], 4-(*N*-acetyl-D-alanyl) amino-4,6-dideoxy-D-glucose [31] and 3,6-dideoxy-3-(4-hydroxybutyramido)-D-galactose [32], as well as *N*-acetyl and *N*-[(*S*)-3-hydroxybutyryl] derivatives of 2,4-diamino-2,4,6-trideoxy-D-glucose (bacillosamine) [28,29,33,35]. In cases where polysaccharides other than *O*-antigens were isolated from encapsulated bacteria, there was no direct evidence that they were constituents of the capsule.

The structure of *O*-specific polysaccharide from lipopolysaccharide of *Pseudoalteromonas marinoglutinosa* KMM 232 (*S*-form) that consists of disaccharide repeating units containing a sulphate group has been described earlier [37]. An unusual structure of acidic *O*-specific polysaccharide was found in one of the recently described species, *Pseudoalteromonas agarivorans* [40], distinct by their stable colony dissociation into *R*- and *S*-form. A distinctive feature of the agarolytic strain KMM 232 is that it forms *R*-type (rough) colonies together with *S*-type (smooth) colonies during its cultivation on solid media. The *R*-form of KMM 232 has traits that are typical characteristics of *R*-bacteria, including *R*-colony formation, loss of flagella, and high sensitivity to antibiotics. The dissociation of *R*- and *S*-forms was observed to be stable for the strain KMM 232 and in other strains of the species *P. agarivorans*. This was the first time *R*- and *S*-form dissociation was described for bacteria of the genus *Pseudoalteromonas* [40].

An acidic *O*-specific polysaccharide containing L-rhamnose, 2-acetamido-2-deoxy-D-galactose, 2,6-dideoxy-2-(*N*-acetyl-L-threonine)amino-D-galactose, and 2-acetamido-2-deoxy-D-mannuronic acid was obtained by mild acid degradation of the lipopolysaccharide of the marine bacterium *Pseudoalteromonas agarivorans* KMM 232 (*R*-form) followed by gel-permeation chromatography. The polysaccharide was subjected to Smith degradation to give a modified polysaccharide with trisaccharide repeating unit containing L-threonine. The initial and modified polysaccharides were studied by sugar analysis and ^{1}H- and ^{13}C NMR spectroscopy, including COSY, TOCSY, ROESY, and HSQC experiments, and the structure of the branched tetrasaccharide repeating unit of the polysaccharide was established as follows (2.3) [41]:

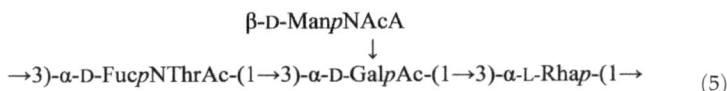

$$\beta\text{-D-Man}p\text{NAcA}$$
$$\downarrow$$
$$\rightarrow 3)\text{-}\alpha\text{-D-Fuc}p\text{NThrAc-}(1\rightarrow 3)\text{-}\alpha\text{-D-Gal}p\text{Ac-}(1\rightarrow 3)\text{-}\alpha\text{-L-Rha}p\text{-}(1\rightarrow \qquad (5)$$

It is noteworthy that one of the polysaccharide components, namely 2,6-dideoxy-2-(*N*-acetyl-Lthreonine) amino-D-galactose, has not been found earlier in nature. It is known that *R*-forms of terrestrial bacteria, unlike *S*-forms lose *O*-specific chains of the lipopolysaccharides and thus attain other properties. A feature of the marine bacterium *P. agarivorans* KMM 232 is that its *S*- and *R*-forms also synthesize lipopolysaccharides, in which *O*-specific polysaccharides have various structures. In the given strain the loss of *O*-specific polysaccharides in the *R*-form was not observed and it was suggested that such variability probably reflects the readiness of the bacterium to adapt to environmental changes. Moreover, it can be shown that Gram-negative marine bacteria substantially differ from terrestrial bacteria in their structural organization and the mechanism by which the cell wall functions [41].

A group of pigmented *Pseudoalteromonas* species [42] is known for their ability to synthesize a variety of pigments (prodigiosin-like, carotenoids and some others) and inhibitory (including antifungal) compounds [43]. Among those red-pigmented bacteria, *Pseudoalteromonas rubra* with the type strain NCMB 1890^T (=ATCC 29570^T were originally isolated from the Mediterranean water off Nice in 1976 by M. Gauthier [44]. The type strain of *P. rubra* has been found to produce an extracellular polyanionic antibiotic that modifies bacterial respiration [45] and cell-bound fatty acids and phospholipids with surface activity [46]. These findings provide evidence of ecophysiological diversification of pseudoalteromonads and on particular remarkable metabolic capacity of *Pseudoalteromonas rubra*, which may play an important role in coexistence and survival of numerous bacterial taxa in marine environments [47].

The structure of the *O*-specific polysaccharide from *P. rubra* type ATCC 29570[T] has been elucidated using ^{1}H and ^{13}C NMR spectroscopy, including 2D COSY, TOCSY, gradient pulse phase sensitive (gNOESY), ROESY, ^{1}H, ^{13}C gradient pulse (gHMQC) and gradient pulse (gHMBC) experiments. It was found that the polysaccharide consisted in 4-keto hexose, 2-acetamido-2,6-dideoxy-D-*xylo*-hexos-4-ulose (Sug, residue B) and two di-*N*-acyl derivatives of uronic acids: 2-acetamidino-3-acetamido-2,3-dideoxy-L-galacturonic acid (residue A) and 2-acetamido-3-(*N*-malyl)amino-2,3-dideoxy-D-glucuronic acid (residue C). The *O*-polysaccharide of *Pseudoalteromonas rubra* ATCC 29570[T] has the structure shown below (Figure 1) [48]. It contains two rarely occurring components, malic acid and 2-acetamido-2,6-dideoxy-D-*xylo*-hexos-4-ulose (Sug). To the best of our knowledge, D-malic acid has been hitherto identified only once in a polysaccharide from *Shewanella algae* BrY [49].

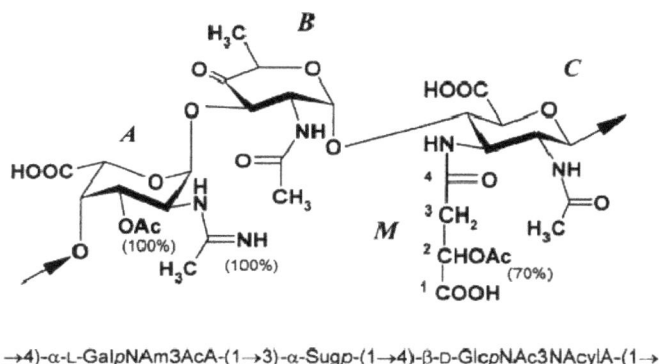

→4)-α-L-GalpNAm3AcA-(1→3)-α-Sugp-(1→4)-β-D-GlcpNAc3NAcylA-(1→

Figure 1. *Pseudoalteromonas rubra* ATCC 29570[T] [48]. Reprinted with permission from Elsevier. M—malic acid residue.

The same keto sugar has been found earlier as a component of capsular polysaccharides from *Streptococcus pneumonia* type 5 [50] and *Vibrio ordalii* O:2 [51] and an *O*-polysaccharides of *Flavobacterium columnare* ATCC 43622 [52] and *Vibrio vulnificus* clinical isolate YJ016 (6, 7) [53].

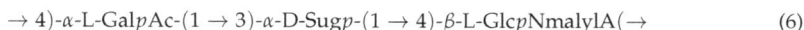

$$\rightarrow 4)\text{-}\alpha\text{-L-Gal}p\text{Ac-}(1 \rightarrow 3)\text{-}\alpha\text{-D-Sug}p\text{-}(1 \rightarrow 4)\text{-}\beta\text{-L-Glc}p\text{NmalylA}(\rightarrow \qquad (6)$$

where Sug is 2-acetamido-2,6-dideoxy-D-*xylo*-hexos-4-ulose, Am is acetimidoyl and malic acid residue (*M*) is *O*-acetylated in ~70% of the units (7).

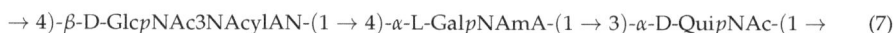

$$\rightarrow 4)\text{-}\beta\text{-D-Glc}p\text{NAc3NAcylAN-}(1 \rightarrow 4)\text{-}\alpha\text{-L-Gal}p\text{NAmA-}(1 \rightarrow 3)\text{-}\alpha\text{-D-Qui}p\text{NAc-}(1 \rightarrow \qquad (7)$$

where QuiNAc stands for 2-acetamido-2,6-dideoxyglucose, GalNAmA for 2-acetimidoylamino-2-deoxygalacturonic acid, GlcNAc3NAcylAN for 2-acetamido-3-acylamino-2,3-dideoxyglucuronamide and acyl for 4-D-malyl (~30%) or 2-*O*-acetyl-4-D-malyl (~70%). The structure of the polysaccharide studied highly resembles that of a marine bacterium *Pseudoalteromonas rubra* ATCC 29570[T] reinvestigated in this work. The latter differs in: (i) the absolute configuration of malic acid (L *vs.* D); (ii) 3-*O*-acetylation of GalNAmA; and (iii) replacement of QuiNAc with its 4-keto biosynthetic precursor.

The polysaccharides of *Pseudoalteromonas rubra* ATCC 29570[T] and *V. vulnificus* CECT 5198 and S3-I2-36 are remarkably similar in structure too [54]. It was found that 2,3-diamino-2,3-dideoxy-D-glucuronic acid (GlcN3NA) exists as an amide and the malic acid is in the L form. Therefore, the polysaccharide of *P. rubra* ATCC 29570[T] has the structure shown in Figure 1, which differs from the polysaccharide structure of *V. vulnificus* CECT 5198 and S3-I2-36 in: (i) the absolute configuration of malic acid (L *vs.* D); (ii) 3-*O*-acetylation of GalNAmA; and (iii) replacement of QuiNAc with its biosynthetic precursor, 2-acetamido-2,6-dideoxy-D-*xylo*-hexos-4-ulose. It can be suggested that both bacteria had originally the same sugar synthesis pathway and glycosyl transferase genes but in *Pseudoalteromonas rubra* the gene for reductase that converts the 4-keto sugar into QuiNAc, has been inactivated by a mutation. Surprisingly, in all these polysaccharides, as in the *O*-polysaccharide of *Pseudoalteromonas rubra*, the mentioned above 4-keto sugar is (1→4)-linked to a β-D-*gluco*-configurated monosaccharides and glycosylated at position 3 by a monosaccharide having the α-L-configuration. When obtained from non-bacterial sources, such keto sugar residues were found to be a component of some saponins from starfish [55,57].

2.4. Genus Plesiomonas

The genus *Plesiomonas* belongs to Enterobacteriaceae family and consists of only one species—*Plesiomonas shigelloides*. Bacteria of this species (previously *Aeromonas shigelloides*) is a ubiquitous, facultatively anaerobic, flagellated, Gram-negative, rod-shaped bacterium which has been isolated from a variety of sources such as freshwater, surface water and many wild and domestic animals, and is particularly common in tropical and subtropical habitats [58].

DNA-DNA hybridization tests showed that all *Plesiomonas shigelloides* strains are closely related to each other thus constituting a separate well defined genus within the family Vibrionaceae. *P. shigelloides* shares biochemical and antigenic properties with Enterobacteriaceae and Vibrionaceae; however, genetically it shows only 8% and 7% similarity, respectively [58]. Infections with *P. shigelloides* have been strongly associated with drinking untreated water [59,60], eating uncooked shellfish or with travel to developing countries [61,62]. Recent studies have suggested that *P. shigelloides* is an opportunistic pathogen in immunocompromized hosts [63] especially neonates [64]. It has been associated with diarrhoeal illness [65] and other diseases in normal hosts as well. *Plesiomonas shigelloides* has been isolated from a variety of clinical specimens including cerebrospinal fluid, wounds and the respiratory tract. Reported cases of meningitis and bacteraemia [64] caused by *P. shigelloides* are of special interest because of their seriousness. *P. shigelloides* causes both localized infections originating from infected wounds and gastrointestinal infections, which can disseminate to other parts of the body [66].

The serotyping scheme of *Plesiomonas shigelloides* proposed by Shimada and Sakazaki [67] and Aldova *et al.* [68] includes 102 *O*-serotypes, some *O*-antigens showing cross-reactivity with antisera directed against lipopolysaccharides (LPS) of *Shigella sonnei*, *Shigella dysenteriae* strains 1, 7 and 8, *Shigella boydi* strains 2, 9 and 13, and *Shigella flexneri* strain 6 [68,69]. Two *P. shigelloides* strains were found to share the structure of *O*-antigens with those of *S. flexneri* and *S. dysenteriae* [70].

Although the antigenic schemes of *P. shigelloides* have been extensively studied with the serological methods mentioned above, the unique structures of *O*-specific polysaccharides are known only for a few strains [70].

Sugar and methylation analyses of native polysaccharides together with one-dimensional ^{1}H and ^{13}C NMR spectroscopy revealed that the two polysaccharides from strains 22074 and 12254 of *P. shigelloides* are identical. The structure of the polysaccharide from strain 22074 was deduced from uronic acid degradation and by NMR spectroscopy where heteronuclear multiple bond connectivity and two-dimensional nuclear Overhauser effect spectroscopy experiments established the pentasaccharide repeating unit as (8):

→ 4)-α-D-Gal*p*A-(1 → 3)-α-D-Glc*p*NAc-α-L-Rha*p*-(1 → 2)-α-L-Rha*p*-(1 → 2)-α-L-Rha*p*-(1 →   (8)

The comparison *O*-PS structure from strains 22074 and 12254 of *Plesiomonas shigelloides* showed the both strains contains a mixture of antigens specific for S. *flexneri* 6 and the common group antigen of S. *flexneri* species and S. *dysenteriae* 1 (see below). This explains the basis of cross-reactivity. Moreover, *P. shigelloides* strains exhibit moderate invasion of Hep-2 cells [69] which suggest that they may cause limited invasion of intestinal epithelial cells, and this is a desirable attribute of a vaccine strain against *Shigella* infection [69]. Since they also share antigens with two major species of *Shigella*, these strains have the potential to give broad protection against shigellosis if used as vaccine strains (9); Structures of the *O*-antigens from *Shigella*, cross-reacting with strains 22074 and 12254 of *Plesiomonas shigelloides*.

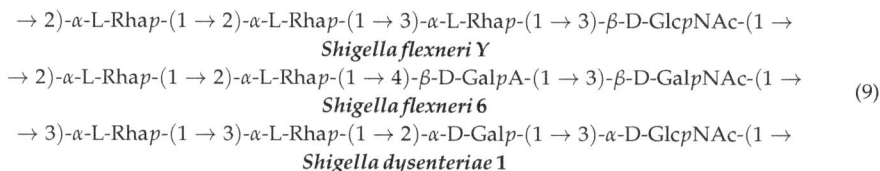

→ 2)-α-L-Rha*p*-(1 → 2)-α-L-Rha*p*-(1 → 3)-α-L-Rha*p*-(1 → 3)-β-D-Glc*p*NAc-(1 →
Shigella flexneri Y
→ 2)-α-L-Rha*p*-(1 → 2)-α-L-Rha*p*-(1 → 4)-β-D-Gal*p*A-(1 → 3)-β-D-Gal*p*NAc-(1 →
Shigella flexneri 6   (9)
→ 3)-α-L-Rha*p*-(1 → 3)-α-L-Rha*p*-(1 → 2)-α-D-Gal*p*-(1 → 3)-α-D-Glc*p*NAc-(1 →
Shigella dysenteriae 1

The structure of the *O*-specific side chain of the lipopolysaccharide (LPS) of *P. shigelloides* O54, strain CNCTC 113/92 has been investigated by NMR spectroscopy, matrix-assisted laser desorption/ionization time of flight mass spectrometry and sugar and methylation analysis. It was concluded that the polysaccharide is composed of a hexasaccharide repeating unit as follows (2.4) [71]:

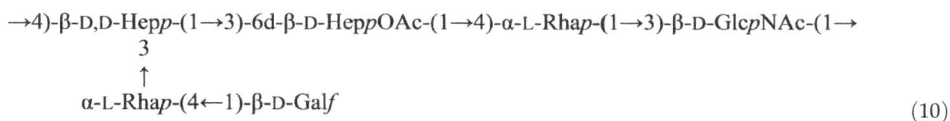

→4)-β-D,D-Hep*p*-(1→3)-6d-β-D-Hep*p*OAc-(1→4)-α-L-Rha*p*-(1→3)-β-D-Glc*p*NAc-(1→
               3
               ↑
α-L-Rha*p*-(4←1)-β-D-Gal*f*   (10)

where   β-D,D-Hep*p*   is   β-D-*glycero*-D-*manno*-heptopyranose   and   6d-β-D-Hep*p*   is 6-deoxy-β-D-*manno*heptopyranose. This structure represents a novel hexasaccharide repeating unit of bacterial *O*-antigen that is characteristic and unique to the *P. shigelloides* strain.

The lipopolysaccharide of *Plesiomonas shigelloides* serotype O74:H5 (strain CNCTC 144/92) was obtained with the hot phenol/water method, but unlike most of the S-type enterobacterial lipopolysaccharides, the *O*-antigens were preferentially extracted into the phenol phase. The poly- and oligosaccharides released by mild acidic hydrolysis of the lipopolysaccharide from both phenol and water phases were separated and investigated by ^{1}H and ^{13}C NMR spectroscopy, matrix-assisted laser-desorption/ionization time-offlight MS (MALDI-TOF) mass spectrometry, and sugar and methylation analysis. The *O*-specific polysaccharide and oligosaccharides consisting of the core, the core with one repeating unit, and the core with two repeating units were isolated. It was concluded that the *O*-specific polysaccharide is composed of a trisaccharide repeating unit with the structure (11) [72]:

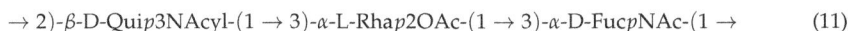

→ 2)-β-D-Qui*p*3NAcyl-(1 → 3)-α-L-Rha*p*2OAc-(1 → 3)-α-D-Fuc*p*NAc-(1 →   (11)

in which D-Qui3NAcyl is 3-amino-3,6-dideoxy-D-glucose acylated with 3-hydroxy-2,3-dimethyl-5-oxopyrrolidine-2-carboxylic acid. The major oligosaccharide consisted of a single repeating unit and a core oligosaccharide. This undecasaccharide contains information about the biological repeating unit and the type and position of the linkage between the *O*-specific chain and core. The presence of a terminal [β-D-Qui*p*3NAcyl-(1→] residue and the [→3)-β-D-Fuc*p*NAc-(1→4)-α-D-Gal*p*A] element showed the structure of the biological repeating unit of the *O*-antigen and the substitution position to the core. The [→3)-β-D-Fuc*p*NAc-(1→] residue has the anomeric configuration inverted compared to the same residue in the repeating unit. The core oligosaccharide was composed of a nonphosphorylated octasaccharide, which represents a novel core type of *P. shigelloides* LPS characteristic of serotype O74. The similarity between the isolated *O*-specific polysaccharide and that found on intact bacterial cells and lipopolysaccharide was confirmed by high resolution-magic angle spin (HR-MAS) NMR experiments.

The structure of the *O*-chain of the lipopolysaccharide (LPS) from *P. shigelloides* strain 302-73 (serotype O1) was determined by chemical analysis, 1D and 2D NMR spectroscopy and MALDI-TOF mass spectrometry. The polysaccharide was constituted by an inear pentasaccharidic repeating unit as follows (12) [73]:

$$\rightarrow 3)\text{-}\alpha\text{-L-PneNAc4OAc-}(1 \rightarrow 4)\text{-}\alpha\text{-L-Fuc}p\text{NAc-}(1 \rightarrow 4)\text{-}\alpha\text{-L-Fuc}p\text{NAc-}(1 \rightarrow 4)\text{-}\alpha\text{-L-Fuc}p\text{NAc-}(1 \rightarrow$$
$$\text{D-QuiNAc4Nb-}(1 \rightarrow$$

(12)

(PneNAc = 2-acetamido-2,6-dideoxy-talose, Hb = *S*-3-hydroxybutanoyl. PneNAc *O*-acetylation was not stoichiometric and was found to be about 75%. The position of the *O*-acetyl group and the amount of acetylation were deduced by NMR spectroscopic analysis. All the monosaccharides included in the repeating unit were deoxyamino sugars, which most probably, together with the presence of *O*-acetyl groups, were responsible for the recovery of the LPS in the phenol layer of the phenol/water extract of dried bacteria cells.

P. shigelloides strain CNCTC 110/92 (O51) was identified as a new example of plesiomonads synthesizing lipopolysaccharides (LPSs) that show preference for a non-aqueous surrounding during phenol/water extraction. Chemical analyses combined with ^{1}H and ^{13}C NMR spectroscopy, MALDI-TOF and ESI mass spectrometry showed that the repeating units of the *O*-specific polysaccharides isolated from phenol and water phase LPSs of *P. shigelloides* O51 have the same structure (13) [74]:

$$\rightarrow 4)\text{-}\beta\text{-D-Glc}p\text{-NAc3NRA-}(1 \rightarrow 4)\text{-}\alpha\text{-L-Fuc}p\text{Am3OAc-}(1 \rightarrow 3)\text{-}\alpha\text{-D-Qui}p\text{NAc-}(1 \rightarrow \qquad (13)$$

containing the rare sugar constituent 2,3-diamino-2,3-dideoxyglucuronic acid (GlcpNAc3NRA), and substituents such as D-3-hydroxybutyric acid (R) and acetamidino group (Am). The HR-MAS NMR spectra obtained for the isolated LPSs and directly on bacteria indicated that the *O*-acetylation pattern was consistent throughout the entire preparation. The ^{1}H chemical shift values of the structure reporter groups identified in the isolated *O*-antigens matched those present in bacteria. It was found that the *O*-antigens recovered from the phenol phase showed a higher degree of polymerization than those isolated from the water phase. A similar behavior of LPS molecules was previously reported for other strains whose LPS was isolated from both phenol and water phases [75]. Therefore the composition of the *O*-repeating units does not seem to be the only factor influencing the physicochemical properties of such LPSs and suggested that the main solubility factor might be conformational rather than compositional.

The lack of structural data concerning a suitable number of *O*-antigen structures prevented us from deducing anything about the structure–activity relationship. However, it is tempting to speculate that the occurrence of deoxy sugars with hydrophobic substituents in all of the *O*-chain structures so far characterized could suggest a method adopted by *P. shigelloides* to adhere to host cells in aqueous environment. Structure determination is the first step into the understanding of the unusual physicochemical properties of LPSs. The possible role of the LPSs associated with an increased hydrophobicity in the pathogenicity of *P. shigelloides* has not been investigated so far. The data herein presented could be used in the future to study the role of such structures for the type of aggregates formed in an aqueous environment and the biological activity of *P. shigelloides* endotoxin.

The core oligosaccha ride is an important contributor in determining the biological and physical properties of the overall lipopolysaccharide and plays a significant role in interactions with the host.

The core oligosaccharide is relatively conserved in its structure and composition compared to the O-chain and can be divided into inner and outer subdomains. The inner core includes unique residues, such as 3-deoxy-D-*manno*-oct-2-ulosonic acid (Kdo) and L-*glycero*-D-*manno*-heptose (Hep) that are characteristic to the LPS. The Kdo residue is located at the reducing end of the oligosaccharide chain and has proven to be critical to the LPS biological activity [76]. At the O-4 position of Kdo there may be one or two Kdo glycosyl residues.

Mass spectrometric studies are now playing a leading role in the elucidation of lipopolysaccharide (LPS) structures through the characterization of antigenic polysaccharides, core oligosaccharides and lipid A components including LPS genetic modifications. The conventional MS and MS/MS analyses together with collision induced dissociation (CID) fragmentation provide additional structural information complementary to the previous analytical experiments, and thus contribute to an integrated strategy for the simultaneous characterization and correct sequencing of the carbohydrate moiety [77].

The structure of the core oligosaccharide moiety of the lipopolysaccharide (LPS) of *Plesiomonas shigelloides* O54 (strain CNCTC 113/92) has been investigated by ^{1}H and ^{13}C NMR, fast atom bombardment mass spectrometry (FAB-MS), MALDI-TOF, monosaccharide and methylation analysis, and immunological methods. It was concluded that the main core oligosaccharide of this strain is composed of a decasaccharide (**??**) [78]:

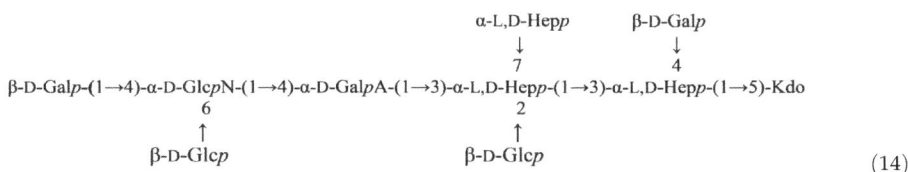

$$
\begin{array}{ccc}
\alpha\text{-L,D-Hep}p & & \beta\text{-D-Gal}p \\
\downarrow & & \downarrow \\
7 & & 4
\end{array}
$$

β-D-Gal*p*-(1→4)-α-D-Glc*p*N-(1→4)-α-D-Gal*p*A-(1→3)-α-L,D-Hep*p*-(1→3)-α-L,D-Hep*p*-(1→5)-Kdo

$$
\begin{array}{ccc}
6 & & 2 \\
\uparrow & & \uparrow \\
\beta\text{-D-Glc}p & & \beta\text{-D-Glc}p
\end{array}
$$

(14)

in which α-L,D-Hep*p* is α-L-*glycero*-D-*manno*-heptopyranose. The nonasaccharide variant of the core oligosaccharide (~10%), devoid of β-D-Glc*p* substituting the α-D-Glc*p*N at position 6, was also identified. The core oligosaccharide substituted at position 4 of the outer core β-D-Glc*p* residue with the single O-polysaccharide repeating unit was also isolated yielding a hexadecasaccharide structure. The determination of the monosaccharides involved in the linkage between the O-specific polysaccharide part and the core, as well as the presence of [→3)-β-D,D-Hep*p*-(1→instead of →3,4)-β-D,D-Hep*p*-(1→] in the repeating unit, revealed the structure of the biological repeating unit of the O-antigen. The core oligosaccharides are not substituted by phosphate residues and represent novel core type of bacterial LPS that is characteristic for the *P. shigelloides* serotype O54. Serological screening of 69 different O-serotypes of *P. shigelloides* suggests that epitopes similar to the core oligosaccharide of serotype O54 (strain CNCTC 113/92) might also be present in the core region of the serotypes O24 (strain CNCTC 92/89), O37 (strain CNCTC 39/89) and O96 (strain CNCTC 5133) LPS.

The first complete structure of a *Plesiomonas shigelloides* core oligosaccharide has been identified, together with the structure of the biological repeating unit of the O-antigen, and the linkage between them. Opinions differ regarding the classification of the genus *Plesiomonas*, because it has some characteristics in common with both Enterobacteriaceae and Vibrionaceae families. A comparison of the 5 S rRNA sequences of a number of Enterobacteriaceae and Vibrionaceae shows that *P. shigelloides* is more related to *Proteus mirabilis* and *Proteus vulgaris* than to any other member of Vibrionaceae tested [79].

The core oligosaccharide of *P. shigelloides* contains the following (2.4) structural element:

$$\begin{array}{c} \alpha\text{-L,D-Hep}p \\ \downarrow \\ 7 \\ \rightarrow\!3)\text{-}\alpha\text{-L,D-Hep}p\text{-}(1\!\rightarrow\!3)\text{-}\alpha\text{-L,D-Hep}p\text{-}(1\!\rightarrow\!5)\text{-Kdo} \end{array} \qquad (15)$$

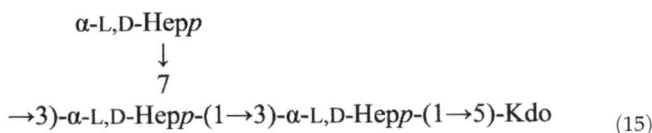

which is present in the majority of characterized enterobacterial and non-enterobacterial core structures.

The LPS of *Plesiomonas shigelloides* serotype O17 is of particular interest since its *O*-antigen structure is identical to that of *Shigella sonnei*, a cause of endemic and epidemic diarrhea and/or dysentery worldwide [80].

The *O*-antigen gene cluster of both *S. sonnei* and *Plesiomonas shigelloides* O17 is located on the plasmid Pinv, apparently acquired by *S. sonnei* from *P. shigelloides* [81,82]. This invasion plasmid is essential for penetration of host epithelial cells and is therefore an important virulence factor [83]. Because of the structural identity of the LPS *O*-specific polysaccharides (*O*-PS) of *S. sonnei* and *Plesiomonas shigelloides* O17, the latter can be used as an immunogenic component of a vaccine against *S. sonnei* [84]. Interpretation of the immunological data and selection of the optimal conjugation conditions require the knowledge of the structure of the LPS core part, which is always present in the O–PS preparations.

Plesiomonas shigelloides O17 LPS contains the same *O*-antigenic polysaccharide chain as a causative agent of dysentery, *Shigella sonnei*. This polysaccharide can be used as a component of a vaccine against dysentery. Core part of the *Plesiomonas shigelloides* O17 LPS was studied using NMR and mass spectrometry and the following structure was proposed (2.4) [85]:

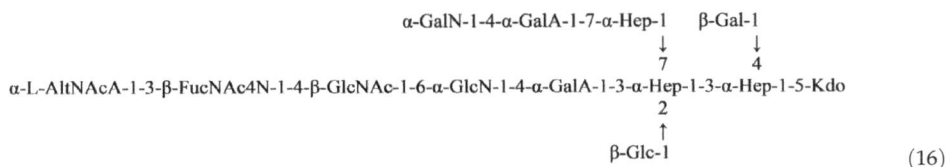

$$\begin{array}{c} \alpha\text{-GalN-1-4-}\alpha\text{-GalA-1-7-}\alpha\text{-Hep-1} \qquad \beta\text{-Gal-1} \\ \downarrow \qquad\qquad\qquad\quad \downarrow \\ 7 \qquad\qquad\qquad\quad 4 \\ \alpha\text{-L-AltNAcA-1-3-}\beta\text{-FucNAc4N-1-4-}\beta\text{-GlcNAc-1-6-}\alpha\text{-GlcN-1-4-}\alpha\text{-GalA-1-3-}\alpha\text{-Hep-1-3-}\alpha\text{-Hep-1-5-Kdo} \\ 2 \\ \uparrow \\ \beta\text{-Glc-1} \end{array} \qquad (16)$$

where Hep is L-*glycero*-D-*manno*-heptose and all sugars, except AltNAcA has the D-configuration.

Overall, the structure of the *Plesiomonas shigelloides* O17 core was similar to that of serotype O54 [78]. The difference being the presence of the additional α-GalN-4-α-GalA fragment on *O*-7 of Hep and the absence of the side chain β-Gal at O-4 of GlcN. Attachment of the *O*-chain in serotype O17 was through *O*-4 of β-GlcNAc, whereas in the serotype O54 it was through *O*-4 of β-Glc replacing β-GlcNAc.

The characterization of the core structure from the LPS of the strain 302-73 (serotype O1) was carried out. The LPS obtained after usual PCP (phenol–chloroform–light petroleum) extraction contained a small number of *O*-chain repeating units. The product obtained by hydrazinolysis was analysed by FTICR-ESIMS LPS was hydrolyzed under mild acid conditions and a fraction that contained one *O*-chain repeating unit linked to a Kdo residue was isolated and characterized by FTICR-ESIMS and NMR spectroscopy. Moreover, after an alkaline reductive hydrolysis, a disaccharide α-Kdo-(2→6)-GlcNol was isolated and characterized. The data obtained proved the presence of an α-Kdo in the outer core and allowed the identification of the *O*-antigen biological repeating unit as well as its linkage with the core oligosaccharide (2.4) [86,87].

The LPS was hydrolyzed under both alkaline and mildly acidic conditions. In both cases, a mixture of oligosaccharides was obtained, which was purified by gel filtration and HPAEC. The oligosaccharides were characterized by chemical analysis, 2D NMR spectroscopy and MALDI-TOF mass spectrometry. A new core structure was found for *P. shigelloides*. In particular, from the analysis of the acid hydrolysed product it was possible to reveal the presence of a of D-*glycero*-D-*talo*-2-octulopyranosonic acid (Ko) residue, which substitutes in part the terminal 3-deoxy-D-*manno*-oct-2-ulosonic acid (Kdo) unit. The Ko residue is not frequently found in core structures.

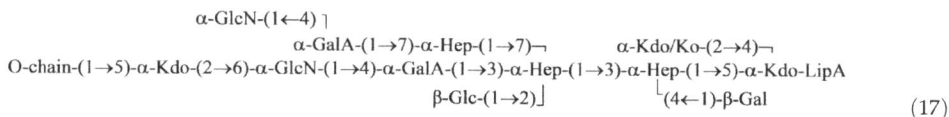

$$
\begin{array}{l}
\alpha\text{-GlcN-}(1{\leftarrow}4)\urcorner \\
\quad\quad \alpha\text{-GalA-}(1{\to}7)\text{-}\alpha\text{-Hep-}(1{\to}7)\urcorner \quad\quad \alpha\text{-Kdo/Ko-}(2{\to}4)\urcorner \\
\text{O-chain-}(1{\to}5)\text{-}\alpha\text{-Kdo-}(2{\to}6)\text{-}\alpha\text{-GlcN-}(1{\to}4)\text{-}\alpha\text{-GalA-}(1{\to}3)\text{-}\alpha\text{-Hep-}(1{\to}3)\text{-}\alpha\text{-Hep-}(1{\to}5)\text{-}\alpha\text{-Kdo-LipA} \\
\quad\quad\quad\quad\quad\quad\quad \beta\text{-Glc-}(1{\to}2)\lrcorner \quad\quad\quad\quad {}^{\llcorner}(4{\leftarrow}1)\text{-}\beta\text{-Gal}
\end{array} \quad\quad (17)
$$

This structure is similar to that of serotype O54 [78] and O17, [85] even if some new features are present in both the inner and outer core. A glucosamine residue was nonstoichiometrically linked to the branching galacturonic acid, and more interestingly, a Ko unit substitutes in part the terminal Kdo residue. The presence of the Ko residue is not frequent in core structures, and to date it has been described as a substitute for Kdo in the LPS of *Yersinia* [88], *Burkholderia* [89], *Acinetobacter* [90], *Serratia* [91]. Finally, this new core oligosaccharide confirmed the lack of a uniform core structure for the unique species of the *Plesiomonas* genus.

2.5. *Genus* Shewanella

Bacteria that are currently classified under the generic name *Shewanella* have been the subject of many scientific studies over at least the last 70 years. To date, this rapidly growing genus contains more than 50 validly described species including both free-living and symbiotic forms. Members of this genus have been isolated from various marine sources, including water, sediments, fish, algae, marine animals and others. Because of their metabolic versatility and wide distribution in a variety of aquatic habitats, *Shewanella* and *Shewanella*-like organisms play a significant role in the cycling of organic carbon and other bionutrients.

The most of the structures of the carbohydrate antigens from these bacteria were reviewed earlier [10,12]. Below is a brief outline of the described structures.

Shewanella oneidensis is a Gram-negative bacterium associated with aquatic and subsurface environments [92]. It can attach to amorphous iron oxides and, in so doing, utilizes the Fe(II)/Fe(III) couple as a terminal electron acceptor during dissimilatory iron reduction.

Capsular polysaccharides (CPS) were extracted from *Shewanella oneidensis* strain MR-4, grown on two different culture media. The polysaccharides were analyzed using ^{1}H and ^{13}C NMR spectroscopy, and the following structure of the repeating unit was established (18) [93]:

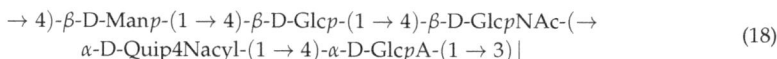

$$
\begin{array}{l}
\to 4)\text{-}\beta\text{-D-Man}p\text{-}(1 \to 4)\text{-}\beta\text{-D-Glc}p\text{-}(1 \to 4)\text{-}\beta\text{-D-Glc}p\text{NAc-}(\to \\
\quad\quad \alpha\text{-D-Qui}p4\text{Nacyl-}(1 \to 4)\text{-}\alpha\text{-D-Glc}p\text{A-}(1 \to 3)\lrcorner
\end{array} \quad\quad (18)
$$

where the residue of 4-amino-4,6-dideoxy-D-glucose (Qui4N) was substituted with different *N*-acyl groups depending on the growth media. All monosaccharides are present in the pyranose form. In the PS from cells grown on enriched medium (trypticase soy broth, TSB) aerobically it was *N*-acylated with 3-hydroxy-3-methylbutyrate (60%) or with 3-hydroxybutyrate (40%), whereas in the PS from cells grown on minimal medium (CDM) aerobically it was acylated mostly with 3-hydroxybutyrate (>90%).

Shewanella spp. MR-4 produces a large quantity of CPS, which gives the cells "smooth" appearance; however, its LPS has no polymeric *O*-chain. The rough type LPS was analyzed using NMR, mass spectroscopy, and chemical methods. Two structural variants (I and II) have been found, both contained 8-amino-3,8-dideoxy-D-*manno*-octulosonic acid and lacked L-*glycero*-D-*manno*-heptose. A minor variant of the LPS contained phosphoramide substituent (2.5) [94]:

Variant I

$$\alpha\text{-GalA-}(1\text{-P}\rightarrow4)$$
$$\downarrow$$
$$\beta\text{-Fru}f\text{-}(2\rightarrow6)\text{-}\alpha\text{-Gal-}(1\rightarrow6)\text{-}\alpha\text{-Gal-}(1\rightarrow3)\text{-}\alpha\text{-Gal-}(1\text{-P}\rightarrow3)\text{-}\alpha\text{-D,D-Hep-}(1\rightarrow5)\text{-}\alpha\text{-8-aminoKdo-}(2\text{-Lipid A}$$

Variant II

$$\alpha\text{-GalA-}(1\text{-P}\rightarrow4)$$
$$\downarrow$$
$$\alpha\text{-D,D-Hep2}PPETN3PN\text{-}(1\rightarrow5)\text{-}\alpha\text{-8-aminoKdo-}(2\text{-Lipid A} \qquad (19)$$

The structure of the *O*-specific polysaccharide from *Shewanella japonica* strain KMM 3601 has been elucidated. The initial and *O*-deacetylated lipopolysaccharides, and a trisaccharide representing the repeating unit, were studied by sugar analysis along with ^{1}H and ^{13}C NMR spectroscopy. The polysaccharide was found to contain a higher sugar, 5,7-diacetamido-3,5,7,9-tetradeoxy-D-*glycero*-D*talo*-non-2-ulosonic acid (a derivative of 4-epilegionaminic acid, 4-eLeg). The following structure of trisaccharide repeating unit was established (20) [95]:

$$\rightarrow 4)\text{-}\alpha\text{-4eLeg5Ac7Ac-}(2\rightarrow4)\text{-}\beta\text{-D-Glc}p\text{A3NAc-}(1\rightarrow3)\text{-}\beta\text{-D-Gal}p\text{NAc-}(1\rightarrow \qquad (20)$$

This polysaccharide contains 5,7-di-*N*-acetyl derivative of the 4-eLeg which was found in nature for the first time. Earlier, the homopolymer of 5-*N*-acetamidoyl-7-*N*-acetyl-derivative of 4-eLeg was identified in the LPS of non-1 serogroup of *Legionella pneumophila* [96].

2.6. *Genus* Aeromonas

Species of the genus *Aeromonas* are common inhabitants of aquatic environments and have been described in connection with fish and human diseases [97,100]. This genus belongs to the family Aeromonadaceae [101,102] and, over the last two decades, the number of recognized species has expanded very rapidly.

A varied clinical picture of *Aeromonas* infections, including gastroenteritis, suggests complex pathogenic mechanisms. Strains of *Aeromonas hydrophila* serogroup O:34 are most common among mesophilic *Aeromonas* species [103], accounting for 26.4% of all isolates, and have been documented as an important cause of infections in humans [104].

The *O*-polysaccharide of *Aeromonas hydrophila* O:34 was obtained by mild-acid degradation of the lipopolysaccharide and studied by chemical methods and NMR spectroscopy before and after *O*-deacetylation. The polysaccharide was found to contain D-Man, D-GalNAc and 6-deoxy-L-talose (L-6dTal) (2.6) [105]:

$$\rightarrow3)\text{-}\beta\text{-D-Gal}p\text{NAc-}(1\rightarrow4)\text{-}\alpha\text{-D-Man}p\text{-}(1\rightarrow3)\text{-}\alpha\text{-L-6d-Tal}p^{\text{I}}2\text{Ac}$$
$$3$$
$$\uparrow$$
$$\alpha\text{-L-6d-Tal}p^{\text{II}}\text{Ac}_{0\text{-}2} \qquad (21)$$

where 6dTal^{I} is *O*-acetylated stoichiometrically at position 2 and 6dTal^{II} carries no, one or two *O*-acetyl groups at any position. Although less common than L-rhamnose and L-fucose, 6-deoxy-L-talose occurs in a number of bacterial polysaccharides and is often present in an *O*-acetylated form. However, to the best of our knowledge, random *O*-acetylation has not been reported for either this or any other monosaccharide component of the lipopolysaccharides.

The core oligosaccharide of *A. hydrophila* (Chemotype III) lipopolysaccharide has been investigated. The studies involved the use of methylation analysis, oxidation with chromium trioxide, partial hydrolysis with acid, periodate oxidation, Smith degradation, and tagging of the reducing end-group. The core is unusual in having 3-acetamido-3,6-dideoxy-L-glucose as a constituent (2.6) [106]:

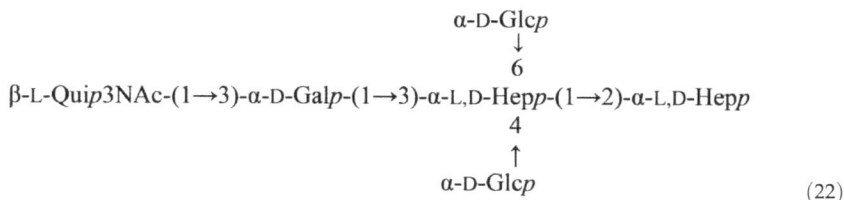

$$\alpha\text{-D-Glc}p$$
$$\downarrow$$
$$6$$
$$\beta\text{-L-Qui}p3\text{NAc-}(1{\rightarrow}3)\text{-}\alpha\text{-D-Gal}p\text{-}(1{\rightarrow}3)\text{-}\alpha\text{-L,D-Hep}p\text{-}(1{\rightarrow}2)\text{-}\alpha\text{-L,D-Hep}p$$
$$4$$
$$\uparrow$$
$$\alpha\text{-D-Glc}p \qquad\qquad (22)$$

A rough strain of *Aeromonas hydrophila*, AH-901, has an *R*-type lipopolysaccharide with the complete core. The following core structure was established by chemical degradations followed by sugar and methylation analyses along with ESIMS and NMR spectroscopy (2.6) [107]:

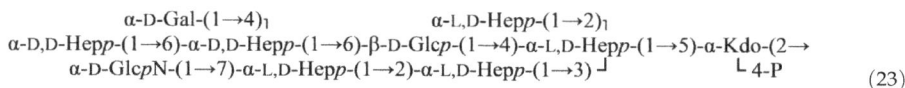

$$\alpha\text{-D-Gal-}(1{\rightarrow}4)_1 \qquad\qquad \alpha\text{-L,D-Hep}p\text{-}(1{\rightarrow}2)_1$$
$$\alpha\text{-D,D-Hep}p\text{-}(1{\rightarrow}6)\text{-}\alpha\text{-D,D-Hep}p\text{-}(1{\rightarrow}6)\text{-}\beta\text{-D-Glc}p\text{-}(1{\rightarrow}4)\text{-}\alpha\text{-L,D-Hep}p\text{-}(1{\rightarrow}5)\text{-}\alpha\text{-Kdo-}(2{\rightarrow}$$
$$\alpha\text{-D-Glc}p\text{N-}(1{\rightarrow}7)\text{-}\alpha\text{-L,D-Hep}p\text{-}(1{\rightarrow}2)\text{-}\alpha\text{-L,D-Hep}p\text{-}(1{\rightarrow}3)\,\lrcorner \qquad\quad \llcorner\,{}_{4\text{-P}}$$
$$(23)$$

where α-D,D-Hep and α-L,D-Hep stand for D-*glycero*- and L-*glycero*-α-D-*manno*-heptose, respectively; Kdo stands for 3-deoxy-D-*manno*-oct-2-ulosonic acid; all monosaccharides are in the pyranose form; the degree of substitution with β-D-Gal is ~50%. Lipid A of the lipopolysaccharide has a 1,4′-bisphosphorylated β-D-GlcN-(1→6)-α-D-GlcN disaccharide backbone with both phosphate groups substituted with 4-amino-4-deoxyarabinose residues.

A. salmonicida is the aetiological agent of furunculosis in salmonid fish, a disease which causes high mortalities in aquaculture. Considerable effort has been devoted to the development of effective vaccines against furunculosis. Very little is known about the role of virulence factors *in vivo* and their role in furunculosis.

It was found, that when grown *in vitro*, *A. salmonicida* strain 80204-1 produced a capsular polysaccharide with the identical structure to that of the lipopolysaccharide *O*-chain polysaccharide. A combination of 1D and 2D NMR methods, including a series of 1D analogues of 3D experiments, together with capillary electrophoresis-electrospray MS (CE-ES-MS), compositional and methylation analyses and specific modifications was used to determine the structure of these polysaccharides. Both polymers were shown to be composed of linear trisaccharide repeating units consisting of 2-acetamido-2-deoxy-D-galacturonic acid (GalNAcA), 3-[(*N*-acetyl-L-alanyl)amido]-3,6-dideoxy-Dglucose {3-[(*N*-acetyl-L-alanyl)amido]-3-deoxy-D-quinovose, Qui3NAlaNAc} and 2-aceacetamido-2,6-dideoxy-D-glucose (2-acetamido-2-deoxy-D-quinovose, QuiNAc) as follows (24) [108]:

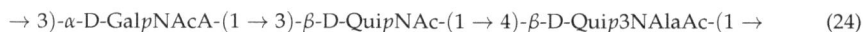

$$\rightarrow 3)\text{-}\alpha\text{-D-Gal}p\text{NAcA-}(1 \rightarrow 3)\text{-}\beta\text{-D-Qui}p\text{NAc-}(1 \rightarrow 4)\text{-}\beta\text{-D-Qui}p3\text{NAlaAc-}(1 \rightarrow \qquad (24)$$

where GalNAcA is partly presented as an amide and AlaNAc represents *N*-acetyl-L-alanyl group. CE-ES-MS analysis of CPS and *O*-chain polysaccharide confirmed that 40%of GalNAcA was present in the amide form. Direct CE-ES-MS/MS analysis of *in vivo* cultured cells confirmed the formation of a novel polysaccharide, a structure also formed *in vitro*, which was previously undetectable in bacterial cells grown within implants in fish, and in which GalNAcA was fully amidated.

To date, a limited number of bacteria have been reported to produce capsular and *O*-chain polysaccharides with identical structures. It appears that this property is not uncommon for fish pathogens and similar findings for *Listonella* (formerly *Vibrio*) *anguillarum* and *V. ordalii* [51,109] have previously been reported. It should be noted that the structures of the CPS and *O*-chain polysaccharide of *L. anguillarum* and *V. ordalii* have recently been re-examined and that the *galacto* configuration of the 2,3-diacetamido-2,3-dideoxy-hexuronic acid in both structures should be revised in favor of the *gulo* configuration.

The core oligosaccharide isolated from the lipopolysaccharide of *Aeromonas salmonicida* subsp. *salmonicida* has been investigated by methylation analysis, NMR spectroscopy (^{13}C and ^1H), oxidation with periodate and chromium trioxide, and Smith degradation (2.6) [110]:

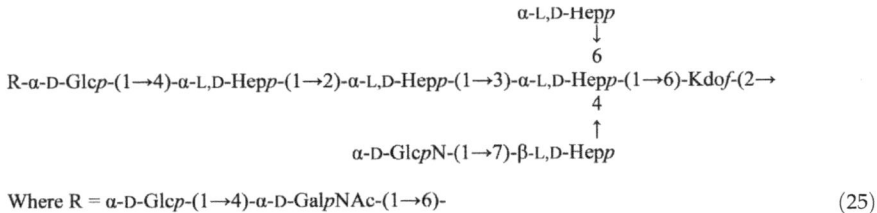

$$\alpha\text{-L,D-Hep}p$$
$$\downarrow$$
$$6$$
$$R\text{-}\alpha\text{-D-Glc}p\text{-}(1{\rightarrow}4)\text{-}\alpha\text{-L,D-Hep}p\text{-}(1{\rightarrow}2)\text{-}\alpha\text{-L,D-Hep}p\text{-}(1{\rightarrow}3)\text{-}\alpha\text{-L,D-Hep}p\text{-}(1{\rightarrow}6)\text{-Kdo}f\text{-}(2{\rightarrow}$$
$$4$$
$$\uparrow$$
$$\alpha\text{-D-Glc}p\text{N-}(1{\rightarrow}7)\text{-}\beta\text{-L,D-Hep}p$$

Where R = α-D-Glc$p$-(1→4)-α-D-Gal$p$NAc-(1→6)- \hfill (25)

The core oligosaccharide structure of the *in vivo* derived rough phenotype of *Aeromonas salmonicida* subsp. *salmonicida* was investigated by a combination of compositional, methylation, CE-MS and one- and two-dimensional NMR analyses and established as the following (2.6) [111]:

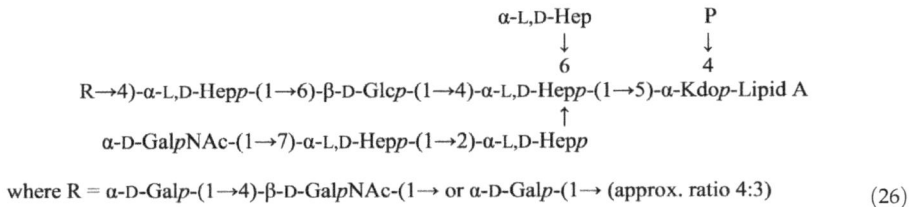

$$\alpha\text{-L,D-Hep} \qquad\qquad P$$
$$\downarrow \qquad\qquad\qquad \downarrow$$
$$6 \qquad\qquad\qquad\quad 4$$
$$R{\rightarrow}4)\text{-}\alpha\text{-L,D-Hep}p\text{-}(1{\rightarrow}6)\text{-}\beta\text{-D-Glc}p\text{-}(1{\rightarrow}4)\text{-}\alpha\text{-L,D-Hep}p\text{-}(1{\rightarrow}5)\text{-}\alpha\text{-Kdo}p\text{-Lipid A}$$
$$\uparrow$$
$$\alpha\text{-D-Gal}p\text{NAc-}(1{\rightarrow}7)\text{-}\alpha\text{-L,D-Hep}p\text{-}(1{\rightarrow}2)\text{-}\alpha\text{-L,D-Hep}p$$

where R = α-D-Gal$p$-(1→4)-β-D-Gal$p$NAc-(1→ or α-D-Gal$p$-(1→ (approx. ratio 4:3) \hfill (26)

Comparative CE-MS analysis of *A. salmonicida* subsp. *salmonicida* core oligosaccharides from strains A449, 80204-1 and an *in vivo* rough isolate confirmed that the structure of the core oligosaccharide was conserved among different isolates of *A. salmonicida*.

While searching for bacteria that cross-react with the recently discovered second causative agent of cholera, *V. cholerae* O139 Bengal [112], six strains of another member of the family Vibrionaceae, *Aerornonas trota*, have been found to agglutinate with specific antiserum to *V. cholerae* O139 in a slide-agglutination test [113]: Polyclonal antiserum to a cross-reactive *A. trota* strain cross-protected infant mice against cholera on challenge with virulent *V. cholerae* O139. The cross-reactive bacteria were not serologically identical, and the antigenic relationship between them was of an a,b-a,c type, where a is the common antigenic epitope and b and c are unique epitopes. Serological and genetic studies suggested that the capsular polysaccharide has the same repeating unit as the *O*-antigen chain [114] and, thus, carries determinants of *O*-specificity.

The structure of the *V. cholerae* O139 capsular polysaccharide has been elucidated as (2.6) [115]:

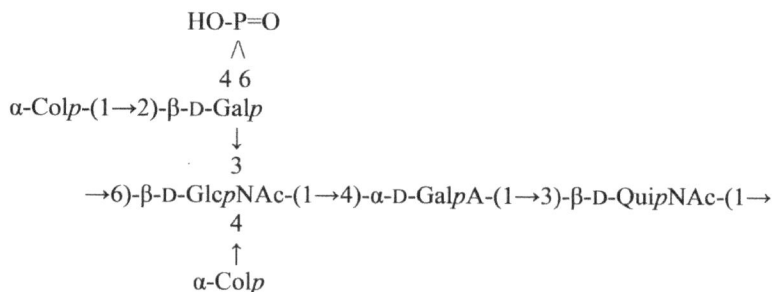

```
                    HO-P=O
                      /\
                     4 6
        α-Colp-(1→2)-β-D-Galp
                      ↓
                      3
    →6)-β-D-GlcpNAc-(1→4)-α-D-GalpA-(1→3)-β-D-QuipNAc-(1→
                    4
                    ↑
                  α-Colp
```

Structure 1

(27)

The presence of 3,6-dideoxy-L-*xylo*-hexose colitose (Col) and a cyclic phosphate diester are the unusual features of this polysaccharide.

The cross-reactive *A. trota* strains produce an *S*-type lipopolysaccharide with a polysaccharide *O*-antigen chain, which has not been chemically analyzed. To reveal a common epitope (or epitopes), which is responsible for the serological cross-reaction between these two microorganisms, the structure of the *O*-specific polysaccharide of *A. trota* strain 1354, which is one of the six cross-reactive strains was determined. On the basis of methylation analysis and NMR spectroscopic studies of the initial and modified, colitose-free polysaccharide, it was concluded that the repeating unit of the *O*-specific polysaccharide has the following structure (28) [116]:

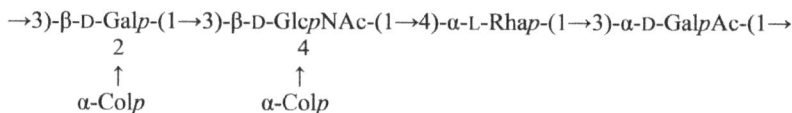

```
  →3)-β-D-Galp-(1→3)-β-D-GlcpNAc-(1→4)-α-L-Rhap-(1→3)-α-D-GalpAc-(1→
              2                    4
              ↑                    ↑
            α-Colp              α-Colp
```

Structure 2

(28)

Mild hydrolysis of the polysaccharide with 48% hydrofluoric acid at 4 °C removed the Col residues completely without significant depolymerization. As a result, a modified polysaccharide was obtained, which lacked colitose but contained the four other sugar constituents of the repeating unit (29):

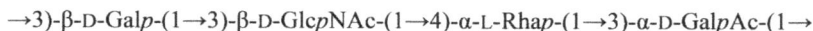

```
  →3)-β-D-Galp-(1→3)-β-D-GlcpNAc-(1→4)-α-L-Rhap-(1→3)-α-D-GalpAc-(1→
```

Structure 3

(29)

Although structurally different, the repeating unit 2 of the *A. trota* *O*-specific polysaccharide has a tetrasaccharide fragment in common with the repeating unit 1 of the capsular polysaccharide of cross-reactive *V. cholerae* O139, which includes Gal, GlcNAc, and two terminal Col residues. It seems likely that the common antigenic epitope is associated with the non-reducing terminal end of the polysaccharide, as was suggested for the oligosaccharide epitopes that determine the blood-group activities of some *Salmonella* and *Escherichia coli* strains [117,118]. Thus, structure 1 corresponds to the biological repeating unit of the *V. cholerae* O139 polysaccharide, and, therefore, its non-reducing terminal tetrasaccharide fragment has the structure 4. With an assumption that the structure 2 also corresponds to the biological repeating unit of the *A. trota* polysaccharide, its non-reducing terminal end should be occupied by the tetrasaccharide fragment 5, which differs from the tetrasaccharide 4 in lacking the cyclic phosphate group only (2.6).

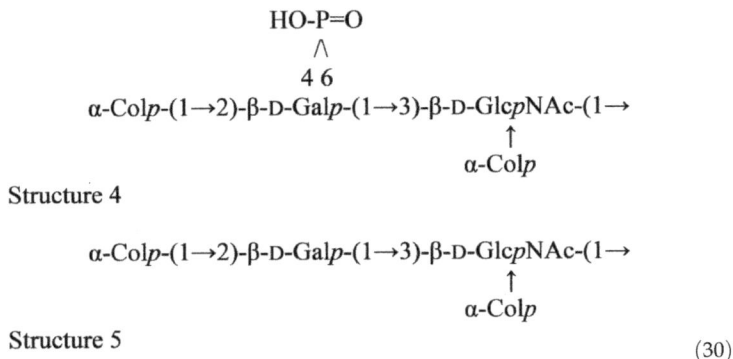

$$\text{HO-P=O}$$
$$\wedge$$
$$4\ 6$$
$$\alpha\text{-Col}p\text{-}(1{\rightarrow}2)\text{-}\beta\text{-D-Gal}p\text{-}(1{\rightarrow}3)\text{-}\beta\text{-D-Glc}p\text{NAc-}(1{\rightarrow}$$
$$\uparrow$$
$$\alpha\text{-Col}p$$

Structure 4

$$\alpha\text{-Col}p\text{-}(1{\rightarrow}2)\text{-}\beta\text{-D-Gal}p\text{-}(1{\rightarrow}3)\text{-}\beta\text{-D-Glc}p\text{NAc-}(1{\rightarrow}$$
$$\uparrow$$
$$\alpha\text{-Col}p$$

Structure 5

(30)

The known cross-reactivity between the strain studied and *Vibrio cholerae* O139 Bengal is substantiated by the presence of a common colitose-containing epitope shared by the O-specific polysaccharide of *A. trota* and the capsular polysaccharide of *V.cholerae*, which is thought to carry determinants of O-specificity.

Aeromonas bestiarum is a member of the bacterial species belonging to the motile aeromonad group that comprises several species such as *A. hydrophila*, *A. sobria*, *A. veronii*, *A. allosaccharophila* and *A. jandaei*, which have been reported as fish pathogens. [119,120]. The results of taxonomic studies revealed that diseases, and thus losses, in commercial carp were mostly caused by strains identified as *A. bestiarum*. However, until now there has been limited knowledge of the compositional diversity of the O-antigenic part of LPS among *Aeromonas* species. Therefore, it appeared purposeful to undertake immunochemical studies of *Aeromonas* strains with the described genomospecies (16S rDNA-RFLP) and their pathogenicity, which then could complete the LPS-based classification data of *Aeromonas* strains. Recently published structural studies of the R-type LPS from *A. hydrophila* strain AH-901 have extended this database [107]. The LPS of the transposone mutant AH-901 of the wild-type strain *A. hydrophila* AH-3 was devoid of the O-chain polysaccharide and contained a complete core with heptoses as the most dominant sugar residues and a lipid A with a diglucosaminyl backbone containing two phosphate groups substituted with 4-amino-4-deoxyarabinoses. Still, the question remains how common this structure of the core region is among motile and non-motile *Aeromonas* species.

The O-specific polysaccharide obtained by mild-acid degradation of *A. bestiarum* 207 lipopolysaccharide was studied by sugar and methylation analyses along with ^{1}H and ^{13}C NMR spectroscopy. The sequence of the sugar residues was determined by ROESY and HMBC experiments. It is concluded that the O-polysaccharide is composed of branched pentasaccharide repeating units (31) [121]:

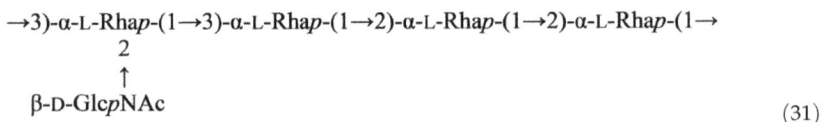

$$\rightarrow3)\text{-}\alpha\text{-L-Rha}p\text{-}(1{\rightarrow}3)\text{-}\alpha\text{-L-Rha}p\text{-}(1{\rightarrow}2)\text{-}\alpha\text{-L-Rha}p\text{-}(1{\rightarrow}2)\text{-}\alpha\text{-L-Rha}p\text{-}(1{\rightarrow}$$
$$2$$
$$\uparrow$$
$$\beta\text{-D-Glc}p\text{NAc}$$

(31)

The determined structure is different from those published for other *Aeromonas* strains. However, the α-L-Rha residue was found in the O-chain polysaccharides of *A. caviae* strains 11212 and ATCC 15468, as one of the components of their pentasaccharide and tetrasaccharide repeating units, respectively [122,123]. Another 6-deoxyhexose residue, 6-deoxy-L-talose, was identified as a dominant component of the *A. hydrophila* O:34 OPS. Interestingly, strains of that serogroup are most common among mesophilic *Aeromonas* species, accounting for 26.4% of all isolates, and have been documented as an important cause of human infections. It is unknown whether this group of isolates is homogeneous with respect to their OPS composition. If some departures from the typical O-antigen structure were found, this could suggest the presence of an immunochemical heterogeneity of the isolates, similar to that observed among *A. salmonicida* strains [105].

Aeromonas caviae is associated with gastrointestinal disease in adults and acute, severe gastroenteritis in children [124]. A number of putative virulence factors have been identified for *A. caviae*, including polar flagella, pili and cytotoxin. Both flagella and pili have been implicated in the adherence of *A. caviae* to human epithelial cells *in vitro*. Some strains of *A. caviae* are able to form biofilms on inert surfaces, a phenomenon attributed to a hyperpiliation of the cells through type IV pili [125]. Less is known about the role of LPS in these processes, although the *flmA* and *flmB* genes of *A. caviae* Sch3N have been implicated in LPS O-chain biosynthesis [126]. As a major cell-surface component, LPS of *A. caviae* has been implicated in the adherence to human epithelial cells and biofilm formation, but the role of LPS in the pathogenesis of *A. caviae*-induced gastroenteritis is not well understood. Comprehensive structural and genetic studies of LPS are essential to determine its etiological role in pathology of the disease.

A. caviae strain 11212 was isolated from the stools of a patient with diarrhea. Sugar analysis, methylation analyses, and a uronic acid degradation together with NMR spectroscopy were the principal methods used in the structural study of the O-polysaccharide from the LPS of this strain. The sequence of the sugar residues could be determined by NOESY and HMBC experiments. It is concluded that the polysaccharide is composed of pentasaccharide repeating units (32) [123]:

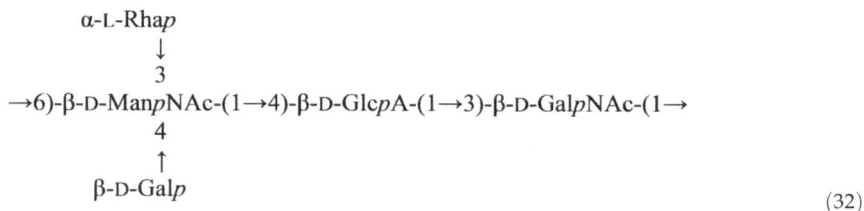

$$
\begin{array}{c}
\alpha\text{-L-Rha}p \\
\downarrow \\
3 \\
\rightarrow 6)\text{-}\beta\text{-D-Man}p\text{NAc-}(1\rightarrow 4)\text{-}\beta\text{-D-Glc}p\text{A-}(1\rightarrow 3)\text{-}\beta\text{-D-Gal}p\text{NAc-}(1\rightarrow \\
4 \\
\uparrow \\
\beta\text{-D-Gal}p
\end{array}
$$

(32)

The O-chain polysaccharide produced by a mild acid degradation of *A. caviae* ATCC 15468 lipopolysaccharide was found to be composed of L-rhamnose, 2-acetamido-2-deoxy-D-glucose, 2-acetamido-2-deoxy-D-galactose and phosphoglycerol. Subsequent methylation and CE–ESIMS analyses and 1D/2D NMR (^{1}H, ^{13}C and ^{31}P) spectroscopy showed that the O-chain polysaccharide is a high-molecular-mass acidic branched polymer of tetrasaccharide repeating units with a phosphoglycerol substituent having the following (33) [127]:

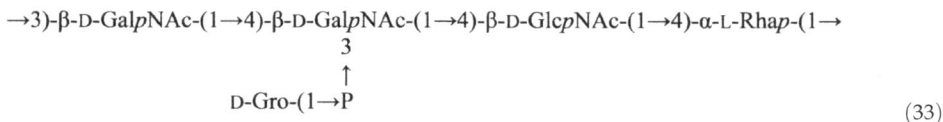

$$
\begin{array}{c}
\rightarrow 3)\text{-}\beta\text{-D-Gal}p\text{NAc-}(1\rightarrow 4)\text{-}\beta\text{-D-Gal}p\text{NAc-}(1\rightarrow 4)\text{-}\beta\text{-D-Glc}p\text{NAc-}(1\rightarrow 4)\text{-}\alpha\text{-L-Rha}p\text{-}(1\rightarrow \\
3 \\
\uparrow \\
\text{D-Gro-}(1\rightarrow\text{P}
\end{array}
$$

(33)

The previously determined structure of the O-chain polysaccharide from *A. caviae* strain 11212 bears no resemblance to the above structure, suggesting the possible need to divide this species into more than one serological group.

Interestingly, the phosphoglycerol moiety identified in the structure of the O-chain polysaccharide of *A. caviae* ATCC 15468 was previously found in the O-chain polysaccharides of *Citrobacter* 016 [128], *Hafnia alvei* strain PCM1207 [129] and *Proteus* species [130], as well as in the exo-polysaccharide produced by *Lactobacillus sake* O-1 and the specific capsular polysaccharide of *Streptococcus pneumoniae* type 45 [131]. It is recognized as an immunodominant epitope, and the cross-reactions between the LPS of *Citrobacter* O16 and *H. alvei* strain PCM 1207 could be attributed to the presence of this shared epitope in their respective O-specific polysaccharide structures.

At present, much research on *Aeromonas* bacteria is focused in epidemiology [132] and immunology [133]. However, since the polysaccharides obtained from many different bacteria are important in the manufacture, distribution, storage and consumption of food products [134], cosmetics and paints, *Aeromonas* polysaccharides are also receiving attention for similar applications.

The *Aeromonas nichidenii* strain 5797 produces an acidic polysaccharide—*Aeromonas* gum. This gum exists as aggregates in aqueous solutions and exhibits a very high viscositythis form. In addition, the gum exists in semi-flexible single chains in cadoxen and dimethyl sulfoxide solutions at room temperature. Structural analysis of this polysaccharide may provide a basis for a better understanding of its use as a gelling agent for food products and for other uses.

This gum was studied by ^{1}H and ^{13}C NMR spectroscopy including 2D COSY, TOCSY, HMQC, HMBC and ROESY experiments after O-deacetylation and Smith degradation. These investigations revealed the presence of an O-acetylated pentasaccharide repeating unit composed of mannose, glucose, xylose and glucuronic acid, and having the following structure (34) [135]:

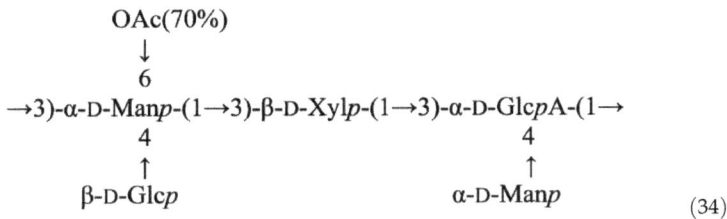

$$
\begin{array}{c}
\text{OAc(70\%)} \\
\downarrow \\
6 \\
\rightarrow 3)\text{-}\alpha\text{-D-Man}p\text{-}(1\rightarrow 3)\text{-}\beta\text{-D-Xyl}p\text{-}(1\rightarrow 3)\text{-}\alpha\text{-D-Glc}p\text{A-}(1\rightarrow \\
\quad\quad 4 \quad\quad\quad\quad\quad\quad\quad\quad\quad\quad\quad 4 \\
\quad\quad \uparrow \quad\quad\quad\quad\quad\quad\quad\quad\quad\quad\quad \uparrow \\
\quad\quad \beta\text{-D-Glc}p \quad\quad\quad\quad\quad\quad\quad \alpha\text{-D-Man}p
\end{array}
\quad\quad (34)
$$

After the O-deacetylation with following Smith degradation of the native gum, the modified polysaccharide building up of linear trisaccharide repeating unit (35) was obtained:

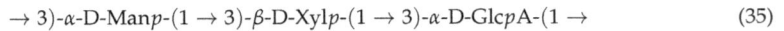

$$\rightarrow 3)\text{-}\alpha\text{-D-Man}p\text{-}(1 \rightarrow 3)\text{-}\beta\text{-D-Xyl}p\text{-}(1 \rightarrow 3)\text{-}\alpha\text{-D-Glc}p\text{A-}(1 \rightarrow \quad\quad (35)$$

Other bacterial polysaccharide gums used in the food industry are xantan gum from *Xantomonas campestris* [136], alginates from *Pseudomonas aeruginosa* [137] and *Azobacter vinelandii* and gellan gum from *Sphingomonas paucimobilis* [138]. Acetylation at position 6 of mannose and the presence of glucose snd glucuronic acid are the only structural similarities of the xantan and aeromonas gums. Gellan gum also has the sugars glucose and glucuronic acid, although the O-acetylation at position 6 is on a glucose residue [139].

2.7. Genus Idiomarina

The bacterial strain KMM 231^T was isolated from a seawater sample taken at a depth of 4000 m from the northwestern Pacific Ocean. This deep-sea strain was found to be Gram-negative, halotrophic, psychrotolerant, heterotrophic and strictly aerobic. On the basis of polyphasic evidence, it was proposed that strain KMM 231 be classified in the new genus, *Idiomarina* gen. nov., as a representative of *Idiomarina zobellii* sp. nov. [140].

The O-polysaccharide was obtained by mild base degradation of the lipopolysaccharide. The following structure of the O-polysaccharide was elucidated by ^{1}H and ^{13}C NMR spectroscopy of the oligosaccharide and base-degraded lipopolysaccharide, including COSY, TOCSY, ROESY, ^{1}H, ^{13}C HSQC, HSQC-TOCSY and HMBC experiments (36) [141]:

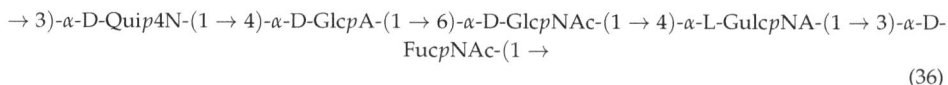

$$\rightarrow 3)\text{-}\alpha\text{-D-Qui}p4\text{N-}(1 \rightarrow 4)\text{-}\alpha\text{-D-Glc}p\text{A-}(1 \rightarrow 6)\text{-}\alpha\text{-D-Glc}p\text{NAc-}(1 \rightarrow 4)\text{-}\alpha\text{-L-Gulc}p\text{NA-}(1 \rightarrow 3)\text{-}\alpha\text{-D-}$$
$$\text{Fuc}p\text{NAc-}(1 \rightarrow$$

(36)

Mild acid degradation of the lipopolysaccharide yielded an oligosaccharide, which represents one repeating unit of the *O*-polysaccharide (37):

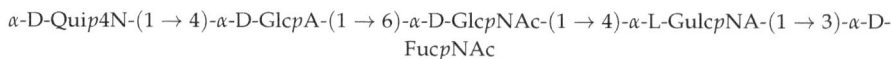

$$\alpha\text{-D-Qui}p4\text{N-}(1 \rightarrow 4)\text{-}\alpha\text{-D-Glc}p\text{A-}(1 \rightarrow 6)\text{-}\alpha\text{-D-Glc}p\text{NAc-}(1 \rightarrow 4)\text{-}\alpha\text{-L-Gulc}p\text{NA-}(1 \rightarrow 3)\text{-}\alpha\text{-D-}$$
$$\text{Fuc}p\text{NAc}$$

(37)

The *O*-polysaccharide is distinguished by the presence of two unusual amino sugars, 4-amino-4,6-dideoxy-D-glucose (D-Qui4N) and 2-amino-2-deoxy-L-guluronic acid (L-GulNA), both having the free amino group. The unexpectedly high acid lability of the glycosidic linkage of 2-acetamido-2,6-dideoxy-D-galactose (D-FucNAc) could be associated with the presence of a free amino group adjacent to the site of attachment of FucNAc to Qui4N. 2-amino-2-deoxy-L-guluronic acid, which has been previously found in nature only in a few bacterial glycopolymers, including the acidic capsular polysaccharides of *Vibrio parahaemolyticus* K15 [142] and the marine bacteria bacteria *Pseudoalteromonas nigrifaciens* KMM 158 [32] and KMM 161 [143], as well as in the cell wall of *Halococcus* sp. strain 24 [144]. Another rare component of the *O*-polysaccharide, 4-amino-4,6-dideoxy-D-glucose, has not been discovered previously with the free amino group but rather carrying various *N*-acyl substituents, including formyl [145], acetyl [146], *N*-acetylglycyl [147], *N*-[(R)-3-hydroxybutyryl]-L-alanyl [148] and other groups.

3. Structure of Carbohydrate Antigens of *Cytophaga-Flavobacterium-Flexibacter* Phylum

3.1. *Genus* Flexibacter

The *Cytophaga-Flavobacterium-Flexibacter* bacteria are represented by a large, somewhat heterogeneous group of filamentous, gliding, Gram-negative bacteria with unusual surface properties [149]. At least seven members of this group are considered to be important fish pathogens. They infect a wide variety of fish species and usually form biofilms, primarily on the tissues associated with the oral cavity. Among these, *Flexibacter maritimus* has recently emerged as a cause of widespread severe mortality and economic losses in farmed marine species worldwide [150].

Flexibacter maritimus, a long rod-shaped, Gram-negative bacterium, has been associated with disease (Flexibacteriosis) in a number of fish species [151] and its economic importance has been related to a cause of cutaneous erosion disease particularly in sea-caged salmonids. In grouper, *Flexibacter maritimus* causes "red boil" disease [152] related to its clinical signs of reduced scales and severe hemorrhage on the body surface, resembling boiled skin and causing a high mortality rate. No effective vaccine has been developed against this pathogen. A clearer definition of the relevant immunoreactive macromolecules of these bacterial fish pathogens is fundamentally important particularly with regard to the mechanisms of pathogenesis and the role of infective biofilms. This information is important for the development of appropriate immunochemical reagents to facilitate speciation and the design of cost-effective, efficacious vaccines. Lipopolysaccharides (LPS, endotoxins) play a role in the pathogenesis of Gram-negative infections and the structural analysis of their antigenic *O*-polysaccharide (*O*-PS) components is important in providing a molecular level understanding of their serological specificities, role in pathogenesis, development of diagnostic agents, and the production of *O*-PS based conjugate vaccines.

An acidic *O*-specific polysaccharide, obtained by mild acid degradation of the *Flexibacter maritimus* LPS was found to be composed of a disaccharide repeating unit built of 2-acetamido-3-*O*-acetyl-4- [(*S*)-2-hydroxyglutar-5-ylamido]-2,4,6-trideoxy-β-glucose and

5-acetamido-7-[(S)-3-hydroxybutyramido]-8-amino-3,5,7,8,9-pentadeoxynonulopyranosonic acid (Sug) having the structure (Figure 2) [153].

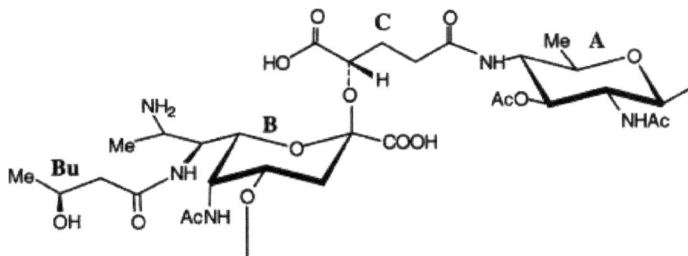

Figure 2. LPS structure of *Flexibacter maritimus* [153]. Reproduced with permission from Wiley-Blackwell.

This *O*-PS contained a new nonulosonic acid derivative, 5-(3-hydroxybutyramido)-7-acetamido-8-amino-3,5,7,8,9-pentadeoxy-β-*manno*-nonulopyranosonic acid, with as yet undetermined configuration at C-8 and tentatively assigned the L-absolute configuration. Moreover, it contains a linkage involving a *R*-2-hydroxyglutaric acid residue reported for the first time as a bacterial polysaccharide component. A similar component, *O*-glycosylated amide linked *R*-malic acid was reported as a component of the *O*-PS from another fish pathogen *Flavobacterium psychrophilum* [154].

3.2. Genus Flavobacterium

The genus *Flavobacterium* includes more than 60 validly described species, isolated from various sources [155]. The pathogenesis of infection with *Flavobacterium* spp. is not well understood; in humans, however, they cause neonatal meningitis, catheter-associated bacteremia, and pneumonia, and have also been associated with some cases of HIV disease [156]. *Flavobacterium* spp. are also characterized by an unusual pattern of antibiotic sensitivity, being resistant to several antimicrobials effective against Gram-negative rods.

Flavobacterium psychrophilum (syn. *Cytophaga psychrophilia, Flexibacter psychrophilus*) is the etiological agent of rainbow trout fry syndrome (RTFS) and bacterial cold water disease, septicemic infections that can cause significant early losses in hatchery-reared salmonids, particularly Rainbow trout (*Oncorhynchus mykiss*) in Europe, and coho salmon (*Oncorhynchus kisutch*) in North America. In the past decade, *Flexibacter psychrophilum* has emerged as a causative agent of severe rainbow trout fry mortality in Europe (RTFS) and is now known to affect salmonids worldwide [157]. The molecular pathogenesis of *Flexibacter psychrophilum* is primarily limited to their exotoxins and plasmids [158]. No vaccine is commercially available for RTFS control and the development of effective, inexpensive, easily administered vaccines and specific diagnostics have become an important goal to reduce losses that occur in immature salmonids. Following a study to differentiate *Flexibacter psychrophilum* from other closely related bacteria using both randomly amplified polymorphic (RAPD)-PCR and polyclonal antibodies, several immunogenic cell surface molecules, including lipopolysaccharides (LPS) that may be involved in pathogenesis were identified as potential vaccine candidates [159]. Recently, several *Flexibacter psychrophilum* surface molecules, including lipopolysaccharide (LPS), have been implicated in its pathogenesis and identified as potential vaccine and diagnostic candidate macromolecules.

The structure of the antigenic *O*-polysaccharide contained in the LPS of *Flexibacter psychrophilum* strain 259-93 was deduced by the application of analytical NMR spectroscopy, mass spectrometry, glycose and methylation analysis, and partial hydrolysis degradations, and was found to be an unbranched polymer of trisaccharide repeating units composed of L-rhamnose (L-Rha*p*), 2-acetamido-2-deoxy-L-fucose (L-Fuc*p*NAc) and 2-acetamido-4-((3S,5S)-3,5-dihydroxyhexanamido)-2,4-dideoxy-

D-quinovose (D-Qui*p*2NAc4NR, 2-*N*-acetyl-4-*N*-((3*S*,5*S*)-3,5-dihydroxyhexanoyl)-D-bacillosamine) (1:1:1) (38) [154]:

$$\to 4)\text{-}\alpha\text{-L-Fuc}p\text{NAc-}(1 \to 3)\text{-}\alpha\text{-D-Quip2NAc4NR-}(1 \to 2)\text{-}\alpha\text{-L-Rha}p\text{-}(1 \to$$
$$\text{where R is } (3S, 5S)\text{-CH}_3\text{-CH(OH)-CH}_2\text{-CH(OH)-CO-}$$
(38)

The occurrence of *N*-acyl derivatives of 2,4-diamino-2,4-dideoxy-D-quinovose (bacillosamine) in bacterial glycans is not unusual. The glycose has been demonstrated to be a constituent of the *O*-antigens of *Fusobacterium necrophorum* [160], *Pseudomonas aurantiaca* IMB 31 [161], *Vibrio cholerae* O:3 and O:5 [162,163], *Pseudomonas aeruginosa* [164], and also in the capsular polysaccharide of *Alteromonas* sp. CMM 155 [31] and a polysaccharide component of *Bacillus licheniformis* [165]. It is of interest that the parent 2,4-diamino-2,4-dideoxy-D-quinovose residue present in the backbone chain of the *O*-PS of *V. cholerae* O:3 LPS [162], shown below, was acylated at the amino group at C-4 by a 3,5-dihydroxyhexanoyl group of undetermined configuration. (3*S*,5*S*)-Dihydroxyhexanoic acid has been found in berries of *Sorbus aucuparia* as the β-D-glucopyranoside of its D-lactone [166]. The 3,5-dihydroxyhexanoic acid in the *O*-PS of *Flexibacter psychrophilum* has the same configuration.

Flavobacterium columnare, formerly referred to as *Flexibacter columnaris* or *Cytophaga columnaris* [155], is a Gram-negative bacterium which causes columnaris disease in warm water fish, a disease that is the second leading cause of mortality in pond raised catfish in the south-eastern United States.

The virulence factors of *Flavobacterium columnare* are relatively unknown, but it has been suggested that, in pathogenesis, adhesion of the bacterium may be related to its surface polysaccharide constituents [167]. This investigation was directed towards characterization of the lipopolysaccharide (LPS) and putative capsule produced by the bacterium, as a first step in identifying their possible role in pathogenesis in fish. In addition, it was considered that characterization of the LPS *O*-polysaccharide (*O*-PS) antigen would provide a structural knowledge basis for the development of a specific antibody diagnostic agent and possible target molecules for a conjugate based vaccine.

The structure of the antigenic *O*-chain polysaccharide of *Flavobacterium columnare* ATCC 43622, a Gram-negative bacterium that causes columnaris disease in warmwater fish, was determined by high-field 1D and 2D NMR techniques, MS, and chemical analyses. The *O*-chain was shown to be an unbranched linear polymer of a trisaccharide repeating unit composed of 2-acetamido-2-deoxy-Dglucuronic acid (D-GlcNAcA), 2-acetamidino-2,6-dideoxy-L-galactose (L-FucNAm) and 2-acetamido- 2,6-dideoxy-D-*xylo*-hexos-4-ulose (D-Sug) (1:1:1) (39) [52]:

$$\to 4)\text{-}\beta\text{-D-Glc}p\text{NAcA-}(1 \to 4)\text{-}\alpha\text{-L-Fuc}p\text{NAm-}(1 \to 4)\text{-}\alpha\text{-D-Sug}p\text{-}(1 \to$$

$$
\begin{array}{ccc}
3 & & 3 \\
\uparrow & & \uparrow \\
\text{OAc} & & \text{OAc}
\end{array}
$$
(39)

It is interesting to note that O3-linked D-Sug was found to be a component of the *O*-PS of the fish pathogen *Vibrio ordalii* serotype O:2 [113], which is the cause of vibriosis among feral and farmed fish and shellfish. The only other reported bacterial source of this glycose is the specific CPS of *Streptococcus pneumoniae* type 5 [50]. However, in the latter polysaccharides, the glycose is found in its β-D-configuration in contrast with the α-D-configuration found in the *F. columnare O*-PS. In agreement with previous studies, we also found that the presence of this 4-ketoglycose in the polymeric structure rendered the *O*-PS unstable under alkaline conditions and even prolonged storage in aqueous solutions at pH 7. A similar result was found in a study of forbeside C, a saponin of *Asterias forbesi* [55], which also has a component D-Sug residue.

3.3. Genus Cellulophaga

The genus *Cellulophaga* belongs to the family Flavobacteriaceae of the phylum Bacteroidetes. It was created to accommodate the heterotrophic aerobic Gram-negative yellow/orange pigmented gliding and agarolytic bacteria of marine origin. Currently this genus comprises six validly described species: *C. algicola*, *C. baltica*, *C. fucicola*, *C. lytica*, *C. pacifica* and *C. tyrosinoxydans* [19]. Data on the *O*-polysaccharide structure of *Cellulophaga* were reported only for *C. baltica* [168] and *C. fucicola* [169] strain NN015860^T isolated from brown alga *Fucus serratus* L., which inhabits the North Sea, Atlantic Ocean.

The *O*-polysaccharide was isolated from the lipopolysaccharide of *Cellulophaga fucicola* and studied by chemical analyses along with ^{1}H and ^{13}C NMR spectroscopy. The following new structure of the *O*-polysaccharide of *C. fucicola* containing 5,7-diacetamido-3,5,7,9-tetradeoxy-L-*glycero*-L*manno*-non-2-ulosonic acid residue (pseudaminic acid, Pse*p*) was elucidated as the following (40):

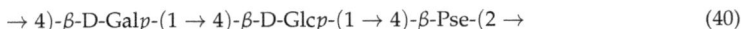

$$\rightarrow 4)\text{-}\beta\text{-}D\text{-Gal}p\text{-}(1 \rightarrow 4)\text{-}\beta\text{-}D\text{-Glc}p\text{-}(1 \rightarrow 4)\text{-}\beta\text{-Pse-}(2 \rightarrow \qquad (40)$$

From the chemical and NMR spectroscopy data it was shown that the repeating unit of this PS from the LPS of *C. baltica* constructed in tetrasaccharide units, containing two D-mannose, 2-acetamido-2-deoxy-D-glucose and D-glucuronic acid residues, and non-stoichiometric quantity of the *O*-acetyl groups (41):

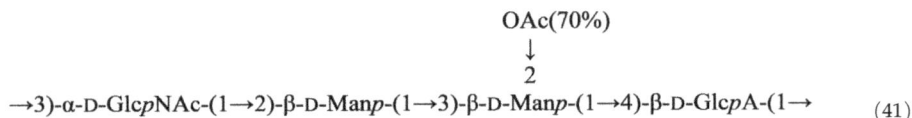

$$OAc(70\%)$$
$$\downarrow$$
$$2$$
$$\rightarrow 3)\text{-}\alpha\text{-}D\text{-Glc}p\text{NAc-}(1\rightarrow 2)\text{-}\beta\text{-}D\text{-Man}p\text{-}(1\rightarrow 3)\text{-}\beta\text{-}D\text{-Man}p\text{-}(1\rightarrow 4)\text{-}\beta\text{-}D\text{-Glc}p\text{A-}(1\rightarrow \qquad (41)$$

The influence of the *O*-acetyl group on the distal sugar residues in the repeating unit was shown.

4. Structure of Carbohydrate Antigens of *Alphaproteobacteria*

4.1. Genus Sulfitobacter

The genus *Sulfitobacter* was established in 1995 for marine gram-negative heterotrophic bacteria isolated from the H_2S/O_2 zone of the Black Sea and includes 10 validly described species. These microorganisms belongs phylogenetically to the cluster *Roseobacter-Ruegeria-Sulfitobacter* of class *Alphaproteobacteria* [19].

The microorganism *Sulfitobacter brevis* KMM 6006 was isolated from the bottom sediments in Chazma Bay (Sea of Japan). The glycopolymer was isolated from this strain was obtained and found to be teichoic acid containing ribitol, glycerine, and N-acetyl-D-glucosamine. The polymeric chain was built up of alternating 1,5-poly(4-N-acetyl-β-D-glucosaminylribitophosphate) and 1,3-poly (glycerophosphate) based on ^{13}C and ^{31}P NMR spectroscopy of the native polymer and the glycoside obtained by its dephosphorylation (42) [170]:

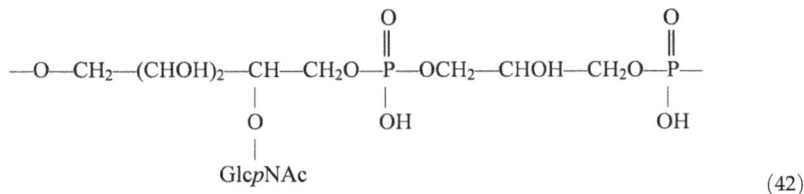

$$
\begin{array}{c}
\quad\quad\quad\quad\quad\quad\quad\quad\quad O \quad\quad\quad\quad\quad\quad\quad\quad\quad\quad O \\
\quad\quad\quad\quad\quad\quad\quad\quad\quad \| \quad\quad\quad\quad\quad\quad\quad\quad\quad\quad \| \\
\text{—O—CH}_2\text{—(CHOH)}_2\text{—CH—CH}_2\text{O—P—OCH}_2\text{—CHOH—CH}_2\text{O—P—} \\
\quad\quad\quad\quad\quad\quad\quad\quad | \quad\quad\quad\quad | \quad\quad\quad\quad\quad\quad\quad\quad | \\
\quad\quad\quad\quad\quad\quad\quad\quad O \quad\quad\quad OH \quad\quad\quad\quad\quad\quad\quad OH \\
\quad\quad\quad\quad\quad\quad\quad\quad | \\
\quad\quad\quad\quad\quad\text{Glc}p\text{NAc}
\end{array}
\qquad (42)
$$

4.2. *Genus* Loktanella

Loktanella rosea, a marine Gram-negative bacterium isolated from sediments of Chazma Bay, Sea of Japan [171]. *L. rosea* is a species nova that belongs to the genus *Loktanella*, which was created in 2004 in order to classify some new heterotrophic Alphaproteobacteria collected from Antartic lakes. *L. rosea* is a mesophilic and chemo-organotroph bacterium with a respiratory metabolism whose growth needs a medium with 1–12% of NaCl.

The LPS from *L. rosea* has been defined through sugar analysis, 2D nuclear magnetic resonance (NMR) and matrix-assisted laser desorption ionization (MALDI) mass spectrometry investigation. A unique highly negatively charged carbohydrate backbone has been identified. The lipid A skeleton lacks the typical phosphate groups and is characterized by two β-GlcNs and an α-galacturonic acid (GalA). This was the first example of a lipid A saccharide backbone in which the α-GlcN-phosphate residue is replaced by a β-GlcN-(1→1)-α-GalA in a mixed trehaloselike linkage (Figure 3).

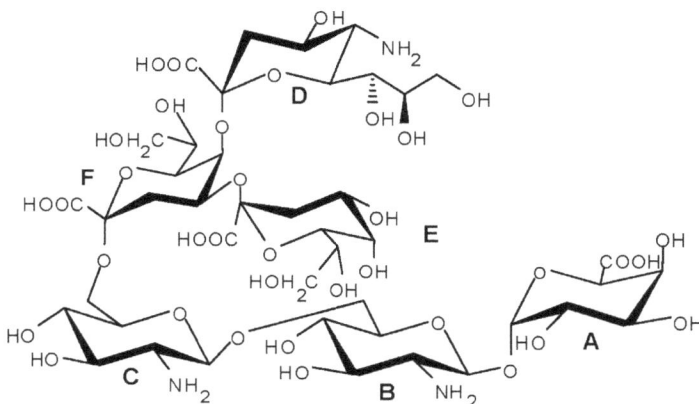

Figure 3. Carbohydrate structure of *Loktanella rosea* [172]. Reproduced with permission from Oxford Univeristy Press.

The core region is built up of three ulosonic acids, with two 3-deoxy-D-*manno*-oct-2-ulosonic acid residues, one of which is carrying a neuraminic acid (Neu). The overall carbohydrate structure is an exceptional variation from the typical architectural skeleton of endotoxins and also implies a very different biosynthesis (43) [172].

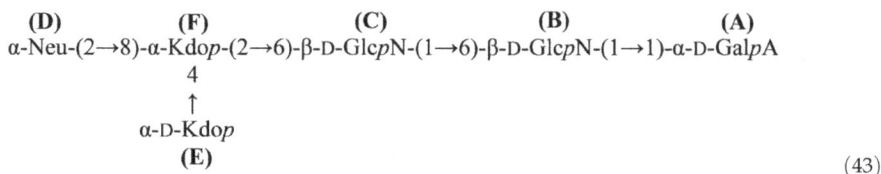

$$
\begin{array}{ccccc}
\textbf{(D)} & \textbf{(F)} & \textbf{(C)} & \textbf{(B)} & \textbf{(A)} \\
\end{array}
$$

α-Neu-(2→8)-α-Kdo*p*-(2→6)-β-D-Glc*p*N-(1→6)-β-D-Glc*p*N-(1→1)-α-D-Gal*p*A

4
↑
α-D-Kdo*p*
(E)

(43)

The lipooligosaccharide (LOS) was found to be characterized by a novel and unique hexasaccharide skeleton comprising: (i) a very small core region exclusively composed of ulosonic sugars and containing an Neu attached to a Kdo unit: α-Neu-(2→8)[α-D-Kdo-(2→4)]-α-D-Kdo-(2→ and; (ii) an exceptional lipid A backbone: β-D-Glc*p*N-(1→6)-β-D-Glc*p*N-(1→1)-α-D-Gal*p*A in which both GlcN residues were present with a β-anomeric configuration. Moreover, it lacked the classical phosphate residues at *O*-4′ and *O*-1, this latter was replaced by an α-GalA linked in a mixed trehalose-like linkage. To the best of our knowledge, this kind of glycosydic linkage was never found in biomolecules; its presence obviously implies profound biosynthetic differences from the canonical LPS lipid A pathway [173].

5. Conclusions

There is an extensive diversity between the chemical structures of the carbohydrate antigens from the different marine bacteria reviewed here. These polymers provide a rich source of uncommon monosaccharides, including higher sugars, and their derivatives having various non-sugar substituents.

In contrast to all LPS structures known to date, LPSs of the *Shewanella* genus contain a novel linking unit between the core polysaccharide and lipid A moieties, namely 8-amino-3,8-dideoxy-D*manno*-octulosonic acid (Kdo8N). The lipooligosaccharide (LOS) from *Loktanella rosea* is characterized by a novel and unique hexasaccharide skeleton among the known LOS structures.

This chemical structural information of carbohydrate-containing biopolymers may be useful in classification of Gram-negative marine bacteria and elaborating the current concepts regarding the organization and mechanisms of functioning of their cell wall.

Subject Index

Pse (pseudaminic acid)-5,7-diacetamido-3,5,7,9-tetradeoxy-L-*glycero*-L-*manno*-non-2-ulosonic acid [169]

Neu (neuraminic acid)-5-amino-3,5-dideoxy-D-*glycero*-D-*galacto*-non-2-ulosonic acid [172]

Acknowledgments: This study was supported in part by the Australian Research Council (ARC) and Advanced Manufacturing Co-operative Research Centre (AMCRC) and by the Russian Foundation for Basic Research Grant 11-04-00781-a and by the Program "Molecular and Cell Biology", Russian Academy of Sciences (RAS).

References

1. Head, IM; Jones, DM; Röling, WFM. Marine microorganisms make a meal of oil. *Nat. Rev. Microbiol* **2006**, *4*, 173–182.
2. Hau, HH; Gralnick, JA. Ecology and biotechnology of the genus *Shewanella*. *Ann. Rev. Microbiol* **2007**, *61*, 237–258.
3. Caroff, M; Karibian, D. Structure of bacterial lipopolysaccharides. *Carbohydr. Res* **2003**, *338*, 2431–2447.
4. Wilkinson, SG. Bacterial lipopolysaccharides—Themes and variations. *Prog. Lipid Res* **1996**, *35*, 283–343.
5. Raetz, CRH; Whitfield, C. Lipopolysaccharide endotoxins. *Annu. Rev. Biochem* **2002**, *71*, 635–700.
6. Kenne, L; Lindberg, B. Bacterial Polysaccharides. In *The Polysaccharides*; Aspinall, O, Ed.; Academic Press: New York, NY, USA, 1983; pp. 287–363.
7. Knirel, YA; Kochetkov, NK. The structure of lipopolysaccharides of Gram-negative bacteria. III. The structure of O-antigens: A review. *Biochemistry (Mosc.)* **1994**, *59*, 1325–1383.
8. Jansson, P-E. The Chemistry of the Polysaccharide Chains in Bacterial Lipopolysaccharides. In *Endotoxin in Health and Disease*; Brade, H, Opal, SM, Vogel, S, Morrison, DC, Eds.; Marcel Dekker: New York, NY, USA, 1999; pp. 155–178.
9. Knirel, YA. O-specific polysaccharides of Gram-negative bacteria. In *Microbial Glycobiology: Structures, Relevance and Applications*; Moran, A, Holst, O, Brennan, P, von Itzstein, M, Eds.; Academic Press: London, UK, 2010; pp. 57–73.
10. Nazarenko, EL; Komandrova, NA; Gorshkova, RP; Tomshich, SV; Zubrov, VA; Kilcoyne, M; Savage, AV. Structures of polysaccharides and oligosaccharides of some Gram-negative marine *Proteobacteria*. *Carbohydr. Res* **2003**, *338*, 2449–2457.
11. Nazarenko, EL. Structure of Carbohydrate Antigens of Some Gram-negative Marine *Proteobacteria*. In *Nanoscale Structure and Properties of Microbial Cell Surfaces*; Ivanova, EP, Ed.; Nova Science Publishers: New York, NY, USA, 2007; pp. 111–144.
12. Leone, S; Silipo, A; Nazarenko, EL; Lanzetta, R; Parrilli, M; Molinaro, A. Molecular structure of endotoxins from gram-negative marine bacteria: An update. *Mar. Drugs* **2007**, *5*, 85–112.
13. Holst, O. Chemical structure of the core region of lipopolysaccharides. In *Endotoxin in Health and Disease*; Brade, H, Morrison, DC, Opal, S, Vogel, S, Eds.; Marcel Dekker: New York, NY, USA, 1999; pp. 115–154.
14. Vinogradov, E; Korenevsky, A; Beveridge, TJ. The structure of the rough-type lipopolysaccharide from *Shewanella oneidensis* MR-1, containing 8-amino-8-deoxy-Kdo and an open-chain form of 2-acetamido-2-deoxy-d-galactose. *Carbohydr. Res* **2003**, *338*, 1991–1997.
15. Vinogradov, E; Korenevsky, A; Beveridge, TJ. The structure of the core region of the lipopolysaccharide from *Shewanella algae* BrY, containing 8-amino-3,8-dideoxy-d-manno-oct- 2-ulosonic acid. *Carbohydr. Res* **2004**, *339*, 737–740.
16. Silipo, A; Leone, S; Molinaro, A; Sturiale, L; Garozzo, D; Nazarenko, EL; Gorshkova, RP; Ivanova, EP; Lanzetta, R; Parrilli, M. Complete structural elucidation of a novel lipooligosaccharide from the outer membrane of the marine bacterium *Shewanella pacifica*. *Eur. J. Org. Chem* **2005**, *2005*, 2281–2291.
17. Silipo, A; Molinaro, A; Nazarenko, EL; Sturiale, L; Garozzo, D; Gorshkova, RP; Nedashkovskaya, OI; Lanzetta, R; Parrilli, M. Structural characterization of the carbohydrate backbone of the lipooligosaccharide of the marine bacterium *Arenibacter certesii* strain KMM 3941[T]. *Carbohydr. Res* **2005**, *340*, 2540–2549.
18. Leone, S; Molinaro, A; Sturiale, L; Garozzo, D; Nazarenko, EL; Gorshkova, RP; Ivanova, EP; Shevchenko, LS; Lanzetta, R; Parrilli, M. The outer membrane of the marine Gram-negative bacterium *Alteromonas addita* is composed of a very short-chain lipopolysaccharide with a high negative charge density. *Eur. J. Org. Chem* **2007**, *2007*, 1113–1122.

19. *Taxonomy Browser*. Available online: http://www.ncbi.nlm.nih.gov/Taxonomy/Browser/wwwtax.cgi accesed on 26 September 2011.

20. Ivanova, EP; Flavier, S; Christen, R. Phylogenetic relationships among marine *Alteromonas*-like proteobacteria: Emended description of the family Alteromonadaceae and proposal of *Pseudoalteromonadaceae* fam. nov., *Colwelliaceae* fam. nov., *Shewanellaceae* fam. nov., *Moritellaceae* fam. nov., *Ferrimonadaceae* fam. nov., *Idiomarinaceae* fam. nov. and *Psychromonadaceae* fam. nov. *Int. J. Syst. Evol. Microbiol* **2004**, *54*, 1773–1788.

21. Ivanova, EP; Bowman, JP; Lysenko, AM; Zhukova, NV; Gorshkova, NM; Sergeev, AF; Mikhailov, VV. *Alteromonas addita* sp. nov. *Int. J. Syst. Evol. Microbiol* **2005**, *55*, 1065–1068.

22. Ivanova, EP; Gorshkova, NM; Mikhailov, VV; Sergeev, AF; Gladkikh, RV; Goryachev, VA; Dudarev, OV; Botsul, AI; Mozherovsky, AV; Slinko, EN; *et al.* Distribution of saprophytic bacteria in the atomic submarine accident zone in Chazhma Bay, Sea of Japan. *Russ. J. Mar. Biol* **2005**, *31*, 65–72.

23. Gorshkova, RP; Isakov, VV; Denisenko, VA; Nazarenko, EL; Ivanova, EP; Shevchenko, LS. Structure of the repeating unit of the *Alteromonas addita* type strain KMM 3600[T] O-specific polysaccharide. *Chem. Nat. Compd. (Russ.)* **2008**, *44*, 549–551.

24. Raguenes, GH; Peres, A; Ruimy, R; Pignet, P; Christen, R; Loaec, M; Rougeaux, H; Barbier, G; Guezennec, JG. *Alteromonas infernus* sp. nov., a new polysaccharide-producing bacterium isolated from a deep-sea hydrothermal vent. *J. Appl. Microbiol* **1997**, *82*, 422–430.

25. Roger, O; Kervarec, N; Ratiskol, J; Colliec-Jouault, S; Chevolot, L. Structural studies of the main exopolysaccharide produced by the deep-sea bacterium *Alteromonas infernus*. *Carbohydr. Res* **2004**, *339*, 2371–2380.

26. González, JM; Mayer, F; Moran, MA; Hodson, RE; Whitman, WB. *Microbulbifer hydrolyticus* gen. nov., sp. nov., and *Marinobacterium georgiense* gen. nov., sp. nov., two marine bacteria from a lignin-rich pulp mill waste enrichment community. *Int. J. Syst. Bacteriol* **1997**, *47*, 369–376.

27. Gorshkova, RP; Isakov, VV; Nedashkovskaya, OI; Nazarenko, EL. Structure of carbohydrate antigens from *Microbulbifer* sp. KMM 6242. *Chem. Nat. Compd. (Russ.)* **2011**, *46*, 837–840.

28. Hanniffy, OM; Shashkov, AS; Senchenkova, SN; Tomshich, SV; Komandrova, NA; Romanenko, LA; Knirel, YA; Savage, AV. Structure of a highly acidic O-specific polysaccharide of lipopolysaccharide of *Pseudoalteromonas haloplanktis* KMM 223 containing l-iduronic acid and -QuiNHb4NHb. *Carbohydr. Res* **1998**, *307*, 291–298.

29. Hanniffy, OM; Shashkov, AS; Senchenkova, SN; Tomshich, SV; Komandrova, NA; Romanenko, LA; Knirel, YA; Savage, AV. Structure of an acidic O-specific polysaccharide of *Pseudoalteromonas haloplanktis* type strain ATCC 14393 containing 2-acetamido-2-deoxy-d and -l-galacturonic acids and 3-(N-acetyl-d-alanyl)amino-3,6-dideoxy-d-glucose. *Carbohydr. Res* **1999**, *321*, 132–138.

30. Muldoon, J; Shashkov, AS; Senchenkova, SN; Tomshich, SV; Komandrova, NA; Romanenko, LA; Knirel, YA; Savage, AV. Structure of an acidic polysaccharide from a marine bacterium *Pseudoalteromonas distincta* KMM 638 containing 5-acetamido-3,5,7,9- tetradeoxy-7-formamido-l-*glycero*-l-*manno*-nonulosonic acid. *Carbohydr. Res* **2001**, *330*, 231–239.

31. Zubkov, VA; Nazarenko, EL; Gorshkova, RP; Ivanova, EP; Shashkov, AS; Knirel, YA; Paramonov, NA; Ovodov, YS. Structure of the capsular polysaccharide from *Alteromonas* sp. CMM 155. *Carbohydr. Res* **1995**, *275*, 147–154.

32. Nazarenko, EL; Zubkov, VA; Shashkov, AS; Knirel, YA; Gorshkova, RP; Ivanova, EP; Ovodov, YS. Structure of the repeating unit of an acidic polysaccharide from *Alteromonas macleodii* 2MM6. *Russ. J. Bioorg. Chem* **1993**, *19*, 740–751.

33. Gorshkova, RP; Nazarenko, EL; Zubkov, VA; Shashkov, AS; Knirel, YA; Paramonov, NA; Meshkov, SV; Ivanova, EP. Structure of the capsular polysaccharide from *Alteromonas nigrifaciens* IAM 13010[T] containing 2-acetamido-2,6-dideoxy-l-talose and 3-deoxy-d-*manno*-octulosonic acid. *Carbohydr. Res* **1997**, *299*, 69–76.

34. Muldoon, J; Perepelov, AV; Shashkov, AS; Nazarenko, EL; Zubkov, VA; Gorshkova, RP; Ivanova, EP; Gorshkova, NM; Knirel, YA; Savage, AV. Structure of an acidic polysaccharide from the marine bacterium *Pseudoalteromonas flavipulchra* NCIMB 2033[T]. *Carbohydr. Res* **2003**, *338*, 459–462.

35. Lindberg, B. Bacterial polysaccharides: Components. In *Polysaccharides: Structural Diversity and Functional Versatility*; Dumitriu, S, Ed.; Marcel Dekker: New York, NY, USA, 1998; pp. 237–273.

36. Gorshkova, RP; Nazarenko, EL; Zubkov, VA; Ivanova, EP; Ovodov, YS; Shashkov, AS; Knirel, YA. Structure of the repeating unit of an acidic polysaccharide from *Alteromonas haloplanktis* KMM 156. *Russ. J. Bioorg. Chem* **1993**, *19*, 327–336.

37. Komandrova, NA; Tomshich, SV; Isakov, VV; Romanenko, LA. Structure of the sulphated *O*-specific polysaccharide of the marine bacterium *Pseudoalteromonas marinoglutinosa* KMM 232. *Biochemistry (Mosc.)* **1998**, *63*, 1200–1204.

38. Rougeaux, H; Guezennec, J; Carlson, RW; Kervarec, N; Pichon, R; Talaga, P. Structural determination of the exopolysaccharide of *Pseudoalteromonas* strain HYD 721 isolated from a deep-sea hydrothermal vent. *Carbohydr. Res* **1999**, *315*, 273–285.

39. Gorshkova, RP; Nazarenko, EL; Isakov, VV; Zubkov, VA; Gorshkova, NM; Romanenko, LA; Ivanova, EP. Structure of the glycerophosphate-containing *O*-specific polysaccharide from *Pseudoalteromonas* sp. KMM 639. *Russ. J. Bioorg. Chem* **1998**, *24*, 839–841.

40. Romanenko, LA; Zhukova, NV; Rhode, M; Lysenko, AM; Mikhailov, V; Stackebrandt, E. *Pseudoalteromonas agarivorans* sp. nov., a novel marine agarolytic bacterium. *Int. J. Syst. Evol. Microbiol* **2003**, *53*, 125–131.

41. Komandrova, NA; Isakov, VV; Tomshich, SV; Romanenko, LA; Perepelov, AV; Shashkov, AS. Structure of an acidic *O*-specific polysaccharide of the marine bacterium *Pseudoalteromonas agarivorans* KMM 232 (R-form). *Biochemistry (Mosc.)* **2010**, *75*, 623–628.

42. Ivanova, EP; Sawabe, T; Lysenko, AM; Gorshkova, NM; Hayashi, K; Zhukova, NV; Nicolau, DV; Christen, R; Mikhailov, VV. *Pseudoalteromonas translucida* sp. nov. and *Pseudoalteromonas paragorgicola* sp. nov., and emended description of the genus. *Int. J. Syst. Evol. Bacteriol* **2002**, *52*, 1759–1766.

43. Holmstrom, C; Kjelleberg, S. Marine *Pseudoalteromonas* species are associated with higher organisms and produce biologically active extracellular agents. *FEMS Microbiol. Ecol* **1999**, *30*, 285–293.

44. Gauthier, MJ. *Alteromonas rubra* sp. nov., a new marine antibiotic-producing bacterium. *Int. J. Syst. Bacteriol* **1976**, *26*, 459–466.

45. Gauthier, MJ. Modification of bacterial respiration by a micromolecular polyanionic antibiotic produced by a marine *Alteromonas*. *Antimicrob. Agents Chemother* **1976**, *9*, 361–366.

46. Kalinovskaya, NI; Ivanova, EP; Alexeeva, YV; Gorshkova, NM; Kuznetsova, TA; Dmitrenok, AS; Nicolau, DV. Low-molecular-weight, biologically active compounds from marine *Pseudoalteromonas* species. *Curr. Microbiol* **2004**, *48*, 441–446.

47. Jensen, PR; Fenical, W. Strategies for the discovery of secondary metabolites from marinebacteria: ecological perspectives. *Annu. Rev. Microbiol* **1994**, *48*, 559–584.

48. Kilcoyne, M; Shashkov, AS; Knirel, YA; Gorshkova, RP; Nazarenko, EL; Ivanova, EP; Gorshkova, NM; Senchenkova, SN; Savage, AV. The structure of the *O*-polysaccharide of the *Pseudoalteromonas rubra* ATCC 29570[T] lipopolysaccharide containing a keto sugar. *Carbohydr. Res* **2005**, *340*, 2369–2375.

49. Vinogradov, E; Korenevsky, A; Beveridge, TJ. The structure of the *O*-specific polysaccharide chain of the *Shewanella algae* BrY lipopolysaccharide. *Carbohydr. Res* **2003**, *338*, 385–388.

50. Jansson, P-E; Lindberg, B; Lindquist, U. Structural studies of the capsular polysaccharide from *Streptococcus pneumoniae* type V. *Carbohydr. Res* **1985**, *140*, 101–110.

51. Sadovskaya, I; Brisson, J-R; Kheu, NH; Mutharia, LM; Altman, E. Structural characterization of the lipopolysaccharide *O*-antigen and capsular polysaccharide of *Vibrio ordalii* serotype O:2. *Eur. J. Biochem* **1998**, *253*, 319–327.

52. MacLean, LL; Perry, MB; Crump, EM; Kay, WW. Structural characterization of the lipopolysaccharide *O*-polysaccharide antigen produced by *Flavobacterium columnare* ATCC 43622. *Eur. J. Biochem* **2003**, *270*, 3440–3446.

53. Senchenkova, SN; Shashkov, AS; Knirel, YA; Esteve, C; Alcaide, E; Merino, S; Tomas, JM. Structure of a polysaccharide from the lipopolysaccharide of *Vibrio vulnificus* clinical isolate YJ016 containing 2-acetimidoylamino-2-deoxy-l-galacturonic acid. *Carbohydr. Res* **2009**, *344*, 1009–1013.

54. Shashkov, AS; Senchenkova, SN; Chizhov, AO; Knirel, YA; Esteve, C; Alcaide, E; Merino, S; Tomas, JM. Structure of a polysaccharide from the lipopolysaccharides of *Vibrio vulnificus* strains CECT 5198 and S3-I2-36, which is remarkably similar to the *O*-polysaccharide of *Pseudoalteromonas rubra* ATCC 29570. *Carbohydr. Res* **2009**, *344*, 1005–1009.

55. Findlay, JA; Jaseja, M; Brisson, J-R. Forbeside C, a saponin from *Asterias forbesi*. Complete structure by nuclear magnetic resonance methods. *Can. J. Chem* **1987**, *65*, 2605–2611.

56. Itakura, Y; Komori, T. Structure elucidation of two new oligoglycoside sulfates, versicoside B and versicoside C. *Liebigs Ann. Chem* **1986**, *1986*, 359–373.

57. Okano, K; Nakamura, T; Kamiya, Y; Ikegami, S. Structure of ovarian asterosaponin-1 in the starfish *Asterias amurensis*. *Agric. Biol. Chem* **1981**, *45*, 805–807.

58. Ruimy, R; Breittmayer, V; Elbaze, P; Lafay, B; Boussemart, O; Gauthier, M; Christen, R. Phylogenetic analysis and assessment of the genera *Vibrio*, *Photobacterium*, *Aeromonas*, and *Plesiomonas* deduced from small-subunit rRNA sequences. *Int. J. Syst. Bacteriol* **1994**, *44*, 416–426.

59. Van Houten, R; Farberman, D; Norton, J; Ellison, J; Kiehlbauch, J; Morris, T; Smith, P. *Plesiomonas shigelloides* and *Salmonella* serotype Hartford infections associated with a contaminated water supply-Livingston County, New York, 1996. *MMWR Morb. Mortal. Wkly. Rep* **1998**, *47*, 394–396.

60. Levy, DA; Bens, MS; Craun, GF; Calderon, RL; Herwaldt, BL. Surveillance for waterborne-disease outbreaks—United States 1995–1996. *MMWR Morb. Mortal. Wkly. Rep* **1998**, *47*, 1–34.

61. Yamada, S; Matsushita, S; Dejsirilert, S; Kudoh, Y. Incidence and clinical symptoms of *Aeromonas*-associated travellers' diarrhoea in Tokyo. *Epidemiol. Infect* **1997**, *119*, 121–126.

62. Rautelin, H; Sivonen, A; Kuikka, A; Renkonen, OV; Valtonen, V; Kosunen, TU. Enteric *Plesiomonas shigelloides* infections in Finnish patients. *Scand. J. Infect. Dis* **1995**, *27*, 495–498.

63. Lee, AC; Yuen, KY; Ha, SY; Chiu, DC; Lau, YL. *Plesiomonas shigelloides* septicemia: Case report and literature review. *Pediatr. Hematol. Oncol* **1996**, *13*, 265–269.

64. Fujita, K; Shirai, M; Ishioka, T; Kakuya, F. Neonatal *Plesiomonas shigelloides* septicemia and meningitis: A case and review. *Acta Paediatr. Jpn* **1994**, *36*, 450–452.

65. Bravo, L; Monte, R; Ramirez, M; Garcia, B; Urbaskova, P; Aldova, E. Characterization of *Plesiomonas shigelloides* from diarrheic children. *Cent. Eur. J. Public Health* **1998**, *6*, 67–70.

66. Korner, RJ; MacGowan, AP; Warner, B. The isolation of *Plesiomonas shigelloides* in polymicrobial septicemia originating from the biliary tree. *Int. J. Med. Microbiol. Virol. Parasitol. Infect. Dis* **1992**, *277*, 334–339.

67. Shimada, T; Sakazaki, R. On the serology of *Plesiomonas shigelloides*. *Jpn. J. Med. Sci. Biol* **1978**, *31*, 135–142.

68. Shimada, T; Arakawa, E; Itoh, K; Kosako, Y; Inoue, K; Zhengshi, Y; Aldova, E. New O and H antigens of *Plesiomonas shigelloides* and their O antigenic relationships to *Shigella boydii*. *Curr. Microbiol* **1994**, *28*, 351–354.

69. Albert, MJ; Ansaruzzaman, M; Quadri, F; Hossain, A; Kibriya, AK; Haider, K; Faruque, SM; Alam, AN. Characterisation of *Plesiomonas shigelloides* strains that share type-specific antigen with *Shigella flexneri* 6 and common group 1 antigen with *Shigella flexneri* spp. ans *Shigella dysenteriae* 1. *J. Med. Microbiol* **1993**, *39*, 211–217.

70. Linnerborg, M; Widmalm, G; Weintraub, A; Albert, MJ. Structural elucidation of the O-antigen lipopolysaccharide from two strains of *Plesiomonas shigelloides* that share a type specific antigen with *Shigella flexneri* 6, and the common group 1 antigen with *Shigella flexneri* spp and *Shigella dysenteriae* 1. *Eur. J. Biochem* **1995**, *231*, 839–844.

71. Czaja, J; Jachymek, W; Niedziela, T; Lugowski1, C; Aldova, E; Kenne, L. Structural studies of the O-specific polysaccharide from *Plesiomonas shigelloides* strain CNCTC 113/92. *Eur. J. Biochem* **2000**, *267*, 1672–1679.

72. Niedziela, T; Dag, S; Lukasiewicz, J; Dzieciatkowska, M; Jachymek, W; Lugowski, C; Kenne, L. Complete lipopolysaccharide of *Plesiomonas shigelloides* O74:H5 (strain CNCTC 144/92). 1. Structural analysis of the highly hydrophobic lipopolysaccharide, including the O-antigen, its biological repeating unit, the core oligosaccharide, and the linkage between them. *Biochemistry* **2006**, *45*, 10422–10433.

73. Pieretti, G; Corsaro, MM; Lanzetta, R; Parrilli, M; Canals, R; Merino, S; Tomas, JM. Structural studies of the O-chain polysaccharide from *Plesiomonas shigelloides* strain 302-73 (serotype O1). *Eur. J. Org. Chem* **2008**, *2008*, 3149–3155.

74. Maciejewska, A; Lukasiewicz, J; Niedziela, T; Szewczuk, Z; Lugowski, C. Structural analysis of the O-specific polysaccharide isolated from *Plesiomonas shigelloides* O51 lipopolysaccharide. *Carbohydr. Res* **2009**, *344*, 894–900.

75. Goethals, K; Leyman, B; Van Den Eede, G; Van Montagu, M; Holsters, M. An *Azorhizobium caulinodans* ORS571 locus involved in lipopolysaccharide production and nodule formation on *Sesbania rostrata* stems and roots. *J. Bacteriol* **1994**, *176*, 92–99.

76. Moll, H; Knirel, YA; Helbig, JH; Zahringer, U. Identification of an alpha-d-Manp-(1→8)-Kdo disaccharide in the inner core region and the structure of the complete core region of the *Legionella pneumophila* serogroup 1 lipopolysaccharide. *Carbohydr. Res* **1997**, *304*, 91–95.

77. Banoub, JH; Aneed, AEl; Cohen, AM; Joly, N. Structural investigation of bacterial lipopolysaccharides by mass spectrometry and tandem mass spectrometry. *Mass Spectrom. Rev* **2010**, *29*, 606–650.

78. Niedziela, T; Lukasiewicz, J; Jachymek, W; Dzieciatkowska, M; Lugowski, C; Kenne, L. Core oligosaccharides of *Plesiomonas shigelloides* O54:H2 (strain CNCTC 113/92). *J. Biol. Chem* **2002**, *277*, 11653–11663.

79. Farmer, JJ, III; Arduino, MJ; Hickman-Brenner, FW. Balows, A, Trüper, HG, Dworkin, M, Wim, H, Schleifer, KH, Eds.; Springer-Verlag: New York, NY, USA, 1992; Volume 3, pp. 3012–3043.

80. Szu, SC; Robbins, JB; Schneerson, R; Pozsgay, V; Chu, C. Polysaccharide-based conjugate vaccines for enteric bacterial infections: typhoid fever, nontyphoid salmonellosis, shigellosis, cholera, and *Escherichia coli* 0157. In *New Generation Vaccines*; Levine, MM, Kaper, JB, Rappuoli, R, Liu, MA, Good, MF, Eds.; Informa Healthcare: New York, NY, USA, 2004; pp. 934–939.

81. Shepherd, JG; Wang, L; Reeves, PR. Comparison of *O*-antigen gene clusters of *Escherichia coli* (*Shigella*) *sonnei* and *Plesiomonas shigelloides* O17: *Sonnei* gained its current plasmid-borne *O*-antigen genes from *P. shigelloides* in a recent event. *Infect. Immun* **2000**, *68*, 6056–6061.

82. Taylor, DN; Trofa, AC; Sadoff, J; Chu, C; Bryla, D; Shiloach, J; Cohen, D; Ashkenazi, S; Lerman, Y; Egan, W. Synthesis, characterization, and clinical evaluation of conjugate vaccines composed of the *O*-specific polysaccharides of *Shigella dysenteriae* type 1, *Shigella flexneri* type 2a, and *Shigella sonnei* (*Plesiomonas shigelloides*) bound to bacterial toxoids. *Infect. Immun* **1993**, *61*, 3678–3687.

83. Watanabe, H; Nakamura, A. Identification of *Shigella sonnei* form I plasmid genes necessary for cell invasion and their conservation among *Shigella* species and enteroinvasive *Escherichia coli*. *Infect. Immun* **1986**, *53*, 352–358.

84. Sayeed, S; Sack, DA; Qadri, F. Protection from *Shigella sonnei* infection by immunisation of rabbits with *Plesiomonas shigelloides* (SVC O1). *J. Med. Microbiol* **1992**, *37*, 382–384.

85. Kubler-Kielb, J; Schneerson, R; Mocca, C; Vinogradov, E. The elucidation of the structure of the core part of the LPS from *Plesiomonas shigelloides* serotype O17 expressing *O*-polysaccharide chain identical to the *Shigella sonnei O*-chain. *Carbohydr. Res* **2008**, *343*, 3123–3127.

86. Pieretti, G; Corsaro, MM; Lanzetta, R; Parrilli, M; Vilches, S; Merino, S; Tomás, JM. Structure of the core region from the lipopolysaccharide of *Plesiomonas shigelloides* strain 302-73 (serotype O1). *Eur. J. Org. Chem* **2009**, *2009*, 1365–1371.

87. Pieretti, G; Carillo, S; Lindner, B; Rosa Lanzetta, R; Parrilli, M; Natalia Jimenez, N; Regue, M; Tomas, JM; Corsaro, MM. The complete structure of the core of the LPS from *Plesiomonas shigelloides* 302-73 and the identification of its *O*-antigen biological repeating unit. *Carbohydr. Res* **2010**, *345*, 2523–2528.

88. Vinogradov, EV; Lindner, B; Kocharova, NA; Senchenkova, SN; Shashkov, AS; Knirel, YA; Holst, O; Gremyakova, TA; Shaikhutdinova, RZ; Anisimov, AP. The core structure of the lipopolysaccharide from the causative agent of plague, *Yersinia pestis*. *Carbohydr. Res* **2002**, *337*, 775–777.

89. Isshiki, Y; Kawahara, K; Zahringer, U. Isolation and characterisation of disodium (4-amino-4-deoxy-β-l-arabinopyranosyl)-(1→8)-d-*glycero*-α-d-*talo*-oct-2-ulopyranosylonate)-(2→4)-(methyl 3-deoxy-d-*manno*-oct-2-ulopyranosid)onate from the lipopolysaccharide of *Burkholdeia cepacia*. *Carbohydr. Res* **1998**, *313*, 21–27.

90. Kawahara, K; Brade, H; Rietschel, ET; Zahringer, U. Studies on the chemical structure of the core-lipid A region of the lipopolysaccharide of *Acinetobacter calcoaceticus* NCTC 10305: Detection of a new 2-octulosonic acid interlinking the core oligosaccharide and lipid A component. *Eur. J. Biochem* **1987**, *163*, 489–495.

91. Vinogradov, EV; Lindner, B; Seltmann, G; Radziejewska-Lebrecht, J; Holst, O. Lipopolysaccharides from *Serratia marcescens* possess one or two 4-amino-4-deoxy-larabinopyranose 1-phosphate residues in the lipid A and d-*glycero*-d-*talo*-oct-2-ulopyranosonic acid in the inner core region. *Chem. Eur. J* **2006**, *12*, 6692–6700.

92. Murray, AE; Lies, D; Li, G; Nealson, K; Zhou, J; Tiedje, JM. DNA/DNA hybridization to microarrays reveals gene-specific differences between closely related microbial genomes. *Proc. Natl. Acad. Sci. USA* **2001**, *98*, 9853–9858.

93. Vinogradov, E; Nossova, L; Korenevsky, A; Beveridge, TJ. The structure of the capsular polysaccharide of *Shewanella oneidensis* strain MR-4. *Carbohydr. Res* **2005**, *340*, 1750–1753.

94. Vinogradov, E; Kubler-Kielb, J; Korenevsky, A. The structure of the carbohydrate backbone of the LPS from *Shewanella* spp. MR-4. *Carbohydr. Res* **2008**, *343*, 2701–2705.

95. Nazarenko, EL; Perepelov, AV; Shevchenko, LS; Daeva, ED; Ivanova, EP; Shashkov, AS; Widmalm, G. Structure of the *O*-specific polysaccharide from *Shewanella japonica* KMM 3601 containing

5,7-diacetamido-3,5,7,9-tetradeoxy-d-*glycero*-d-*talo*-non-2-ulosonic acid. *Biochemistry (Mosc.)* **2011**, *76*, 791–796.

96. Knirel, YA; Senchenkova, SN; Kocharova, NA; Shashkov, AS; Helbig, JH; Zähringer, U. Identification of a homopolymer of 5-acetamidino-7-acetamido-3,5,7,9-tetradeoxy-d-*glycero*-d*talo*- nonulosonic acid in the lipopolysaccharides of *Legionella pneumophila* non-1 serogroups. *Biochemistry (Mosc.)* **2001**, *66*, 1035–1041.

97. Austin, B; Adams, C. Fish Pathogens. In *The Genus Aeromonas*; Austin, B, Altwegg, M, Gosling, PJ, Joseph, S, Eds.; Wiley: Chichester, UK, 1996; pp. 197–244.

98. Figueras, MJ. Clinical relevance of *Aeromonas. Rev. Med. Microbiol* **2005**, *16*, 145–153.

99. Saavedra, MJ; Guedes-Novais, S; Alves, A; Rema, P; Tacao, M; Correia, A; Martinez-Murcia, AJ. Resistance to β-lactam antibiotics in *Aeromonas hydrophila* isolated from rainbow trout (*Oncorhynchus mykiss*). *Int. Microbiol* **2004**, *7*, 201–211.

100. Saavedra, MJ; Figueras, MJ; Martinez-Murcia, AJ. Updated phylogeny of the genus *Aeromonas. Int. J. Syst. Bacteriol* **2006**, *56*, 2481–2487.

101. Martinez-Murcia, AJ; Benlloch, S; Collins, MD. Phylogenetic interrelationships of members of the genera *Aeromonas* and *Plesiomonas* as determined by 16S ribosomal DNA sequencing: Lack of congruence with results of DNA-DNA hybridizations. *Int. J. Syst. Bacteriol* **1992**, *42*, 412–421.

102. Yanez, MA; Catalan, V; Apraiz, D; Figueras, MJ; Martinez-Murcia, AJ. Phylogenetic analysis of members of the genus *Aeromonas* based on *gyrB* gene sequences. *Int. J. Syst. Evol. Microbiol* **2003**, *53*, 875–883.

103. Janda, JM; Abbott, SL; Khashe, S; Kellogg, GH; Shimada, T. Further studies on biochemical characteristics and serologic properties of the genus *Aeromonas. J. Clin. Microbiol* **1996**, *34*, 1930–1933.

104. Janda, JM; Guthertz, LS; Kokka, RP; Shimada, T. *Aeromonas* species in septicemia: Laboratory characteristics and clinical observations. *Clin. Infect. Dis* **1994**, *19*, 77–83.

105. Knirel, YA; Shashkov, AS; Senchenkova, SN; Merino, S; Tomas, JM. Structure of the O-polysaccharide of *Aeromonas hydrophila* O:34; a case of random O-acetylation of 6-deoxy-l-talose. *Carbohydr. Res* **2002**, *337*, 1381–1386.

106. Banoub, JH; Shaw, DH. Structural investigations on the core oligosaccharide of *Aeromonas hydrophila* (chemotype III) lipopolysaccharide. *Carbohydr. Res* **1981**, *98*, 93–103.

107. Knirel, YA; Vinogradov, E; Jimenez, N; Merino, S; Tomás, JM. Structural studies on the R-type lipopolysaccharide of *Aeromonas hydrophila. Carbohydr. Res* **2004**, *339*, 787–793.

108. Wang, Z; Larocque, S; Vinogradov, E; Brisson, J-R; Dacanay, A; Greenwell, M; Brown, LL; Li, J; Altman, E. Structural studies of the capsular polysaccharide and lipopolysaccharide O-antigen of *Aeromonas salmonicida* strain 80204-1 produced under *in vitro* and *in vivo* growth conditions. *Eur. J. Biochem* **2004**, *271*, 4507–4516.

109. Sadovskaya, I; Brisson, J-R; Mutharia, LM; Altman, E. Structural studies of the lipopolysaccharide O-antigen and capsular polysaccharide of *Vibrio anguillarum* serotype O:2. *Carbohydr. Res* **1996**, *283*, 111–127.

110. Shaw, DH; Hart, MJ; Lüderitz, O. Structure of the core oligosaccharide in the lipopolysaccharide isolated from *Aeromonas salmonicida* ssp. salmonicida. *Carbohydr. Res* **1992**, *231*, 83–91.

111. Wang, Z; Li, J; Vinogradov, E; Altman, E. Structural studies of the core region of *Aeromonas salmonicida* subsp. *salmonicida* lipopolysaccharide. *Carbohydr. Res* **2006**, *341*, 109–117.

112. Albert, MJ. *Vibrio cholerae* O139 Bengal. *J. Clin. Microbiol* **1994**, *32*, 2345–2349.

113. Albert, MJ; Ansaruzzaman, M; Shimada, T; Rahman, A; Bhuiyan, NA; Nahar, S; Qadri, E; Islam, MS. Character-ization of *Aeromonus trota* strains that cross-react with *Vibrio cholerae* O139 Bengal. *J. Clin. Microbiol* **1995**, *33*, 3119–3123.

114. Waldor, MK; Mekalanos, JJ. *Vibrio cholerae* O139 specific gene sequences. *Lancet* **1994**, *343*, 1366.

115. Knirel, YA; Paredes, L; Jansson, P-E; Weintraub, A; Widmalm, G; Albert, MJ. Structure of the capsular polysaccharide of *Vibrio cholerae* O139 synonym Bengal containing d-galactose-4,6-cyclophosphate. *Eur. J. Biochem* **1995**, *232*, 391–396.

116. Knirel, YA; Senchenkova, SN; Jansson, P-E; Weintraub, A; Ansaruzzaman, M; Albert, MJ. Structure of the O-specific polysaccharide of an *Aerornonas trota* strain cross-reactive with *Vibrio cholerae* O139 Bengal. *Eur. J. Biochem* **1996**, *238*, 160–165.

117. Anderson, M; Carlin, N; Leontein, K; Lindquist, U; Slettengren, K. Structural studies of the O-antigenic polysaccharide of *Escherichia coli* 086, which possesses blood-group B activity. *Carbohydr. Res* **1989**, *185*, 211–223.

118. Perry, MB; MacLean, LL. Structure of the polysaccharide *O*-antigen of *Salmonella riogrande* O:40 (group R) related to blood group A activity. *Carbohydr. Res* **1992**, *232*, 143–150.

119. Kozinska, A; Figueras, MJ; Chacon, MR; Soler, L. Phenotypic characteristics and pathogenicity of *Aeromonas* genomospecies isolated from common carp (*Cyprinus carpio* L.). *J. Appl. Microbiol* **2002**, *93*, 1034–1041.

120. Kozinska, A; Guz, L. The effect of various *Aeromonas bestiarum* vaccines on non-specific immune parameters and protection of carp (*Cyprinus carpio* L.). *Fish Shellfish Immunol* **2004**, *16*, 437–445.

121. Turska-Szewczuk, A; Kozinska, A; Russa, R; Holst, O. The structure of the *O*-specific polysaccharide from the lipopolysaccharide of *Aeromonas bestiarum* strain 207. *Carbohydr. Res* **2010**, *345*, 680–684.

122. Wang, Z; Liu, X; Dacanay, A; Harrison, BA; Fast, M; Colquhoun, DJ; Lund, V; Brown, LL; Li, J; Altman, E. Carbohydrate analysis and serological classification of typical and atypical isolates of *Aeromonas salmonicida*: A rationale for the lipopolysaccharide-based classification of *A. salmonicida*. *Fish Shellfish Immunol* **2007**, *23*, 1095–1106.

123. Linnenborg, M; Wildmalm, G; Rahman, MM; Jansson, P-E; Holme, T; Qadri, F; Albert, MJ. Structural studies of the *O*-antigenic polysaccharide from an *Aeromonas caviae* strain. *Carbohydr. Res* **1996**, *291*, 165–174.

124. Barer, MR; Millership, SE; Tabaqchali, S. Relationship of toxin production to species in the genus *Aeromonas*. *J. Med. Microbiol* **1986**, *22*, 303–309.

125. Bechet, M; Blondeau, R. Factors associated with the adherence and biofilm formation by *Aeromonas caviae* on glass surfaces. *J. Appl. Microbiol* **2003**, *94*, 1072–1078.

126. Gryllos, I; Shaw, JG; Gavin, R; Merino, S; Tomas, JM. Role of flm locus in mesophilic *Aeromonas* species adherence. *Infect. Immun* **2001**, *69*, 65–74.

127. Wang, Z; Liu, X; Li, J; Altman, E. Structural characterization of the *O*-chain polysaccharide of *Aeromonas caviae* ATCC 15468 lipopolysaccharide. *Carbohydr. Res* **2008**, *343*, 483–488.

128. Kocharova, NA; Thomas-Oates, JE; Knirel, YA; Shashkov, AS; Dabrowski, U; Kochetkov, NK; Stanislavsky, ES; Klolodkova, EV. The structure of the *O*-specific polysaccharide of *Citrobacter* O16 containing glycerol phosphate. *Eur. J. Biochem* **1994**, *219*, 653–661.

129. Jachymek, W; Czaja, J; Neidziela, T; Lugowski, C; Kenne, L. Structural studies of the *O*-specific polysaccharide of *Hafnia alvei* strain PCM 1207 lipopolysaccharide. *Eur. J. Biochem* **1999**, *266*, 53–61.

130. Kolodziejska, K; Perepelov, AV; Zablotni, A; Drzewiecka, D; Senchenkova, SN; Zych, K; Shashkov, AS; Knirel, YA; Sidorczyk, Z. Structure of the glycerol phosphate-containing *O*-polysaccharides and serological studies of the lipopolysaccharides of *Proteus mirabilis* CCUG 10704 (OE) and *Proteus vulgaris* TG 103 classified into a new *Proteus* serogroup, O54. *FEMS Immunol. Med. Microbiol* **2006**, *47*, 267–274.

131. Moreau, M; Richards, JC; Perry, MB; Kniskern, PJ. Structural analysis of the specific capsular polysaccharide of *Streptococcus pneumoniae* type 45 (American type 72). *Biochemistry* **1988**, *27*, 6820–6829.

132. Janda, JM; Abbou, SLJ; Janda, M; Abbott, SL. Evolving concepts regarding the genus *Aeromonas*: An expanding panorama of species, disease presentations, and unanswered questions. *Clin. Infect. Dis* **1998**, *27*, 332–997.

133. Crivelli, C; Demarta, A; Peduzzi, R. Intestinal secretory immunoglobulin A (sIgA) response to *Aeromonas* exoproteins in patients with naturally acquired *Aeromonas diarrhea*. *FEMS Immunol. Med. Microbiol* **2001**, *30*, 31–35.

134. Iager, F; Reicher, F; Ganter, JLMS. Structural and rheological properties of polysaccharides from mango (*Mangifera indica* L.) pulp. *Int. J. Biol. Macromol* **2002**, *31*, 9–17.

135. Xu, X; Ruan, D; Jin, Y; Shashkov, AS; Senchenkova, SN; Kilkoyne, M; Zhang, L. Chemical structure of aeromonas gum—Extracellular polysaccharide from *Aeromonas nichidenii* 5797. *Carbohydr. Res* **2004**, *339*, 1631–1636.

136. Garcia-Ochoa, F; Santos, VE; Casas, JA; Gomes, E. Xanthan gum: Production, recovery, and properties. *Biotechnol. Adv* **2000**, *18*, 549–579.

137. Lattner, D; Flemming, H-C; Mayer, C. ^{13}C-NMR study of the interaction of bacterial alginate with bivalent cations. *Int. J. Biol. Macromol* **2003**, *18*, 81–88.

138. Gacesa, P. Alginates. *Carbohydr. Polym* **1988**, *8*, 161–182.

139. Sutherland, IV. Microbial polysaccharides from Gram-negative bacteria. *Int. Dairy J* **2001**, *11*, 663–674.

140. Ivanova, EP; Romanenko, LA; Chun, J; Matte, MH; Matte, AR; Mikhailov, VV; Svetashev, VI; Huq, A; Maugel, T; Colwell, RR. *Idiomarina* gen. nov., comprising novel indigenous deep-sea bacteria from the Pacific Ocean, including descriptions of two species, *Idiomarina abyssalis* sp. nov. and *Idiomarina zobellii* sp. nov. *Int. J. Syst. Evol. Microbiol* **2000**, *50*, 901–907.

141. Kilcoyne, M; Perepelov, AV; Tomshich, SV; Komandrova, NA; Shashkov, AS; Romanenko, LA; Knirel, YA; Savage, AV. Structure of the *O*-polysaccharide of *Idiomarina zobellii* KMM 231[T] containing two unusual amino sugars with the free amino group, 4-amino-4,6-dideoxy-d-glucose and 2-amino-2-deoxy-l-guluronic acid. *Carbohydr. Res* **2004**, *339*, 477–482.

142. Torii, M; Sakakibara, K; Kuroda, K. Occurrence of 2-amino-2-deoxy-hexuronic acids as constituents of *Vibrio parahaemolyticus* K15 antigen. *Eur. J. Biochem* **1973**, *37*, 401–405.

143. Gorshkova, RP; Nazarenko, EL; Zubkov, VA; Ivanova, EP; Gorshkova, NM; Isakov, VV. Structure of the *O*-specific polysaccharide from *Pseudoalteromonas nigrifaciens* KMM 161. *Biochemistry (Mosc.)* **2002**, *67*, 810–814.

144. Reistad, R. 2-Amino-2-deoxyguluronic acid: A constituent of the cell wall of *Halococcus* sp., strain 24. *Carbohydr. Res* **1974**, *36*, 420–423.

145. Vinogradov, EV; Shashkov, AS; Knirel, YA; Kochetkov, NK; Tochtamysheva, NV; Averin, SP; Goncharova, OV; Khlebnikov, VS. Structure of the *O*-antigen of *Francisella tularensis* strain 15. *Carbohydr. Res* **1991**, *214*, 289–297.

146. Leslie, MR; Parolis, H; Parolis, LAS. The structure of the *O*-antigen of *Escherichia coli* O116:K⁺:H10. *Carbohydr. Res* **1999**, *321*, 246–256.

147. Parolis, H; Parolis, LAS; Olivieri, G. Structural studies on the *Shigella*-like *Escherichia coli* O121 *O*-specific polysaccharide. *Carbohydr. Res* **1997**, *303*, 319–325.

148. Katzenellenbogen, E; Romanowska, E; Kocharova, NA; Knirel, YA; Shashkov, AS; Kochetkov, NK. The structure of glycerol teichoic acid-like *O*-specific polysaccharide of *Hafnia alvei* 1205. *Carbohydr. Res* **1992**, *231*, 249–260.

149. Nakagawa, Y; Sakane, T; Suzuki, M; Hatano, K. Phylogenetic structure of the genera *Flexibacter*, *Flexithrix*, and *Microscilla* deduced from 16S rRNA sequence analysis. *J. Gen. Appl. Microbiol* **2002**, *48*, 155–166.

150. Bernadet, JF. Immunization with bacterial antigens: *Flavobacterium* and *Flexibacterium* infections. *Dev. Biol. Stand* **1997**, *90*, 179–188.

151. Handlinger, J; Soltani, M; Percival, S. The pathology of *Flexibacter maritimus* in aquaculture species in Tasmania, Australia. *J. Fish Dis* **1997**, *20*, 159–169.

152. Ostland, VE; LaTrace, C; Morrison, D; Ferguson, HW. *Flexibacter maritimus* associated with bacterial stomatitis in Atlantic salmon smolts reared in net-pens in, British Columbia. *J. Aquat. Anim. Health* **1999**, *11*, 35–45.

153. Vinogradov, E; MacLean, LL; Crump, EM; Perry, MB; Kay, WW. Structure of the polysaccharide chain of the lipopolysaccharide *from Flexibacter maritimus*. *Eur. J. Biochem* **2003**, *270*, 1810–1815.

154. MacLean, LL; Vinogradov, E; Crump, EM; Perry, MB; Kay, WW. The structure of the lipopolysaccharide *O*-antigen produced by *Flavobacterium psychrophilum* (259-93). *Eur. J. Biochem* **2001**, *268*, 2710–2716.

155. Bernardet, JF; Segers, P; Vancanneyt, M; Berthe, F; Kersters, K; Vandamme, P. Cutting a Gordian knot: Emended classification and description of the genus *Flavobacterium*, emended description of the family Flavobacteriaceae, and proposal of *Flavobacterium hydatis* nom. nov. (basonym, *Cytophaga aquatilis* Strohl and Tait 1978). *Int. J. Syst. Bacteriol* **1996**, *46*, 128–148.

156. Manfredi, RA; Nanetti, A; Ferri, M; Mastroianni, A; Coronado, OV; Chiodo, F. *Flavobacterium* spp. organisms as opportunistic pathogens during advanced HIV disease. *J. Infect* **1999**, *39*, 146–152.

157. Ostland, VE; McGrogan, DG; Ferguson, HW. Cephalic osteochondritis and necrotic sceritis in intensively reared salmonids associated with *Flexibacter psychrophilus*. *J. Fish Dis* **1997**, *20*, 443–451.

158. Dalsgaard, I. Virulence mechanisms in *Cytophaga psychrophilia* and other *Cytophaga*-like bacteria pathogenic for fish. *Annu. Rev. Fish Dis* **1993**, *3*, 127–144.

159. Crump, EM; Perry, MB; Clouthier, SC; Kay, WW. Antigenic characterization of the fish pathogen *Flavobacterium psychrophilum*. *Appl. Environ. Microbiol* **2001**, *67*, 750–759.

160. Hermansson, K; Perry, MB; Altman, E; Brisson, J-R; Garcia, MM. Structural studies of the *O*-antigenic polysaccharide of *Fusobacterium necrophorum*. *Eur. J. Biochem* **1993**, *212*, 801–809.

161. Knirel, YA; Zdorovenko, GM; Veremeychenko, SN; Lipkind, GM; Shashkov, AS; Zakharova, IY; Kochetkov, NK. The structure of the *O*-specific polysaccharide chain of *Pseudomonas aurantiaca* IMB31 lipopolysaccharide. *Russ. J. Bioorg. Chem* **1988**, *14*, 352–358.

162. Chowdhury, TA; Jansson, P-E; Lindberg, B; Lindberg, J. Structural studies of the *Vibrio cholerae* O:3 O-antigen polysaccharide. *Carbohydr. Res* **1991**, *215*, 303–314.

163. Hermasson, K; Jansson, P-E; Holme, T; Gustavsson, B. Structural studies of the *Vibrio cholerae* O:5 O-antigen polysaccharide. *Carbohydr. Res* **1993**, *248*, 199–211.

164. Knirel, YA; Vinogradov, EV; Shashkov, AS; Wilkinson, SG; Tahara, Y; Dmitriev, BA; Kochetkov, NK; Stanislasky, ES; Mashilova, GM. Somatic antigens of *Pseudomonas aeruginosa*: The structure of O-specific polysaccharide chains of the lipopolysaccharide from *P. aeruginosa* O1 (Lanyi), O3 (Habs), O13 and O14 (Wokatsch), and the serologically related strain NCTC 8505. *Eur. J. Biochem* **1986**, *155*, 659–669.

165. Zehavi, U; Sharon, N. Structural studies of 4-acetamido-2-amino-2,4,6-trideoxy-d-glucose (*N*-Acetylbacillosamine), the *N*-acetyl-diamino sugar of *Bacillus licheniformis*. *J. Biol. Chem* **1973**, *248*, 432–435.

166. Tschesche, R; Hoppe, H-J; Snatzke, G; Wulff, G; Fehlhaber, H-W. On parasorboside, the glycosidic precursor of parasorbic acid, from berries of Mountain Ash. *Chem. Ber* **1971**, *104*, 1420–1428.

167. Ofek, I; Doyle, RJ. *Bacterial Adhesion to Cells And Tissues*; Chapman & Hall: London, UK, 1994; pp. 1–16.

168. Tomshich, SV; Komandrova, NA; Widmalm, G; Nedashkovskaya, OI; Shashkov, AS; Perepelov, AV. Structure of an acidic O-specific polysaccharide from *Cellulophaga baltica*. *Russ. J. Bioorg. Chem* **2007**, *33*, 91–95.

169. Perepelov, AV; Shashkov, AS; Tomshich, SV; Komandrova, NA; Nedashkovskaya, OI. A pseudoaminic acid-containing O-specific polysaccharide from a marine bacterium *Cellulophaga fucicola*. *Carbohydr. Res* **2007**, *342*, 1378–1381.

170. Gorshkova, RP; Isakov, VV; Shevchenko, LS; Ivanova, EP; Denisenko, VA; Nazarenko, EL. Structure of teichoic acid from the marine proteobacterium *Sulfitobacter brevis* KMM 6006. *Chem. Nat. Compd. (Russ.)* **2007**, *43*, 643–647.

171. Ivanova, EP; Zhukova, NV; Lysenko, AM; Gorshkova, NM; Sergeev, AF; Mikhailov, VV; Bowman, JP. *Loktanella agnita* sp. nov. and *Loktanella rosea* sp. nov., from the north-west Pacific Ocean. *Int. J. Syst. Evol. Microbiol* **2005**, *55*, 2203–2207.

172. Ierano, T; Silipo, A; Nazarenko, EL; Gorshkova, RP; Ivanova, EP; Garozzo, D; Sturiale, L; Lanzetta, R; Parrilli, M; Molinaro1, A. Against the rules: A marine bacterium, *Loktanella rosea*, possesses a unique lipopolysaccharide. *Glycobiology* **2010**, *20*, 586–593.

173. Raetz, CRH; Reynolds, CM; Trent, MS; Bishop, RE. Lipid A modification systems in Gram-negative bacteria. *Annu. Rev. Biochem* **2007**, *76*, 295–329.

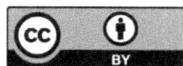

MDPI AG
St. Alban-Anlage 66
4052 Basel, Switzerland
Tel. +41 61 683 77 34
Fax +41 61 302 89 18
http://www.mdpi.com

Marine Drugs Editorial Office
E-mail: marinedrugs@mdpi.com
http://www.mdpi.com/journal/marinedrugs